A DICTIONARY OF PUBLIC HEALTH

A DICTIONARY OF

PUBLIC

HEALTH

John M. Last

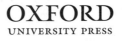

UNIVERSITY PRESS

2007

OXFORD
UNIVERSITY PRESS

Oxford University Press, Inc., publishes works that further
Oxford University's objective of excellence
in research, scholarship, and education.

Oxford New York
Auckland Cape Town Dar es Salaam Hong Kong Karachi
Kuala Lumpur Madrid Melbourne Mexico City Nairobi
New Delhi Shanghai Taipei Toronto

With offices in
Argentina Austria Brazil Chile Czech Republic France Greece
Guatemala Hungary Italy Japan Poland Portugal Singapore
South Korea Switzerland Thailand Turkey Ukraine Vietnam

Published by Oxford University Press, Inc.
198 Madison Avenue, New York, New York 10016

www.oup.com

Oxford is a registered trademark of Oxford University Press.

Library of Congress Cataloging-in-Publication Data

Last, John M., 1926–
A dictionary of public health / John Last.
   p. ; cm.
ISBN-13 978-0-19-516090-1
ISBN 0-19-516090-8
1. Public health—Dictionaries. 2. Medical care—Dictionaries.
[DNLM: 1. Public Health—Dictionary—English. WA 13 L349 2006] I. Title.
RA423.L37 2006
362.1003—dc22   2006002499

1 3 5 7 9 8 6 4 2

Printed in the United States of America
on acid-free paper

CONTENTS

PREFACE

Public health is the art and science of promoting and protecting good health, preventing disease, disability, and premature death, restoring health when it is impaired, and maximizing the quality of life when health cannot be restored. Public health requires collective action by society; collaborative teamwork involving physicians, nurses, engineers, environmental scientists, health educators, social workers, nutritionists, administrators, and other specialized professional and technical workers; and an effective partnership with all levels of government. The definitions and discussions of public health and related concepts on pp 306–307 offer further insight into the breadth, depth, and scope of this domain. The horizons are far flung, the boundaries are ill defined, the interfaces with other institutions of society and with other disciplines and professions are numerous.

Many aspects of public health have specialized vocabularies. Communicable disease control, epidemiology, genetics, nutrition, toxicology, social work, sanitation and public health engineering, environmental sciences, administration, and other specialized fields all have their own languages. It is necessary for all public health workers to understand these languages and timely to provide a reference source for the essential components of this vocabulary, a place where all who need to understand the meaning can find definitions and explanations of about 5,000 words and phrases that public health workers use to communicate information on the concepts, methods, ideas, theories, beliefs, and values of the diverse aspects of public health sciences and practice.

Like everyday speech, technical vocabularies grow, evolve, and change rapidly, so dictionaries can never be truly current. While I have been compiling this dictionary, new concepts and new words and phrases to describe them have come upon the scene and familiar ones have acquired new meanings. Meanwhile, others fall into disuse, are overtaken by events, become obsolete. This has happened in aspects of public health science and practice, including HIV surveillance, environmental health, veterinary epidemiology and animal health; in molecular genetics; in systematic reviews; and in behavioral and social sciences. I have done my best to keep in touch with these shifting frontiers, and I have retained some obsolete terms that readers encounter in old books and journals, as well as some that have only historical interest.

Some definitions are accompanied by an explanation and discussion, occasionally approaching the detail of a short encyclopedia article. Others are just a bald definition, in glossary style. Further information is available at Web sites that appear with some definitions. There are brief biographical accounts of historically significant people who have contributed to the advance of public health, and information on nationalities and dates of most of the people whose names are mentioned. These features are intended to encourage browsing, as well as use of the book for reference purposes.

Using descriptions and discussions in the textbooks, monographs, journals, and reference works listed in the bibliography and assisted by colleagues in several countries, I composed definitions for several thousand words and phrases culled from the indexes, tables of contents, texts, and glossaries in textbooks, monographs, official reports, and journals of public health, basing my interpretation on their implied meanings from the contexts in which they are used. I have tried to interpret, adapt, paraphrase, rewrite, and sometimes clarify and simplify existing definitions, often adding explanations, comments, and brief discussions. I circulated draft definitions to the associate editors and to other correspondents who volunteered their help, inviting them to review and edit my work at each stage. This was an iterative process, leading to second, third, fourth, fifth, and sixth drafts and this final version. At each stage I dropped some items and added others. All the definitions are based on established understanding of the meaning of the terms, but the wording is my own. I have tried not to plagiarize existing definitions, but I have adopted almost unchanged a few that originally appeared in the *Dictionary of Epidemiology*.

John M. Last
Oltawa, Canada
2006

ACKNOWLEDGMENTS

The associate editors and correspondents suggested additions and deletions, kept me focused, corrected egregious errors, and restrained my occasional intemperate remarks (public health is entwined with politics, and public health politics can be partisan). I am beholden to them all for innumerable substantive contributions and valuable comments. Of course I take responsibility for the final work, especially for its defects. In addition to the associate editors and correspondents, many others contributed ideas, amendments, comments, or corrections. They include Onyebuchi Arah, Maureen Birmingham, Ruth Bonita, Devra Breslow, Lester Breslow, Claire-Lise Chaignat, Dominique Charron, Denis Daumerie, Charles Delacollette, Peter Drotman, Guy Eslick, Marie-Laure Granchamp Charles Guest, Max Hardiman, Basil Hetzel, David Heymann, Steven Jonas, Alex Kalache, Maurice King, David Last, Dorothyanne Last, Rebecca Last, Christina Mills, Debra Nanan, Desmond O'Byrne, Christopher Park, David Pencheon, Philippe Petit, George Pickett, Alan Schapira, Vergil Slee, Daniel Tarantola, Damien Thuriaux, Carla Troy, Emmanuelle Tuerlings, Kaat Vandemaelen, David Waltner-Toews, Elizabeth White, Brenda Wilson, and Stéphane With.

I am grateful to other colleagues in the World Health Organization and other United Nations agencies, and in Health Canada, local public health departments in Ottawa and Kingston, Ontario, in the Canadian Public Health Association, and in the Department of Epidemiology and Community Medicine at the University of Ottawa, who have discussed informally with me the meaning of the words and phrases we use in our work and in some instances took part in what were in effect focus group discussions that helped to set the boundaries, clarify my thoughts, and to provide ideas that formed the basis for definitions and discussions in this dictionary. Jonathan Last helped me to organize my electronic files. I have had much help from Carrie Pedersen and from the production editor Rosanne Hallowell at Oxford University Press, excellent copy-editing by Phyllis Jankowski and fact-checking by Kerry Doyle, as well as help from Sylvie Desrochers, Fay Draper, and Mariella Peca in the Department of Epidemiology and Community Medicine at the University of Ottawa. Without all this help, this dictionary would be a poor thing indeed. The work was done in my home office, and drafts were printed at the University of Ottawa. My wife Wendy Last read the entire first and second drafts and added cross-references and sustained me throughout the long labor. I thank her especially, and everyone else who helped me.

J.M.L.

SI UNITS

Base and dimensionless SI units

Physical quantity	Name	Symbol
length	metre	m
mass	kilogram	kg
time	second	s
electric current	ampere	A
thermodynamic temperature	kelvin	K
luminous intensity	candela	cd
amount of substance	mole	mol
*plane angle	radian	rad
*solid angle	steradian	sr

*dimensionless units

Derived SI units with special names

Physical quantity	Name of SI unit	Symbol of SI unit
frequency	hertz	Hz
energy	joule	J
force	newton	N
power	watt	W
pressure	pascal	Pa
electric charge	coulomb	C
electric potential difference	volt	V
electric resistance	ohm	Ω
electric conductance	siemens	S
electric capacitance	farad	F
magnetic flux	weber	Wb
inductance	henry	H
magnetic flux density (magnetic induction)	tesla	T
luminous flux	lumen	lm
illuminance	lux	lx
absorbed dose	gray	Gy
activity	becquerel	Bq
dose equivalent	sievert	Sv

Decimal multiples and submultiples to be used with SI units

Submultiple	Prefix	Symbol	Multiple	Prefix	Symbol
10^{-1}	deci	d	10	deca	da
10^{-2}	centi	c	10^2	hecto	h
10^{-3}	milli	m	10^3	kilo	k
10^{-6}	micro	μ	10^6	mega	M
10^{-9}	nano	n	10^9	giga	G
10^{-12}	pico	p	10^{12}	tera	T
10^{-15}	femto	f	10^{15}	peta	P
10^{-18}	atto	a	10^{18}	exa	E
10^{-21}	zepto	z	10^{21}	zetta	Z
10^{-24}	yocto	y	10^{24}	yotta	Y

Conversion of units to SI units

From	To	Multiply by
in	m	2.54×10^{-2}
ft	m	0.3048
sq. in	m^2	6.4516×10^{-4}
sq. ft	m^2	9.2903×10^{-2}
cu. in	m^3	1.63871×10^{-5}
cu. ft	m^3	2.83168×10^{-2}
l(itre)	m^3	10^{-3}
gal(lon)	l(itre)	4.546 09
miles/hr	m s^{-1}	0.477 04
km/hr	m s^{-1}	0.277 78
lb	kg	0.453 592
g cm^{-3}	kg m^{-3}	10^3
lb/in^3	kg m^{-3}	$2.767\ 99 \times 10^4$
dyne	N	10^{-5}
poundal	N	0.138 255
lbf	N	4.448 22
mmHg	Pa	133.322
atmosphere	Pa	$1.013\ 25 \times 10^5$
hp	W	745.7
erg	J	10^{-7}
eV	J	$1.602\ 10 \times 10^{-19}$
kW h	J	3.6×10^6
cal	J	4.1868

A DICTIONARY OF PUBLIC HEALTH

A

abandonment 1. Negligent or malicious breaking off of an asymmetrical or dependency relationship, as between physician and patient or between parent(s) and dependent child(ren). 2. A philosophical term for absence of a source of moral or ethical authority external to the self.

abatement Reduction or preferably elimination of public health hazards or nuisances such as environmental pollutants, noxious smells, excessive noise. Abatement is often an important activity in public health departments. It may require enforcing legislation or regulations and facilitation by technical means.

abduction 1. Illegal removal of a child or other dependent person from the family or legally designated provider of care. 2. A method of reasoning that arrives at the most logical inference after considering all the available evidence, then decides which solution is the best fit. This is used in artificial intelligence and is the basis for evidence-based diagnosis.

abiotic transformation Literally, a biologically important chemical transformation in the absence of living organisms. An example is formation of stratospheric ozone from oxygen, catalyzed by solar ultraviolet radiation.

ABO blood groups Classification of blood types based on presence of agglutinogens A, B, both, or neither in red blood corpuscles. Blood may also have Rhesus (Rh) agglutinogen, an enzyme that causes red blood cells to clump together. Blood transfusions require that donor and recipient blood groups are compatible at least for these agglutinogens. See also BLOOD GROUPS and RHESUS FACTOR (RH FACTOR).

aborigines The indigenous inhabitants of a colonized country. They often have high incidence and prevalence rates of multiple social and health problems and reduced life expectancy when their habitat, culture, and way of life are disrupted and drastically changed by colonial and postcolonial occupation. Common health problems of these populations include self-destructive conduct such as substance abuse, alcoholism, adolescent suicide, and metabolic disorders related to the transition from a traditional hunter-gatherer diet to high carbohydrate, fat, and salt intake, leading to ADIPOSITY, non-insulin-dependent diabetes, hypertension, gout, etc.

abortion Expulsion from the uterus of a fetus before it is viable, i.e., before 20 weeks' gestation and/or 500 grams fetal weight. This occurs naturally to an estimated 20% to 30% of conceptions as a consequence of death or severe damage to the fetus caused by disease, environmental agents, ingested toxins, or other suspected and unknown factors; or it may be artificially induced by the action of a pregnant woman, a lay person, or health care professional. Most of the half million annual maternal deaths in the world, predominantly in low-income countries, are due to infection and sepsis following botched, often self-induced abortions. See also MATERNAL MORTALITY.

abortion laws Most organized jurisdictions have enacted legislation or evolved legal practices determined by common law precedents, specifying the circumstances, if any, under which it is legally permissible to terminate a pregnancy by inducing and performing an abortion. In many countries abortion laws discriminate against poor, uneducated women in that they are less able to negotiate their way through legal, bureaucratic, and health service obstacles or gain access to available facilities elsewhere.

abscissa The horizontal or X axis of a graph; the vertical or Y axis is the ORDINATE, and the two axes are the CARTESIAN COORDINATES.

absolute risk The probability that a specified event will occur in a specified population, in contrast to the RELATIVE RISK of the event, which compares absolute risks in different populations.

absolute risk approach A disease-control method based on the observation that proportional reduction in risk for given absolute reductions in RISK FACTORS is independent of the level of the risk factor. For instance, reducing systolic blood pressure by 10 mm Hg produces the same percentage reduction in risk of heart attack or stroke at all levels of pretreatment blood pressure. The benefits of reducing such risk factors depend mainly on the absolute risk of disease, not on the pretreatment levels of specific risk factors. This contrasts with risk factor management based on a threshold for each factor (e.g., blood pressure, cholesterol level) above which a treatable abnormality (hypertension, hyperlipidemia) is deemed to be present. Absolute risks are strongly influenced by unmodifiable risk factors, such as age, sex, and prior history of disease, and are expressed as percent probabilities of disease occurrence within specified time horizons, usually 5 or 10 years. Under the absolute risk approach, the decision to treat elevated blood pressure or serum cholesterol depends on the estimated overall level of risk, rather than the level of any single risk factor. Implementing an absolute risk approach may imply substantial changes to public health strategies and to the circumstances in which allocation of resources for preventive medication is justifiable.

absorption The process of taking a substance into a fluid medium, e.g., by dissolving it or by transforming it chemically. This occurs when airborne gases diffuse through alveoli and after digestion, involving biochemical transformation and transport via the circulatory system.

abstinence Refraining from action, continence, particularly refraining from activities regarded as pleasurable by those who indulge, including sexual activity, drinking alcohol, and smoking. Some groups advocate abstinence from sexual intercourse as the preferred method of avoiding teenage pregnancy and sexually transmitted diseases. This is effective when conscientiously adhered to, but admonitions to be chaste can be unrealistic if social and cultural pressures are ignored or when aimed at powerless girls and women, or if the strength of the sexual impulse in uninhibited youth is overlooked. It is an inappropriate approach in cultures in which girls and women lack autonomy and control of the HIV/AIDS pandemic is a priority, as in Sub-Saharan Africa and other low-income countries.

academic freedom The right of scholars to study and report on any problem that their curiosity and conscience dictate, without fear of retribution. This right may be infringed when studies are paid for by governments, industries, or faith-based groups that exert their authority to suppress, censor, or alter findings, forbid certain lines of inquiry, or interfere with the dissemination of results. Such infringement can harm personal and population health, for instance when a pharmaceutical corporation suppresses findings that cast doubt on the safety or efficacy of drugs, and when governments influenced by security concerns, commercial lobby groups, ideology, or political pressure impede dissemination of impartial objective information, such as about aspects of environmental health or human reproduction. Academic freedom also may be perverted by vocal or aggressive ideologues within or outside the academic community who may use it to promote a specific cause. Public health scientists conducting clinical trials and evaluating environmental risks have been among victims of infringed academic freedom.

acceptable daily intake (ADI) Syn: reference dose. The acceptable daily intake is the estimated daily intake for humans, including sensitive subgroups (e.g., children), that is not likely to cause harmful effects during lifetime exposure. ADIs are generally used with reference to health effects other than cancer, for which there may be a threshold for inducing adverse effects.

acceptable risk A risk that has significantly smaller and/or fewer detrimental consequences than the potential hazards of alternative courses of action. Environmental regulations such as those of the US ENVIRONMENTAL PROTECTION AGENCY define acceptable risk as a lifetime exposure level to known carcinogens that does not increase cancer risk by an amount varying from more than 1 chance in 1 million to 1 in 10,000 or higher, depending on the substance or factor. This definition is used when establishing a cleanup goal for hazardous waste sites. However, the loose and variable criteria for what constitutes "acceptable" make it essential to specify the context in which the term is used. In a broader context, the definition of an acceptable risk depends on who is assessing the risk. There is an ethical difference depending on whether a risk is self-imposed or imposed by others and who stands to gain or lose as a result of the assessment.

accessibility Openness, the quality of being approachable, available in practice, to clients, users of a health care system. Accessibility is one of the criteria used to assess the quality of a health care system or a public health service and should be distinguished from availability, which means that a service exists but does not consider whether potential patients or clients actually are able to use it. The term also describes the ability to comprehend the language of the health care provider and the physical distance between providers and potential users of health care services.

access to information The process of locating and using information gathered by public officials and often also those in the private sector. One characteristic of an open democratic society is that citizens are able to find out what elected and appointed officials are saying and doing about issues of concern. Some officials may prefer secrecy and may close ranks against outsiders, revealing as little as possible about their actions and reasons for their decisions. Public health officials are not immune from the tendency of officialdom to withhold information that ought to be in the public domain. They may mean well and may believe they have sound political reasons for this behavior, but citizens increasingly have enforced their right to know by means of access to information legislation.

accident An unplanned, unanticipated event leading to damage, injury, or death, commonly classified according to the site of occurrence (traffic, workplace, domestic, recreational). For such events involving road transport the preferred term is TRAFFIC CRASH, which avoids the implication of a random event. Epidemiological study often identifies predictable determinants and causal factors that could be controlled to reduce or eliminate many risks of injury and premature death, especially those in the workplace and those involving traffic.

acclimatization The process of physiological and psychological adjustment to unaccustomed climatic conditions that initially are perceived to be extreme: too hot, too cold, too humid. A similar process of adaptation to social and cultural conditions, ACCULTURATION, may occur also when individuals relocate in another country or locality. Either process can have adverse effects on health because of poor physiological adjustment to altogether different climatic conditions or exposure to pathogens to which there is no acquired immunity, or for other reasons.

accommodation 1. The living space of a person, family, or group of people. 2. Variation in the aperture of the iris and the shape of the lens of the eye induced by ocular muscles, enabling clarity of vision under varying conditions of light and distance of the eye from the object visualized.

accountability The state of being answerable for decisions and actions; a criterion that can be used as an indicator of how well a health care system functions. In clinical and public health practice, professional staff are usually called to account for their actions only when things have gone badly wrong, as in tort claims and malpractice suits. Accountability is not usually part of audit or evaluation procedures. Elected or appointed officials seeking ways to reduce costs of local public health services (and therefore reduce taxes) may overemphasize financial accountability and disregard the absence of diseases as evidence that control measures are effective.

accreditation The process used to confer and periodically renew official recognition upon an institution or service in the health care, educational, and some other sectors of society. Medical schools, schools and programs of public health, hospitals, community clinics, etc., undergo this exhaustive, even exhausting, process, involving collection and analysis of detailed statistics on all aspects of the structure, activities, and as far as possible the outcomes of the activities of staff in the institutions being considered for accreditation, usually at 5- or 7-year intervals.

acculturation Adoption and assimilation by a person or social group of the cultural customs, traditions, practices, and behavior of what previously had been for them an alien culture. This process may slowly proceed over several generations or may be abrupt; in the latter case it may be accompanied by social and familial disruption that, depending on circumstances, can have adverse or beneficial effects on population and personal health. Adverse effects can arise from unfamiliarity with the health care system and public health regulations of the new country.

accuracy The degree to which a measurement or an estimate based on measurement represents the true value of the attribute being measured. Not to be confused with PRECISION or VALIDITY.

acetone A colorless, volatile liquid with a characteristic odor, formed by denaturation of fats. It is produced as an abnormal metabolic product in DIABETES, starvation, etc., and used industrially as a solvent.

acetylcholinesterase An enzyme required to hydrolyze acetylcholine, a neurotransmitter that transmits signals at neuromuscular junctions and between neurons in the brain. This enzyme is essential for the normal function of muscles, including vital respiratory, as well as voluntary, muscles. If its action is blocked, muscles become paralyzed and rigid, causing asphyxia and death. When acetylcholine accumulates, toxic effects may include muscle spasms, followed by paralysis, hypersalivation, respiratory distress, and death. Some acetylcholinesterase inhibitors are absorbed through the skin and through the exoskeleton of arthropods and are effective NERVE GASES and INSECTICIDES. Occupational exposure to insecticides, such as MALATHION and PARATHION, containing acetylcholinesterase inhibitors caused many fatal episodes until these and similar insecticides were withdrawn from the market or their use restricted and carefully controlled. Deaths occasionally still occur among farmers and gardeners.

acid aerosol A colloid atmospheric suspension of liquid or solid acidic particles, as in SMOG, that irritates and inflames respiratory epithelium and causes permanent damage if exposure is prolonged. Atmospheric acid aerosols are due to solution in water vapor or fog of gaseous sulfur and nitrogen oxides from natural or, more often, anthropogenic sources, generally combusted fossil fuel.

acid-fast stain Special staining solution such as ZIEHL-NEELSEN STAIN that is used to detect the presence of MYCOBACTERIA, such as *Mycobacterium tuberculosis*, in sputum, other body fluids, or tissues; called acid-fast stain because the stain is taken up by the capsule of the microorganism and retains its color when washed in a weak solution of hydrochloric or other acid.

acid precipitation (mist, fog, rain) Syn: acid deposition. Atmospheric ACID AEROSOLS are removed by wet deposition (rain, snow, mist, fog) or dry deposition of particles on vegetation. This is harmful to aquatic and terrestrial ecosystems, to the fabric of many buildings, and to the human respiratory system, aggravating and perhaps causing chronic bronchitis and emphysema in populations living in smoky industrial areas. This is a serious environmental and public health problem in many urban communities with heavy traffic and industry. See also SMOG.

acquired immunodeficiency syndrome (AIDS) The clinical stage of infection with the HUMAN IMMUNODEFICIENCY VIRUS (HIV), characterized by destruction of immune defense mechanisms; reduced numbers of T-4 lymphocytes; susceptibility to opportunistic infections, including *Pneumocystis carinii* pneumonia, tuberculosis, and uncommon viral (cytomegalovirus) and fungal infections such as *Candida albicans* affecting the alimentary, respiratory, and genital systems; rare malignancies such as Kaposi's sarcoma; and other manifestations. Modern treatment can prolong survival considerably, but ultimately AIDS is usually fatal. It is among the worst pandemics ever to afflict humanity. As of 2005, more than 42 million people have been infected with HIV and more than 12 million have died of AIDS since the disease was identified in the early 1980s. Sub-Saharan Africa has been badly affected: in many communities entire generations of young sexually active adults have been devastated. The incidence is rising sharply in India, China, and southeast Asia. See http://www.unaids.org for current information, estimates of incidence and death rates, global and regional control programs, local initiatives, and many other details.

acrolein A petroleum by-product; a yellowish liquid used in the manufacture of plastics and synthetic fibers. Also present in tobacco smoke. It is a potent mucous membrane irritant.

acroosteolysis A condition caused by prolonged occupational exposure to VINYL CHLORIDE, in which bone density is pathologically reduced in the extremities, i.e., fingers and toes. It may also be associated with RAYNAUD'S DISEASE.

acrylonitrile A colorless, volatile, highly reactive liquid with many industrial uses, e.g., in the manufacture of acrylic fibers, rubberized compounds. It is an ingredient of tobacco smoke. It is highly toxic in that it may release cyanide. It is mutagenic in vitro, carcinogenic in animals, and a possible human carcinogen.

actinic keratosis Precancerous epidermal thickening and scaly lesions caused by exposure to solar radiation, occurring especially in fair-skinned people. The occurrence of these lesions is an indication for avoidance of excessive exposure to solar radiation and requires treatment before they progress to basal or squamous cell skin cancer.

actinic radiation The component of solar radiation consisting mainly of ultraviolet radiation. It stimulates photochemical and oxidative DNA damage. Acute exposure causes sunburn, followed by sun tan in susceptible persons, and chronic or intermittent acute exposure leads to benign and malignant skin lesions, e.g., melanoma and nonmelanoma skin cancer and cataracts.

action research The use of observational study or experiment, preferably a carefully designed controlled study, in social services or a health care system or service to evaluate the effects of changes in methods, procedures, activities, resource allocation, etc.

activated charcoal A preparation of charcoal that can adsorb toxicants, e.g., narcotics, chlorine gas. It is used in water filtration devices to remove organic chemical contaminants from drinking water and as an antidote in industrial accidents or self-poisoning, but its efficacy is questionable.

active immunity Immunity induced by development of antibodies following initial exposure and immunologically protective response to alien antigens on re-exposure. This may be lifelong or transient. It happens after exposure to many common infectious pathogens encountered in childhood, e.g., in the days before measles vaccine became available, infection with the measles virus and, currently, active immunity to measles following measles vaccine. See also IMMUNITY and PASSIVE IMMUNITY.

activism The policy and practice of taking energetic action to right perceived wrongs that afflict society or a particular group. Activism is commonly directed to causes such as improving facilities for persons with physical impairments and has often played an honorable role in public health reforms but can have a negative aspect when an influential group promotes a cause that may have unfavorable public health implications, such as the National Rifle Association's successful blocking of much gun control legislation in the United States. See also ADVOCACY.

activities of daily living (ADL) scale A scale for recording a person's functional capability based on answers to questions about mobility, self-care, grooming, and ability to dress, wash, keep house, shop for food; originally developed and described in 1957 by the American physician Steven Katz and others. The ADL scale and many modifications assign a numerical score to physical ability and outcomes of interventions for persons with known or suspected disabilities, such as those caused by arthritis. The ADL scale is used to assess health status and to evaluate progress and response to treatment.

activity limitation Restriction or inhibition of a usual activity considered to be essential for independent living, e.g., dressing, bathing, food shopping. This can be due to disease, injury, or treatment, e.g., prescribed bed rest, splints, etc. Its extent is assessed by clinical examination and/or questionnaire.

activity status index A simple set of 12 questions on physical activity and function developed at Duke University, Durham, North Carolina, that assesses ability to walk, run, do housework, take part in strenuous sports, etc. The questions are available at http://www.cebp.nl/media/m119.pdf.

actuarial statistics Statistical data on mortality, life expectancy, or risk of death in a defined population. When this population comprises the policyholders of a life insurance corporation, commonly used to calculate insurance premium rates, it is, of course, a selected group, not representative of the national population as a whole. Comprehensive national data are preferable.

actuary A demographer, mathematician, accountant, or other professional person who specializes in compiling and analyzing statistical data on mortality, to compile official statistics, set premium rates for life insurance, or for research on aspects of vital and health statistics.

ACT UP Acronym for AIDS Coalition to Unleash Power, an activist advocacy group that seeks to enhance control measures against the HIV/AIDS epidemic by aggressive public action. There are ACT UP chapters in New York, San Francisco, several other US cities, and in Paris, London, and elsewhere. The group offers advice and support to persons with HIV/AIDS. ACT UP has compiled a graphic record about deceased victims of AIDS. See http://www.actuporalhistory.org/.

acupuncture A form of traditional medicine practiced in China for about 4,000 years, in which fine needles are inserted through the skin at specific sites and gently manipulated. Acupuncture is based on the theory that this form of manipulation corrects imbalances in the life forces that are responsible for most ailments. Research by neurophysiologists in modern China and elsewhere has demonstrated that acupuncture can have two physiological actions, release of endorphins and sensory overload, either or both of which can relieve pain and sometimes can be an effective form of anesthesia. Toward the end of the 20th century, acupuncture became a popular form of alternative therapy in Europe and America for chronic conditions such as arthritis.

acute Referring to a disease or condition, this means sudden in onset, loosely used to mean severe; referring to exposure, short-term and intense. See also and contrast CHRONIC.

acute radiation syndrome (injury) A condition that affected ATOMIC BOMB survivors and those close to nuclear reactor accidents. Severity varies with exposure. Above 500 cGy there is bone marrow depression, hemorrhagic gastroenteritis, and death within 2 weeks. Exposure to as much as 200 cGy causes gastrointestinal symptoms, increasing debility, leukopenia, thrombocytopenia, gastrointestinal hemorrhage, and death in most cases within a few weeks. Lower exposure levels have lower immediate mortality rates but cause chronic debility; alopecia; and malignant disease of the brain, hematopoietic tissues, or kidneys, with a latent period of 5 to 20 years or more.

adaptation The process of physiological adjustment to environmental conditions. Organisms best able to adjust to a changed environment have enhanced prospects for survival and an advantage in propagating themselves. Adaptation explains the development of antibiotic-resistant strains of microorganisms, pesticide-resistant insects, and insecticide-resistant weeds, and is a central principle of evolutionary biology. Thus the word "adaptation" also refers to the evolutionary changes that proceed over the course of many generations of an organism.

adaptive strategy In behavioral science, the actions taken by individuals or groups in response to an environmental or a social challenge.

addiction Pathological dependence on a substance or compulsion to act in a particular manner, inability to limit use of a mood-modifying or consciousness-altering substance, such as a licit or illicit drug, or alcohol, or to compulsively gamble. The cardinal symptom of addiction is withdrawal symptoms when the supply is disrupted, and a common feature is the inadequacy of voluntary control over the addictive behavior. This may be a psychological or psychotic process, or a feature of a physiological or pharmacological state of dependence on a substance, such as nicotine or alcohol, or a narcotic or mood-modifying drug, such as opium, heroin, or cocaine. A new behavioral addiction is compulsive use of computers for time-consuming Internet chatting, computer games, or other activities.

additive An ingredient that is added to foods, fluids, and other substances, such as metallic alloys, to confer a special property, such as resistance to deterioration, brighter color, added strength. By implication, the additive is present in small or even trace amounts, and should have only beneficial effects and no undesirable consequences. Assessing the effects on health of FOOD ADDITIVES is an important feature of food and nutrition science.

adduct A substance produced in or introduced into the body and incorporated into cells by covalent bonding with DNA or other molecules. Many carcinogens form adducts with DNA.

adenovirus A group of viruses first isolated from human adenoid tissue, responsible mainly for acute respiratory disease; also other conditions, such as gastroenteric disease, conjunctivitis.

adherence Health-related behavior that abides by the recommendations of a health care professional or the investigator in a research project. The word "adherence" is preferred by some who consider the alternative, COMPLIANCE, to imply coercion or excessive authoritarianism.

adiabatic process In meteorology, a steady-state system in which heat neither enters nor leaves a defined zone or region but ambient temperature increases as atmospheric pressure rises, and decreases as atmospheric pressure falls. This accounts for temperature changes with altitude. The process is relevant in AEROSPACE MEDICINE, for instance in the design of high-flying passenger aircraft in which cabin air pressure helps to maintain air temperature at high altitudes, as well as the atmospheric concentration of oxygen and other gases at physiologically necessary levels.

adiposity Overall expansion of body fat, often with depletion of muscle mass, physical strength, and agility. It should be distinguished from OBESITY, which is expansion of body mass involving fat tissue, muscles, and viscera. Adiposity is common in affluent societies, where it is usually confused with and called "obesity." Adiposity is a disorder of lifestyle, whereas obesity often runs in families and may be genetically determined.

adjustment 1. A general term for the physiological and psychological process of adapting to environmental conditions 2. The emotional process of adapting to particular social circumstances. 3.

A summarizing procedure for comparing two or more sets of data, such as mortality rates in different populations, that minimizes the effects of factors, such as age composition, other than the particular difference, such as causes of death, for which the experience of the populations are being compared. Adjustment for age differences is usually performed with rates, proportions, relative risks, using one of the mathematical procedures of direct or indirect STANDARDIZATION.

administration Management, supervision, and evaluation of an organization, institution of society, service, social system, or component of the health care system. This is the usual way most organizations conduct their affairs and fulfill their purpose. The distinction between administration and MANAGEMENT is ill-defined, but administration is said to be concerned with broad policy, whereas management is the manner in which policies are executed. When the word is capitalized ("the Administration") it is a generic term for the leaders of the governing party of the nation. The word is part of the title of government agencies in the health and other sectors of many countries.

adolescence The phase of the human life cycle between child and adult, characterized by physical growth (increase in height, muscle mass, bone strength and density, and weight) and development of sexual maturity. It is a time of heightened vulnerability to many environmental and emotional hazards. The age span of adolescence varies. It begins on average 2 years earlier in females than in males. Thus, it ranges from about 11 to 17 for females, 13 to 19 for males. It occurs at younger ages everywhere than in generations 100 years ago, which is usually attributed to improved nutrition.

adolescent behavior Many adolescent behavior patterns are, perhaps subconsciously or instinctively, aimed at enhancing sexual attractiveness and/or self-image or are a response to peer pressure. Some of these behavior patterns are hazardous to health. These include sexual experimentation and promiscuity; experimentation with mood-modifying substances such as tobacco, alcohol, and illicit drugs; driving cars and motor cycles at excessive speed; and taking extreme risks in many forms of outdoor adventures.

adolescent health Adolescence, a time of physical growth, physiological change, psychological and psychosexual development, is a period of heightened vulnerability to disease and injury that justifies deploying health services to enhance health and minimize adverse outcomes. However, many adolescents who perceive themselves to be healthy rarely or never use health care services unless they are injured or ill, so physicians who see them at such times are advised to use the opportunity to screen for high-risk conditions and to counsel about healthy behavior.

adoption 1. The formal legal process whereby ADOPTIVE PARENTS assume responsibility to provide necessities of life (shelter, clothing, food) for a dependent child who is not their common offspring, generally an emotionally bonding, as well as a legally binding, procedure. 2. Less formally, the term applies to the process of accepting a person, or a concept or document, e.g., adoption of the minutes of a previous meeting. 3. In sociology and educational psychology, the word describes how individuals accept new ideas and concepts, and individuals are classified as early or late adopters, according to their willingness or otherwise to accept innovations.

adoptive parent(s) Adult(s) usually unrelated by blood ties who assume legally conferred authority and responsibility for the upbringing and well-being of one or more child(ren).

adsorption In physical chemistry and physiology, the process whereby molecules adhere to a surface membrane, rather than being taken into the tissue or substance beneath that membrane.

adult A mature human. The age of maturity is variously defined, by anatomical characteristics (completion of growth, closure of epiphyses, etc) and by legal criteria that vary among different jurisdictions and for different purposes, e.g., capacity to drive a car, vote, serve in armed forces, marry without parental consesnt, obtain contraceptive advice without parental consent, purchase cigarettes or alcohol, and attend entertainments for adults only. See also AGE OF CONSENT.

adulterants Substances added deliberately or inadvertently to food or milk, e.g., to dilute it or alter its flavor. Most adulterants are undesirable, harmful, or dangerous; some are illegal. When they are legally permissible, in most jurisdictions their nature and concentration must be stated.

advance directives Syn: LIVING WILL. A formal written statement setting out a person's wishes in the event of incapacitating illness such as stroke, ALZHEIMER'S DISEASE. Advance directives may include information such as do-not-resuscitate orders and instructions about preferred methods of disposal of the body after death. It is important to ensure the legal force of an advance directive because without this, family members, physicians, nurses, and "right to life" activists in some jurisdictions can intervene and may gratuitously prolong terminal illness and suffering.

adverse reaction An unwanted or undesirable consequence of a diagnostic, preventive, or therapeutic regimen or procedure, e.g., immunization against childhood infections. Compare and contrast SIDE EFFECT, which is an unwanted but not necessarily undesirable consequence.

advertising Bringing to public notice a service, product, or system by displaying it on billboards, publishing it in the press, or announcing it in electronic media. From the public health perspective, advertising may be a means to achieve a desirable end, such as ensuring vaccination of vulnerable infants, or an undesirable end, such as unhealthy dietary habits or driving too fast.

advocacy Arguing and/or acting in support of a particular cause, policy, group of people, etc. This is a major activity of many public health associations and local health departments, some of which designate individuals who have demonstrated proficiency in this role. See LOBBYIST.

Aedes A widespread genus of Culex mosquitoes, many of which can be disease vectors, e.g., for dengue, yellow fever, viral encephalitis, and viral hemorrhagic fevers. Typically, members of this genus are peridomestic in habitat and can breed in small bodies of water, such as puddles left by tropical rainstorms, small pools of water inside car tires, etc.

aeration Passage of a gas, such as atmospheric air or oxygen, through water, a chemical solution, or sewage sludge to agitate the fluid, and/or encourage solution of the gas in the fluid. Aeration is an important feature of sewage treatment, during which many fecal pathogens are rendered harmless. See also BIOCHEMICAL OXYGEN DEMAND.

aerobic exercise A physiological term for vigorous physical activity at a level that is just compatible with the capacity of a particular individual's cardiovascular and respiratory systems to exchange oxygen and carbon dioxide while maintaining without distress an accelerated heart rate and respiration rate. This varies according to an individual's fitness and physical training

aerobics A form of systematic exercises that aims to enhance health by achieving a sustained increase in expenditure of energy and oxygen uptake. Participants in aerobics often judge when they have achieved this state by the perception of elevated heart rate and breathing frequency. They also may experience mood elevation attributable to release of endorphins. This may lead to "addictive" or compulsive maintenance of an aerobics regimen. The benefits of aerobics include improved physiological function and increased longevity when the activity is sustained over many years.

aerodynamic particle size The size of a sphere of uniform density that has the aerodynamic properties of a specified particle. This particle size determines the period of time that a small body can remain suspended in the atmosphere. Depending on mass and air movement, prolonged atmospheric suspension is possible for particles ranging from 25 to 50 microns, but larger particles (200 microns or more) with low density can remain suspended in the atmosphere for many hours under suitable conditions. Particles smaller than 10 microns can be inhaled into the bronchi, and particles smaller than 2.5 microns, such as silica dust in mines, can penetrate to and lodge in alveoli.

aerosol 1. Suspension in a gaseous medium of solid or liquid particles. The particle size required for prolonged suspension is related to the density of the particles, but particles less than 1 to 2.5 microns in diameter can remain suspended indefinitely. 2. A liquid or solid substance in particle form, packed under high pressure and released as a fine mist that remains suspended in the atmosphere for a prolonged period when the pressure of the package is suddenly reduced.

aerospace medicine The branch of medical specialization that focuses on the health of air crews and passengers in aircraft and space vehicles and their support personnel. Aerospace medicine emphasizes applied physiology and physiological adaptation to changes in atmospheric pressure and gravitational forces. Exposure to volatile toxic fumes from aviation fuel is another concern. The interfaces with public health include many aspects of PREVENTIVE MEDICINE and detection and control of dangerous contagious diseases that can be transported from one country to another by air crew, passengers, or insect vectors carried by long-distance aircraft.

affect The feelings or emotional state of an individual and the influence of this on behavior.

affective disorders A large class of disorders of mood or emotional conditions, including BIPOLAR DISORDER, DEPRESSION, POST-TRAUMATIC STRESS DISORDER, and abnormal mood states sometimes associated with SUBSTANCE ABUSE and drug dependency. Collectively these conditions comprise a large proportion of the GLOBAL BURDEN OF DISEASE.

affective domain A term used mainly in educational psychology and health education that refers to the aspect of mental function concerned with feelings and emotions.

affirmative action A practice adopted in the Eisenhower administration in the 1950s and later implemented under US civil rights legislation, intended to ensure that members of disadvantaged groups, i.e., women in some walks of life, AFRICAN AMERICANS, other VISIBLE MINORITIES, and persons with disabilities, were not discriminated against but instead were given preference in hiring and in access to the quota of places available for university-level education. One consequence that has not been achieved to the degree that was hoped for is significant improvement in the health experience of disadvantaged minorities.

aflatoxins A class of mycotoxins produced by a mold (*Aspergillus flavus*) that has carcinogenic and hepatotoxic properties. They usually occur as a contaminant in foodstuffs such as peanuts. Many are also acutely toxic. They may be killed and the toxin inactivated by irradiating foodstuffs.

African American A citizen or resident of the United States whose ancestry can be traced to Africa. A term intended to avoid the pejorative associations of words such as "negro" and "black." An estimated 10 to 12 million slaves of African origin came involuntarily to the Americas in the Portuguese, Spanish, Dutch, French, and British colonial periods and in the first eight decades of the United States. Their original gene pools, predominantly from west and east Africa, have been mixed with those of their European slave owners, and their cultural ties with Africa have been lost or distorted, but some genetic traits, e.g., tall stature of some lineages and the SICKLE CELL TRAIT, have persisted. African Americans are underrepresented among the best educated professional classes in the United States and overrepresented among the lowest socioeconomic groups and in prisons. They have shorter life expectancy and higher death rates than white and Hispanic Americans from stroke, hypertension, diabetes, and violence. Their access to health-promoting, disease-preventing, diagnostic and therapeutic services is overall disproportionately inadequate. An approximate equivalent term is Afro-Caribbean, but these are not minority groups in their own country as African Americans are in the United States, and their health indicators usually are superior to those of African Americans.

after-burner A high temperature combustion chamber or aircraft engine component in which residual products of prior combustion undergo further, more complete combustion. The aim is to enhance the efficiency of combustion and minimize the toxic or malodorous emission products generated in earlier phases of an industrial process or operation of an internal combustion engine.

agar A protein gel that is widely used as a culture medium for bacteria.

age The duration of time a person has lived. Age is conventionally defined from the time of birth, which counts as zero, and is measured in completed years of life. For some purposes, age is measured from conception, and sometimes it may be convenient to use units shorter than a year.

ageism Discrimination or prejudice against persons on the basis of their age.

agency An organization that exists for a specific purpose, usually established by and accountable to a national, regional, or local government. The word appears as part of the title of numerous government organizations, such as AGENCY FOR INTERNATIONAL DEVELOPMENT, AGENCY FOR TOXIC SUBSTANCES AND DISEASE REGISTRY.

Agency for Healthcare Research and Quality The agency of the US Department of Health and Human Services that oversees publicly funded health care. It monitors and conducts surveillance of many aspects of health care. Among other activities, this agency is responsible for the work of the US PREVENTIVE SERVICES TASK FORCE. Information for health professionals and for the general public can be accessed at http://www.ahrq.gov/.

Agency for International Development Abbreviated as AID, or preferably USAID. The US government agency that administers and disburses foreign aid in the form of material, professional and technical support, primarily aimed at low-income developing countries. For details and current activities, see http://www.usaid.gov/.

Agency for Toxic Substances and Disease Registry A US federal government agency that is administered by the CENTERS FOR DISEASE CONTROL AND PREVENTION and is concerned with control and prevention of exposure to hazardous substances, especially in hazardous waste sites. The role, functions, scope, current activities, and interactions with other government agencies can be seen at http://www.atsdr.cdc.gov/atsdrhome.html.

Agenda 21 A set of goals proposed at the United Nations Conference on Sustainable Development (the Rio Summit) in 1992 and adopted by 178 countries. Many of the goals of Agenda 21 are relevant to population and public health. For details, see http://www.unep.org/Documents/Multilingual/Default.asp?DocumentID=52.

agent (of disease) A pathogenic organism, dietary ingredient, chemical substance, or physical condition of the environment that is necessary for disease to occur if the agent is present, present in excess, or in some circumstances, if it is absent or deficient.

Agent Orange The trade name of a broad-leaf herbicide comprising 50% 2,4-D–butyl ester and 50% 2,4,5-T–butyl ester that was used in aerial spraying of tropical forests in Vietnam, with the aim of reducing cover for Vietnamese forces against whom American troops were waging war in the 1970s. Known health effects of the dioxin contaminants in this family of herbicides include CHLORACNE and CANCER. There is limited evidence of spina bifida and other birth defects in offspring of exposed adults. Toxic levels of DIOXINS and/or other ingredients in this herbicide are a suspected cause of a high incidence of serious birth defects among exposed Vietnamese and a high incidence of neoplasia among Vietnam veterans and their offspring.

age of consent A precisely defined age, albeit an age that varies among jurisdictions such as states in the United States, European nations, and Canadian provinces; varies between the sexes; and varies according to the purpose for which it is defined. Males are regarded as able to consent on their own behalf at younger ages than females in some cultures and for some aspects of law, but an exception is marriage laws, where the female legal age for marriage is 12 years in some jurisdictions but older for males. It is important for public health officials to be familiar with local laws regarding consent to participate in preventive or therapeutic interventions, especially when these apply to intimate personal matters, such as contraceptive advice for unmarried teenage girls.

age-specific rate The rate at which an event or a condition is observed in a specific age group. The numerator is the number of eligible events or conditions observed in that age group, the denominator is the amount of person-time (or number of persons) in that age group at risk of the eligible event or condition, with both events and person-time or populations being counted for the same time period. Classification of data into specified age groups and enumeration of numerators and denominators in each age group is required for calculation of age-specific rates.

age standardization Syn: age adjustment. Mathematical procedures for adjusting rates in two or more populations with differing age structure so as to adjust for rate differences among them that are or could be attributable to the effect of age differences, rather than other factors. Direct and indirect methods are available, involving mathematical calculations. For a description of the direct method, see http://www.cdc.gov/nchs/datawh/nchsdefs/ageadjustment.htm. See also STANDARDIZATION.

agglomerate (*n*) A collection of solid particles that adhere to one another, or a substance that aggregates into an ill-defined clump.

aggregation 1. Assembly of particles, generally in dry, stable form, i.e., an aggregate, such as coal gas production from coal. A similar process in liquids leads to COAGULATION or FLOCCULATION. 2. Summation into a single set of data previously arranged in several sets.

aggression Behavior characterized by anger, hostile thoughts, words, and actions toward others, manifest in speech, tone of voice, body language, outward expressions of anger or rage, threatened or actual physical violence, sometimes communal or collective violence. Aggressive conduct often harms the health of other individuals, and group aggression can harm entire groups or communities. Aggression in attacks on and defense of territory or during invasion of another group's territory is a frequent behavioral trait of animals and humans. It is not regarded as a human instinct but may have some survival value and may play a role in courtship. Aggression is a determinant of several common public health problems, e.g., various forms of DOMESTIC VIOLENCE and some traffic crashes as well as WAR and TERRORISM.

aging In biology, the process of growing older. Organs and tissues age, apparently because the clones of cells that constitute them have finite life spans. In demography and vital statistics, AGING OF THE POPULATION refers to a population in which there is an increasing proportion of persons in older age groups. See also SENESCENCE.

aging of the population The demographic trend toward higher proportions of middle-aged and older persons with lower proportions of children and young adults that occurs when birth rates decline without a corresponding decline of death rates in infancy and childhood, over a period of a generation or more. Early in the 21st century, populations almost everywhere in the world are aging, and in some, notably in Western and Eastern Europe, the process has advanced to the extent that the total population would also decline in the absence of immigration. The important effects of aging of the population are economic and social. The proportion of dependent elderly people rises, including old people living alone without close kin to care for them, which produces a need for larger numbers of long-term care facilities for infirm elderly.

agricultural workers Persons who work in the agricultural sector may be settled or migratory workers and may be exposed to various environmental safety and health risks, e.g., exposure to hazardous equipment, adverse weather, toxic pesticides, irritant or allergenic dusts, pollens, etc. Migratory and transient agricultural workers (and their dependent children) are especially vulnerable because they may be exposed in one setting and fall ill in another; the nature and level of exposure often are difficult to determine, and they often have limited or no access to health care.

agro-ecosystem An ecosystem composed of agricultural regions. The aim is as far as possible to maintain a biological balance, by returning nutriment to the soil in the form of treated human and animal waste, and to avoid excessive use of pesticides or fertilizers. Until the development of large scale machine-operated agriculture, almost all agricultural regions in the world were ecologically sustainable although of course susceptible to droughts, floods, etc. The ecological sustainability of many modern agricultural developments is questionable because it is often dependent on use of artificial fertilizers. However, traditional agro-ecosystems such as paddy fields were hospitable to vector-borne diseases such as malaria and schistosomiasis.

agronomy Land management aimed at enhancing agricultural productivity; the art and science of soil and crop management that are the underlying principles of agriculture and are therefore critical in sustaining life-supporting ecosystems.

AIDS See ACQUIRED IMMUNODEFICIENCY SYNDROME.

Aid to Families with Dependent Children (AFDC) A federal social assistance program operated by the Office of Family Assistance in the Administration for Children and Families of the Department of Health and Human Services. It is managed at state level and is intended for families who lack the material resources to care for their children and children deprived of parental support living at home. See http://www.acf.dhhs.gov/programs/afdc/afdc.txt for details.

air bag A safety device intended to protect occupants of automobiles from injury in traffic crashes. It was developed as an alternative to seat belts, which some automobile drivers and passengers would not or could not tolerate. External impact and/or sudden deceleration releases and inflates the air bag, which softens the force of impact during a traffic crash. The explosive force of the rapidly inflating air bag can cause injury to small children, short adults, and pregnant women. Evaluation has demonstrated that seat belts provide a higher degree of protection from death and serious injury in traffic crashes, and use of both seat belts and air bags provides the highest degree of protection.

airborne Pertaining to microorganisms, particles below a specified size, and DROPLET NUCLEI that are small enough to remain suspended in the atmosphere for long periods, during which they may be inhaled and cause disease or lung damage. The specified size varies with density and environmental conditions. Particles from 25 to 50 microns can remain suspended for long periods; particles smaller than 2.5 microns can penetrate to the alveoli of the lungs.

air emissions Release or discharge of a pollutant from a stationary source, such as a furnace stack or agricultural feedlot, or a mobile source, such as the exhaust pipe of an automobile.

air mass A term for an ill-defined but meteorologically significant region of the atmosphere, such as a region of very high humidity and electrical charge that could be associated with tornado formation, or a region with high levels of pollution or SMOG. See also AIR SHED.

air monitoring Collection of indoor and/or outdoor air samples and examination for atmospheric air pollutants, including gases and suspended particles, to assess and report on air quality. It may be conducted on a continuous or intermittent basis, using several varieties of instruments to monitor for specific toxic substances, particulate matter, etc.

air pollutants Gases, fumes, suspended aerosols, smoke, mist, vapor, or radioactive, biologically active, or malodorous substances or any combination of these that contaminates ambient air.

air pollution Contamination of ambient outdoor or indoor air by harmful gases, noxious fumes or vapors, solid suspended particulate matter, or some combination of these, commonly caused by emission products of combusted fuels of industrial, domestic, and/or automobile origin. All of these adversely affect human health. See also SMOG.

air quality criteria The ambient levels of air pollutants and exposure times above which there may be adverse or harmful consequences

Air Quality Index An arbitrarily defined scale used by weather forecasters (e.g., in radio and television broadcasts) that assigns a score for air quality, based on the quantity of suspended particulate matter, irritant or toxic gases such as sulfur dioxide, and the "pollen count" of allergenic grasses and weeds. Improved criteria for a valid and reproducible air quality index are a research priority because this would be a useful aid in deciding whether persons with compromised respiratory or cardiovascular systems should venture outdoors. Currently, lack of consistency from one jurisdiction to another reduces the value of this indicator.

air quality standards The estimated ambient levels of air pollutants and exposure times above

which there may be adverse or harmful consequences and for which laws or regulations require compliance. In practice, air quality standards are exceeded frequently and government actions generally do not go beyond public advisories such as recommending that infants, the elderly, and persons with chronic cardiorespiratory problems should remain indoors until air quality improves with a change of weather or wind. See also NATIONAL AMBIENT AIR QUALITY STANDARDS.

air sampling Collection for analysis of samples of air from a workplace or from weather stations that may or may not collect air of comparable quality to that which prevails in inhabited regions of the same locality. The air may be collected while it is moving or still, intermittently short term, or continuously. Samples can be analyzed for many varieties of contaminants and normal ingredients.

air shed Syn: air basin. A region where topography and prevailing weather conditions limit air movement, leading to stagnation of air masses. An air shed may transcend political boundaries, leading to problems of air pollution control when the pollution originates in one nation and affects citizens of another, e.g., air pollution from the Ohio basin affects southern Ontario.

Al-Anon An organization allied to ALCOHOLICS ANONYMOUS that provides social support to family members of people with ALCOHOL DEPENDENCE.

ALARA Acronym for "as low as reasonably achievable," a standard for radiation and chemical exposure that is advocated for many diagnostic and therapeutic purposes, as well as industrial exposures.

alastrim A mild form of SMALLPOX, a disease now presumed to be eradicated and extinct.

albinism A genetically determined metabolic defect causing absence of melanin pigment. This produces a characteristic appearance of pink skin, red eyes, and white hair. Albinism is associated with heightened sensitivity to actinic radiation. Persons with albinism (albinos) may be targets for discrimination.

alcohol Unqualified this word usually refers to ethyl alcohol or ethanol, a colorless volatile liquid with the formula C_2H_5OH, which is the active ingredient in alcoholic beverages and can also be used as a solvent and fuel. Alcoholic drinks have been used in some form by almost all human societies since antiquity, sometimes in religious rituals or orgiastic rites but usually as a recreational drink. Most people can tolerate alcohol intake in moderation, but a small proportion become addicted, and everyone experiences impaired judgment and dexterity when the blood alcohol concentration rises above a critical level. The same word can also refer to methyl alcohol, or methanol ("rubbing alcohol"), which is a dangerous neurotoxin if ingested. See also BREATHALYZER and IMPAIRED DRIVING.

alcohol abuse Excessive consumption of alcohol, especially when it is habitual or frequently repeated and associated with impaired capacity to function in the family and society, operate a motor vehicle or moving machinery, etc.

alcohol addiction See ALCOHOL DEPENDENCE.

alcohol dependence Syn: alcohol addiction, alcoholism. Physiological and/or psychological dependence upon alcohol consumption, in which the affected person cannot function effectively without recourse to alcohol and experiences withdrawal symptoms when denied access to alcohol. The features include a daily alcohol intake equivalent to 75 grams or more, morning drinking, deterioration of ability to perform usual work, and, in advanced stages, neurological impairment, memory loss, hepatic cirrhosis, vitamin deficiencies such as of thiamine (caused when alcohol replaces balanced nutritional intake), and often downward social mobility. There are associated psychosocial consequences, including loss of job, domestic violence, family breakup. There is controversy about the nature of alcohol dependence: is it inherited or acquired, a psychiatric disturbance, a metabolic dependency, a consequence of habituation, a response to environmental stresses and stimuli? It sometimes appears to have characteristics of all of these.

alcoholic A person with ALCOHOL DEPENDENCE, i.e., one who is dependent upon or addicted to alcohol. A word that often is used pejoratively.

Alcoholics Anonymous (AA) A worldwide voluntary self-help movement founded in 1935 by two men with long-term alcohol dependency. AA members provide mutual support to encourage one another to abstain from alcohol, using a BUDDY SYSTEM and regular gatherings in which AA members describe their experiences and the actions they take to avoid alcohol use. AA meetings somewhat resemble those of evangelical religious services, although AA members may have no adherence to any specific faith or formal religious belief system. For more information see http://www.alcoholics-anonymous.org.

alcohols A large class of chemical compounds composed of carbon, hydrogen, and oxygen, some of which are liquids and others solids, and many of which are widely used in everyday society and in industry. The best known is ETHYL ALCOHOL (C_2H_5OH), or ethanol. This is the active ingredient in alcoholic beverages, used in virtually all human societies throughout history as a stimulant, mood modifier, and sedative. Other common compounds include methanol, i.e., METHYL ALCOHOL (wood spirits or methylated spirits), which is used as a solvent, and butyl and propyl alcohols, which have important industrial uses.

aldehydes A family of organic chemical compounds containing the -CHO combination, formed by oxidation of an alcohol. Many aldehydes, including acetaldehyde, the first metabolite of alcoholic beverages, are toxic, some dangerously so.

aldicarb An anticholinesterase pesticide in the carbamate family, used to spray crops such as potatoes. Aldicarb (or metabolic products) can cause gastrointestinal and other cholinergic symptoms if it contaminates food or water supplies.

aldrin A volatile white crystalline chlorinated hydrocarbon INSECTICIDE that acts by disrupting the insect's nerve impulses and is toxic to humans; it is absorbed through the skin, and absorption causes irritability and depression. It has been banned in most developed countries.

algae Single or multicellular predominantly aquatic plant organisms. In sewage treatment, algae are used for biological filtration. Under some circumstances they form a symbiotic relationship with pathogenic organisms such as *Vibrio cholerae*.

algal bloom Profuse exuberant growth of algae, often at the expense of other living things in the affected ecosystem, that can choke waterways and make water unfit for drinking and irrigation. Some algal blooms produce toxins that concentrate as they move up the food chain.

algorithm A systematic process consisting of an ordered sequence of stages in which each stage is determined by the outcome of the stage that preceded it. The word commemorates the Arab mathematician Mohammed Ibn Musa Al-Khowarismi (c. 780–850), who was one of the founders of algebra. An algorithm can be displayed visually in the form of a FLOW CHART.

alienation Estrangement or withdrawal from society or family. This may be a manifestation of a mental disorder or of social or political disaffection. When it occurs in a family or social group, it may include rejection of health care, and this can have adverse health implications for members of the family or social group other than those who feel directly alienated.

alkaloids A large class of organic chemicals containing nitrogen compounds, usually of plant origin, that includes therapeutically important hypnotics, analgesics, psychoactive drugs, etc.

alkyl nitrates Important compounds in this group include nitroglycerin and ethylene glycol. Their adverse effects on health include cardiovascular and neurological dysfunction.

allele Alternative forms of the same gene that occupy the same locus on a chromosome.

allergen A substance, generally a protein, that induces ALLERGY, i.e., causes an allergic reaction.

allergic rhinitis Syn: hay fever. An allergic inflammatory process affecting the upper respiratory tract, causing redness, swelling, and profuse mucosal discharge from the nose, often accompanied by conjunctivitis.

allergy A malfunction of antigen-antibody interaction associated with inflammatory changes in mucosal tissues that may have localized or generalized clinical manifestations, including ASTHMA, hay fever, urticaria (hives), and, most seriously, a life-threatening anaphylactic reaction. Allergic reactions afflict most people from time to time, and some people all or most of the time.

allocative efficiency A term used by health economists to describe the degree to which resources are allocated efficiently. The economic analysis may or may not take ethical issues into account, and equitable resource allocation is as important as economic efficiency. See also EFFICIENCY.

allopathic medicine The prevailing form of conventional or orthodox medical practice, based as far as feasible on formally arrived-at diagnostic categories of conditions that are treated on the basis of best available evidence for efficacy of therapeutic measures. Early in the 21st century it is increasingly in transition into EVIDENCE-BASED MEDICINE.

Alma-Ata Declaration The document resulting from a conference sponsored by WHO and UNICEF in 1978 at Alma-Ata in what was then the Soviet Union. It proclaimed a health policy calling for HEALTH FOR ALL the people of the world and for equitable treatment of all people, based on community participation, healthy environments, and primary health care. The Alma-Ata Declaration has been one of the guiding principles of WHO policies since that time. See http://www.who.int/hpr/NPH/docs/declaration_almaata.pdf for the text of the Declaration.

almoner A British term, now almost obsolete, for the hospital official who dispensed alms to indigent patients. The functions of the almoner broadened to include a considerable component of SOCIAL WORK, especially after the foundation of the NATIONAL HEALTH SERVICE. Almoners now are trained social workers, and are officially so designated in the United Kingdom.

alpha error Type I error; the error of rejecting a true null hypothesis, i.e., declaring that there is a significant difference among data sets when in reality there is not.

alternative medicine, therapy A general term for forms of diagnosis and treatment to which people may turn in preference to orthodox or allopathic medicine. These include CHIROPRACTIC, HERBAL REMEDIES, ACUPUNCTURE, HOMEOPATHY, hypnotherapy, faith healing, and a great many others. Aspects with origins in traditional and folk medicine have stood the test of time and include many remedies with empirically demonstrated efficacy. Alternative medicine is popular with people with chronic conditions for which orthodox medicine offers no cure and not much relief, such as chronic arthritis, multiple sclerosis, and intractable asthma. Most varieties of alternative medicine are harmless and at least spare their users the hazardous side effects of modern pharmaceutical preparations, but they can be harmful if they have untoward side effects or if they are used by people for whom orthodox medicine offers a certain cure or more effective therapy.

altruism An aspect of human values, altruism is a moral and ethical motivation to help and aid others for reasons that are not self-interest, often at the cost of some self-sacrifice. It motivates charity, donating blood, organs for transplantation, etc. It is observed in some animals, e.g., dolphins, and may have evolutionary importance for humans. It is probably a learned behavior, not an instinct. Altruism has been implicit in the work of healing professions since ancient times and along with "enlightened self-interest" it is a motive for the more historically recent activities of public health and the professional groups who practice it.

aluminosis A relatively benign form of pneumoconiosis due to inhalation of aluminum dust.

aluminum (Al) A silvery-gray metallic element widespread in nature as alumino-silicate (bauxite), from which it is extracted by electrolysis. Its strength and light weight have made aluminum the preferred metal for aircraft construction. It has been suggested that aluminum toxicity may be incriminated in the pathogenesis of ALZHEIMER'S DISEASE, but this is unproven.

alveolitis 1. Inflammation of the alveoli of the lungs, often a precursor of pneumonia. 2. The same term describes inflammation of a tooth socket.

Alzheimer's disease A degenerative brain disease characterized by memory loss and dementia that is an increasingly common cause of disability and death among older people. It was identified by the German neurologist Alois Alzheimer (1864–1915). It has characteristic pathological features, including anatomical changes and amyloid deposits in the brain. Its cause is unknown, but genetic factors, aberrant metabolism of copper and/or aluminum, other dietary or metabolic factors, and age-related vascular degeneration have been proposed. Its prevalence rises with age, from 2% to 3% at age 65 years to 25% to 30% at age 85 years. In societies with aging populations and many elderly people who lack strong family support systems, the need for custodial institutional care presents challenging social and economic problems. Numerous support groups exist in many countries. Information about US resources is available at http://www.alzheimers.org/.

Amanita phalloides An extremely poisonous mushroom that causes progressive and irreversible hepatic and renal necrosis. It is said to have been used to kill her enemies by the Florentine Lucretia Borgia (1480–1519) and before her by the Roman empress Messalina (22–48 CE).

amaurosis Blindness caused by damage to the optic nerve, usually due to disease or injury.

ambient relating to the immediately surrounding environment.

amblyopia Impaired vision due to lesions in the visual cortex, usually of congenital origin.

ambulatory care Literally, medical care of persons who are able to walk in and out of a clinic. The care may be primary, episodic, or part of continuing care for an existing condition. Typically, physicians providing ambulatory care are working under time pressure, which is unfortunate if it leaves no time for initiatives aimed at opportunistic early disease detection.

amebiasis Infection with amebae, which cause chronic dysentery, occasionally amebic abscess of the liver and rarely meningitis or brain abscess. This very common fecal-oral infection is transmitted in contaminated water or food. Amebae are ubiquitous in water supplies in many low-income countries but are killed by boiling the water before drinking it or using it for cooking.

American Association of Retired Persons (AARP) A large national organization in the United States that advocates on behalf of Americans in the older age groups, roughly 55 years and older. There are equivalent organizations in most other nations in the Organization for Economic Cooperation and Development (OECD), i.e., upper-income nations. See http://www.aarp.org.

American Board of Preventive Medicine The examining body of the AMERICAN BOARDS that is responsible for examining candidates and reassessing practitioners who seek certification or recertification in the specialty of preventive medicine. See http://www.abprevmed.org/ for further information.

American Boards In the United States, the supervisory bodies in each of the specialties in medicine that set the standards, administer assessment procedures, i.e., formal examinations and periodical reassessment of specialized physicians, certifying fitness to practice that specialty. Professionals who have fulfilled the requirements of a specialty board are described as "board certified." In other English-speaking nations, i.e., United Kingdom, Australia, Canada, etc., and elsewhere in the world, comparable systems of specialized colleges fulfill this role, and many also act as professional organizations for members of the relevant specialty.

American College of Preventive Medicine The US professional college for physicians who have fulfilled the requirements for certification in the specialty of preventive medicine. The closest British equivalent is the Faculty of Public Health of the Royal Colleges of Physicians of the United Kingdom, which has similar standards that are generally considered somewhat more rigorous. Royal Colleges or a specialized "faculty" of a Royal College perform this function in Australia, New Zealand, and Canada, and comparable bodies exist in many other countries. See http://www.acpm.org for details.

American Conference of Governmental Industrial Hygienists A body that represents public health workers in industry. Its activities include its role in setting standards for THRESHOLD LIMIT VALUES (TLVs), the levels of occupationally related exposures to toxic and potentially toxic chemicals encountered in workplaces. See http://www.acgih.org/home.htm for details.

American Indian Syn: Native American. A person whose ancestry includes aboriginal or pre-Columbian inhabitants of North, Central, or South America. Various terms are used in parts of the Americas. In the United States, the official term is

Native American. In Canada, the official term is First Nations people. Members of such groups generally have lower life expectancy and other unfavorable health indicators compared with those of the colonizing ethnic groups in the same localities.

American Medical Association (AMA) The principal professional organization for licensed physicians in the United States. It is an academic society concerned with professional standards of competence and integrity that has branches in all states, holds national and regional annual scientific meetings, publishes journals and a newspaper for its members, is a lobbying and negotiating group in dealings with governments and insurance providers, and speaks for the medical profession in many interactions with the general public, consumer groups, and the like. For details and publications, including the *Journal of the American Medical Association (JAMA)*, see http://www.ama-assn.org.

American National Standards Institute (ANSI) A private, nonprofit organization that aims to ensure uniformly high quality in a wide range of scientific and commercial activities including many in the health sector. Information about this institute is available at http://www.ansi.org/default.aspx.

American Public Health Association (APHA) The US organization, founded in 1872, that serves professional groups engaged in every branch of public health science and practice. It is an academic professional society that holds annual national and many regional meetings and an activist advocacy and lobbying group with the federal and state governments. It publishes a monthly journal, the *American Journal of Public Health*, and a monthly newspaper, *The Nation's Health*, for its members, and some important books used all over the world, notably the *Control of Communicable Diseases Manual (CCDM)*. The broad scope and reach of public health science and practice are apparent from the large number of sections that make up the constituency of the APHA. Its activities and those of its sections can be found at http://www.apha.org. There are similar organizations of public health workers in many other countries.

American Sign Language (ASL) A means of communication by hand and finger signals and movements for the hearing impaired (and others not necessarily deaf) that enables deaf people to communicate. ASL is used worldwide by the hearing impaired, regardless of the local spoken language.

Ames test A screening test for mutagenic activity using strains of *Salmonella typhimurium* unable to synthesize histidine. Mutagens produce strains of *S. typhimurium* that can synthesize histidine. The test was developed by Bruce Ames (b. 1928), an American molecular geneticist.

amines A large class of organic substances derived from ammonia in which one of the hydrogen atoms has been replaced by a hydrocarbon consisting of or containing aliphatic amines. Some of these compounds are malodorous, and this loose descriptive term is often used pejoratively for any substance that smells bad. The term is therefore preferably avoided.

amino acid The basic chemical compound that when assembled with others forms proteins. Amino acids are the building blocks of proteins. The 64 codons of the genetic code allow the use of 20 different amino acids in the synthesis of proteins.

ammonia (NH_3) Colorless alkaline gas with a suffocating pungent odor, produced by bacterial decomposition of proteins, purines, urea, etc. It is manufactured and widely used industrially as the basis for many other compounds and can be a cause of industrial gas poisoning.

amniocentesis A procedure performed by perforating the amniotic sac with a needle and aspirating a small quantity of amniotic fluid. This diagnostic test is used at or soon after 15 weeks' gestation to identify defects such as genetic abnormalities of the fetus, by growing cells from this fluid in a culture medium for 2 weeks, then examining these cells microscopically in search of cytological abnormalities. The procedure may risk fetal damage and induced abortion, especially in unskilled hands.

amosite A form of ASBESTOS, found mainly in South Africa, with a high iron content and also containing aluminum and magnesium silicates. It is considered to be a particularly hazardous form of asbestos. Exposure to amosite asbestos is associated with high risks of asbestosis, lung cancer, and mesothelioma.

amphetamines The generic name for a family of synthetic central nervous system stimulant compounds that induce wakefulness, alertness. They are used for this purpose by people seeking to remain alert during long periods of sleeplessness. However, they also induce hyperexcitability, suppress appetite, and can cause psychotic symptoms resembling paranoia. Therefore, they must be used cautiously. Prolonged use can induce addiction. Some amphetamines have been used therapeutically to treat narcolepsy and attention deficit disorder. Illicit variants, usually methamphetamine or closely related derivatives, known as "speed" or CRYSTAL METH are easily manufactured and are widely used in underground cultures, and increasingly among others such as young people in rural communities.

amphibole Bisilicate mineral, a common form of ASBESTOS.

amyl nitrite A volatile liquid producing fumes that dilate coronary arteries, thus enhancing blood flow to the heart muscle. It is used to relieve the ischemic pain (angina pectoris) produced by myocardial ischemia. It has been used as an adjuvant sexual stimulant, mainly by homosexual men, although its efficacy for this purpose is dubious, and there may be health risks.

anabolic steroids Synthetic steroid hormones that have some masculinizing effects, building muscle mass, enhancing body strength and athletic performance. They are popular with competitive athletes and bodybuilders, but their use is prohibited in many competitive sports because of the unfair advantage they confer on users and the associated risks to health. If used by adolescents, they may cause premature closure of epiphyses and stunted growth. In adults, they may cause testicular atrophy, baldness, and increased risk of cardiovascular disease and sudden death. See http://www.nida.nih.gov/Infofacts/Steroids.html for more information.

anal sex Sexual intercourse consisting of insertion of the penis through the anal sphincter into the partner's rectum. This form of intercourse is used mainly by male homosexuals and sometimes by heterosexual couples to avoid risking pregnancy or vary sexual pleasure. It can be a way to transmit sexually transmitted diseases, including HIV infection. See also BAREBACK.

analysis of variance Syn: ANOVA. A set of statistical methods for assessing the contribution of independent variables to the mean value of a continuous dependent variable. The procedure consists of identifying the total variability, summing the squares of differences from the overall mean value, and using complex calculations or a table that allows for the number of degrees of freedom, testing the statistical significance of the independent variables.

analytic study A general term for a study that aims to establish causal relationships among sets of categorical variables, such as exposure to defined health hazards and disease outcomes related to these exposures. Examples include cross-sectional, case control, and cohort studies.

anaphylaxis Extreme sensitivity to an ALLERGEN, clinically manifest as acute-onset swelling of mucosal tissues including the trachea, where it causes life-threatening obstruction of the airway.

Anatomic Therapeutic Chemical (ATC) classification An international systematic standard for pharmaceutical drugs that groups them according to the organ or tissue on which they act, their mode of action, and their chemical composition. The ATC uses a unit of measurement, the defined daily dose (DDD). The World Health Organization endorses the use of ATC/DDD, but it emphasizes that this does not necessarily imply approval of any specific ATC drugs.

androgens Steroid hormones that exert a masculinizing influence. Testosterone is the principal one, secreted by the testes, but both men and women secrete androgens in the suprarenal glands. The illicit use of androgens and related steroids as performance-enhancing substances by athletes has tainted many professional and amateur sports. Moreover, such use is a serious health risk because it can induce cardiovascular disease and sudden death in apparently fit and healthy athletes.

anecdotal evidence Evidence derived from medical (or lay) histories, unsupported by objective data. Anecdotal evidence can be an important indicator of need for further study. This may be an ANECDOTAL STUDY, such as the medical histories of a series of cases of a rare condition, and may in turn suggest further investigation, such as a CASE CONTROL STUDY. Examples include the case history series that preceded the first epidemiological studies of malignant neoplasm of the vagina in young women caused by prenatal exposure to diethylstilbestrol (DES) and of hemangiosarcoma of the liver in workers exposed to vinyl chloride. Anecdotal evidence influences policy making when politicians play on emotions aroused by publicizing a single case to promote a particular cause, such as investing in costly diagnostic equipment.

anecdotal study A semiformal or formal research project that relies on ANECDOTAL EVIDENCE. In the health sector this may consist of a collection of medical case histories. In some fields of science, e.g., sociology and anthropology, anecdotal study is formalized with rules and PROTOCOLS that are often rigorous to determine the way the evidence is collected, analyzed, and interpreted. See also QUALITATIVE ANALYSIS.

anemia Abnormally low hemoglobin concentration in the blood. This can arise from several common causes. 1. IRON DEFICIENCY ANEMIA is caused by iron loss (e.g., due to chronic bleeding from peptic ulcer, menstrual disorders, intestinal parasites such as hookworm) and/or inadequate iron intake, or metabolic disorders that disrupt dietary iron uptake. 2. Destruction of red blood corpuscles caused by HEMOLYSIS, as in SICKLE CELL ANEMIA, chronic MALARIA, or other diseases that cause hemolysis. 3. Diseases affecting blood-forming tissues in the bone marrow, i.e., aplastic and hypoplastic anemia, either primary diseases or secondary conditions, e.g., to malignant disease such as leukemia. 4. Megaloblastic or pernicious anemia, a specific disease caused by vitamin B_{12} deficiency. 5. Numerous other miscellaneous causes. The level at which anemia is considered clinically significant and requiring treatment, formerly set at 10 mg/100 mL blood, is now usually set at 9 mg/100 mL.

angel dust The street name for phencyclidine hydrochloride (PCP), an illicit hallucinogenic drug that can cause schizophrenia-like behavior, delirium, coma, and death of users. It is easily synthesized and circulates widely among young people seeking a cheap thrill. Its use is a public health problem because it creates a high-risk group for drug-induced mental illness.

angina Also called angina pectoris or angina of effort, this is usually a severe cramp-like pain in the chest, often radiating to the neck, jaw, and left arm, associated with exertion and relieved by rest. Variations in distribution and severity of the pain are common. It is caused by myocardial ischemia, i.e., ischemic or coronary heart disease. It may be a premonitory sign of acute myocardial infarction and is often regarded as an indication for coronary arterial bypass surgery. In French, the word *angine* without a qualifying adjective means painful sore throat, as does Vincent's angina in English. This is an occasional potential source of confusion.

angiosarcoma A dangerous malignant condition associated with exposure to VINYL CHLORIDE. It often affects the liver but can occur in any organ or tissue.

anilines A class of liquid organic chemical compounds of carbon, hydrogen, and nitrogen that are the basis for many dyes, pharmaceutical substances, and plastics. Many of these compounds are toxic, and some are carcinogenic.

animal bites Many animals will bite or scratch an attacker when threatened, and predators use their teeth to catch and kill their prey. When humans are bitten, the bite often becomes infected unless carefully cleansed and disinfected. The danger is acute and potentially life-threatening if the animal has RABIES. Other diseases acquired after animal bites or scratches include cat scratch disease, rat bite fever, and, rarely, tularemia and plague.

animal model Study of a disease or its determinants that is conducted with laboratory animals, using conditions, processes, etc., that mimic as far as feasible those occurring in humans. Animal models can facilitate the study of pathogenesis and experimental treatments that are not possible with living humans, whether healthy or sick.

animal rights movement A political and moral protest movement that developed in Britain, Europe, and the United States in the 19th century and is primarily concerned with protecting animals from harmful experimentation. In its extreme, militant form, the movement may involve terrorist acts against medical and biological scientists, destruction of laboratories, and release of laboratory animals that may expose the public to danger from pathogens or toxic chemicals. Concern for well-being and welfare of domestic animals, and for humane care of experimental animals, is a moral and ethical obligation, but the animal rights movement sometimes takes this to excessive lengths.

animal testing Animals have been widely used for many years to test vaccines, pharmaceutical drugs, cosmetics, etc. This is a legal requirement under the US Food and Drugs Act and similar legislation in most other nations. The ethical constraints are specified in the regulations of research-granting agencies and internationally by the Council for International Organizations of the Medical Sciences, which has published guidelines on the ethical treatment of animals.

animal welfare Protection of domestic and experimental animals is safeguarded by legislation and regulation intended to prevent cruelty and undue suffering. In the United States, the European Union countries, and many others, legislation reinforces ethical guidelines formulated and regulated by research-granting agencies to protect animals used in research, and legislation also regulates the welfare of domestic and farm animals.

anisakiasis Invasive infection of the intestinal walls by larvae of nematode worms of the genus *Anisakis*, causing granulomatous swellings and symptoms resembling peptic ulcer.

anomie (Fr, derived from Gr) Absence of accepted social standards and values, a condition that can affect an individual or a society. A term used by the French social scientist Emile Durkheim (1858–1917) in his classic work *Suicide* (1897).

anonymous HIV testing A procedure in HIV testing, in which the identity of the tested individual is withheld or in which all personal identifying information is stripped from the specimen before it is submitted for testing. Disclosure of a positive test result for HIV infection can have serious adverse consequences for employment, eligibility for insurance policies, social life, etc. Thus, there are advantages for individuals to retain the right to keep secret the fact that they have tested positive. This can be achieved by anonymous-linked HIV testing, in which the identity of individuals with positive results can be ascertained only by reference to an identifying code number and only the individual concerned knows the number. Another form of anonymous HIV testing is used in SEROPREVALENCE surveys, in which the blood samples are stripped of all personal identifiers. This is anonymous-unlinked HIV testing.

Anopheles The genus of mosquitoes that are vectors for MALARIA and for some other diseases. Female anopheline mosquitoes require blood meals for their eggs to mature. Malaria parasites pass the sporogenous phase of their life cycle in the female mosquito's gut and body cavity. Anopheline mosquitoes have a life span of 2 to 3 weeks, which is long enough for malaria parasites to complete the mosquito phase of their life cycle in climates with ambient temperatures above about 24°C.

anosmia Loss of the sense of smell. This can occur as a consequence of various neurological disorders, damage to the olfactory sensory nerve endings in the vault of the nose, sensory overload, and blocking of sensory input by toxic damage to the olfactory nerve endings, caused by certain poisonous gases and fumes, such as HYDROGEN SULFIDE. Thus, it can be a dangerous, even occasionally life-threatening condition.

anoxia Relative or absolute lack of oxygen. Absolute lack of oxygen to vital organs (brain, heart) for longer than a few minutes is fatal; relative lack of oxygen causes CYANOSIS due to raised concentration of reduced hemoglobin in the blood, imparting a bluish color to the skin.

ANSI Acronym for AMERICAN NATIONAL STANDARDS INSTITUTE.

antagonism The interaction of opposing forces. The situation in which two or more factors acting together produce an effect that is less than the sum of each acting independently; in absolute or complete antagonism, the effects cancel each other out so the result is no change at all or a steady state. Contrast SYNERGISM.

antecedent causes of death The condition(s) that led to or precipitated the immediate cause of death, as recorded on a DEATH CERTIFICATE. For example, myocardial ischemia caused by coronary artery disease is an antecedent cause of heart failure (the immediate cause of death), where the underlying cause is coronary arterial atherosclerosis.

antenatal Literally, before birth; pertaining to the provision of services for pregnant women and for their unborn children.

antenatal care The monitoring methods and procedures for pregnant women that are routine in societies with good-quality health care services and systems. These include assessing the mother's health and obstetric fitness (adequacy of the pelvis for vaginal delivery, absence of anatomical and pathological abnormalities); routine regular surveillance throughout pregnancy to detect departures from normal blood pressure, hemoglobin level, renal function, etc., and monitoring the health and development of the fetus.

anthracite A hard, high-quality variety of coal that burns at higher temperatures and emits fewer toxic products and contaminants such as heavy metals than does lower-grade coal.

anthracosis The variety of pneumoconiosis caused by inhalation and deposition in the lungs of respirable particles of coal dust; an occupational disease of coal miners, commonly known as BLACK LUNG because at autopsy the lungs are black and the condition causes chronic cough with black sputum. Coal dust containing silica, commonly found in many coal mines, causes the more severe condition of silicoanthracosis (also called anthracosilicosis).

anthrax A bacterial disease of animals and humans caused by *Bacillus anthracis*. The organism can gain entry to the body via the skin, where it causes cutaneous anthrax; from skin lesions it may invade the body to cause septicemia or pneumonia. An alternative and far more dangerous route of entry is by inhalation or ingestion of anthrax spores. This causes a form of contagious pneumonia or gastroenteritis that has a very high case fatality rate. The anthrax bacillus has been used as a terrorist weapon and could be a weapon in BIOLOGICAL WARFARE. For further information, see http://www.bt.cdc.gov/agent/anthrax/.

anthropogenic Literally, man-made, of human origin.

anthropology The scientific study of human beings. Physical anthropology is concerned with anatomical structure and function, usually in a comparative sense in which structure and function of humans and other primates and sometimes other vertebrate species are compared. This science has provided insights into human evolution and is applied in aspects of ERGONOMICS. Social and cultural anthropology are concerned with the structures, functions, traditions, customs, religions, laws, etc., of a group or community whose characteristics are studied and analyzed. Understanding and application of cultural anthropology are essential to public health workers who deal with ethnic groups such as recent and sometimes long-established immigrants, so this subject is part of the core curriculum in many schools of public health. The specialty of forensic anthropology aims to discover incriminating evidence of wrongdoing in cases of violent death, e.g., from the mass graves of massacre victims, and has provided plots for many crime novels.

anthropometry The techniques and methods used to assess the dimensions of humans (height, weight, proportional size of limbs, ratio of fat to muscle, etc.).

antibiotic Syn: antimicrobial. A class of substances produced by living organisms, such as plants and fungi, capable of killing or inhibiting the growth of pathogenic bacteria. The word *antibiotic* first appeared in English in 1829, applied not to biology or microbiology but to a school of philosophy that differentiated life from living,. The modern usage was coined in 1944 by the Australian medical scientist Howard Florey (1898–1968) to describe the properties of penicillin.

antibiotic resistance The clinical phenomenon in which a previously efficacious antibiotic fails to work because the pathogens the antibiotic is designed to destroy have developed metabolic or other defenses against the antibiotic. Antibiotic resistance is becoming a serious global public health problem. Exposure of pathogens to low doses of antibiotics in the environment, antibiotic use to promote healthy growth in animal husbandry, and other nontherapeutic uses foster the development of resistant strains of pathogens. The phenomenon of antibiotic resistance is proof of Darwin's theory of evolution.

antibody The central feature of the body's immunological defense mechanism is the protein molecule that is modified or formed in the body in response to the stimulus provided by an alien antigen or antigenic substance, usually a protein. Antibody formation occurs principally in the lymphatic tissues and T-lymphocytes, whose action is disrupted by retroviruses such as HIV. It is the central feature of the body's immunological defense mechanisms.

antidepressant A mood-modifying drug that reverses or relieves the symptoms of depression.

Because depression is common and suicide is an occasional end result, effective antidepressant drugs, notably selective serotonin reuptake inhibitors (SSRIs), can contribute significantly to personal and population health. If the antidepressant is also a sedative, it may make the condition worse. Premature cessation of treatment with an antidepressant can cause a relapse into profound, potentially suicidal depression.

antigen A substance, e.g., protein, polysaccharide, glycolipid, living tissue, or organ, that is alien to the body and induces a specific immune response and ANTIBODY production when introduced, e.g., by an invading microorganism, inhalation, ingestion, injection of foreign protein, etc.

antihistamines A class of drugs that block or inhibit the effect of histamine on the body. They act by antagonizing the effect of histamine receptors in mucosa, skin, smooth muscle cells, and mucous glands, thus suppressing the symptoms of hay fever, urticaria, and other allergic conditions; some antihistamines inhibit nausea and vomiting. Many have side effects such as drowsiness and slowed reflexes that impair the capacity to drive a car or operate moving machinery.

antimalarial A drug, for example quinine and its derivatives, used to treat malaria. Antimalarials act by destroying or inhibiting growth or reproduction of the malaria parasite. Unfortunately, malaria parasites have developed resistance to many antimalarial drugs. See http://www.cdc.gov/travel/malariadrugs.htm for current recommendations.

antimicrobial drugs Drugs that kill microorganisms or inhibit their growth and reproduction.

antimony (Sb) An element classified as semimetallic, blue-white in color, used in alloys to harden lead and tin, e.g., to make blocks of print for linotype printing machines and in compound form in paints and pigments. Its toxicity resembles that of arsenic but is less serious; it causes dermatitis, and inhaled dust causes a form of pneumoconiosis.

antiretroviral drugs A class of therapeutic agents used to treat HIV and retard the onset and progression of AIDS. The first of these was ZIDOVUDINE.

antisepsis The process of minimizing contamination with pathogenic organisms by using toxic chemicals to kill the organisms. Until the discoveries by 19th century bacteriologists of the causal relationship of bacterial infection to sepsis, i.e., purulent inflammation, no systematic actions were taken to reduce or prevent the risk of contamination of wounds by pathogenic organisms, although pioneers such as IGNAZ SEMMELWEIS and OLIVER WENDELL HOLMES applied empirical observations to advocate hand-washing to reduce the risk of puerperal sepsis. Antisepsis was established in 1859 by the British surgeon JOSEPH LISTER for surgical operations and obstetrics. See also ASEPSIS.

antiseptic A substance used to achieve antisepsis. The early varieties, such as carbolic acid spray used by Joseph Lister, were either toxic or not highly effective or both. Well-known modern examples include tincture of iodine, methyl alcohol, hydrogen peroxide, and sundry vegetable preparations. Lysol is used as an environmental antiseptic.

antiserum A contraction of antitoxic serum. A biologically active preparation of human or animal serum containing specific antitoxins or antibodies, thus providing PASSIVE IMMUNITY.

antisocial behavior Actions or a tendency to actions that are not in the public interest or that may harm others, e.g., vandalism, bullying, habitually aggressive driving, speeding.

antitoxin A substance such as a serum or medication that inhibits or prevents the action of a toxin. Examples include tetanus and diphtheria antitoxins, which prevent the harm that would otherwise be done by the toxins these organisms produce.

anxiety An emotional state characterized by agitation, unease, restlessness, or fear, for which there is no perceptible cause. Anxiety disorders are a common form of neurosis that cause much unhappiness and consume great quantities of professional time and huge amounts of money for psychopharmaceutical agents to treat them or at least to relieve the symptoms.

Apgar score A composite index devised by the American pediatrician Virginia Apgar (1909–1974) to evaluate neonatal status by assigning a numerical score of 0 to 2 for heart rate, respiratory rate, skin color, muscle tone, and response to stimuli, i.e., a total score ranging from 0 to 10. The lower the score, the poorer the prognosis is for the infant.

APHA American Public Health Association; public health associations in other jurisdictions beginning with "A" (Australia, Alabama, Alaska, Arkansas, Alberta, etc).

applied research A loosely used term that can mean research carried out as a by-product of routine service or research done for an explicit pragmatic purpose.

appropriate health technology A term popularized by aid workers in low-income countries that describes diagnostic and therapeutic facilities and services that are economically sustainable.

aquaculture Farming of aquatic organisms, e.g., mollusks, fish, certain root vegetables such as water chestnuts. Rice production in paddy fields could also be described as aquaculture, at least in its early stages. Although efficient, aquaculture may foster the spread of some water-borne pathogens.

aquifer A porous water-bearing permeable stratum of rock, gravel, or sand or an underground water-course. The water in underground aquifers may or may not be potable, i.e., be free of or contaminated by pathogens. It sometimes has a high content of dissolved sodium, calcium, or magnesium salts.

arbovirus Arthropod-borne virus, a large family of viruses characterized by the epidemiological feature that all are transmitted by an arthropod vector such as mosquito, blackfly, or tick. The diseases they cause tend to have distributions dependent upon the seasonality of the arthropod vector. Many arbovirus species survive in the vector during periods of hibernation or overwintering.

arc welding A method of fusing metals together by using an electric current to generate incandescent heat that melts the metals at their junction. Arc welding produces high concentration of ultraviolet radiation and toxic metal fumes. Arc welders must use goggles or a visor that is impermeable to UV radiation to prevent serious ocular damage, but they usually lack protection from toxic fumes, which can lead to occupational disease.

ARDS Acute respiratory distress syndrome; a common, serious, often fatal condition especially among infants and children in low-income countries. See also SEVERE ACUTE RESPIRATORY SYNDROME (SARS).

area sampling A method of probability sampling in which a region designated for study is divided into parts (usually according to readily identifiable geographical features and with roughly comparable populations); the parts are numbered and sampled according to a recognized sampling method, such as use of a table of random numbers.

ariboflavinosis Severe deficiency of riboflavin (vitamin B_2). The vitamin is plentiful in milk and eggs, so the condition can occur among VEGANS. Deficiency causes angular stomatitis, dermatitis, and ocular lesions, an interstitial keratitis.

Aristotle (384–322 BCE) This ancient Greek philosopher, student of Plato, established the rules of formal logic and influenced scientific thought for 1,000 years, until empirical observations refuted his faulty theories about biology, reproduction, the composition of matter, etc.

arithmetic mean A measure of central tendency, computed by adding all the values in the set and dividing by the number of values in the set. See also AVERAGE.

armed services The sector of society, usually tax-supported, that is responsible for defending the nation against hostile adversaries, commonly divided into land, sea, and air forces. Members of the armed services are usually carefully assessed for physical fitness. In most nations they have access to a higher degree of preventive medical services than do most civilians, and in some nations they are entitled to medical care at public expense.

aromatic hydrocarbons A class of organic hydrocarbon compounds characterized by the presence of one or more benzene derivatives, i.e., a ring-shaped arrangement of at least five (usually six) carbon atoms. The compounds with one or more benzene rings in their structure include BENZENE, TOLUENE, and XYLENE. They are toxic and irritant, and benzene is a carcinogen.

arsenic (As) Metalloid element used in alloys and in chemical compounds to make pigments and (formerly) medicinal compounds, including Paul Ehrlich's MAGIC BULLET used in the early 20th century to treat syphilis. It is both an acute and a chronic poison, with very high toxicity; favored by some notorious criminal poisoners and writers of detective fiction.

arsenicals A class of chemicals containing arsenic compounds, with many industrial, commercial, and even medicinal uses. Arsenic and many of its compounds are poisonous, and some are carcinogens.

arsine A colorless gas produced by hydrogenating arsenic compounds and sometimes by digestion of certain fungi in sewage. It is toxic and even lethal at high concentrations. Mild and moderate exposure causes hemolysis and liver damage.

artesian aquifer The water in a subsurface stratum of a geological composition that permits flow. Water in the aquifer is under pressure and may escape to the surface as a spring; if a pipe or tube well is inserted into it, the water flows or can be pumped to the surface. Artesian water often has a high concentration of dissolved salts, but it is usually free of pathogens because these have been filtered out or destroyed by other soil organisms. Artesian water is widely used for irrigation, watering of live stock, and is usually potable, i.e., suitable for human consumption without further treatment despite the frequently high mineral and salt content. Sometimes it contains salts such as magnesium sulfate that have physiological or therapeutic impact.

arthritis Literally, inflammation of joints. Arthritis is the most common cause of physical disability among older people and thus is a large public health problem. Degenerative arthritis occurs the most frequently, but rheumatoid arthritis is relatively common in younger people.

arthropod A common name for any member of the phylum Arthropoda, which includes insects, spiders, crustaceans, and myriopods, characterized by segmented bodies, exoskeletons, and, depending on the species and genus, appendages that may include six, eight, or more limbs, antennae, and wings. Arthropods are by far the most numerous of all animal species. Many are important disease vectors and some can directly cause diseases, e.g., by venomous bites.

arthropod-borne diseases A large, heterogeneous group of conditions, of viral, rickettsial, bacterial, protozoal, or metazoal origin that share the epidemiological feature of transmission by an arthropod vector such as a mosquito, tick, sandfly, or blackfly. Transmission may be mechanical, the pathogen simply using the arthropod to travel to a susceptible host, as flies transmit fecal-oral infection or trachoma. However, transmission of arthropod-borne diseases usually is biological; that is, the pathogen undergoes a portion of its life cycle in the arthropod vector, as, for example, malaria parasites do. In the case of some, including many virus diseases (arbovirus diseases), the transmission cycle may include a period of "hibernation" of both the arthropod and the pathogen during cool or dry seasons, known as OVERWINTERING.

artificial insemination In mammals, including humans, fertilization of an ovum by sperm other than by sexual intercourse. The sperm may be supplied by the husband or male partner of the woman and injected vaginally; or the sperm may be supplied by a donor of known identity or an anonymous donor, and injected vaginally; IN VITRO FERTILIZATION is another method, in which sperm and ovum are brought together in laboratory conditions and implanted in the woman's uterus after fertilization occurs. There are considerable and complex public health and ethical issues and problems associated with each of these methods, as well as implications for the offspring when the sperm is anonymously donated.

asbestos A fibrous mineral substance, chemically a bisilicate. It is nonflammable, chemically inert, and an efficient insulator against heat and electrical charge. The common varieties include CHRYSOTILE ASBESTOS ("white asbestos") and AMPHIBOLES, including crocidolite ("blue asbestos") and AMOSITE. Asbestos was widely used as a seemingly inert insulating material for more than 100 years, until its harmful effects were recognized. All forms of asbestos are biologically active. Inhaled asbestos fibers cause irreversible progressive pulmonary fibrosis. They are also confirmed carcinogens, causing carcinoma of the lung and mesothelioma of the pleura and peritoneum.

asbestosis The form of PNEUMOCONIOSIS caused by inhalation of asbestos fibers, characterized by its relentlessly progressive destruction of lung structure and function. This crippling and ultimately fatal occupational disease of asbestos workers is also an environmental disease in asbestos mining and refining communities, where inhaled asbestos dust can affect children and even domestic and wild animals. Occupational and environmental regulations lagged a long way behind the rising incidence of fatal asbestosis and asbestos-induced cancers, but strict regulations and adequate compensation for affected workers and others are now relieving the problem.

ascariasis Infection with the nematode roundworm *Ascaris lumbricoides* or one of its relatives.

ascertainment The formal process of identifying and delineating the dimensions of a health problem such as endemic infectious disease in a specified community or region.

ascorbic acid (vitamin C) A water-soluble organic chemical that occurs naturally in fruits and vegetables. Vitamin C is required for several biochemical processes to function normally. These include tyrosine metabolism, which controls adrenal gland function among other things, and metabolism of bone and cartilage. Deficiency of ascorbic acid or vitamin C causes SCURVY.

asepsis Absence of pathogenic organisms. The process of achieving asepsis by eliminating or at least minimizing contamination with pathogenic organisms. Asepsis relies on thorough cleaning, hand-washing, and scrupulously cleaning of the operating environment. The aim is to exclude all pathogenic microorganisms to eliminate potential bacterial sepsis. This is the method of infection control first advocated and applied in obstetrics by IGNAZ SEMMELWEIS and OLIVER WENDELL HOLMES and routinely used in modern surgical practice.

aspartame An artificial sweetener; claimed to expose users to fewer adverse health effects than saccharin, although the evidence is sparse.

aspergillosis A severe mycotic disease affecting the lungs, with inflammatory and allergic features, caused by inhaling fungus spores that occur, for example, in moldy hay.

aspermia A condition in which semen contains no spermatozoa or contains only dead and decomposed spermatozoa. The causes include vasectomy and diseases of the testes, e.g., fibrosis following mumps orchitis, high doses of ionizing radiation, exposure of testicles to severe heat, exposure to toxic chemicals such as DIBROMOCHLOROPROPANE (DBCP).

asphalt A tarry solid form of coal that occurs naturally and also is manufactured; used in road surfacing. Its fumes include polycyclic aromatic hydrocarbons (PAHs) and some carcinogens.

asphyxiant A chemical that causes asphyxia, e.g., by blocking the uptake of oxygen, such as happens when oxygen is displaced by an inert gas such as carbon dioxide, or when carbon monoxide or cyanide compounds bind hemoglobin, preventing it from accepting oxygen molecules in inspired air.

aspirin Acetyl salicylic acid. The chemical has powerful anti-inflammatory properties that make it an effective agent to relieve pain and reduce fever. It also helps to inhibit blood clotting, so in small daily maintenance doses it is an effective way to reduce the risk of vascular and coronary thrombosis.

assay A trial, experiment, or routine procedure to ascertain the composition, concentration, or strength of a substance, chemical compound, or contaminant.

assessment A formal process of evaluation of a process or system, preferably quantitative but sometimes necessarily qualitative. Examples include clinical assessment and assessment of the efficacy of preventive and therapeutic regimens.

assimilation 1. Part of the process of digesting food. 2. In social demography, the process by which an ethnic or culturally distinct group is absorbed into another group, often losing part or all of its distinguishing cultural characteristics in the process.

association Literally, a connection. Several meanings are relevant in public health 1. In epidemiology, statistical dependence of one phenomenon or variable upon another but not necessarily indicating a causal relationship. 2. A group that shares a common purpose or interest; usually capitalized when it is part of the name of an organization. 3. A mental or emotional connection between two or more concepts or ideas ("association of ideas").

Association des Épidémiologistes de Langue Française (ADELF) The principal professional organization for epidemiologists whose working language is French.

Association of Schools of Public Health The organization that serves schools of public health, and is a clearing house for information, for instance about curricula. See http://www.asph.org for details.

Association of State and Territorial Health Officials The professional organization for health officers in the states and territories of the United States. See http://www.astho.org/ for details.

Association of Teachers of Preventive Medicine The organization of academic staff who teach in medical schools, schools of public health, etc., in the United States and Canada with some members in other countries. Although not large, this organization has taken important initiatives, including sponsorship of the PREVENTIVE SERVICES TASK FORCE, which established guidelines for the conduct of clinical and community-based preventive interventions such as screening procedures. In 2006, the name was changed to Association for Prevention Teaching and Research. See http://www.atpm.org for details.

assortative mating Choice of sexual partners on the basis of similarity of social background, culture, education, etc., i.e., couples of similar phenotype and possibly genotype, thus nonrandom mating.

assumption A fundamental belief or tenet that is taken for granted and requires no proof or reconfirmation when it forms a basic premise in logical reasoning. See also OCCAM'S RAZOR.

asthma A recurrent, chronic disease of the lungs characterized by generalized narrowing of small airways due to swelling of the epithelium of bronchi and bronchioles, causing severe dyspnea, wheezing, and paroxysmal cough. Asthma is often associated with ALLERGIES, but environmental determinants are also important. Environmental tobacco smoke and ambient air pollution can cause new-onset asthma in children. It is often familial, suggesting a genetic basis, and linked to seasonal environmental allergens (pollens, grasses, etc.) and to irritant atmospheric contaminants (environmental tobacco smoke, industrial pollutants, smog, very cold air). The prevalence of asthma has approximately doubled in the last 20 to 30 years for reasons that have not yet been satisfactorily explained.

asylum 1. A refuge or place of safety, and in an abstract sense the assurance of safety for persons or groups who have been threatened with harm. 2. An alternative term for a refuge for the mentally or physically infirm and for a custodial MENTAL HOSPITAL (now obsolete usage).

asylum seekers A term, sometimes used pejoratively, to describe REFUGEES from war or political persecution. Such people are frequently treated harshly, including being forced to live in camps and enduring conditions such as restricted human rights and lack of health care and education for dependent children.

atavism Recurrence of disease or constitutional characteristics of ancestors in descendent members of a family tree.

ataxia Impaired coordination and balance caused by various neurological disorders affecting the cerebellum or peripheral nervous system.

atherosclerosis Syn: atheroma. A disorder due to accumulation of low-density lipid deposits in the intimal lining of arteries that leads to narrowing, plaque formation, and eventually to blockage of the lumen of the arteries, associated with loss of elasticity (arteriosclerosis or "hardening of the arteries" and arterial aneurism). When the plaques are dislodged from arterial walls, they produce emboli. When the coronary arteries are affected, coronary occlusion is a common outcome, and when arteries supplying the brain are affected, cerebral thrombosis, cerebral embolus, or cerebral hemorrhage (stroke) can occur. Thus, atherosclerosis is the underlying pathogenesis of two leading causes of death.

athlete A person who has undertaken training or exercises to become proficient in physical activities such as competitive sports (athletics). Athletes are generally healthier and enjoy greater longevity than do nonathletes, but depending on the nature of the sports they practice, their competitiveness and violence, the accompanying trauma, stress on bones, joints and soft tissues, or their use of performance-enhancing drugs such as steroids, they may be exposed to a range of risks of injury and even premature death. The specialty of SPORTS MEDICINE has developed many health-promoting and injury-avoiding methods to cater to athletes' needs.

athlete's foot A fungus infection of the feet, usually caused by dermatophytosis, that causes inflammation, itching, burning, and often an unpleasant odor. It is very common, highly infectious, and usually acquired by contact with surfaces, such as in communal changing rooms. It usually responds to fungicidal creams or ointments, but reinfection is common.

atmosphere The gaseous envelope surrounding the earth, made up of nitrogen (about 78%), oxygen (about 21%), and trace amounts of many other gases and vapors, including argon, carbon dioxide, water vapor, etc. Other planets in the solar system also have atmospheres, i.e., gaseous envelopes, but their composition is entirely different and not compatible with life as we know it.

atmospheric chemistry The branch of meteorology concerned with the chemical composition of the atmosphere and with the chemical and photochemical processes that occur in the atmosphere. Monitoring atmospheric chemistry is an important function of national environmental agencies because of concern about the concentration of acid aerosols, toxic pollutants, and possible terrorist threats.

atomic bomb The first-generation nuclear weapons, developed and tested during World War II, and used with devastating loss of life and destruction of urban infrastructure on Hiroshima, Japan, on August 6, 1945, then 2 days later on Nagasaki. Subsequently many more atomic bombs were built and tested, until they were superseded by more deadly hydrogen bombs using nuclear fusion. All contaminate the environment with radioactive fallout and therefore are a serious long-term danger to population health. Personnel involved in atomic bomb tests have subsequently had high incidence of and death rates from malignant diseases. See also NUCLEAR WEAPON.

atomic bomb survivors The atomic bombs dropped on Hiroshima and Nagasaki had a combined death toll of more 200,000 including many thousand immediate deaths from burns, blast, and acute radiation exposure. During subsequent decades there has been a continuing toll of deaths from radiation-related leukemia, brain, thyroid, and bone cancer and other malignant diseases among the survivors.

attack rate The cumulative incidence rate of a condition in a particular population or group of people such as patients admitted to a hospital. The population is often poorly defined. Although commonly used, the term is often vague because neither the size of the "population at risk" nor the time dimension is known or precisely enumerated.

attention deficit hyperactivity disorder (ADHD) A commonly diagnosed condition of grade (primary) school children, characterized by restlessness, disruptive conduct, and inability to concentrate on the lessons that a classroom teacher is attempting to impart. The associated factors, which may or may not be causes, include intelligence below or above the level at which lessons are pitched; emotional disturbance, sometimes associated with disordered family dynamics; boredom; and impaired hearing or vision. Accurate diagnosis and suitable intervention are essential, rather than prescription of drugs such as stimulants or tranquilizers, which can be addictive and/or have adverse effects. ADHD can affect people of all ages, not only children.

attenuation The process of weakening, dilution, diminution, or reduction (preferably elimination) of harmful effects of a pathogenic organism or its antigens or metabolic products, used in the preparation of vaccines.

attitude A relatively stable favorable or unfavorable feeling or belief about a concept, person, or object, usually regarded as less firmly rooted than VALUES, although the distinction is ill-defined. Attitudes can often be inferred by observing behavioral responses to sensory stimuli and can be measured with an attitude scale. See also VALUES.

attitude scale A survey instrument, usually made up of questions or statements to which a range of alternative responses, e.g., degree of agreement with leading statements, is possible.

attitude survey A community-based or sometimes an institutional-based study in which selected individuals are asked to provide answers to questions aimed at assessing their beliefs, values, or attitudes to an issue, problem, or concept. The questions, best presented orally rather than in a self-completed questionnaire, may be open-ended or may provide a series of alternatives, e.g., statements with which respondents are asked to indicate their agreement or disagreement.

attributable risk The rate or proportion of a disease or other outcome of interest among exposed persons in a defined population that can be attributed to an exposure of interest. Subtle variations can be calculated by using one of several available epidemiological methods.

attributable risk in the exposed The risk or proportion of cases of a disease or other outcome of interest among exposed persons in a defined population that can be attributed to an exposure of interest. The term implies a risk, i.e., a probability, but attributable risks are often expressed more loosely as proportions or fractions of the total risk of interest that can be attributed to exposure. For protective exposures, risk may be associated with the absence of exposure and measured by prevented risk (or fraction).

attrition Literally rubbing or wearing away; in follow-up studies of a population, the loss of study subjects for whatever reason.

audiology The clinical assessment or scientific study of hearing.

audiometry Instrumental measurement of hearing acuity that identifies and detects hearing loss at all sound wave frequencies required for a full range of hearing.

audit An examination or review of a process, by implication often a searching review, especially when carried out by an officially constituted authority. See also MEDICAL AUDIT.

authority Legitimate power, decision-making capacity, and the means to cause others to obey. The word applies both to the abstract quality and to the individual or organization in command.

autism A developmental disorder in which infants and children exhibit severe learning disability, inability to form social and emotional bonds and other inappropriate emotional responses, and sometimes extraordinary proficiency in a specific field, such as music or mathematics. This last, high-functioning form is known as Asperger's syndrome, after the Austrian pediatrician Hans Asperger (1906–1980) who identified it. Enhanced interest in this disorder resulted from media attention in the 1990s and led to more frequent diagnosis, but information on prevalence and long-term course of the condition probably is unreliable. A suggested causal association with infant immunizations was refuted by epidemiological studies.

autoclave A device that sterilizes surgical instruments, dressings, etc., by steam heating under pressure. It is an effective, efficient system that kills all or almost all pathogenic organisms.

autoimmune diseases A heterogeneous group of diseases, some of obscure etiology, including rheumatoid arthritis and ulcerative colitis, characterized by development of antibodies that attack the host's cells and tissues. For descriptions and details, see http://www.niaid.nih.gov/publications/autoimmune/autoimmune.htm and http://www.niaid.nih.gov/final/immds/immdeff.htm.

automation Control of the stages of an industrial or manufacturing process by means of electronic signals. Automation has both positive and negative consequences for workers. It can reduce or eliminate exposure to hazardous work processes, but unless there are built-in safeguards, the process can continue even after a worker has been injured on the job. Workers may also experience loss of self-esteem and low morale if they perceive themselves to be equated with "cogs in the machine" by managers of the industrial processes.

autonomic nervous system The portion of the nervous system, including the cerebellum, much of the brainstem, and a network of neural plexuses in the thorax and abdomen, that controls vital functions, including heart beat, respiration, the muscular contractions of the alimentary tract, etc.

autonomy Free will; self-governing, ability of a person or a group to choose a course of action. Autonomy is a basic human right and is one of the principles of BIOETHICS.

autopsy Anatomical and microscopic examination of a dead body aimed at discovering the cause of death and/or other associated conditions. Literally the word means "seeing with one's own eyes." Some prefer the word "necropsy," but etymology accords equal rank to both words.

autosome Any chromosome other than X or Y, the sex chromosomes.

auxiliary personnel A general administrative term for all categories of personnel in health care services other than those with professional qualifications.

average Arithmetically, the result of aggregating all the values in a set and dividing by the number of units in the set to yield a value in the center of the set. This is the arithmetic mean, one of the MEASURES OF CENTRAL TENDENCY. In practice, the concept of the "average" is often ill-defined, meaning ordinary, usual, common, or an arbitrarily imagined concept, such as the average man or the average salary.

avian influenza A lethal strain of the influenza virus designated H5N1 that began to affect poultry in Southeast Asia in 2003. It is transmissible to humans and has a high case fatality rate. Evidence on human-to-human transmission is equivocal. It can be carried over long distances by migratory birds. It is a potential causal agent for dangerous human epidemics. Information on the status of this disease is available at http://www.who.int/csr/disease/avian_influenza/en/ and http://www.cdc.gov/flu/avian/.

Avicenna or Abu Sina (980–1037) Persian philosopher, scientist, physician, whose *Canon of Medicine* gathered and augmented the existing medical knowledge of his time. This was a link between Greek and Roman medicine and physicians who began to advance empirical medical knowledge and formulate new theories of disease causation in the European renaissance.

avoidable risk The risk of disease at some unspecified future period that could be avoided by a specified shift to a more favorable exposure distribution of recognized risks. For example, the risk of disease and premature death from smoking-related diseases could be reduced by reduction of smoking rates.

axiom A generally accepted and perhaps self-evident principle, maxim, or rule, based on empirical observations, logical analysis of evidence, or universal experience.

axis 1. One of the two dimensions of a graph. 2. The central core of an organ or an organism. 3. The central (usually imaginary) line through the center of an object. 4. The conceptual framework of a classification system in disease taxonomy.

Ayurvedic medicine An ancient Indian traditional form of medical practice based on balance of body systems that uses dietary measures, herbal remedies, yoga. It also invented surgical techniques, for instance to manage bladder stones.

AZT See ZIDOVUDINE.

B

baby boom The surge in the number of births that followed the return of peace after the end of World War II in many of the combatant nations is known as the baby boom. It lasted from 1946 to the early 1960s and was attributable to restoration of intact marriages and new marriages, associated with rising prosperity and optimism about the future. As these birth cohorts reached adult life and started families of their own, there was an "echo of the baby boom" with another surge in the numbers of births in the years from the early 1970s to the early 1990s.

Baby Doe case A legal test case in the United States in 1982 involving an infant born with severe Down syndrome and esophageal atresia whose parents refused surgical intervention. Although the baby died before court-ordered intervention was possible, the publicity prompted federal and state legislation in the United States aimed at protecting newborns from abuse attributable to parental or medical neglect and similar legislation in several other countries. Several other cases identified as "Baby Doe," either of liveborn but gravely disabled infants or of severely malformed and sometimes nonviable fetuses, for instance with anencephaly, have been subjects of similar court cases in the United States.

bacillus Rod-shaped bacterium, a term originally applied to all bacteria with this shape, but now confined to a single genus of spore-forming organisms, one of which is *Bacillus anthracis*, the causative organism of ANTHRAX.

backache, back pain A common diagnostic and therapeutic problem in occupational and family medicine, which causes much discomfort and lost time from work and costs industry and insurers heavily. This ill-defined condition is a significant clinical and public health problem. Workers required to move heavy weights often sustain muscle and ligament strains and sprains, and it is not uncommon for pain to persist for months or even years. Education and training on ergonomic ways to lift heavy weights can help to reduce the problem. Precise diagnosis may be elusive and may be complicated by the occurrence of backache as a feature of malingering. There may be little or no physical evidence on radiological or other examination, but the pain and stiffness can be debilitating. Women with similar symptoms may have their condition attributed to a gynecological cause, and persons of both sexes may be unjustly accused of malingering.

background level The usual concentration or intensity of a substance, agent, or event in the environment in the absence of perturbations associated with exceptional circumstances. An example is the environmental level of ionizing radiation from terrestrial and cosmic sources in the absence of radiation accidents.

bacteria Plural of bacterium, the general name for a very large class of single-celled organisms that occur in nature. A few hundred varieties of bacteria out of a total of many millions can cause disease in humans, i.e., are pathogenic. Some, including commensal organisms in the intestinal tract and nitrogen-fixing bacteria in the soil, are essential to healthy human life, and others, such as bacteria that cause fermentation, have great economic importance. Most others are harmless. Bacteria subsist on organic matter, living or dead, and most can reproduce rapidly. Some can survive in adverse environments for prolonged periods in spore form. Bacteria are classified according to their shape: the COCCUS (plural: cocci) is spherical, the BACILLUS (plural: bacilli) is rod-shaped, the spirillum (plural: spirilla) is corkscrew-shaped. Some bacteria aggregate in clumps; some are motile. A useful distinction of pathogenic bacteria is the reaction to GRAM STAIN.

bacterial infection An infection caused by bacteria. The GRADIENT OF INFECTION is very wide, ranging from acute, fulminating, life-threatening, to symptomless subclinical, and the epidemiological and public health significance similarly varies. From the public health perspective, the most important infections are mild, subclinical, and symptomless conditions that do not restrict ability to move about and mingle with others yet can be transmitted and cause more serious disease in susceptible contacts. The same applies to infections caused by other varieties of pathogens.

bactericide A substance that kills bacteria, rather than merely preventing their reproduction. Some antibiotics, as well as many disinfectants, act this way.

bacteriologist A practitioner or research-oriented scientist of BACTERIOLOGY. Local public health departments either have bacteriologist(s) on staff or have a collaborative working relationship with bacteriologists in a public health laboratory.

bacteriology The scientific study of BACTERIA, involving their identification, classification, growth, reproduction, cytogenetics, immunology, and pathogenicity. This is one of the essential sciences of public health practice and made enormously important contributions that led to dramatic improvement in health in the century from roughly 1850 to 1950. In the early 20th century, when it became feasible to identify and eventually to visualize viruses, the science of bacteriology merged with virology, the study of viruses. MICROBIOLOGY is the term for the specialty dealing with the scientific study of all varieties of microorganisms.

bacteriophage Syn: phage. A family of viruses that destroy ("eat") bacteria, including many pathogenic species. Before the discovery of antibiotics, development of bacteriophage as a therapeutic weapon was a research priority, but although some of this was promising, the main use for bacteriophage since antibiotics became available has been in research on the molecular biology of genes. The rising frequency of antibiotic-resistant bacteria has led to some resurgence of interest in bacteriophage, but practical applications are elusive. More information and reference to additional sources can be found at http://www.bacteriophage .com/.

bacteriostatic A substance that prevents reproduction of pathogenic bacteria but does not kill them. Some antibiotics are bacteriostatic, rather than bactericidal. Their efficacy depends on the action phagocytes that destroy pathogenic bacteria, which cannot proliferate to attack the host.

baffle, baffler A device to change the direction or reduce the velocity of fluid or vapor passing through an effluent or emission discharge system of an industrial plant or waste disposal facility.

baffle chamber A part of the exhaust system of a furnace, fitted with metal or ceramic plates at an angle with the movement of emissions, where coarse particulate matter settles, so it is not discharged into the environment and can be gathered and disposed of safely in other ways.

bagassosis A form of pneumoconiosis caused by inhalation of the dust and organic matter contained in bagasse, the fibrous and dusty residue of sugar cane, which is used as biomass fuel and causes severe air pollution when it is burned; bagassosis is an occupational disease of sugar cane workers and their families.

BAL (British anti-Lewisite) See DIMERCAPRO PANOL.

balneology The scientific study of medicinal benefits of baths, hot springs, mineral waters, etc.

Bamako Initiative A strategic approach to health care, infrastructure and resource development, and capacity building, and the provision of essential drugs and their rational use in primary health care, especially for mothers, infants, and children, worked out at a conference convened jointly by WHO and UNICEF in Bamako, Mali, in 1987. Although originally the emphasis was on maternal, infant, and early child care, the goals broadened in response to changing needs, such as the impact of the HIV/AIDS epidemic. Many relevant documents on the Bamako Initiative and related activities can be accessed at http://www.un .org/issues/docs/d-child.asp.

Bangkok Charter At the 6th World Congress on Health Promotion held in Bangkok in 2005, the delegates agreed on significant revisions of the OTTAWA CHARTER FOR HEALTH PROMOTION, and created the Bangkok Charter for Health Promotion in a Globalized World. For details and discussion, see http://www.who.int/healthpromotion/conferences/6gchp/en.

bareback A colloquial and street language term that originally meant unprotected anal sexual intercourse, in particular between disclosed seroconcordant HIV-positive male sexual partners. The word has been generalized to mean unprotected anal sex, regardless of HIV status and sexual orientation. This behavior is most common among persons with low self-esteem and those who are casual about sexual relationships and indifferent to or deliberately engage in extreme risk-taking behavior, a pattern that has serious implications for HIV/AIDS control programs.

barefoot doctor Village-level primary health care practitioner in China from the 1949 revolution until after the cultural revolution, now superseded by more fully trained rural health care workers. They provided first aid, basic health care, health education, maternal and child care, and advice on nutrition. In other countries, e.g., Iran and Guatemala, similar systems of health care, mainly in rural regions, are or were staffed by primary care workers with similar roles and levels of training.

barium (Ba) A heavy metal derived from barytes, barium sulfate, used in pigments, fireworks, and as a radiopaque solution or paste in contrast media radiography. Soluble compounds of barium, e.g., those used in fireworks, are poisonous and occasionally cause childhood poisoning.

Barker hypothesis Syn: thrifty phenotype hypothesis. A hypothesis proposed in 1990 by the British epidemiologist David Barker (b. 1939) that intrauterine growth retardation, low birth weight, and premature birth have a causal relationship to the origins of hypertension, coronary heart disease, and non-insulin-dependent diabetes, in middle age. Barker's hypothesis derived from a historical cohort study that revealed a significant association between the occurrence of hypertension and coronary heart disease in middle age and premature birth or low birth weight. The hypothesis is not supported by evidence from low-income countries, where intrauterine growth retardation and low birth weight are common but hypertension and coronary heart disease are less prevalent than in high-income countries. The evidence is presented in Barker's book *Fetal and Infant Origins of Adult Disease* (1992).

barograph An aneroid BAROMETER that records variations in atmospheric pressure on a revolving drum so that trends such as the speed of pressure changes can be tracked.

barometer An instrument to measure atmospheric pressure. A mercury barometer is a glass tube sealed at the top from which air has been evacuated; atmospheric pressure pushes the mercury column up the tube to a height that indicates the air pressure. An aneroid BAROMETER uses a corrugated metal vacuum drum, so the surface of the drum moves in and out as the air pressure changes; a system of levers transfers these movements to a pointer on a circular dial graduated in increments of atmospheric pressure, usually measured in kilopascals.

barotrauma Injury attributable to sudden change in air pressure, e.g., aviators performing aerobatics with rapid changes of altitude, scuba divers rising too quickly to the surface, releasing gases dissolved in blood and body tissues, causing the dangerous, painful, and sometimes lethal condition called the BENDS. Other manifestations of barotrauma include rupture of the ear drum and hemorrhage into paranasal sinuses and the globe of the eye.

barrier contraceptive A contraceptive that works by imposing a physical barrier between sperm and ovum, e.g., CONDOM, DIAPHRAGM, cervical cap, and FEMALE CONDOM. Other forms of barrier contraceptive include foams, jellies, and sponges, usually impregnated with spermicides. See also CHEMICAL CONTRACEPTIVE and CONTRACEPTION.

barrier nursing Syn: bedside isolation. Nursing care of a contagious patient in an otherwise open hospital ward, comprising rigorous antisepsis, the use of gowns, gloves, masks, and adjacent facilities for hand-washing before and after attending to the patient, all intended to minimize the risk of CROSS-INFECTION. Modern hospital design has made barrier nursing obsolete, except in emergencies, e.g., wars or natural disasters when many injured and sick persons may have to be crowded together in makeshift accommodation.

basal cell carcinoma Syn: rodent ulcer. A common variety of skin cancer that occurs on skin exposed to solar radiation. Head and neck lesions are common, especially in fair-skinned people, and the incidence is rising on intermittently exposed areas (upper trunk in males and females, lower leg in females). It commonly spreads locally and erodes through the dermis to underlying tissues unless treated, but rarely metastasizes.

basal metabolic rate The minimum energy required by the body to sustain metabolism, measured by oxygen consumption and expressed in kilojoules per square meter of body surface.

base pair Two nucleotide bases on DNA molecules that can pair in only one way, adenine with thymine, and guanine with cytosine.

baseline data The set of data collected at the beginning of a period of study. Cf: BENCHMARK.

basic health care Term applied to simplified health care services proposed for use in low-income countries, consisting of essential preventive vaccinations; health education; primary care; prenatal, postnatal, and infant care; and primary care-level medical, surgical, and obstetric care.

basic medical sciences Syn: Preclinical sciences. A term applied to anatomy, physiology, biochemistry, pathology, microbiology, genetics, pharmacology, epidemiology, and related sciences that are a prerequisite to thorough understanding of clinical and public health sciences.

basic reproductive rate The number of infections produced, on average, by one infectious case in the early stages of an epidemic when HERD IMMUNITY is low or zero and virtually all persons in the exposed population are susceptible. A term used in infectious disease epidemiology; the word "rate" is a misnomer because there is no precise or consistent time element.

bat The mammalian order *Chiroptera* in which specialized limbs have membranes that act like wings. Bats have public health significance because some blood-feeding species can carry the rabies virus, with or without apparent adverse effect, and can also carry and transmit other pathogens, e.g., histoplasmosis. Insectivorous bats reduce the prevalence of mosquitoes and other insect pests near houses, and their presence is sometimes encouraged for this reason.

bat rabies Empirical evidence suggests that at least some species of bats can carry the rabies virus without actually getting rabies. They apparently excrete the virus in feces and can transmit it to other animals in saliva. Speleologists working in caves frequented by large numbers of bats have occasionally been reported to get rabies, allegedly by inhalation of airborne rabies virus, but probably by invasion of the virus through skin abrasions.

battered child syndrome A severe form of CHILD ABUSE (DOMESTIC VIOLENCE) first identified by pediatric radiologists who observed x-rays of children with multiple limb and rib fractures at varying stages of healing, indicating that the fractures had occurred at different times, and therefore it was likely that they had been inflicted deliberately during repeated assaults. See also SHAKEN BABY SYNDROME. Public health nurses participate in surveillance and control measures.

battering, battery Violence causing serious bodily harm, thus the crime "assault and battery."

When it occurs in a family, such as spousal or child battery, it is a serious form of DOMESTIC VIOLENCE, a known but often unrecognized public health problem.

battery 1. A chemical device for storage of electrical charge. Several varieties have public health importance. The conventional automobile battery uses lead plates and sulfuric acid; lead poisoning is an occupational hazard of workers with these, notably battery-breakers who dismantle used batteries to recover the lead. Mercury and cadmium batteries can release toxic amounts of mercury and cadmium into the environment when combusted in an incinerator. 2. A violent assault. See BATTERING.

Bayesian inference A form of reasoning widely used in CLINICAL EPIDEMIOLOGY. It begins with description of the facts before exposure or intervention under investigation and adds fresh information gathered during the course of study to yield probabilities of the state of affairs after the exposure or intervention. It does not use conventional statistical significance tests but relies on methods of estimating levels of uncertainty around parameter estimates, referred to as credible intervals or uncertainty intervals. The name honors the English clergyman, gambler, and amateur mathematician Thomas Bayes (1702–1761), whose posthumously published *Essay Towards Solving a Problem in the Doctrine of Chance* (1763) set out the principles of this form of statistical inference.

BCG vaccine The vaccine against tuberculosis prepared from live attenuated bovine tubercle bacilli using a method developed by the French microbiologists Léon Calmette (1863–1933) and Camille Guérin (1872–1961) in the late 1920s. Initial trials had catastrophic results because of contamination with virulent strains of tubercle bacilli and other organisms, but further trials demonstrated the safety and efficacy of BCG vaccine, and it has been widely used since the 1940s, now especially as part of vaccination regimens in low- and middle-income countries.

beat knee Bursitis or subcutaneous cellulitis in the region of the kneecap, caused by prolonged kneeling and abrasions that become inflamed and infected, characteristically an occupational injury of underground miners working in confined spaces.

becquerel (Bq) The SI unit of radioactivity, a measure of the amount of a radioactive substance that produces one disintegration per second. The name honors the French physicist Antoine Henri Becquerel (1852–1908), and supersedes the CURIE: $1\,Bq = 2.7 \times 10^{-11}$ curies.

bed blocker A slang or jargon term for a patient occupying an acute short-stay hospital bed for a prolonged period to the exclusion of other, and perhaps more acutely ill, patients. The term usually has a derogatory implication, which is unfair because almost all such patients occupy hospital beds for reasons beyond their control.

bed occupancy A statistical measure of the activity of a hospital, expressed as the percentage of occupied beds to available beds. Hospital administrators and financial managers strive to achieve a high bed occupancy, but the unpredictability of illness and injury requires that beds should be available if possible at all times. It is not a rate because there is no set time dimension.

behavior The manner in which persons or groups conduct themselves, that may be indicative of thoughts, feelings, moods, emotions, motivation, etc. An observable response to a stimulus or an action that has a specific frequency, duration, and purpose, whether conscious or subconscious. To some extent, human behavior is innate and universally expressed, as in the joy of marriage festivals and the grief of bereavement, and to some extent, it is environmentally and culturally determined, particularly in the context of group behavior. This is mobilized to enhance good health by means of purposeful exercises in schools, public gatherings, and television programs. See also HEALTH BEHAVIOR.

behavior modification A method of changing an individual's conduct based on manipulating environmental conditions in order to evoke different stimulus-response reactions from those of past experience, for instance associating unpleasant stimuli with compulsive gambling aims to discourage the addiction.

behavioral diagnosis Systematic description and analysis of health-related behaviors that can affect the outcome of health educational programs. See also PRECEDE-PROCEED MODEL.

behavioral epidemic An epidemic attributable to the power of suggestion rather than to an agent, such as an infectious pathogen or noxious substance. It is manifest in aberrant behavior, such as convulsions or fainting fits of pupils in a school, or historically as "dancing mania" that occurred in medieval Europe. Sometimes it has physical features, such as skin rashes. "Epidemic" is an apt word because the condition spreads by direct contact: word of mouth. Radio or television can provoke epidemics, e.g., of suicidal conduct if a character in a popular television program commits (fictional) suicide. Episodes of communal or national passion, such as lynchings and genocidal massacres provoked by a demagogue leader or group, in which former friends and working colleagues turn against their neighbors, such as occurred in the former Yugoslavia in the 1990s, are a particularly dangerous form of behavioral epidemic.

behavioral epidemiology The study of individual and group habits, customs, and behaviors in relation to health outcomes. See also SOCIAL EPIDEMIOLOGY, which deals with almost identical problems and uses the same or very similar methods and procedures.

behavioral medicine The application of behavioral science theory and techniques to prevention and treatment of disease, disability, and premature death. It is applied in HEALTH PROMOTION programs and in the treatment of cardiovascular disease and hypertension and in psychotherapy. See also PRECEDE-PROCEED MODEL.

behavioral objective A term used primarily in educational theory and practice to specify the aim of an educational program or method in terms of how the learner is expected to behave at the end of the educational process. For example, a behavioral objective of an educational program aimed to improve safety in the workplace would be that workers will know how to use, and will use, equipment such as hard hats, ear protectors, and eye-protecting goggles.

behavioral risk factors These are common risk factors associated with ways people behave. They include taking insufficient exercise, eating to excess, smoking, overindulgence in alcohol and other mood-modifying substances, reckless driving, and aggressive and violent conduct toward others, all of which are associated causally with disease, injury, and premature death. See also RISK-TAKING BEHAVIOR.

behavioral sciences The study of the behavior of individuals or groups, notably in the sciences of PSYCHOLOGY, SOCIOLOGY, and ANTHROPOLOGY.

bejel A childhood syphilitic infection with *Treponema pallidum* that is not sexually transmitted but spreads via infected mucous discharges, commonly from mother to infant or child to child.

belief 1. A statement or proposition that is accepted by a person or group as being true. 2. An abstract concept, such as a religious faith or a set of CORE VALUES involving virtues such as truth-telling, integrity, or concern for the well-being of others, often outwardly manifest in behavior.

belief system The combination of all conceptual understanding about the nature of the world and the individual's place in it, together with spiritual or supernatural beliefs. This combination shapes traditional and modern theories about the nature and causes of disease and helps to determine individual and societal responses to preventive and therapeutic regimens.

bell-shaped curve The graphic representation of the NORMAL (GAUSSIAN) DISTRIBUTION in which a variable is symmetrically distributed on either side of a central value.

benchmark A measurement or point of reference at the beginning of an activity, such as a survey, or the evaluation or research project, that is used for comparison with subsequent measurements of the same variable. Alternatively, a benchmark is an acceptable standard in evaluation, e.g., of air quality or performance of staff members in an organization.

benchmark dose The amount of a substance, usually a toxicant, that causes a specific increase, usually 5% or 10%, in frequency or severity of a health outcome.

bends Syn: BAROTRAUMA. So named by those exposed to this occupational risk of working for long periods under increased atmospheric pressure because if the pressure is reduced too rapidly, gases, principally nitrogen, dissolved in synovial fluid, are released as bubbles, causing excruciating pain that causes the sufferer to bend over, doubled up in agony. The condition can be fatal or cause permanent damage if bubbles are released in blood vessels in the brain or heart.

beneficence The ethical principle of doing good. This means doing good because it is the morally correct course of action, not doing good as a charitable act. It is one of the primary motives for public health action, whether the action is carried out for the public good, the benefit of others, or from enlightened self-interest, which may motivate actions intended to eliminate or control a danger to health, such as a nidus of infection or a hazardous workplace. Some ethicists define it as the duty to do good and avoid doing harm to other people, which includes acting to promote the interests of others and acting to protect the weak and vulnerable. It includes also the duty of advocacy, as in the *amicus curiae* (friend of the court) role in legal actions in which public or personal health has been harmed.

benefit-cost ratio The ratio of quantifiable benefits to actual or estimated costs expressed in monetary terms. It is used to assess the economic feasibility or success of a health program. It varies over a wide range. For instance, the cost of preventing dangerous contagious childhood diseases, such as measles, diphtheria, and poliomyelitis, is a few cents per child, whereas the monetary cost of caring for a case may be many thousands of dollars. The cost to society of preventing premature deaths from traffic crashes, coronary heart disease, or lung cancer (if it could be computed) might be several thousands of dollars per "prevented premature death," but this may be considerably less than the value in goods and services of the productive period of lives lengthened. The term cost-benefit ratio is more often used.

bentonite A form of silica clay first found in deposits at Fort Benton, Wyoming, that has been widely used industrially because of its impermeability, strength, and insulating properties. Its uses include linings for hazardous waste storage and chemical waste dumps. Bentonite miners have a high prevalence of silicosis.

benzene Aromatic hydrocarbon, C_6H_6 is the basic member of a large family of compounds; it is a colorless, volatile, flammable liquid, widely used industrially as a solvent and to synthesize many benzene-based industrial chemicals. It is highly toxic and a known carcinogen associated with increased risk of acute myeloid leukemia among persons with high-level exposures.

benzidine An aromatic amine that, like β-naphthylamine, is a carcinogen. It is an industrial dyestuff and has been used in a colorimetric test for occult blood in feces, but the false-positive rate is unacceptably high.

benzo-α-pyrene Sometimes called benzapyrene. A confirmed animal carcinogen produced by combustion of coal, biomass, tobacco, and other carbon-based fuels of organic origin. It was identified as an ingredient of the tarry residue from combusted pipe tobacco and shown to cause malignant change when painted on rabbit skin in a series of classic experiments by the British pathologist Ernest Kennaway (1881–1958). It is an ingredient of combusted carbon in urban air pollution and also occurs in trace amounts in foods that have been burned or charred during cooking.

benzodiazepines A class of pharmacologically active synthetic chemicals with hypnotic, sedative, and tranquilizing properties that are among the most widely prescribed medications. They are mild and have few serious side effects, but dependency and withdrawal symptoms are common.

benzol The name originally given to benzene by the German chemist Justus Freiherr von Liebig

(1803–1873), who discovered it. It has many important chemical derivatives, notably the aniline dyes, many of which have the same carcinogenic properties as benzene.

beriberi A disease caused by deficiency of vitamin B (thiamine) that is prevalent in parts of south and southeast Asia. It occurs among persons whose diet is deficient in thiamine for other reasons, e.g., because of dietary disruption associated with chronic alcoholism. It was a common and serious disease among prisoners of war held by the Japanese in Asia in World War II. Its features include edema and peripheral neuritis and, in severe cases, heart failure. It is prevented and cured by dietary intake of adequate amounts of thiamine.

Berkson's bias A form of SELECTION BIAS that causes hospital cases and controls in a CASE CONTROL STUDY to be systematically different from one another because the combination of exposure to risk and occurrence of disease increases the likelihood of being admitted to the hospital. This produces a systematically higher exposure rate among hospital patients, so it distorts the ODDS RATIO. The bias was described by the American statistician Joseph Berkson (1899–1982).

berm 1. Low-lying flat land beside a river that is inundated when the water level rises. If the berm is contaminated by human or animal waste or toxic chemicals, these contaminants can enter the river during floods or periods of high water. 2. A gently sloping ramp between road and sidewalk that can be negotiated by a wheelchair.

Bernard, Claude (1813–1878) French physiologist who formulated the principle of homeostasis, the physiological self-corrective mechanism that "automatically" seeks to restore the normal internal bodily environment when it is disrupted. Bernard's concepts remain relevant in studies of the physiological basis of many environmental health problems.

Bernoulli distribution The probability distribution associated with two mutually exclusive and exhaustive outcomes, e.g., survival or death, first described by the Swiss mathematician Daniel Bernoulli (1700–1782). A Bernoulli variable is one that has only two possible values.

Bertillon classification The first numerical taxonomy of disease in which all disease entities were arranged in "chapters" according to their anatomical and/or pathological basis, the precursor of the INTERNATIONAL CLASSIFICATION OF DISEASES (ICD). It was developed by the French vital statistician and demographer Jacques Bertillon (1851–1922), who is better known for developing

fingerprinting as a reliable way to identify individuals, especially criminals.

berylliosis Syn: beryllium disease. A chronic granulomatous condition consequent on exposure to beryllium dust, causing interstitial pulmonary fibrosis, lymphadenopathy, progressive debility, and sometimes cancer (beryllium is a confirmed animal carcinogen).

best practices The consensus of expert panels regarding acceptable organization, staffing, and provision of services by a public health agency, medical clinic, hospital, or other health care facility. The criteria for "best practices" are sometimes called BENCHMARKS; they are among the items examined during the ACCREDITATION process.

beta error Type II error; the error of not rejecting the null hypothesis, i.e., declaring that a difference does not exist when in fact it does.

beta particle, beta radiation High-energy ionized electrons emitted by the spontaneous disintegration of the nuclei of radioactive elements or induced nuclear disintegration in particle accelerators.

betel nut A palm nut that, when crushed and chewed, releases alkaloids and tannin that are a stimulant, making betel a rival of tobacco as a leading form of substance abuse in south Asian countries. It is carcinogenic, addictive, and largely responsible for oral cancers being among the leading forms of cancer in those countries. Betel nut is often mixed with tobacco, spices, and ash to make paan, which is also addictive and carcinogenic. The juice is bright red, and the profuse salivation induced by betel juice leads to spitting that leaves a highly visible residue.

Beveridge, William (1879–1963) English economist and social administrator who wrote a paper on social insurance for the British government, published in 1942, the darkest period of World War II for the British. The Beveridge Report was the blueprint for the NATIONAL HEALTH SERVICE (NHS) and its social security provisions enacted in 1948 by the UK Labour government.

Bhopal A city in central India that was the site of one of the worst environmental disasters of modern times. In 1984, an accident at a Union Carbide plant released large quantities of methyl isocyanate (a chemical used to synthesize carbamate pesticides) into the neighborhood around the factory. More than 40,000 and perhaps as many as 300,000 people were poisoned, and more than 2,000 people died almost instantly. Many survivors were left with serious residual disability, including blindness and paralysis of voluntary muscles.

bias Systematic distortion of results or findings from the true state of affairs, or any of several varieties of processes leading to systematic distortion. In everyday usage, "bias" often implies the presence of emotional and/or political prejudices that influence conclusions and decisions. These prejudices may occur in public health sciences, for instance in epidemiology as a consequence of a CONFLICT OF INTEREST, but any of several other factors often account for the presence of bias. Epidemiologists have identified more than 20 varieties of bias, but several of these are variations of fundamental flaws in design, methods, procedures, or logical reasoning. The most common types include SELECTION BIAS, OBSERVER BIAS, bias due to CONFOUNDING, and bias due to ERRORS OF LOGICAL REASONING. Several of the biases encountered in epidemiological and social science investigations may include more than one of these unless investigators exercise great care with methods, design, and procedures. Other causes are systematic variation of measurements and/or statistical summary measures (means, rates, measures of association, etc.) and flaws in study design, data collection and analysis, or interpretation of the evidence.

bibliometrics A term used in quantitative studies of peer-reviewed scientific publications, dealing with measurement of the spread and impact of information published in scientific media, based on the statistical analysis of information in sources such as the *Index Medicus* and *Science Citation Index*. Bibliometric studies help to evaluate the effectiveness of scientific research as an instrument of public health policy.

bilharzia Syn: schistosome. The species of blood flukes (flatworms) identified and described by the German tropical disease specialist Theodor Bilharz (1829–1862). The flukes pass the first phase of their life cycle in freshwater snails and, after an intermediate stage as free-living cercarial worms, invade the human or animal (e.g., water buffalo) host through the skin, then migrate to blood vessels in the mucosa of the bladder or bowel, depending upon the species. There they cause the debilitating and often ultimately fatal disease SCHISTOSOMIASIS, which afflicts tens of millions of people in Egypt, other African and Middle Eastern nations, central and south America, and south and southeast Asia.

Billings, John Shaw (1838–1913) An American physician and public health specialist. He established the NATIONAL LIBRARY OF MEDICINE, compiled a medical dictionary, designed the Johns Hopkins University medical school, and helped to recruit its founding team of leading physicians, surgeons, and medical scientists.

bills of mortality The written records maintained in medieval parish registers in England of baptisms and deaths, containing a statement of the cause of death, used in early vital statistical analyses, notably by the English merchant and amateur scientist JOHN GRAUNT (1620–1674), who is often described as the founding father of VITAL STATISTICS. Similar church-based vital records were established about the same time, in the 15th or early 16th century, in Sweden and France. All such parish records are a valuable resource in studies of HISTORICAL DEMOGRAPHY.

binary variable A variable with only two possible values, zero and one, or on/off.

binomial distribution A probability distribution associated with two mutually exclusive outcomes, e.g., death or survival, presence or absence of a specific finding in laboratory or other investigations. The BERNOULLI DISTRIBUTION is a special case of the binomial distribution.

bioaccumulation Progressively increasing concentration of a substance in the organs or tissues of organisms at successive stages of the food chain, or in an organism (including humans) when the rate of absorption or uptake exceeds the rate of excretion or metabolism.

bioactivation The conversion in an organism or human body of a supposedly inert substance into a biologically active substance. An example is the conversion of polycyclic aromatic hydrocarbons to highly reactive diol epoxides that react with and damage DNA.

bioassay Biological assay; quantitative assessment of the potency of a chemical or biological substance by observing and measuring its effects on cells, tissues, living organisms, or humans.

bioavailability The characteristic of a substance, such as a pharmaceutical preparation or toxic chemical compound, that enables it to interact with enzymes or other bodily ingredients in normal metabolic processes.

biochemical oxygen demand (BOD) An indicator of water pollution based on the amount of oxygen taken up by microorganisms that decompose organic waste matter in water. It is calculated by storing a sample of water containing a known amount of oxygen for 5 days at 20°C. The oxygen content is measured again after this time. A high BOD indicates the presence of a large number of microorganisms, which suggests a high level of pollution.

biochemistry The branch of chemistry concerned with the study of compounds that occur in living organisms, with their synthesis, interactions, metabolism, secretion, excretion, etc.

biocide A substance that kills living organisms.

bioconcentration Increase in concentration of chemicals or biological substances as a consequence of active uptake from media, usually water, into biological systems, such as microorganisms, plankton, water weeds, or other marine or terrestrial plants, often with progressively increasing concentration as the compound moves through the food chain.

biodegradable The capacity of substances, such as paper and plastics, to decompose physically and/or chemically as a result of the action of living organisms, usually microorganisms.

biodiversity This means richness and variety of all life forms from microorganisms to complex multicellular plant and animal species, including humans, that occupy an ecosystem. The word can be applied to all the life forms that occupy the global ecosystem or to any subdivision of it. Biologists believe diversity enhances ecosystem health, including human health. Agricultural methods that encourage monoculture are vulnerable to plant diseases that can destroy an entire crop, whereas biologically diverse crops are inherently likely to contain genetic strains resistant to specific plant pathogens, so the ecosystem of which they are part is more robust.

bioengineering Syn: biomedical engineering. 1. Analysis of mechanical aspects of bodily functions, especially muscle action. This is the scientific basis for many methods and techniques of ERGONOMICS. 2. Machinery that can replicate and perform bodily functions, such as moving paralyzed muscles. Applications of engineering science and technology to augment or replace malfunctioning or nonfunctioning bodily systems. These include prosthetic limbs, cardiac pacemakers, and an ingenious and sophisticated array of electronic equipment to substitute for sensorimotor defects, such as paralyzed limbs, loss of vision, loss of hearing. 3. The use of biological methods to manufacture drugs, medications, and diverse substances useful in industry.

bioenvironmental vector control Control measures against vector-borne diseases that rely on a combination of predator species and altering the environment and ecosystems in order to eliminate or minimize the abundance and distribution of vectors. Examples include draining swamps to eliminate the habitat of mosquito larvae, introduc-

tion of predators or pathogens inimical to vector species, and releasing sterile male or genetically modified male mosquitoes that lead to population collapse of mosquitoes. Approaches that rely on introduced predator species have undesirable unintended consequences if the predators become established in and take over an ecological niche. They may then become pests themselves.

bioethics This means biological ethics, or the ethics of living things, often called medical ethics, or biomedical ethics. It is the philosophical discipline concerned with the distinctions between right and wrong and with the moral basis for decision making in medicine and its basic sciences and specialized fields, including public health. Several philosophical approaches are defined. Virtue-based ethics is founded on virtues such as altruism, integrity, truthfulness, prudence, compassion, fairness, or impartiality in judging situations. Principle-based ethics is founded on four principles: respect for autonomy, beneficence, nonmaleficence, and justice or equity, i.e., impartial and equal treatment for all. Duty-based or deontological ethics follows courses of action dependent upon moral values, usually set by religious beliefs. Bioethics is the preferred term for this scholarly and practical pursuit because philosophers and ethicists are concerned about ethical problems beyond the boundaries of medicine and the biomedical sciences.

biofeedback 1. The use of electronic devices to monitor autonomic bodily functions, such as heart rate, respiration, and bowel and bladder activity, accompanied by conscious efforts to modify these functions. 2. A therapeutic method based on enhancing awareness of one's own physiology and procedures to achieve control of high blood pressure, reactions to stress, etc.

biogas Flammable gas, e.g., methane, generated by biological decomposition of organic matter, usually biomass and/or animal and human excreta. This has been a successful and efficient source of fuel energy for heating and cooking in Chinese villages for many years.

biohazard A biological or chemical agent or substance that is harmful or endangers life; this includes pathogenic organisms, their cultures, and tissue, hospital dressings, used hypodermic needles, etc., that are contaminated with blood or other body fluids, designated as hazardous waste. Sometimes physical environmental factors or conditions such as high levels of ionizing radiation are described as biohazards, although the warning symbols or logos used to identify biohazards and ionizing radiation are quite different.

biological assessment of concentration Use of living organisms, commonly bacteria such as coliforms, to derive an estimate of the level of a substance, such as sugar in a test solution.

biological control See BIOENVIRONMENTAL VECTOR CONTROL.

biological marker See BIOMARKER.

biological monitoring Monitoring of the environmental concentration of toxic or noxious substances based on their effect on biological systems. The proverbial canary in the mine shaft is an example. An important method is examination of blood or tissue samples for signs of the effects of exposure to toxic substances, e.g., environmental lead compounds.

biological parent Syn: birth parent. A parent, mother or father, who has contributed half the chromosomes and genes to an individual, as contrasted with an adoptive parent, who is genetically unrelated to that individual.

biological warfare The use of pathogenic organisms as weapons in armed conflict and/or the deliberate destruction of public health defenses against pathogens, such as water purification systems, as was done in Iraq in the 1992 Gulf War. This is an ancient practice, recorded in medieval wars when infected corpses were catapulted over the walls of a besieged city or flung into wells. Blankets infected by smallpox patients were used by colonizing Europeans to infect indigenous populations in the Americas. In the world wars of the 20th century, combatants on both sides experimented with strains of anthrax, bubonic plague, and other contagious pathogens, but their use was limited to a few experiments, for example, by the Japanese in their war against China in the late 1930s and early 1940s. Since the 1950s, several nations, including the United States, the United Kingdom, and the former Soviet Union, are known to have continued experiments, ostensibly to develop effective countermeasures, but perhaps also to determine whether such weapons would have strategic value. Biological warfare presents a very serious public health problem, especially if combined with deliberate destruction of public health infrastructure and withholding of medical supplies and similar countermeasures. See also BIOTERRORISM and WEAPONS OF MASS DESTRUCTION (WMD). For more details, see http://www.sis.nlm.nih.gov/Tox/biologicalwarfare.htm.

biology The scientific study of living organisms, concerned with their structure, function, growth and development, reproduction, evolution, interrelationships with other organisms, etc. It is an es-

sential basic science of all aspects of public health work.

biomagnification A form of BIOACCUMULATION in which the digestive and/or metabolic processes of the organisms through which a chemical compound migrates lead to increased concentration in successive host species greater than the arithmetical sum of the amounts absorbed from organisms lower in the food chain. An example is the increasing concentration of fat-soluble compounds, such as PCBs, DDT, and mercury, in the livers of plankton, fish, fish-eating birds, and animals.

biomarker A cellular or molecular indicator of exposure, health effects, or susceptibility that can be used to measure the absorbed, metabolized, or biologically effective dose of a substance, the response to the substance, including susceptibility and resistance, idiosyncratic reactions, etc.

biomass All the organic matter, vegetable, animal, insect, microorganisms, living and dead, in a region or in the world as a whole. Biomass thus means more than just material of plant origin. The word is usually used to describe the total mass of specific kinds of living things, e.g., trees, insects, microorganisms, and occasionally all kinds collectively. The biomass of microorganisms is the largest single component and outweighs vertebrate biomass by several orders of magnitude.

biomass fuel This is vegetable matter such as wood or agricultural waste that is burned as fuel for cooking and heating. It often generates copious amounts of smoke and fumes that can cause indoor and environmental air pollution. In many low-income countries, inhalation of smoke and fumes from combusted biomass fuel is a common and serious public health problem. See also INDOOR AIR POLLUTION.

biome An ecosystem comprising plants and animals.

biomedical ethics See BIOETHICS.

biometry Literally, measurement of life or living things. A word coined by the British biologist and mathematician Karl Pearson (1857–1936), who used the word to mean the application of statistical methods in the study and analysis of biological processes. The word was modified slightly in the title of the journal *Biometrika* that Pearson founded. Pearson and Francis Galton (1822–1911) played major roles in the foundation of biometry, or biostatistics.

biomimicry A term used by the American naturalist Janine Benyus in *Biomimicry* (1997) to describe features of plants and animals that maximize efficient interaction with the ecosystem, and to advocate human use of similar design features in dwellings, appliances, and equipment that replicate natural systems.

biophile A term applied to all the naturally occurring elements essential to the life of plants and animals. These include carbon, hydrogen, nitrogen, oxygen, phosphorus, sulfur, chlorine, iodine, bromine, calcium, magnesium, potassium, sodium, iron, manganese, copper, and vanadium.

biophilia A word used by the American ecologist Edward O. Wilson (b.1929) to describe the affinity of different living species for one another and specifically the interdependent bond, as well as the affinity, between humans and other species of plants and animals. Wilson makes explicit the role of biophilia in maintaining sustainable global ecosystems and population health.

biopsychosocial (adj) A word that describes the interaction of biological, psychological, and social determinants of health and risk factors for disease. This conceptual field led to the rise of the science of PSYCHONEUROIMMUNOLOGY, which identifies and studies ways in which bodily functions are influenced by psychological and social factors. Its importance in clinical preventive medicine is acknowledged, but existing knowledge seldom suffices for effective interventions. It has been a useful concept in psychosomatic and family medicine.

biorhythm Cyclic variation in physiological function, including circadian rhythm, the wake-sleep cycle, and the menstrual cycle. Diurnal rhythms presumably respond to variations of incident sunlight. Biorhythms, such as the menstrual cycle, respond to buildup of hormone levels, but the actual mechanism responsible for this is not known in detail.

biosocial A word familiar to readers of the venerable *Journal of Biosocial Science*, meaning the combined influence of biological and social determinants of health and disease. Original articles in this journal deal also with psychological factors, so in practice the meaning is indistinguishable from the meaning of BIOPSYCHOSOCIAL.

biosphere The regions of the earth occupied by life forms, comprising a layer of land, sea, and air about 20 to 30 km deep, in which all known life forms are concentrated.

biostatistics The application of statistics to biological and medical problems. This is one of the basic sciences of public health, applied in the analysis of vital and health statistics and in the use of statistical tests for associations, correlation, significance levels, etc., in epidemiology, toxicology, environmental health sciences, and all other public health sciences.

biota A collective name for all the plant and animal life forms in a region or the entire world.

biotechnology Technology based on the properties and actions of living organisms. Examples include the use of microorganisms in fermentation of milk to produce cheese and sugar solutions of many varieties to produce alcohol.

bioterrorism A form of TERRORISM, indiscriminate violent hostile acts against the general population, that employs biological agents, such as pathogenic organisms or their spores, cultures or toxic products, or even infected persons, to spread dangerous contagious disease in an indiscriminate manner among the general population. Because it threatens the health of the public, bioterrorism is a potentially serious public health problem. In 2001–2002, episodes of bioterrorism occurred in the United States aimed against congressional leaders. See also TERRORISM.

biotransformation The process of biochemical changes of complex organic compounds in a living organism, e.g., conversion of sugars and glycogen into energy that is stored as fats.

biotype A group of organisms that have a common genotype.

bipolar disorder Syn: manic-depressive illness. An emotional disorder in which wide mood swings occur. There is a strong familial tendency, which may be genetically determined. Its public health significance arises from the risk of suicide or self-harm that occurs with a mood swing into deep depression and sometimes also from the conduct of persons with acute mania.

bipyridyls A family of organic chemical herbicides, including PARAQUAT, that are highly toxic to humans if ingested. Other bipyridyls, e.g., diquat, used for aquatic weed control, are less toxic.

birds Vertebrates characterized by beak, feathers, and reproduction by means of eggs hatched outside the body. This is a very diverse group, some of which carry diseases transmissible to humans. Examples of bird-to-human disease transmission include PSITTACOSIS, ORNITHOSIS, HISTOPLASMOSIS, WEST NILE VIRUS, AVIAN INFLUENZA, and several varieties of viral encephalitis transmitted to humans by mosquito vectors. Some migratory species traverse large tracts of the earth, but generally they do not carry diseases over long distances.

birth Syn: parturition. Delivery of an infant capable of independent existence, an event that occurs naturally when the cervix is fully dilated, at which stage the uterine, abdominal, and pelvic muscles expel the fetus from the uterus. Independent existence of an infant is possible after it has reached 28 weeks' gestation and is considered viable (although it is now common for infants of lower gestational age treated in neonatal intensive care to survive). See also CHILDBIRTH.

birth certificate The official legal document that records details of a live birth, i.e., date, place of birth, the sex of the baby, parents' identity, and additional information, such as birth order, birth weight, and whether the birth was medically attended and vaginal or cesarean. Birth certificates are the source for vital statistics on birth rates, infant and neonatal mortality rates, and various other statistical data.

birth cohort The component of the population born during a specified period, generally a year, sometimes a 5- or 10-year period. The birth year identifies the birth cohort when persons born during a specified period are studied as they achieve age-defined or date-defined intervals.

birth control A euphemism for advocacy and use of contraception, occasionally perceived as pejorative because the word "control" in this context may convey the notion of coercion by an authoritarian government or other external authority. However, the birth control movement rarely had government support in its early days. It evolved from beginnings in the mid-19th century and gathered momentum with the teachings of MARGARET SANGER, MARIE STOPES, and others, aided by loosening of restrictions on access to and sale of contraceptives coinciding with wider use of sex education. It played an important part in enhancing women's health status in the first half of the 20th century and subsequently. See also CONTRACEPTION.

birth defect Any structural or functional anomaly manifesting at any age and due to genetic or environmental causes acting before birth. The term does not specify the nature of the defect, whether it is due to genetic or chromosomal aberrations or damage to the fetus caused by disease such as the rubella virus or a toxic chemical. Whether this lack of precision about the meaning of the term is desirable or not depends on the context. There is uncertainty about whether some conditions, for instance autism, should or should not be classified as birth defects.

birthing center A setting, usually outside or separate from a hospital, designed for pregnant women to go for labor and childbirth, generally staffed by nurse-midwives rather than medically qualified obstetricians, and as far as possible devoid of the features that critics describe as the "medicalizing" of childbirth.

birth interval The period of time that elapses between the birth of one offspring and the birth of the next offspring of the same mother.

birth order The number of an offspring in a sibship, counting the first as 1, the second as 2, and so on, usually including only live births. In demographic studies, stillbirths and miscarriages are sometimes also counted because their number may be medically and/or socially relevant.

birth rate The number of live births in a defined administrative jurisdiction, in a calendar year divided by the midyear population of the jurisdiction, with the customary multiplier of 1,000 to produce a whole number rather than a decimal or fraction.

birth spacing The time interval between successive births to a mother, one of the significant variables in the study of human fertility.

birth weight The weight of an infant at birth, an important indicator of health status. The birth weight of a normal full-term infant is usually in the range 3,000 to 4,000 grams. Low birth weight, usually caused by prematurity, or various diseases, is birth weight below 2,500 grams. See also INTRAUTERINE GROWTH RETARDATION.

bis (chloromethyl) ether (BCME) A volatile, colorless liquid produced by the reaction of methyl alcohol, formaldehyde, and anhydrous hydrogen chloride, used in the manufacture of a range of important substances, including ion-exchange resins, bactericides, and pesticides. BCME and related chemicals, such as chloromethyl methyl ether (which has similar industrial uses), are powerfully carcinogenic, causing lung cancer after occupational exposure to the fumes. Workers engaged in manufacture and use of these substances must therefore wear respirators.

bisphenol A A plastic monomer that is an endocrine disrupter. In male animals (and possibly humans) it has a feminizing action, and in females it causes early onset of maturation.

black box A slang or jargon term for something whose inner workings are unknown or that cannot be examined to find out how the process works; a way to study a problem in which the methods, procedures, etc., are not described, explained, or perhaps even fully understood. Inferences, if any, from the findings relate only to the empirical observations.

black box epidemiology The use of observational epidemiological methods and inference to arrive at conclusions about cause-effect relations between risk factors and disease outcomes without necessarily understanding or attempting to explain detailed causal mechanisms or the pathogenesis of the specific disease that is being studied. The investigation of cholera in London in the 1850s by JOHN SNOW was an early example of black box epidemiology.

Black Death The name given to the catastrophic pandemic that struck Europe in 1347 to 1350 and caused the death of an estimated one third of the population. The descriptions of cases and their modes of death and such other evidence as exists indicate that the cause of this pandemic was almost certainly bubonic, pneumonic, and septicemic PLAGUE. The infestation of many dwellings by large numbers of rats favored the occurrence of zoonotic plague, and its spread to humans was favored by propinquity and filthy living conditions. Speculating about other possible causes is a pastime of epidemiologists with an interest in history. Anthrax and epidemic streptococcal septicemia and several other diseases have been proposed as alternative causes of the pandemic.

black lung Syn: ANTHRACOSIS. An occupational disease of coal miners, this is a variety of pneumoconiosis caused by inhalation of coal dust, leading to chronic bronchitis and emphysema, associated with silicosis if the coal is contained in or adjacent to strata of silica-bearing rock, and sometimes complicated by tuberculosis. The chronic cough is accompanied by expectoration of black sputum (coal-dust stained), and at autopsy the lungs are black. It has long been a common cause of chronic disability and premature death among coal miners in many parts of the world, although its ravages have been reduced in recent years by improved working conditions in many mining communities.

black magic A term loosely descriptive of witchcraft, generally used when referring to occult practices of tribal communities in preliterate cultures and some segments of other cultures.

blackout: Syn: drop attack. Transient loss of consciousness. There are many possible causes, including medical conditions such as epilepsy and heart block, ingestion or inhalation of many varieties of neurotoxic substances, e.g., alcohol, anesthetic agents, volatile solvents, and several illicit substances. It becomes a public health problem when the person who suffers from it drives a car or machinery, endangering others as well as himself or herself.

blackwater fever A dangerous manifestation of malaria, usually malignant tertian malaria caused by *Plasmodium falciparum*, associated with extensive destruction of red blood corpuscles and resulting hemolysis, with renal excretion of hemolyzed corpuscles, urine that is dark brown, renal failure, high fever, delirium, and often a fatal outcome.

bladder cancer A malignancy of the epithelial lining of the bladder; often associated with exposure to occupational, environmental carcinogens, such as aniline dyes and heavy machine oils, and also with tobacco smoking.

blasting The use of explosives, e.g., dynamite, to break up rocks in quarries and mines. This is a dangerous activity that exposes workers to risk of death or injury from the explosion, hearing loss caused by the percussive force of the explosion, and longer term chronic respiratory disease, such as PNEUMOCONIOSIS caused by inhalation of dust following blasting operations.

bleach An oxidizing substance, so called because it causes color to fade from cloth. Bleaching agents such as hydrogen peroxide and solution of sodium hypochlorite are used as disinfectants, for instance, in NEEDLE EXCHANGE PROGRAMS.

blindness Syn: amaurosis. Loss of eyesight, a serious impairment and disability often leading to handicap. Several causes of blindness are preventable, and these have considerable public health importance. Their causes and control have been studied by epidemiologists, nutritionists, etc. These include XEROPHTHALMIA, caused by vitamin A deficiency; TRACHOMA, an infection caused by *Chlamydia trachomatis* transmitted by flies or child-to-child contact; ONCHOCERCIASIS (RIVER BLINDNESS), caused by a filarial worm carried by the blackfly vector; and CATARACT, due to opacity of the lens, an age-related condition that is aggravated by excessive exposure to solar or other forms of radiation. Several categories of blindness are recognized. Total blindness means complete inability to see, i.e., to distinguish light from darkness. Legally blind means inability to read letters or symbols on a visual acuity chart and important or significant signals, such as traffic lights. Partial blindness can be due to several conditions, e.g., scotoma, in which there are defects in the visual field. Color blindness is an inherited disorder due to absence or defective production of one or more of the retinal pigments required for color perception.

block 1. A research design in which specified groups (blocks) are randomly selected for study. 2. An identifiable geographical region, e.g., a city block, that is the smallest unit for statistical tabulation of data in a census. See also CENSUS TRACT.

block grant A financial disbursement of money to an agency or a research group without explicit demands or requests regarding the manner in which the money should be spent.

block(ed) randomization See RANDOM ALLOCATION.

blood The fluid that circulates in all animals, comprising pale yellow liquid protein PLASMA in which are suspended ERYTHROCYTES (red cells) that transport oxygen, leukocytes (white cells) that provide antibodies to guard against disease, and PLATELETS required for clotting. Blood is pumped by the heart through arteries, arterioles, and capillaries to the organs and limbs, returns in the veins and then via the heart to the lungs, where the erythrocytes that give it its color release carbon dioxide and take up oxygen. It is a vehicle for infection in syphilis, other diseases, and a target in malaria, septicemia, and many other diseases, a fact underscored since transfused blood was found to be a vehicle for the transmission of dangerous new diseases, including HIV and hepatitis C. Blood is essential to life. It can be transfused from one person to another only after careful testing to ensure compatibility. In addition to its clinical and public health importance, blood has philosophical and symbolic significance, for it is equated with identity, inheritance, emotions, and spiritual values. See also BLOOD GROUPS.

blood bank A place for the assessment, screening, collection, storage, and provision of blood and blood products for transfusions to sick and injured persons in need of this service. The most important functions of blood banks are accurate typing of collected blood, precise matching of donor blood to the blood group of potential recipients, and screening for HIV and other diseases. Some blood banks also conduct research on aspects of hematology and blood transfusion.

blood-borne diseases A class of infections in which the pathogenic agent circulates in the blood or is harbored in other body fluids, and is transmitted when infected blood or other body fluids are conveyed in some manner to an uninfected susceptible person. Blood-borne diseases include HUMAN IMMUNODEFICIENCY VIRUS, most SEXUALLY TRANSMITTED DISEASES, several varieties of viral hepatitis, and tropical infections including MALARIA, TRYPANOSOMIASIS, etc. An important activity of blood banks is to screen donors for evidence of blood-borne diseases.

blood-brain barrier Although the brain, like all body organs and tissues, is sustained by blood that circulates through its tissues, some pathogenic organisms are incapable of invading vital parts of the brain, in particular, the cerebrospinal fluid. Other pathogens, including the bacteria that cause MENINGOCOCCAL DISEASES, and under certain circumstances dangerous infectious pathogens such as MYCOBACTERIUM TUBERCULOSIS and several common viruses, penetrate this blood-brain barrier and cause MENINGITIS. The blood-brain barrier is of variable value in blocking chemical toxicants. For instance, lipid-soluble molecules are readily taken up.

blood donors Persons who donate blood for transfusion and/or preparation of blood products such as concentrates used to treat hemophilia. The British political economist Richard Titmuss (1907–1973) described blood donation by voluntary unpaid donors in Britain as a form of high ALTRUISM. In some countries, blood donors are paid, which appeals to people in desperate need, prisoners in penal institutions, and the like. Persons in low-income countries also have a financial incentive to donate blood. For various reasons, these may not always be suitable blood donors. Before effective screening tests were developed, transfusions of blood from infected donors was a frequent route of infection with HIV/AIDS and HEPATITIS B and C for many people in North America, Europe, Australia, New Zealand, and elsewhere, causing serious epidemics.

blood groups Humans belong to one of several genotypes that can be identified by the blood groups to which they belong. The main blood groups are designated A, B, AB, and O, and are further subdivided into RHESUS (RH) FACTOR positive and negative, M and N, and several others that have been identified. The frequency of these groups varies geographically and among ethnic groups, reflecting migrations in earlier eras and differential survival rates according to genetically determined susceptibility to lethal epidemic and endemic diseases, including plague, smallpox, and influenza in earlier generations, for which blood groups are a marker.

blood lipids See LIPIDS.

blood matching, typing See BLOOD BANK.

blood pressure The action of the heart as a pump forces blood along the great vessels and into progressively smaller vessels, against the elastic counterforce of arterial walls and the hydraulic resistance to its flow as the arteries get smaller. Obviously, blood is under pressure. This pressure is measured with a sphygmomanometer by the height of a column of mercury in a vacuum tube, or an aneroid instrument applying the same principle, using an inflatable cuff wrapped around the upper arm, and listening to the variation in sounds as the pressure of the cuff falls when it is deflated. Adult blood pressure has a NORMAL DISTRIBUTION in populations. This should not be confused with the optimal distribution for good health. It is on average about 120 mm Hg systolic and 70 mm Hg diastolic. High blood pressure, or HYPERTENSION, is among the most common global public health problems. The fundamental cause remains the topic for much research, but much is known about empirical associations, e.g., with electrolyte (salt) intake, low birth weight, obesity, emotional stress, physical inactivity.

blood transfusion See BLOOD BANK and BLOOD GROUPS.

blue-collar worker A term that originated in the United States to describe unskilled and semiskilled manual workers, such as those on factory assembly lines. See also WHITE-COLLAR WORKER.

Blue Cross-Blue Shield A private sector, non-profit hospital and medical insurance program originally set up in the United States and now with subsidiaries or comparable private sector insurance corporations in many other countries. See http://www.bcbs.com/ for information and details.

board certified A health professional who has passed the relevant examinations for admission to the ranks of a specialty or specialized branch of the health profession in the United States.

board of health The officially designated group of people, usually comprising both professional and lay members, charged with responsibility for overseeing the provision and conduct of public health services. Boards of health are sometimes elected and sometimes appointed by higher officials, such as state governors, mayors, etc. They exercise fiscal and political control over local public health departments, and sometimes are unfortunately prone to political and ideological influence.

body burden The concentration or amount of an agent or substance that accumulates in tissues and/or body fluids after repeated exposure, often detectable on examination by suitable means.

body fluids A term that includes blood, tears, sweat, serous and mucous secretions from all bodily orifices, saliva, urine, and semen. In clinical usage, the term refers to body fluids that can transmit infections, which tears and sweat rarely do.

body image The concept of physical appearance a person has. This may bear little or no relationship to a person's actual appearance to others. For example, a slender adolescent girl or young woman may perceive herself to be fat and overweight, and her perception of her body image may lead her to embark on a drastic dietary regimen, as happens in anorexia nervosa. Similarly, an overweight person may have a body image of being slim and graceful that contrasts with the reality, which may lead to denial of obesity and the need to undertake a low-calorie diet.

body mass index (BMI) Syn: Quetelet index, named for the Belgian polymath LAMBERT ADOLPHE JACQUES QUETELET (1796–1874). The body weight in kilograms divided by the square of the height in meters. This anthropometric measure is an indicator of fatness and obesity. It correlates closely with skinfold thickness and density of the body. The desirable range is 20 to 25. Above 25 is overweight, and above 30 is obesity. BMI below the lower end of the acceptable range indicates undernutrition. The BMI has been regarded as a reliable predictor of susceptibility to coronary heart disease, but the ratio of waist-to-hip circumference may be a better predictor.

body politic Any group of people who are governed by any means. As used by the English philosopher Thomas Hobbes (1588–1679) in *Leviathan* (1651), it meant all persons subject to "the sovereign power of the commonwealth." In modern politics and public health practice, it means all the persons, sectors of society, and social institutions in the population served, by implication the population of the nation or an administrative region of it.

boiler workers Industrial work with boilers carries several kinds of occupational hazards. The manufacture of boilers traditionally has been an extremely noisy procedure, and many boiler makers have occupationally induced deafness. Maintenance involves working with insulating material, including until recently asbestos, so ASBESTOSIS and MESOTHELIOMA have been risks. Cleaning out scale (precipitated salts) from inside boilers carries a risk of PNEUMOCONIOSIS.

bomb calorimeter A device for measuring the calorific content of foodstuffs by completely combusting them in a closed chamber.

bond 1. A binding agreement, such as a legal contract. 2. In chemistry, the union of two or more elements or molecules. 3. More generally, the union of two or more substances, as in the process of welding, or by means of a bonding agent or adhesive. 4. An emotional tie between people.

bonding 1. Forming a strong and lasting relationship, as in mother-infant bonding and the "team spirit" that develops among members of a company of people engaged in an interest or activity that they conduct collectively, such as a sporting contest, theatrical performance. Bonding can affect behavior, including aspects that influence health, e.g., by imposing group or peer pressure to use or refrain from using tobacco or other substances, forms of sexual activity. 2. Causing two substances, materials, etc., to adhere strongly together, generally using a bonding agent or adhesive, which may contain a volatile solvent that can sometimes be harmful if inhaled.

bone marrow The richly vascularized tissue that occupies the cavities inside skeletal bones. It is an essential blood-forming organ responsible for producing erythrocytes, platelets, and some varieties of leukocytes. At birth, these cavities are filled entirely with blood-forming myeloid tissue (red marrow), but in later life the marrow in the limb bones is replaced by fat (yellow marrow). Samples of bone marrow are extracted for examination by aspiration through a wide-bore needle or by trephine and used for transplants in some otherwise lethally malignant conditions.

boolean A branch of mathematical logic named for its inventor, the English mathematician George Boole (1815–1864). Boolean logic is a set of postulates that delineates the logical basis for inclusion or exclusion of entities in sets. See also VENN DIAGRAM.

booster An inoculation, or series of inoculations, with an antigenic substance that enhances the antibody titer, that is, the level of acquired immunity, consequent upon the original inoculation. Because antibody titer often declines with time, booster doses are required to maintain a sufficient level of immunity to provide protection from infection.

borderline psychosis A term used loosely to describe conditions in which there are symptoms suggestive of schizophrenia or other psychosis but not loss of contact with reality. Persons with this diagnosis should be carefully monitored because they often deteriorate and sometimes harm themselves and/or others.

boreal Of or pertaining to the geographical north, as in boreal forest, aurora borealis. Some vector-borne diseases have a boreal distribution.

Borrelia burgdorferi The spirochete that causes LYME DISEASE, transmitted by an arthropod vector, usually a tick.

botulism A form of FOOD POISONING caused by ingesting the toxin of *Clostridium botulinum* due to anaerobic growth of this organism typically in foodstuffs such as potted vegetables or meats that have been prepared without adequate hygienic precautions. The food in which the organism grows may smell and taste "bad," but the toxin itself is tasteless. Sporadic cases occur mainly among members of culturally defined communities fond of home-prepared potted meats. Botulinus toxin has been identified as a potential weapon in BIOTERRORISM. The botulinus toxin is sometimes used therapeutically and as the proprietary preparation Botox in cosmetic surgery.

bovine spongiform encephalopathy (BSE) Syn: mad cow disease. A degenerative brain disease of cattle, a TRANSMISSIBLE SPONGIFORM ENCEPHALOPATHY, caused by a PRION that probably originated as the prion responsible for scrapie in sheep and was transmitted to cattle when cattle feed fortified with animal protein produced from slaughtered sheep became popular. The large epidemic of mad cow disease in the United Kingdom in the 1980s has been followed by a smaller epidemic of variant CREUTZFELDT-JAKOB DISEASE (vCJD) among humans, almost certainly caused by ingesting beef containing the prion responsible for spongiform degeneration. Outbreaks and isolated cases of BSE and vCJD have been reported in France, Canada, the United States, and Japan, and in 2004, a seemingly identical disease was reported in a goat. Feeding animal parts, whether raw or rendered, to domestic animals has been banned, and testing feed cattle for evidence of BSE is mandatory in most nations. The BSE epidemic and uncertainty about possible transmission to other animals and to humans are among the major challenges facing veterinary and human public health in the early 21st century. Current information and links are at http://www.cdc.gov/ncidod/dvrd/bsc/.

braille The system of tactile reading and writing invented by Louis Braille (1809–1852), a blind French music student, when he was about 15 years old. Braille is based on the positions of six raised dots on stiff paper or cards, derived from a French military night signaling method. The original system used the raised dots to represent alphabet letters. It was subsequently expanded to include numbers, mathematical symbols, and musical scores.

brain cancer A general term for several varieties of neoplasm, often loosely used to include nonmalignant meningioma, but strictly speaking, referring to aggressive, invasive malignant conditions such as astrocytoma or metastatic cancer. These malignant neoplasms can affect all age groups. Some epidemiological evidence implicates environmental agents.

brain death A condition in which electroencephalographic recording reveals no evidence of brain activity at the cortical level. Autonomic centers in the base of the brain may continue to function, as in the persistent vegetative state, or the heart may continue to beat under the influence of autonomic conduction tissue in the heart. When brain death precedes organ death, organs, e.g., kidneys, liver, heart, may be harvested for transplantation surgery.

brain development The brain develops from ectodermal and mesodermal tissue, beginning early in fetal life. Aberrations of development include NEURAL TUBE DEFECTS, anencephaly, spina bifida, hydrocephalus, etc., some of which appear to be a consequence of FOLIC ACID deficiency.

brainstem The anatomical region between the cerebral cortex and cerebellum, which are above it, and the spinal cord, which is below it, that contains many vital centers responsible for control of essential functions e.g., respiration, that normally proceed automatically. For this reason, brainstem lesions are often life-threatening.

brainstorming An intense unstructured discussion and often argument among relevant experts aimed at developing or advancing ideas about a problem that can sometimes lead to new or more effective ways to tackle the problem.

BRCA-1, BRCA-2 Two genes isolated and identified in 1994 and 1995 that are associated with heightened susceptibility to breast cancer, although they are responsible for only a small proportion of breast cancers. Women with mutations in either of these genes have a 56% to 85% risk of getting breast cancer at a relatively young age. BRCA-1 is also associated with increased susceptibility to ovarian cancer. Screening tests are available for these genes, but the tests have been patented, and a royalty fee must be paid for using them, and suitable strategies and tactics to deal with the presence of either gene present clinical and ethical challenges.

bread A carbohydrate foodstuff prepared from cereals, such as wheat, barley, and rye, that dates from at least Neolithic times; it is used in one form or another by almost all human societies and is a basic dietary component of people everywhere. Because it is baked and usually eaten dry, it seldom carries pathogens, but the grain flour of which it is made can be contaminated, e.g., with ERGOT, or toxic chemicals. These can cause food-borne epidemics, as in Pont-Saint-Esprit in France in 1950.

breakbone fever A popular name for DENGUE FEVER, which causes severe limb pain.

breakpoint 1. In chlorination of drinking water, the amount or concentration of chlorine required to destroy pathogenic bacteria, such as coliform organisms 2. In helminth epidemiology, the mean worm load below which helminth mating frequency is too low to maintain reproduction, leading to a decline and eventual disappearance of infection from the population.

breast cancer The highest incidence female cancer, now second to lung cancer as a cause of female cancer death in countries where women adopted cigarette smoking in the second half of the 20th century. The incidence varies widely, being highest in rich industrialized nations. The high incidence among women of zero and low parity suggests a relationship to hormonal influences. A high-calorie diet and adiposity are associated with increased incidence. Breast feeding has a protective effect. Epidemiological and animal studies have identified many other risk factors, but none offer convincing promise of interventions aimed at reducing incidence rates.

breast cancer screening Several procedures are advocated for population SCREENING aimed at the early detection of breast cancer. BREAST SELF-EXAMINATION is widely advocated and used, but evaluation reveals disappointing results. MAMMOGRAPHY, employing low-penetration radiographs (x-rays), has demonstrated convincingly its efficacy in early detection that leads to effective intervention. Thermography, which measures the infrared radiation emitted from breast tissue, is based on the premise that cancerous tissue is warmer than normal breast tissue, but this has unacceptably high false-positive and false-negative rates. Only mammography has been shown by randomized controlled trials to be effective in reducing breast cancer mortality.

breast feeding Nutritionally, breast milk is the most suitable food for human infants because it is the right composition to meet physiological and developmental needs; undergoes subtle changes in composition and content as infants develop; requires no preparation; and is usually available on demand in a healthy woman with normal breasts and nipples. Most nutritionists and pediatricians recommend breast feeding for 6 months. Fashions, fastidiousness about exposing breasts in public in modern urban society, and economic demands of employment may discourage breast feeding. Disincentives may arise from the blandishments of infant formula manufacturers who have sometimes used dubious advertising methods to promote their products and to imply that breast feeding is a sign of social inferiority, is unglamorous, and will damage a woman's figure. Advertisers do not mention the possible hazards of formulas, such as the risk of malnutrition and gastrointestinal infection. However, some diseases, including hepatitis B and HIV, can be transmitted from mother to infant by breast milk from an infected mother.

breast milk Unqualified, this term refers to human breast milk, secreted by the mammary glands from late pregnancy until the natural or induced termination of lactation. The composition of breast milk changes from watery colostrum with a high carbohydrate content during the perinatal period to denser fluid with a higher content of fat and protein during the postnatal period. Breast milk has several obvious advantages over artificial formula feeds, notably that it is stored naturally at body temperature under sterile conditions, as well as being the naturally correct composition.

breast self-examination A popular and widely used practice encouraged by many physicians, preventive medicine specialists, women's groups, cancer societies, and the media, said to enhance the prospects for early detection of breast cancer. Unfortunately, recent careful evaluations have failed to demonstrate the efficacy of breast self-examination.

breathalyzer A device to detect the presence and concentration of alcohol, using a colorimetric method in which the concentration of alcohol or its metabolic products in exhaled air causes differential color changes in a potassium chromate mixture. The concentration of alcohol in exhaled air correlates with blood alcohol concentration in a ratio of 2,100:1. The color change in breathalyzers is set to show when blood alcohol concentration exceeds the legal limit. In most of the United States and in many other countries, this is 0.08%. Advocates for stronger measures against alcohol-impaired driving seek reduction to 0.05%, which is the legal limit in some countries. The breathalyzer is widely used by police forces to detect alcohol-impaired drivers. Evidence from breathalyzer tests is admissible in most law courts. Refusal to take a breath test is commonly accepted as prima facie evidence of the driver's admission of alcohol impairment.

British Medical Association (BMA) The professional society for British doctors, founded in 1832, that is both a political and an academic organization. It serves the interests of members of the medical profession, and the people of Great Britain, advising the government and the public about medical matters. It publishes a weekly general medical journal, the *British Medical Journal*, and a large number of specialized journals. See http://www.bma.org.uk for details.

British National Formulary A UK-published list of approved drugs and medications, listing their generic and proprietary names, pharmacological action, dosage, indications, contraindications, side effects, and reported adverse reactions. This is produced and maintained up to date in collaboration by the British Medical Association and the Royal Pharmaceutical Society of Great Britain. See http://www.bnf.org/bnf/ for details. Many nations produce such lists, usually in collaboration with the pharmaceutical manufacturers, and publish frequent revisions. Other examples include the US Pharmacopeia and National Formulary (see UNITED STATES PHARMACOPEIA) and the WHO's ESSENTIAL DRUGS AND MEDICINES list.

British thermal unit (BTU) The quantity of heat required to raise 1 pound of water 1°F, equal to 1055.06 joules. Although obsolete and superseded by the SI unit the JOULE, the BTU is still used in some public health engineering applications.

bromodichloromethane This is a TRIHALOMETHANE industrial chemical and environmental pollutant that occurs in chlorinated drinking water. It is a confirmed animal and suspected human carcinogen.

bronchiolitis Inflammation of the bronchioles, often a serious acute illness, which may be due either to pathogenic organisms or to exposure to irritant gases or fumes or severe SMOG episodes. In the latter instance, bronchiolitis is a common cause of death.

bronchitis Inflammation of the bronchi and usually of the adjacent parts of the respiratory tract (trachea, bronchioles) causing cough, expectoration of sputum, and often fever and malaise. It may be acute or chronic. Chronic bronchitis often leads to EMPHYSEMA. It is a very common disease, often associated with environmental, occupational, or lifestyle factors, such as smoking and/or with recurrent bouts of respiratory infection.

brownfield A parcel of land that is the scene of past industrial development and has been left in a degraded, often polluted, condition that renders it unfit for agriculture or for human housing. The British term, industrial waste site, perhaps conveys more clearly the nature of the human and environmental problem, its cause, and the settings in which it occurs.

brucellosis A communicable disease caused by *Brucella* organisms, occurring in goats, cows, and some other domestic animals, transmitted to humans in milk or by direct contact. The name of the organism and the disease honors the memory of the discoverer, the British pathologist David Bruce (1855–1931). In humans, brucellosis often causes an indolent remittent illness with recurrent fever and debilitation. The illness that made the British pioneer of modern nursing, FLORENCE NIGHTINGALE (1820–1910), bedridden after her return from the Crimean War until her death several decades later was probably brucellosis.

bubonic plague The dangerous contagious disease acquired by humans from fleas that have been infected with blood sucked from infected rats. It causes high fever, gross swelling of lymph glands in the groins and axillae (known as buboes), skin rash, and debilitation and is often fatal. This was almost certainly the disease called the BLACK DEATH in medieval Europe. It can occur sporadically but often it is highly contagious, requiring UNIVERSAL PRECAUTIONS for medical and nursing care.

buddy system A method of encouraging people to care for one another, such as for several isolated old people to stay in touch by means of daily phone calls or visits or for patients with AIDS, so that departures from usual state of health can more readily be detected and dealt with promptly. A buddy system is used in some dangerous occupations by workers who observe each other's exposure to hazards and can take rapid action if required.

budget The statement of finances setting out in a balance sheet all sources of income and the expenditures, with itemized listing of the nature of each. Often there is also a statement of predicted sources of income and expenditure for the forthcoming fiscal period, as well as for the immediately past or completed fiscal period. Accountants and financial managers use various methods to prepare budgets, but the one essential feature common to all is a statement that seeks to reconcile and account for all monetary flows for whatever reason. Preparation and balancing of budgets preoccupy elected and appointed public servants. See also RESOURCE ALLOCATION.

buffer 1. Something that weakens the force of impact or stabilizes the action of an acid or alkaline chemical compound; the word has many industrial applications, e.g., "buffer zone" and "buffer storage" in solid waste disposal. 2. In computing, a memory storage device.

building code The regulations applicable to construction of all accommodations intended for occupancy, whether residential or public. These include many clauses based on established public health sciences and practice, e.g., about lighting, ventilation, space per person, provision of facilities for cooking, sanitation, waste disposal, etc., as well as explicit rules relating to fire safety. Details vary, but principles are similar in most jurisdictions. See also MODEL STANDARDS.

built environment A general term covering residential, industrial, and public buildings, roads, and services, such as water supplies, electrical wiring, and sewerage, in HUMAN SETTLEMENTS.

bulimia An eating disorder of psychogenic origin, most often occurring in adolescent girls and young women, that is characterized by alternative gorging and induced vomiting of food. It may occur in BEHAVIORAL EPIDEMIC form among adolescent school girls who attempt to mimic the appearance of fashion models or very thin popular entertainers.

bullying A form of interpersonal violence mainly among school children in which an individual or a group picks on and directs abusive behavior and often physical violence against a vulnerable individual, often one who is physically and/or intellectually distinguishable from the rest of the group. Bullying can be a serious health risk for the victim, who is often physically harmed or may be driven to self-harm, even suicide.

bund A wall or inert barrier at the boundaries of a landfill site or toxic waste dump.

burden of disease The amount of ill health from a given cause (disease, injury, cause of disease, or risk factor) in a population of interest. It is usually expressed as lost healthy years (or months). The World Health Organization conducted a major study of the global burden of disease that led to important publications (http://www.who.int/healthinfo/bodproject/en/index.html). See also DISABILITY-ADJUSTED LIFE YEARS (DALYs) and HEALTH GAP INDICATORS (MEASURES).

bureau A general name applied to an office, agency, or organization, usually signifying official designation and/or governmental status, e.g., Bureau of Health Professions.

bureaucracy A management system in which power derives from office rather than from birthright or political connections. The word is often used pejoratively to describe governmental organizations in which managerial tasks are specialized and divided among many individuals, but bureaucracy flourishes in the private sector as well as in government departments, because it is a necessary feature of large and complex organizations. It is often criticized because it can be cumbersome, it may be difficult or impossible to identify decision makers and person(s) responsible for action, and sometimes it may be susceptible to corruption.

Burkitt's lymphoma A malignant lymphoma first identified in East Africa, where the British surgeon Denis Burkitt (1911–1993) observed that its distribution coincided with that of malaria-carrying anopheline mosquitoes, and thus recognized that the condition was probably caused by an agent transmitted by mosquitoes. This agent was found to be a herpes virus, the EPSTEIN-BARR VIRUS, which has been detected in more than 95% of cases.

burnout A condition of emotional exhaustion that rather commonly afflicts overworked persons, e.g., health professionals, attributable to the combination of long hours, inadequate rest and relaxation, demanding clients, and often unsympathetic supervisors. A treatment often advocated is a long vacation, followed, if possible, by a change of duties on returning to work, although this often is unrealistic and there are no formal trials confirming its efficacy.

burns A frequent cause of industrial and domestic injury, classified as first, second, and third degree burns according to severity. Third degree burns, i.e., burns that cause skin loss, are life threatening if they involve more than 30% to 40% of the body surface. Prevention of burns is an important priority of industrial hygiene services, and emergency treatment is an essential feature of FIRST AID services. Mass burns may occur in major industrial accidents, terrorist attacks, etc., and require prolonged heavy use of specialized intensive care services and facilities.

bursitis Inflammation of a bursa, i.e., the fluid-filled sac that serves as a lubricating cushion between a joint and the overlying skin. Inflammation is commonly of occupational origin. Examples include BEAT KNEE, housemaid's knee, and tennis elbow.

butadiene A gaseous compound used in the manufacture of plasticized rubber products. It is toxic, can form an explosive mixture with air, and is stored in fatty tissue but has a relatively brief half-life. It is less toxic than other compounds in the same chemical family, such as styrene.

buzz groups Small informal discussion groups, usually of three to five people formed by participants at a conference, aimed to ensure maximum participation and sharing in decision making. Members of buzz groups are usually not given an agenda of items to discuss but are encouraged to single out one or two points mentioned in earlier phases of the conference and seek to resolve problems that relate to these points.

bylaws A formal set of written rules developed to deal with the many contingencies that can arise in an organization, a professional association, a workplace, etc. It usually covers the range of situations that commonly occur; sets out duties, rights, sanctions that may be invoked in the event of violation of specific bylaws; and specifies the procedure to be followed in the event that the bylaws need to be modified.

byssinosis An obstructive lung disease, a form of PNEUMOCONIOSIS, occurring as an occupational hazard among persons who work with unprocessed cotton; it is caused by inhalation of cotton dust.

C

cachexia A condition of severe weight loss, generalized weakness, and wasting, often accompanied by impaired immune function and mental sluggishness. The causes include cancer, starvation as in famine, chronic infection (e.g., advanced tuberculosis), and anorexia nervosa.

cadmium (Cd) Silvery-white metallic element, used in corrosion-resistant electroplating, in batteries, and in control rods for nuclear reactors. As an environmental and industrial poison, cadmium has been responsible for several epidemics of renal damage associated with osteoporosis and osteomalacia, e.g., ITAI-ITAI DISEASE in Japan.

caesium See CESIUM.

caffeine A bitter-tasting alkaloid extracted from COFFEE beans, tea leaves, or kola nuts, or synthesized. It is a diuretic and central nervous system stimulant. As the active ingredient of coffee, it is consumed worldwide. Weak epidemiological evidence has raised suspicions that caffeine or, more likely, other complex organic substances occurring in coffee are carcinogenic. It may also be a risk factor for coronary occlusion or more broadly for cardiovascular disease.

Cairo Declaration Several statements have been issued after international meetings in Cairo. These include a declaration by Allied leaders in World War II in 1943, a declaration on human rights in the Islamic world in 1990, and—the most relevant to public health—the Cairo Declaration that was affirmed by most of the delegates to the 1994 United Nations International Conference on Population and Development (see http://www.un.org/popin/icpd/conference/bkg/egypt.html).   Points emphasized in this Cairo Declaration deal with sustainable development; reproductive health and family planning; services addressing domestic violence, gender equality, and empowerment of women; control of sexually transmitted diseases; health promotion and reduction of morbidity and mortality; and resource mobilization. The conference developed an action plan that has been partly implemented in some countries.

caisson disease See DECOMPRESSION SYNDROME.

calcium (Ca) An essential element that in compound form provides density for bones and teeth and is an integral part of several essential enzyme systems and metabolic processes. Calcium ions play a critical role in neuromuscular excitability. Hypocalcemia causes tetany.

calibration Adjustment of a measuring instrument using an accepted standard so that the distribution of measurements or readings from the instrument agrees with the accepted standard. Everyday examples include adjusting clocks to national time signals and odometers in automobiles to measured distances on highways. It is good practice to check all laboratory instruments periodically against accepted standards and recalibrate them as necessary.

calorie A measure of energy expenditure. The amount of energy (as heat) required to raise the temperature of 1 gram of water by 1° Celsius at a pressure of one standard atmosphere. The calorie has been replaced by the SI unit the JOULE, but calorie measure remains popular and widely used.

calorific value The calorific values of various foodstuffs are the criteria used by dieticians when composing nutritious and well-balanced diets containing all the essential ingredients, i.e., proteins, fats, carbohydrates, vitamins, and minerals. A BOMB CALORIMETER measures calorific values.

calorimeter An instrument for measuring calorie value, consumption, combustion. Several types exist, e.g., to measure quantity of heat generated by physical activity, and the BOMB CALORIMETER to measure the calorific value of foodstuffs.

Campylobacter A motile spiral microorganism that causes abortion in some mammals and that in humans causes acute enteritis with epidemiological features similar to those of SALMONELLOSIS. This may be acquired directly from animals, usually pets; by consuming undercooked meat or food or milk; or rarely from food handlers.

Canadian Institute for Health Information The Canadian national agency that collects, collates, analyzes, and interprets health-related statistics in Canada, comparable to the US NATIONAL CENTER FOR HEALTH STATISTICS. The range of its activities and electronic versions of its reports are available at http://www.cihi.ca.

Canadian Institute for Scientific and Technical Information An approximate Canadian equivalent of the NATIONAL LIBRARY OF MEDICINE in the biomedical science fields; it is a repository for all scientific publications in Canada. It is a very large paper and electronic collection that includes reference works and serial publications in the natural and physical sciences and engineering, as well as in the biological and biomedical sciences. Many of the works it houses are accessible at http://cisti-icist.nrc-cnrc.gc.ca/cisti_e.html.

Canadian Institute of Health Research (CIHR) The approximate Canadian equivalent of the National Institutes of Health. Its advisory bodies set health and biomedical research policies, including those dealing with ethical concerns, and assign priorities and allocate funds to research programs, national centers of excellence, research projects, and personnel grants for scholars. Details are available at http://www.cihr-irsc.gc.ca/.

Canadian mortality data base A computerized data base on all deaths recorded in Canada, maintained continuously since 1950. All death certificates are permanently stored on microfiche, and the relevant information on them is extracted into machine-readable form to permit RECORD LINKAGE. The national record linkage system enables causes of death to be related to relevant occupational, environmental, and medical information in long-term HISTORICAL COHORT STUDIES.

Canadian Public Health Association (CPHA) The national not-for-profit organization for all public health workers in Canada. Like the AMERICAN PUBLIC HEALTH ASSOCIATION and similar organizations in many other nations, it promotes public health education, seeks to protect and promote the health of the nation's people, and is an advocacy group and a professional organization that publishes a scientific journal and a newsletter for its members. It also engages in international public health work in developing countries and the former Soviet satellite nations. For more details, see http://www.cpha.ca/.

Canadian Task Force on Preventive Health Care Formerly known as the Canadian Task Force on the Periodic Health Examination, this expert committee was established in 1974 to assess the evidence on efficacy of routine physical examinations. It broadened in scope to consider and evaluate a wide range of screening procedures and preventive interventions. Its contributions include the concept of the HIERARCHY OF EVIDENCE and definitive evaluations of a wide range of SCREENING procedures. It has produced many reports, which are available at http://www.ctfphc.org/. It was the model for the US PREVENTIVE SERVICES TASK FORCE.

cancer A malignant neoplasm that occurs when disruption of cellular growth causes cells of an organ or tissue to develop and reproduce abnormally. Cancer cells typically invade and destroy healthy tissue and organs adjacent to the original primary site and metastasize to distant sites. The terminology signifies the affected tissue. A cancer of epithelial cells is called a CARCINOMA. Cancer in epithelial glands is an adenocarcinoma. Cancer of endothelial (e.g., skeletal, connective, or circulatory tissue) is a sarcoma, often using a term identifying the site with the suffix "sarcoma," e.g., osteosarcoma, fibrosarcoma, lymphosarcoma. The rate of growth, degree of invasiveness, and tendency to spread to organs and tissues remote from the site of origin (to metastasize) vary greatly. The histopathologic findings are a prognostic clue: rapidly growing and metastasizing cancers typically have cells that appear microscopically undifferentiated and of widely varying size and appearance, but this is not always true. Molecular BIOMARKERS are analyzed to assess prognosis and guide treatment choices. Cancer is common. The lifetime probability of getting cancer (other than nonmelanoma skin cancer) is 35% to 40%, and the probability of dying of cancer is 20% to 25%. Many cancers are treatable, and many can be completely cured or prevented. Changes in behaviors and lifestyles can reduce risk, for instance refraining from tobacco use and avoiding excessive sun exposure or using sunblock and wearing protective hats and clothing. Occupational cancer risks can be reduced by eliminating or minimizing exposures to known carcinogenic chemicals and ionizing radiation.

cancer registry A REGISTRY of cancer cases in a defined jurisdiction, a state, province, or nation. Ideally, the registry collects information about every diagnosed case. The information comes from pathologic, radiologic, postoperative, and other diagnostic reports and from death certificate diagnoses. In many jurisdictions, it is transmitted routinely to the cancer registry without formal notification of patients or next of kin that information about them has been collected. In this respect, cancer registries follow the rules of a census bureau, and all who work in the registry with personal data must swear an oath of secrecy. In some nations in the European Union, this is an insufficient safeguard of personal privacy, and patients must give informed consent for the relevant information to be transmitted to the cancer registry. Inevitably, some decline to release personal information, thus defeating one of the purposes of the registry, comprehensive population coverage, a necessity for epidemiological study of rare cancers. Cancer registries have provided valuable information and statistical data for many studies of cancer causes and control, such as regional, occupational, and other variations in incidence and survival rates in relation to treatment methods.

candidiasis Fungus infection caused by organisms of the *Candida* species that can affect the mouth, vagina, anal region, or gut, mainly in elderly, debilitated, or immunocompromised persons, such as those with AIDS.

cannabis Syn: cannabinol. The alkaloid psychoactive ingredient in MARIJUANA that when inhaled or ingested causes a state of relaxation and euphoria. Cannabis use may become habitual, but it is not an addictive substance comparable to nicotine, heroin, or cocaine, and there is no convincing evidence that cannabis use causes serious or irreversible central nervous system damage. Chronic use in youth may be associated with lack of motivation, but it is doubtful this is a causal relationship. However, cannabis may be used in social settings in which dangerous illicit drugs are also circulated and used, so impressionable users, notably teenagers, may adopt dangerous drug habits. Cannabis use impairs judgment, so driving a car or operating machinery can be hazardous. Marijuana smoke contains carcinogens similar to those in tobacco. Its use for management of chronic pain is increasingly recognized, and it is legally available for this purpose in some jurisdictions. See MARIJUANA.

canning A method of preservation for fruit, meat, milk, and other foodstuffs that includes heat sterilization, often addition of preservatives, coloring, and flavor enhancing agents, vitamins, and sealing the finished product in a glass, plastic, or metal container. If properly done, canning can preserve food for many years. The main health risks arise from contamination of home canned foods by pathogens such as the spores of *Clostridium botulinum*, and rarely from lead or antimony poisoning if unsuitable compounds containing these or other toxic metals are used as sealants.

capacity 1. In lay usage and the physical sciences, the number of persons a public space can accommodate, the volume of a container, the ability to carry an electric current. 2. In psychology and medicine, the legal and intellectual capability to comprehend issues and make decisions required to sign or affirm a last will and testament or other legally important documents is described as testamentary capacity, encompassed in the phrase "of sound mind" that is sometimes part of the preamble to an affidavit or will. The same word describes physical and intellectual capability to operate a motor vehicle or other machinery that becomes dangerous to the operator and others if the capability is impaired by disease, drugs, or alcohol.

capacity building A term used mainly in INTERNATIONAL HEALTH meaning development of health systems in low-income countries. It includes activities directed at upgrading technical and professional skills and establishing and/or strengthening infrastructure in the health, education, and social sectors, usually with financial, as well as technical and professional, assistance from donor nations and nongovernmental organizations. The aims include closing the INGENUITY GAP.

capital cost Investment in buildings or equipment that once made will produce a tangible and lasting result and will not need to be repeated on an ongoing or recurring basis, in contrast to operating costs, which include the cost of maintenance, upkeep, and refurbishment.

capitation A method of payment for services based on the number of persons registered as potential users of the service, rather than on fees for each item of service rendered.

capture–mark–recapture method A method, derived from wildlife biology, of estimating the size of a study population that makes use of overlapping, incomplete, but intersecting sets of data, to derive reasonably accurate numerators and denominators for epidemiological study. If two independent sources are available, α is the number of cases found in both sources, β is the number found only in the first source, and γ is the number found only in the second source, the maximum likelihood population estimate is the product of the total found in each source divided by the total found in both sources, that is, $(\alpha+\beta) \times (\alpha+\gamma) \div \alpha$. If three or more sources are available, log linear methods are used to model the degree of dependency among the sources. The method is especially useful in studies of elusive and ill-defined populations, such as sex workers, homeless people, and migratory agricultural laborers.

carbamate insecticides A group of insecticides that work by blocking the enzyme acetylcholine esterase. They are environmentally toxic but less so than ORGANOPHOSPHATE INSECTICIDES.

carbaryl The most widely used carbamate insecticide, considered the safest, with low systemic and cutaneous toxicity for humans, with rapidly reversible cholinesterase inhibition.

carbon cycle The metabolic pathway of carbon molecules, mainly as carbohydrate compounds (i.e., cellulose polysaccharides, glucose, glycogen) from plants to herbivores to carnivores, and the transpiration and respiration of carbon dioxide and oxygen. This term should not be used to describe combustion of carbon-based fuels because this is not a cycle but leads to progressive environmental accumulation of carbon combustion products.

carbon dioxide (CO_2) Colorless inert gas, a product of fermentation and respiration, and the raw material of PHOTOSYNTHESIS. It is a major component of industrial and automobile emissions and consequently of GREENHOUSE GASES. It has wide industrial uses as an inert fire extinguisher, a coolant in nuclear reactors, and as a refrigerant ("dry ice"). It is an asphyxiant when its atmospheric concentration prevents the intake of oxygen to sustain life.

carbon disulfide A common industrial solvent, a volatile liquid that produces heavier than air fumes that cause toxic encephalopathy, peripheral neuropathy, and impaired spermatogenesis.

carbon monoxide (CO) A colorless, odorless gas, an emission by-product when carbon-based fuels are incompletely combusted. It is used industrially in the manufacture of steel and as a fuel (COAL GAS). It selectively binds to hemoglobin to form CARBOXYHEMOGLOBIN, preventing uptake of oxygen and therefore asphyxiation. Inhaled carbon monoxide causes accumulation of toxic concentrations, leading to industrial and domestic accidents, and is sometimes a method of suicide.

carbon sinks Environmental and ecosystem components that absorb or metabolize atmospheric carbon dioxide. They include phytoplankton in surface layers of ponds, lakes, and oceans; oceans themselves, which dissolve atmospheric CO_2; and trees and other plants containing CHLOROPHYLL that metabolize CO_2. Some geological formations can also absorb atmospheric CO_2.

carbon tetrachloride Tetrachloromethane. A solvent and cleaning agent formerly used in dry cleaning but found to be a liver and kidney toxin; now designated as an industrial poison and a possible human carcinogen.

carboxyhemoglobin A compound of hemoglobin produced by bonding with carbon monoxide. Because this is a chemically stable bond, it prevents hemoglobin from performing its function of oxygen transport, causing asphyxiation. Carbon monoxide also bonds with heme moieties in myoglobin and cytochromes and blocks their function in oxygen storage and energy generation, thus contributing to its toxicity. Carboxyhemoglobin imparts a bright pink color to the skin.

carcinogen An agent that causes cancer. The INTERNATIONAL AGENCY FOR RESEARCH ON CANCER (IARC) identifies specific chemical, physical, and biological cancer-causing agents, dietary factors, and genetic predisposing factors. Common carcinogens include ionizing radiation, combustion products of tobacco and biomass fuels, some hormones and related steroids, some industrial chemicals and pharmaceuticals, and certain dietary ingredients. The IARC classifies carcinogens into four categories (with two subcategories). Group 1 are agents known to be carcinogenic to humans. Group 2A are agents probably carcinogenic to humans. Group 2B are agents that are possibly carcinogenic. Group 3 are agents unclassified with regard to human carcinogenesis. Group 4 are agents probably not carcinogenic to humans. The risk of cancer can be reduced but not eliminated by avoiding or minimizing exposure to known carcinogens. Comprehensive current lists of confirmed human carcinogens are available from the IARC, the American Cancer Society, the UK Department of Health and Human Services, and several other sources. For example, see http://www-cie.iarc.fr/monoeval/crthall.html and http://ntp.niehs.nih.gov/ntp/roc/toc11.html.

carcinogenesis The pathological process by which cancer occurs. Some aspects of the process remain unknown, but a simplified explanation is that disruption of DNA causes cells to disobey the signals responsible for differentiation, cell division, and programmed cell death. The process begins with initiation, which is an irreversible transformation of cellular growth regulation that establishes unregulated growth, usually associated with genetic or chromosomal damage caused by a carcinogenic agent. The next stage is promotion, whereby an agent causes initiated cells to divide abnormally. This is followed by progression, the transition of initiated cells to a phase of unregulated growth and invasiveness, often with metastases and pleomorphism, i.e., variation of cell size, nuclear shape, etc. Usually the process is irreversible but rarely it may spontaneously cease, and the pace with which it advances can vary widely. It can be arrested and sometimes reversed by radiotherapy or chemotherapy.

carcinoma Malignant neoplasm of any epithelial tissue is called a carcinoma. It is the most common form of malignant neoplasm. Sometimes the word is loosely used to describe all malignancies, and derivative words such as CARCINOGEN describe agents that can cause any form of malignant neoplasm. The characteristics of carcinoma include local tissue destruction, invasiveness, and distant metastases.

carcinoma in situ A carcinoma that is localized to the site of its origin, has not invaded or destroyed surrounding tissues, has not spread to more distant sites, and is usually amenable to cure, e.g., by localized excision. An example is early carcinoma of the cervix.

cardiopulmonary resuscitation (CPR) Emergency method of restoring heart beat and respiration when these have been interrupted briefly. It is administered by mouth-to-mouth breathing and firm rhythmic pressure on the sternum over the pericardial region repeated at 2- to 3-second intervals. When available, as in most hospitals, "paddles" to administer electric shocks may be used in attempts to restore sinus rhythm if the ventricles are fibrillating.

cardiovascular disease A term covering all forms of disease of the heart and blood vessels. It is a useful rubric in disease classification systems and in publicity campaigns to draw attention to the magnitude of the public and personal health problem caused by this group of conditions that collectively are responsible for almost half of all deaths in industrialized countries, but its failure to indicate anything about causes or control reduces its value in public health and disease-prevention programs. The two largest components are CORONARY HEART DISEASE and HYPERTENSION. Another important, albeit numerically smaller, group is congenital heart disease. Rheumatic heart disease was prevalent in industrial nations until the middle of the 20th century but has receded since, although it still occurs in some low-income countries and in deprived regions of affluent countries. See also GLOBAL BURDEN OF DISEASE.

care The health and social services provided to individuals and populations. In public health, "care" means services to preserve, protect, and restore good health.

caregiver Any person, usually a family member, friend, or less often a health professional, who cares for a dependent sick person or persons, emphasizing compassionate personal care.

caries Syn: Dental caries, tooth decay. Erosion of dental enamel is a very common dental health problem, associated with high carbohydrate dietary intake (especially sugar) that encourages decay-producing oral bacteria, and poor oral hygiene. Fluoride is required for formation of strong and healthy dental enamel, so fluoride deficiency increases the tendency to dental caries.

carpal tunnel syndrome A common chronic disorder of the median nerve that occurs as an occupational disease of keyboard operators or is associated with conditions, including pregnancy, diabetes, hypothyroidism. The occupational disease is treated by adjusting the position of office workers' hands on computer keyboards and sometimes splinting.

carrier 1. A person or animal who harbors a specific infectious agent, usually does not have any symptoms or signs of the disease the agent causes, yet can transmit the disease agent to others. 2. A genetic carrier is a person who carries a gene that is transmissible to subsequent generations, where it is expressed as manifest abnormality. The carrier's phenotype may not show any evidence of genetic abnormality. 3. An insurance carrier provides reimbursement of part or all of medical or hospital expenses for health insurance policy holders.

carrying capacity The number of people that a nation, a region, or the planet can sustain. There is uncertainty about the earth's carrying capacity. Optimists believe there is abundant unused capacity; pessimists believe the human population has already exceeded its carrying capacity. See also SUSTAINABLE DEVELOPMENT.

Cartesian coordinates A system for locating the position of a point or variable by reference to its position on two or three axes, each of which intersects at right angles to the other(s). In a two-dimensional graph, these are usually called the X and Y axes. The distance of the variable from the X axis is called the ordinate, and the distance from the Y axis is the abscissa. The coordinates are named in honor of the French mathematician and philosopher René Descartes (1596–1650).

cartogram A diagrammatic map that presents statistical information visually. This may be done in various ways, the best known of which is a CHOROPLETH MAP, in which regions are color-coded or differentially shaded according to the prevalence or incidence of the factor(s) displayed.

case 1. An instance of a disease. 2. A jargon term, generally considered dehumanizing, for a person diagnosed or otherwise identified as having a condition of interest. 3. The term describing the dispute between parties involved in a legal action in a court of law.

case, collateral A case that occurs in a place contiguous with or geographically adjoining that in which case(s) have been the subject of epidemiological investigation. A collateral case may therefore signal extension of the range of an epidemic.

case conference In public health practice this usually means a meeting of members of several professional experts in relevant specialties and disciplines that is convened to deal with a specific and sometimes complex public health problem, such as provision of housing for families who have lost their home in a fire or identifying the optimum way to support a family of destitute children whose parents lack the resources to care for them.

case control study The epidemiological method of investigation of a condition of interest that compares the history of exposure to specified risks among cases to exposure among persons who resemble the cases in other respects but do not have the condition of interest, the CONTROLS. This widely used method has yielded much valuable information about many serious diseases. It is especially useful in the study of rare conditions. It is standardized medical history taking extended to a specified population of persons with the condition of interest and comparison of facts in these medical histories with facts in the history of persons who do not have the condition of interest. However, case control studies can be flawed by several possible sources of BIAS, e.g., due to inappropriate selection of controls or differing quality and quantity of information about past exposures of cases and controls, and by many kinds of uncontrolled CONFOUNDING variables.

case definition The criteria used to establish a specific diagnosis. These criteria vary according to the nature of the disease and the purpose for which the case definition is used. When a specific pathogenic organism or pathological process is implicated, unequivocal diagnostic tests are usually available. With diseases such as multiple sclerosis, a scoring system is used, based on points for each of several diagnostic features, each of which is a common feature of the disease but none of which alone is sufficient for diagnosis. The SYNDROMIC APPROACH TO TREATMENT is mostly used in surveillance and control of dangerous epidemics because screening and diagnostic tests are rarely if ever feasible. Moreover, it is more important to identify all possible, as well as probable, cases, especially with contagious diseases.

case fatality rate The proportion of the cases of a condition of interest who die of the condition within a specified period of follow-up after diagnosis and/or medical intervention, often expressed as percentages of deaths in a 1-year or 5-year period.

case-finding 1. In communicable disease control, locating, identifying, and assessing persons who have had intimate or close contact with a diagnosed case of contagious disease, such as tuberculosis and sexually transmitted diseases; also identification and assessment of persons who may have been exposed to contaminated food in an outbreak of food poisoning. Ethical issues may arise when case-finding involves invasion of privacy. See also CONTACT TRACING. 2. In clinical practice, especially in primary care, opportunistic case-finding in the course of routine medical examinations for other purposes yields new cases of conditions such as hypertension, diabetes, cancer, etc., leading to earlier intervention than would otherwise occur. Case-finding is preferred, rather than SCREENING, as the optimal way to detect hypertension.

case law This is law based on resolution of a legal dispute that establishes a precedent that is upheld through the highest court in the nation and is thenceforth followed in similar cases. This is the basis for some public health law and regulations, for example those dealing with some aspects of environmental pollution. See also PUBLIC HEALTH LAWS.

case load The number and variety of patients or clients served by a clinic or health care facility. Also the number of patients or clients of an individual health care professional. Case loads vary widely according to demand, supply, accessibility, specialty, presence of GATEKEEPERS, season, economic and social conditions, and other factors. See also CATCHMENT AREA.

case management The method, often a formal protocol, for care of persons identified as having cases of specific conditions, such as notifiable communicable diseases, cancer at specified sites, etc.

case mix The range of diagnostic and/or treatment categories that make up the CASE LOAD of a physician, other health care provider, clinic, or hospital.

case report A descriptive account of a case of a condition of interest, providing details of all the relevant circumstances, occasionally providing a basis for inferences about causes and possible methods of control that could be applied in the future.

case study An account of a person's health problem or of a problem situation that purports or aspires to be comprehensive and contains all the information needed to make a rational decision about the actions required to achieve an optimum outcome. It may provide the basis for a formal report, perhaps one intended for publication.

caste The hereditary groups into which members of some cultures, notably the Hindus of Indian society, have traditionally been divided. Persons within the same caste may be considered socially equal with one another and often differ in social status, prestige, religious observance, income, occupation, opportunity, and health experience from persons in other castes. In the past there has been little social intercourse or marriage across caste boundaries, but the sharp division of Indian society into many subgroups has begun to break down in urban areas of modern industrial India under pressure from educational, media-driven, and political forces. The implications of this trend for population health include the potential for reducing the gaps in health experience. Some aspects of the caste system can be discerned in other societies, e.g., among the hereditary aristocracy in Europe and the wealthiest families and prominent sports and media stars in modern industrial and commercial society in the United States and in other apparently egalitarian societies.

casual contact transmission This is transmission by way of a person who has had transient, rather than close or ongoing, contact with an active case of a transmissible disease.

casualty A person injured in an accident or in armed combat. Also formerly the name of the hospital department where casualties are received, i.e., the emergency department.

casuistry 1. A method of decision making in BIOETHICS based on a combination of prior moral beliefs, usually with a foundation in religious faith, and their application in cases with similar features to those of the case under consideration. 2. A method of reasoning in which conclusions are based on data from individual case(s). For this reason, conclusions may not be generalizable.

CAT scan Syn: CT scan. See COMPUTED AXIAL TOMOGRAPHY.

cat-scratch disease A bacterial infection with fever, malaise, and lymphadenopathy, usually due to *Bartonella* infection and acquired from a bite, scratch, or even just licking, of a cat.

cataract An opacity in the ocular lens, associated with aging, also with exposure to actinic radiation, and an occupational disease of workers exposed to infrared radiation, such as smelter workers. Removal of cataracts is among the earliest surgical operations. It has been practiced by traditional African healers who used tools such as sharp thorns. In modern Western nations with large proportions of elderly people, cataract surgery has become very common, often done as an outpatient or day-hospital procedure.

catastrophe theory A branch of mathematics dealing with prediction of large changes in the total system that can be a result of small changes in a critical variable that is part of the system. Certain epidemics, gene frequencies, and behavioral phenomena, such as the spread of rumors, may follow the mathematical rules of this theory.

catastrophic illness The term used mainly in the United States for a serious and complex condition that requires highly specialized and therefore costly treatment and aftercare, which generate personal expenses often far in excess of those covered by public services or the reimbursements available through private sector insurance COVERAGE.

catchment area 1. The topographically defined region that potentially or actually supplies water to a reservoir. 2. The region from which persons come to receive health and other services. The size and population of this can vary greatly, depending on the nature of the service. Thus, the catchment area and population for accident and emergency services may differ in both size and distribution from those of regional cancer centers.

cathode rays The stream of electrons emanating from the negative pole (cathode) of a vacuum tube when an electric current is passed through it. At very high voltages, cathode rays emit high-energy x-rays, i.e., ionized radiation. At lower voltages, such as in TV screens and computer monitors, low-energy x-rays are produced but are blocked by lead in the glass screen.

cattle Gregarious hoofed animals (ungulates) that have been domesticated since humans transformed from a society of hunter-gatherers to one that pastured cattle, goats, and sheep about 8,000 to 10,000 BCE. Cattle are the main source for milk, meat, and leather in many human communities. Grazing cattle transform ecosystems, and human contact with cattle leads to disease risks, including parasitic infections such as SCHISTOSOMIASIS and beef TAPEWORM. Infections such as ANTHRAX, MEASLES, INFLUENZA, and TUBERCULOSIS probably evolved in ecosystems that brought humans and cattle into close continuing contact. A new disease, BOVINE SPONGIFORM ENCEPHALOPATHY, or "mad cow disease," began to occur in epidemic form after cattle feed was fortified with animal residue containing the prion causing SCRAPIE in sheep.

Caucasian Syn: white. Strictly speaking, an ethnographic term for a person of Indo-European or European "race" but in practice often a vague, sometimes emotive designation. In multicultural and multiracial societies, the term can cause controversy about the concept of "race" as an acceptable descriptive term. Although used in some official statistics, the designation "Caucasian" has little or no credibility in scientific discourse.

causal inference The method of logical reasoning that seeks to use all available facts to arrive at a conclusion about the relationship of particular causes to their effects. This is the main method of reasoning in the public health sciences, especially epidemiology. It was discussed in a seminal monograph by Mervyn Susser, *Causal Thinking in the Health Sciences* (1973), and in many later articles and monographs. See also HILL'S CRITERIA and LOGIC.

causality Syn: causation. The study of relationships between causes and effects based on CAUSAL INFERENCE from available sources of information, such as empirical observations and evidence, preferably based on objective scientific studies. In public health, much evidence often comes from epidemiological studies. These mostly yield circumstantial evidence but as human experiments are often impractical or considered unethical, epidemiological evidence may be the best or the only evidence available. The study of causality goes considerably further in applications of causal inference that rely on logical assembly and assessment of all pertinent information, perhaps supported by in vitro laboratory studies and other sources of evidence. For instance, when searching for the causal pathogen responsible for a communicable disease, investigators may use the HENLE-KOCH POSTULATES, although these do not necessarily help.

cause In general, something that produces an effect. In medicine and public health it is customary to distinguish necessary cause, sufficient cause, and proximal cause and distal cause. A necessary cause is one without which a condition cannot occur, e.g., *Mycobacterium tuberculosis* is the necessary cause of tuberculosis; a sufficient cause is the occurrence of environmental, behavioral, and/or other factors, e.g., poverty and malnutrition that promote the disease. A proximal cause is an immediate precipitating factor, e.g., exposure to ultraviolet radiation is a proximal cause of skin cancer. A distal cause is more remote, e.g., the presence of ozone-destroying substances in the atmosphere that lead to penetration of higher levels of ultraviolet radiation flux.

cause of death See DEATH CERTIFICATE.

cause-specific rate The incidence or death rate from a specific cause such as cancer or coronary heart disease. Cause-specific incidence and death rates for cancer are further classified by the site of the cancer to yield rates for common cancers, such as lung, breast, prostate, and colon.

CD-4 cells T-helper white blood cells responsible for production of immune globulin that protects against virus infections. Other cells, including - CD-3 and CD-8, play a role in this process. These cells are receptors for and are attacked by HIV, and their number is an indicator of the progress of HIV infection to frank AIDS.

cease and desist order In public health law, a legally enforceable requirement to comply with a written notice with respect to health and safety standards, e.g., about food handling, disposal of waste products. Failure to comply is punishable in law by heavy fines and/or imprisonment.

celibacy The status of a person who refrains from sexual activity with others, permanently (e.g., for reasons motivated by religious beliefs) or temporarily (because of circumstances such as sex segregation during an expedition or while in an institution). Celibate persons are not at risk for sexually transmitted diseases or pregnancy.

cell The biological unit comprising nucleus, cytoplasm, and usually other components such as mitochondria that differentiates into many kinds of specialized tissues to form the organs and architectural units of the body. It is the site of many kinds of metabolic interchange and is vulnerable to many kinds of malfunction associated with pathogenesis and diseases.

cell-mediated immunity Immunity that results primarily from stimulation of T-helper cells.

censoring A term used in biostatistics to describe loss of cases to follow-up or observations of unknown value at one or both ends of a distribution of a set of data.

census A periodic enumeration of the population, primarily intended to collect information to identify eligible voters, tax payers, and sometimes to identify people eligible for military service, and incidentally many other useful facts, e.g., about housing conditions. The earliest census was probably carried out about 1500 BCE in ancient Egypt. Censuses were used by the Romans and have been conducted at 10- or 5-year intervals in almost all industrial nations for more than 100 years. Censuses provide much information for public health services, e.g., identifying proportions of single-parent mother-led families,

and localities with high proportions of isolated old people living alone, who may be at high risk of health problems. Public health nursing and other services can be targeted at the vulnerable people who live in such localities. In some countries record linkage systems and privacy laws permit relating census data to hospital discharge and death certificate data, providing a useful additional tool for health policy and epidemiological research studies.

census tract A term used mainly in the United States meaning a defined region, usually in an urban area, that is usually the smallest geographically identifiable region for enumeration in a census.

center of excellence An academic and research setting, usually an integral part of a university, school of public health, or comparable center of advanced study, that is identified and recognized by peers and funding agencies as a place where outstanding original work has been done, is being done, and is expected to continue to be done in the future. To some extent, centers of excellence are defined by the reputation they acquire, but governmental and other funding agencies may seek deliberately to establish them. Examples in the latter category include the specialized research units established with long-term funding by the UK Medical Research Council, and the clinical research center of the US National Institutes of Health.

Centers for Disease Control and Prevention (CDC) The US federal government facility based mainly in Atlanta, Georgia, that provides investigative and educational facilities in most branches of public health sciences, serving the United States and much of the rest of the world in epidemic investigation, laboratory study of emerging pathogens, etc. The CDC has conducted many important original investigations of communicable and noncommunicable diseases. It has several specialized centers, including National Centers for Birth Defects, Chronic Disease Prevention and Health Promotion, Environmental Health, Health Statistics, HIV, STD and Tuberculosis, Injury Prevention and Control, Immunization Programs, the Epidemiology Program Office, and the Public Health Program Office. Details of CDC's activities are available at http://www.cdc.gov. See also EPIDEMIC INTELLIGENCE SERVICE.

central death rate The computed or estimated death rate at the center of an age range of a population, for instance the death rate of a national population in the age range 20 to 29 years or 65 to 74 years. For many purposes this could be misleading, but it is often used to describe the child mortality rate, especially in low-income countries.

central tendency The grouping of numerical data about a value at or near the midpoint of the overall distribution. Three common measures of central tendency are mean, median, and mode. See also MEASURES OF CENTRAL TENDENCY.

centrifuge A machine that separates solid particles suspended in a fluid medium into components according to their mass, accelerating the process of sedimentation by applying rotational forces to a container, e.g., a centrifuge tube, so the most dense particles sink rapidly to form the deepest layer, with successive layers of progressively lower density above them.

cercaria The larval stage of trematode worms such as schistosomes. These are tiny tadpole-shaped, free-swimming creatures that invade and develop in the tissues of the intermediate hosts, freshwater mollusks, from which they emerge and become free-swimming again when developed to the stage when they can invade the definitive host, warm-blooded mammals such as humans.

cerebral palsy A general term for a class of neurological conditions manifest at or soon after birth due to brain damage caused by transient interruption of the blood supply to the brain with anoxia sufficient to produce lasting neural deficit. This can take many forms, including spastic paralysis of voluntary muscles, loss of coordination, impaired control of sphincters of bladder and/or bowel, and mental impairment. The causes include birth trauma, compression of the umbilical cord, and possibly some toxins. Cerebral palsy can be considered a public health problem because some causes are preventable, and many with the condition require lifelong care and social assistance.

certainty In philosophy and science, a fact or concept that is established beyond all possibility of doubt, for example that all humans die. Science advances by using observation, experiment, and logical reasoning, i.e., inductive and deductive logic, to refute previously accepted "certainties" and replace them with new, more valid certainties.

certificate of need A document issued by a federal, state, or local government agency to confirm approval for a health care institution or facility to construct a new building, invest in expensive equipment, or provide medically insured services specified on that particular certificate. The same term also describes the form used by public health workers, social workers, school teachers, etc., to record details setting out reasons an individual or a family may require social assistance.

certification 1. Completion of an official form or document for statutory and/or legal purposes, as in certification of birth, marriage, annulment, divorce, and death, certifiable insanity, etc. 2. Completion of educational and/or other requirements to practice a profession such as medicine, nursing, or law that is open only to legally qualified practitioners. BOARD CERTIFICATION is certification by a specialty board, such as the American Board of Preventive Medicine.

cervical smear Syn: Pap (Papanicolaou) smear, named for its originator, the Greek physician Georges Papanicolaou (1883–1936). Cytological examination for cervical cancer detects abnormalities indicating precancerous or cancerous changes in the cells of the cervix of the uterus. Most authorities recommend that routine cervical smears begin within 3 years of sexual activity or at age 21 years, whichever comes first, thereafter every 1 to 2 years until after menopause and with three successive negative smears. This is a valid test for abnormal cells if properly done and a reliable screening test for early cancer of the cervix.

cervicitis Inflammation of the cervix of the uterus, a condition often associated with inadequate sexual hygiene. The symptoms include vaginal discharge, discomfort, and pain on intercourse. The causes include sexually transmitted diseases, postpartum ulceration of cervical lacerations, etc.

cesarean section Extraction of the fetus through an abdominal incision, rather than by vaginal delivery. The name derives from the apocryphal story that Julius Caesar was delivered this way. The indications for cesarean section include obstructed labor (e.g., because of pelvic malformation) or central placenta previa. Increasingly, the operation is performed to hasten delivery, to deliver neonates at times convenient to the attending obstetrician, or to spare women the pain and after effects of vaginal delivery.

cesium (Cs) An alkaline metallic element used in photoelectric cells. Radioactive cesium is a product of postnuclear radioactive decay, and its presence in the environment is an indicator that leakage from a NUCLEAR REACTOR has occurred, e.g., levels were very high in the region of the radioactive plume north and west (downwind) from the CHERNOBYL nuclear reactor.

cesspool, cesspit An obsolete method of sewage disposal consisting of a pond or pit into which sewage is dumped. It is occasionally still used in some low-income countries. It is malodorous and a potential nidus of fecal-oral disease transmission. Although some digestion of its contents does occur, there is no provision for outflow, such as with septic tanks or larger water-carried sewage disposal systems. Other health hazards of cesspools include overflow and flooding.

cestodes A large class of flatworms that includes segmented TAPEWORMS, many of which parasitize humans and other mammals. These parasites are attached to the intestinal lining of their host by a head bearing hooks and/or suckers to hold it in place. They absorb nourishment through their entire body surface, thereby depriving their host of this. Most have male and female sex organs in every segment. They produce huge numbers of eggs excreted in their host's feces, and usually have a primary host that is a predator of a secondary host in which the cestode passes an early phase of its life cycle. Cestodes include the beef and pork tapeworms.

Chagas disease Syn: American trypanosomiasis. A chronic disease elucidated by the Brazilian physician Carlos Chagas (1879–1934), who investigated the disease and died of it. The cause is a hemoflagellate intracellular protozoan, *Trypanosoma cruzi*. It is transmitted by blood-feeding bugs that roost inside houses in endemic regions of South and Central America and is transmissible in blood transfusions. Improved housing and vector control programs are successfully eliminating it from many formerly endemic areas. A tropical diseases program of WHO, UNICEF, and the World Bank aims to eliminate Chagas disease by 2010. For details, see http://www.who.int/trd/diseases/chagas/default.htm.

chain reaction A series of chemical, biochemical, or nuclear reactions that once begun continues inexorably and usually cannot be stopped or interrupted. The term is used mainly to describe the process of nuclear reactions in nuclear power plants and nuclear weapons.

chakara Also chakra. In Ayurvedic medicine, the armamentarium of some 500 herbal and other remedies that were originally described and their effects recorded by Chakara, an Indian leader and innovator of this medical system, about 200 CE.

chance See RANDOM.

chancre The painless cutaneous sore, usually on the genitals, that is the presenting sign of early infection with SYPHILIS, beginning as a localized raised red swelling then ulcerating, at which stage innumerable treponemas of syphilis are present in the exudate, so it is maximally infectious.

chancroid Painful ulcerating genital lesion(s) caused by *Haemophilus ducreyi*, a sexually transmitted disease.

change agent A person, team, group, or media method, such as radio or television, that facilitates behavior change for health improvement by mobilizing sociological and/or psychological factors, to raise vaccination rates, reduce cigarette smoking by teenagers, enhance contraceptive use, etc.

chaos theory A branch of mathematics discovered in 1963 by the American meteorologist Edward Lorenz (b. 1917) to explain how small perturbations in a system can have far-reaching consequences. These cannot be predicted using conventional mathematical models and require application of complex innovative methods. Chaos theory may apply to biological processes, such as the course of metastases in some cancers, and has proved useful in scenarios of possible future disease patterns in relation to changing climates.

charcoal Carbonized wood or other organic matter that has been partially burned or roasted to rid it of water and can be used as a fuel that is comparatively smokeless and therefore, when properly combusted, contributes less atmospheric pollution than does raw wood.

charitable foundations See FOUNDATIONS.

charity Beneficence toward others, especially those in financial and other need, often leading to the provision of alms, financial aid, and services of various kinds, notably health-related services. Many charitable FOUNDATIONS focus on health needs, including provision of enhanced public health services. An example is the MARCH OF DIMES, which was founded with the explicit aim of raising funds for the treatment and prevention of poliomyelitis and relied almost entirely on donations of small sums of money by individuals for operating costs, rather than large, often posthumous bequests of capital that produce income for annual disbursements to worthy causes. See also ALTRUISM.

chart 1. A visual display of information or a map 2. Jargon for MEDICAL RECORD, derived from the fact that a temperature chart is often the first page of hospital medical records.

chastity Sexual continence, i.e., refraining from sexual contact with all others except a legal or otherwise acknowledged spouse. Not to be confused with CELIBACY but like celibacy a state that minimizes risk of sexually transmitted disease, provided the sex partner is also chaste.

chelating agents Chemicals that reduce differences in solubility of nonfatty and fatty substances. Chelating agents are used therapeutically to treat lead and other heavy metal poisoning by forming excretable compounds. In industry, they may cause occupational dermatitis.

chelation 1. The formation of an organic chemical compound in which a heavy metal is part of a ring complex. 2. A process that enhances mixing of fatty and nonfatty ingredients in an industrial process or in the preparation of foods.

chemical contraceptive A contraceptive that relies on chemical action to kill the sperm or ovum, rather than acting as a physical barrier to union of sperm and ovum. Examples include spermicidal foam or jelly. Some can become irritants of vaginal epithelium.

chemical dependency Strictly speaking, physiological or pharmacological dependence on a chemical substance, such as a psychoactive drug, that a user relies upon. Failure to take doses of the drug can lead to the occurrence of WITHDRAWAL SYMPTOMS.

chemical hazard A chemical substance that is hazardous to health if persons are exposed. Many such chemicals have been identified, and TIME-WEIGHTED AVERAGES, MAXIMUM ALLOWABLE CONCENTRATIONS, etc., have been established for many of these.

chemical weapons One category of WEAPONS OF MASS DESTRUCTION, chemical weapons were used in World War I and by several military forces later, despite international conventions to ban them. They include poisonous gases, such as chlorine, mustard gas, phosgene, and sarin, and food contaminants, such as ricin and botulinus toxin, that are deliberately introduced into foodstuffs, such as flour, with the intention of harming people. The definition is broadened to include substances such as napalm, the modern and far more deadly equivalent of burning sulfur and pitch that were used in some ancient wars. Some chemical weapons, e.g., sarin gas, have been used in terrorist attacks in recent years.

chemist 1. A person who studies and/or applies the science of chemistry. 2. The British term for a PHARMACIST.

CHEMLINE A computerized data base of information about chemical substances maintained by the NATIONAL LIBRARY OF MEDICINE until 1998 when it, and TOXLINE, a similar data base of toxic substances, were merged with MEDLINE. The information previously available in these two data bases was subject to royalty payments by the National Library of Medicine, whereas MEDLINE and web search engines such as Google are just as informative and are free. For information, see http://nnlm.gov/ner/nesl/9709/toxlit.html.

chemoprevention A method of disease prevention by long-term, usually lifelong, medication to modify risk factors. Examples include use of therapeutic agents to reduce blood pressure and serum cholesterol levels. It is an expensive disease prevention strategy, applicable only in high-income countries, but it is among the most effective methods of preventing complications of hypertension and coronary heart disease or disease progression.

chemoprophylaxis The use of antibiotics to prevent the occurrence of clinical infections or the progression of infection to disease. The term also describes the use of natural or synthetic compounds to prevent cancer development, e.g., TAMOXIFEN to prevent breast cancer.

chemotherapy The use of chemicals or antibiotics to treat an infection, a malignancy, or other condition with the aim of curing it or preventing its further progress. The principal varieties of chemotherapy are antibiotics to control and preferably eliminate pathogens and cancer chemotherapy. Cancer chemotherapy uses cytotoxic drugs, often in combinations that can destroy immune cells, as well as cancer cells, making replacement immune therapy necessary.

Chernobyl An industrial city in Ukraine in which nuclear reactors to generate electric power were constructed by the Soviet Union. In 1986, one of these reactors was the site of a nuclear accident that spread radioactive contamination in a wide plume mainly to the northwest, the direction of the prevailing wind. There were several immediate deaths of acute radiation sickness and, in the aftermath, several hundred deaths of radiation-related malignant diseases. An increased incidence of malignant diseases among the exposed population has been observed and is expected to persist for 20 to 30 years.

chi square (χ^2) test A family of statistical tests used to determine whether two or more sets of data or populations differ significantly from one another, based on comparing observed with expected distributions of the sets of data and calculating the statistical probability that the differences could be due to chance alone, using the chi square mathematical distribution. The test requires counts of data, often based on probability samples, or the comparison of distribution of data in a sample to a predetermined standard. Two frequently used chi square tests are those of Pearson and the MANTEL-HAENSZEL TEST.

chickenpox An infectious disease that most commonly occurs in childhood, caused by the varicella-zoster virus, HERPES VIRUS 3. It causes mild fever and a generalized vesicular rash that does not leave residual scars unless vesicles become infected. Most children recover completely and rapidly. However, the varicella-zoster virus apparently remains dormant and can reactivate later in life to cause HERPES ZOSTER, a varicella-like rash usually confined to a distribution of a single dermatome that is acutely painful often for a prolonged period of months, even years.

chigger The larval stage of an arthropod mite, of which about 50 species attack humans and livestock. The main vector-borne disease for this group is SCRUB TYPHUS.

child abuse Maltreatment of children, which includes physical violence, such as beating, forcible confinement, sexual molestation, assault, and psychological maltreatment. The term also includes neglect and failure to provide the necessities of life (food, shelter, clothing). The legal upper age limit defined as "childhood" varies from 14 to 18 years. Child abuse is notifiable to law enforcement and/or child protection agencies in most industrial nations. Studies often show that adults who have abusive behavior were abused when they were children.

childbirth Complete delivery of a viable infant from the uterus of the mother followed by expulsion of the placenta, without specifying whether the delivery is vaginal or by cesarean section. Childbirth is usually a normal, natural, albeit often strenuous and painful experience for the mother, but there are risks of complications due to malposition of the fetus, hemorrhage, postpartum infection, toxemia of pregnancy, etc. Preventing complications and minimizing the risks is a high priority of antenatal and postnatal care conducted by family physicians, nurse-midwives, maternal and child health services, perinatologists, and obstetricians.

child care A general term for health-related, social, and educational services directed to the health and well-being of children, and more specifically the range of health-promotion and disease-prevention services for children. In many jurisdictions, e.g., the European Union, New Zealand, and the Canadian province of Quebec, child care is a tax-supported service provided at least partly by government agencies.

child guidance services A range of educational, counseling, social, psychological, and protective services that are provided in some jurisdictions to assist children, and their parents, experiencing learning or social problems. Usually linked with educational services, sometimes with correctional services.

child health services Health services for children, usually SCHOOL HEALTH SERVICES, sometimes an extension of MATERNAL AND CHILD HEALTH services, sometimes both.

child mortality rate The mortality rate in children aged from 1 to 4 years. This is a type of central death rate. Alternatively, it is the probability of dying between the first and fifth birthday. In low- and middle-income countries, these rates can be estimated using data from DEMOGRAPHIC AND HEALTH SURVEYS or from SAMPLE REGISTRATION SYSTEMS because vital registration systems are not usually sufficiently complete to allow direct measurement. Given the uncertainty of such estimated rates, it is wise to confirm their provenance and to interpret them cautiously. Mortality rates in this age range are a sensitive indicator of vulnerability to nutritional deficiencies and childhood infections. See also UNDER 5 MORTALITY RATE.

child protection acts Most industrialized nations and some developing countries have enacted legislation aimed to protect infants and children by helping to ensure that they are provided with the necessities of life (shelter, clothing, food); to protect them from exploitation as bonded laborers, prostitutes, etc.; and to ensure that they receive adequate health care and education.

child-resistant package A method of packaging pharmaceutical preparations in a screw-top container that requires firm downward pressure at the same time as a rotational movement to undo the cap and get to the contents. While this method of packaging is child resistant, it may also be resistant to the efforts of elderly, arthritic, and other disabled persons to open the container and get to the pills inside.

child survival The proportion of liveborn infants who survive through the middle years of childhood, a potentially useful indicator of population health level. It is variously defined as survival past the age of 5 years and survival past the age of 10 years, and because of the uncertainty about definition of the duration of survival, the term is preferably avoided.

child welfare agencies As the name implies, these are agencies concerned with the welfare of children. Although they fulfill an essential service in safeguarding the interests of children, they may be obliged to operate according to regulations that can separate children from their parents with the end result that instead of healing wounded families, child welfare agencies occasionally open the wounds further.

Chinese medicine China has had organized civilized societies since at least the 4th millennium BCE, and some aspects of its medical beliefs and practices date to that distant time. Chinese herbal medicine and ACUPUNCTURE both originated in the 3rd millennium BCE with several beliefs about causes and control of disease based at least partly on the concepts of *yin* (dark, moist, soft, female) and *yang* (light, dry, hard, and male), i.e., beliefs about the quality and character of people and the diseases they experienced. Herbal remedies had the additional advantage of a basis in empirical observations and some, e.g., GOSSYPOL for male contraception and the rauwolfia alkaloids for high blood pressure, have withstood modern pharmacological scrutiny that identified active ingredients and found a rational basis for their efficacy.

chiropody The term used mainly in the British Commonwealth for the specialty of PODIATRY, the diagnosis and treatment of disorders of the feet such as bunions, corns, calluses.

chiropractic A form of alternative medicine based on the theory that many diseases are caused by misplacement of vertebrae and can be relieved by manipulating the spine. Since it was founded in 1895 by an American merchant D. D. Palmer (1845–1913), chiropractic has evolved from an unorthodox practice with unusual beliefs about the causes of many diseases regarded as quackery by allopathic physicians, toward a mainstream position of respectability. Chiropractic treatment costs are reimbursed by most medical and hospital insurance programs, and orthopedic surgeons and physiatrists mostly agree that chiropractic methods of manipulation are an effective treatment for the symptoms of whiplash injury, some other post-traumatic conditions, etc.

Chlamydia The organisms that cause TRACHOMA (*C. trachomatis*); PSITTACOSIS (*C. psittaci*); chlamydial pneumonia and bronchitis (*C. pneumoniae*); and also urethritis and vaginitis, which are sexually transmitted forms of *C. trachomatis.*

chloracne A disfiguring lumpy red skin eruption resembling very bad acne affecting mainly the face and torso, attributable to relatively high-level exposure to PCBs, FURANS, or DIOXINS. Severe cases have permanent disfiguring skin scarring.

chloramphenicol One of the early broadspectrum antibiotics, used extensively in the late 1950s until its bone marrow toxicity was recognized. Despite this it remains a treatment of choice for some rickettsial infections including TYPHUS FEVER and for epidemic meningitis.

chlordane A cyclodiene pesticide in the same family as aldrin and dieldrin, absorbed through the skin, highly toxic and, for this reason, no longer approved for use in the United States but still used, like many other toxic pesticides, in some low-income countries.

chlordecone With the trade name Kepone, this powerful pesticide was briefly manufactured in a plant in Virginia for about 3 years from 1973 to 1975. Industrial hygiene was inadequate, and there was considerable environmental contamination. Workers exposed to chlordecone experienced bizarre neurological symptoms, including ataxia, visual and speech disorders, toxic psychosis, and also aspermia or severe oligospermia causing infertility. Chlordecone, and a related chemical pesticide trade named Mirex, also are powerfully carcinogenic. Both are now banned.

chlorinated hydrocarbons The general name for a large class of organic chemicals including many of great commercial importance, i.e., pesticides, solvents, TRIHALOMETHANES, etc. They are formed by substitution of one or more hydrogen atoms by chlorine in a hydrocarbon and have chemical structures ranging from relatively simple to very complex. They include methyl and methylene chloride, chloroform, and carbon tetrachloride. Many are widely used in industry. They include some highly toxic chemicals, carcinogens, and ENDOCRINE DISRUPTERS.

chlorination The process of water treatment involving infusion of chlorine gas or a chlorine compound such as chloramine into drinking water in order to kill pathogenic organisms such as coliforms that would otherwise be present and would cause disease if ingested. This is an effective method of purifying water for drinking and use in swimming pools. Some protozoal and other water-borne pathogens are resistant to chlorination but can be removed by appropriate filtration methods. However, if the organic content of the water is very high, some of the chlorine binds with organic substances to produce potentially harmful compounds, including TRIHALOMETHANES, which can be carcinogenic.

chlorine (Cl) A greenish gas, used in liquid solution as a disinfectant, e.g., for swimming pools, and bleach. During World War I, it was used to make chloroethane and MUSTARD GAS, two poisonous gases, in an early instance of chemical warfare.

chlorofluorocarbons (CFCs) A class of chemicals that have been widely used industrially as solvents and refrigerants. They were long believed to be inert and environmentally innocuous. However, CFCs are capable of degrading stratospheric ozone and thus are identified as one of the principal ozone-destroying substances responsible for attenuation of the stratospheric ozone layer and for increased penetration of harmful ionizing ultraviolet radiation to the biosphere.

chloroform A TRIHALOMETHANE, used in 1847 as an anesthetic agent by the Edinburgh obstetrician James Young Simpson (1811–1870) and soon afterward by the London physician JOHN SNOW (1813–1858), who administered it to Queen Victoria to relieve pain during the birth of her two youngest children. After that it was widely used for several decades until superseded by safer anesthetic agents. Like other trihalomethanes, it is a liver poison and a carcinogen.

chloromethyl ethers A family of widely used industrial solvents, many of which are strongly carcinogenic and require special precautions such as use of protective clothing and sometimes respirators by workers handling them.

chlorophyll The green pigmented protein compound that occurs in all plants, including single-cell phytoplankton, and metabolizes carbon dioxide with the production of oxygen, i.e., it is the essential enzyme that drives the CARBON CYCLE. Thus, chlorophyll is a vitally important substance to all life on earth.

chloroprene A flammable solvent used in the manufacture of neoprene rubber. Human exposure is by skin absorption and inhalation. It causes respiratory irritation and adverse effects on the central nervous system, liver, and kidneys. It is a mutagen and impairs spermatogenesis.

chloroquine An aminoquinoline QUININE derivative that was successfully and widely used for malaria prophylaxis during and after World War II, until widespread chloroquine resistance of malaria parasites (plasmodia) greatly reduced its value.

chlorpyrifos A widely used insecticide that is environmentally persistent and believed to be relatively free of adverse toxic effects on humans and other mammals. However, there are some concerns about developmental neurotoxicity related to prenatal or infant exposure.

chocolate An alkaloid refined from cacao seeds, originally native to Central America and used by priests in pre-Columbian religious rituals; chocolate took Europeans by storm when brought back to Spain on Columbus's third voyage. Soon it was used everywhere in confectionary and drinks. It

may be the most widely used confectionary in the world. It is not addictive like nicotine but some people ("chocoholics") experience periodic cravings. It induces feelings of comfort among many who consume it. Excessive consumption can contribute to obesity because of the high calorie content of most chocolate confectionary. It has no adverse health effects, and there is some evidence that dark chocolate helps to provide protection from coronary heart disease.

cholera An acute bacterial enteric disease that causes profuse watery diarrhea with fluid and electrolyte loss, prostration, collapse, and often death unless treated by replacement of fluid and electrolytes, which reduces case fatality rates to about 1%. The 19th century pandemics caused widespread loss of life. Cholera is endemic in parts of south and southeast Asia, and since the early 19th century it has spread around the world in a series of pandemics, the latest of which is designated the seventh cholera pandemic, which spread to South America in 1991. Until oral rehydration therapy was developed, cholera had very high case fatality rates, especially among debilitated and undernourished people. See http://www.who/int/topics/cholera/en/ for current information on outbreaks and global status.

cholesterol A sterol that occurs in animal tissues in several lipids, categorized as LOW DENSITY LIPOPROTEINS (LDL) and HIGH DENSITY LIPOPROTEINS (HDL). An excess of LDL is associated with destructive changes in the arterial lining with deposition of atheromatous plaques, e.g., in coronary arteries, where they promote thrombosis and myocardial infarction. However, dietary intake of cholesterol may enhance a sense of well-being, and a sharply reduced cholesterol intake or use of drugs to lower serum cholesterol may be associated with depressed mood, anger, and violent behavior, although the evidence for a causal relationship to mood changes is weak.

chorionic villus sampling A method of screening used in early pregnancy consisting of a percutaneous transabdominal biopsy of chorionic tissue to test for evidence of fetal chromosomal abnormalities. The procedure carries a small risk of inducing miscarriage.

choropleth map A map in which regions with differing occurrence rates of conditions of interest (e.g., cancer) are visually distinguished by different color or shading corresponding to rates at which the designated conditions have occurred in each region during the period of observation.

Christian Science A sect of Christianity founded by an American chronic invalid, Mary Baker Eddy

(1821–1910), that rejects medical, surgical, obstetric, and preventive interventions such as immunizations. Christian scientists rely on faith in the power of Jesus Christ to protect them. Their relevance to public health is that they may acquire or transmit dangerous communicable diseases (measles, poliomyelitis, tuberculosis, etc). Otherwise, their beliefs are potentially harmful mainly to themselves and dependent members of their families.

chromatography A method of separating organic compounds in a mixture by transporting it in solution through a specially prepared filter that differentially absorbs the component compounds. This is the basis for some diagnostic tests, such as those based on the polymerase chain reaction.

chromium (Cr) Silver-gray metallic element used in alloys. An essential trace element in glucose metabolism. Exposure to chromium fumes during smelting or electroplating causes ulceration of mucosal surfaces, e.g., nasal mucosa.

chromosome The component of the cell nucleus consisting of strands of genetic material (DNA). In humans there are normally 46 chromosomes, 23 from each parent. Chromosomal aberrations and deletions or additions are associated with various BIRTH DEFECTS and cancers, especially leukemia (some evidence suggests their importance in most types of cancer). Each chromosome contains many individual genes. Mapping these genes has been the subject of intense research since the 1990s, notably in the HUMAN GENOME PROJECT.

chronic Prolonged, long-lasting, long-term, often but not necessarily implying incurable. The US National Center for Health Statistics defines a chronic condition as one of 3 months or greater duration, but some self-limiting conditions, for instance adolescent acne and herpes zoster, may continue for considerably more than 3 months before eventually subsiding completely.

chronic bronchitis Long-term or permanent cough with sputum indicative of inflammatory changes in the respiratory tract and often breathlessness. The condition is an outcome of chronic exposure to respiratory irritants, notably tobacco smoke or urban air pollution, often aggravated by recurring respiratory infections. With right-sided heart failure as a terminal consequence, it is a common cause of severe disability and premature death among lifelong cigarette smokers. See also CHRONIC OBSTRUCTIVE PULMONARY DISEASE (COPD).

chronic disease Any disease that is long-lasting or permanent. In practice, chronicity is often defined as an illness episode of 6 weeks' duration or more, but this is misleading if a prolonged illness of finite duration, such as an attack of herpes zoster, is placed in the same category as a long-term disease or disorder that does not eventually resolve or respond to treatment but gets worse, such as chronic bronchitis or multiple sclerosis.

chronic disease control The strategies and tactics that can be deployed to identify, prevent, or minimize effects of the diverse range of conditions of public health importance not caused by transmissible agents. Many are better described as NONCOMMUNICABLE CONDITIONS (DISEASES). The principal diseases for which preventive measures can be used include cancer, cardiovascular disease, emphysema and some degenerative diseases of the central and peripheral nervous systems and of bones and joints. Strategic and tactical approaches include early detection by SCREENING or CASE-FINDING, disease-specific interventions such as regulation of diet and insulin for diabetes and health-promotion programs such as exercise and diet regimens for obesity and cardiovascular disease.

chronic fatigue syndrome Debilitating recurrent or continuous lack of energy, often with other symptoms, such as sleep disorders, muscle weakness, vague aches, and pains. There may be low-grade fever, headaches, photophobia, and fleeting muscle pains. Laboratory test results usually are normal. The condition may appear as a sequel to infectious MONONUCLEOSIS or other viral infections, but often there are no specific precursor diseases. Various explanations have been offered. A CLINICAL ECOLOGY theory postulates an environmental cause and attributes the condition to MULTIPLE CHEMICAL SENSITIVITIES, an alleged reaction to unspecified manmade chemicals. No convincing evidence supports this theory. Some skeptical physicians regard this condition as the modern equivalent of "neurasthenia" of the early 20th century and "chlorosis" of the 18th and 19th centuries.

chronic obstructive pulmonary disease (COPD) Syn: chronic bronchitis and emphysema. A debilitating disease of the respiratory system, characterized by cough, sputum, shortness of breath, and often other features such as weight loss; it may be caused by environmental or occupational exposures, recurrent infection, but most often by long-term cigarette smoking.

chronic toxicity tests Tests for chronic toxicity, including cumulative effects and for evidence of potential carcinogenicity, mutagenicity, and teratogenicity. They are conducted on animals, and results must be interpreted with caution because some human mutagens and teratogens do not have comparable effects on animals such as the small rodents customarily used for testing.

chronobiology The scientific study of bodily rhythms or "biological clocks," such as circadian rhythm, the menstrual cycle, and the programmed onset of sexual maturation.

chrysotile asbestos White asbestos, alleged to be less dangerous than other forms of asbestos, but incriminated in ASBESTOSIS, MESOTHELIOMA, and LUNG CANCER.

cigarette Cigarettes are made by enclosing TO-BACCO in a cylinder of chemically impregnated paper that smolders, rather than burns, when ignited. Smokers inhale the fumes and smoke to obtain the desired dose of the highly addictive drug NICOTINE. By the early 20th century, this had become the main mode of tobacco use. The invention of machines to mass produce cigarettes and heavy promotion by tobacco manufacturers during World War I (1914–1918) made the custom of cigarette smoking ubiquitous among men by the 1920s. Aided by advertising, cigarette smoking spread increasingly among women in Western nations by the 1940s. Evidence of the causal connection of cigarette smoking to lung cancer began to appear in the 1950s, after German precursor studies published in the late 1930s. By the 1990s, resistance to cigarette smoking in public places had begun to transform society in North America, parts of the European Union, Australia, and New Zealand, but it remains popular among youth, especially poorly educated females, and is rapidly spreading in low- and middle-income nations. Strong public health action is needed if nations are to reduce and eventually eliminate cigarette smoking and, preferably, all forms of tobacco use. See also FRAMEWORK CONVENTION ON TOBACCO CONTROL.

cigarette smoke Tobacco smoke contains a large variety of toxic substances including several known carcinogens, respiratory irritants, cardiovascular toxins. Two varieties of tobacco smoke are MAINSTREAM SMOKE, which is directly inhaled and harms the smoker, and SIDESTREAM SMOKE, which harms those nearby who are exposed to its irritant effects on respiratory and conjunctival mucosa or obliged to breathe it. If tobacco had first been marketed after the mid-20th century, it would never have passed mandatory premarketing toxicity tests that existed by that time. Beginning in the last quarter of the 20th century, local ordinances in the United States and national laws in many other Western nations restricted smoking in public places, reducing or eliminating previ-ously ubiquitous cigarette smoke in restaurants, etc., that was a health risk for chronically exposed workers. See also INVOLUNTARY SMOKING.

ciguatera fish poisoning Food poisoning due to a toxin produced by a dinoflagellate and algae that are the diet of tropical reef fish. Concentration increases up the marine food chain to larger fish. Neurological and gastrointestinal symptoms appear about an hour after a meal containing these fish.

cinchona Syn: Peruvian bark. A tree native to South America from which the alkaloids QUININE and quinidine are extracted. Pre-Columbian civilizations in Central and South America discovered the efficacy of cinchona infusions to control malaria and relieve symptoms of fever from other causes, and European colonists brought this knowledge to Europe in the 15th century.

CINDI An acronym for Children in Distress, primarily a network of African nongovernmental organizations with a major focus on children orphaned by the HIV/AIDS pandemic. See http://www.cindi.org.za. The initial letters formerly were used by the Center for Integration of Natural Disaster Information, operated by the US National Geological Survey and focused mainly on earthquakes, hurricanes etc. CINDI also stands for COUNTRYWIDE INTEGRATED NONCOMMUNICABLE DISEASE INTERVENTION.

cinnabar Mercury sulfide, a bright red pigment used for many centuries in paints and dyestuffs. Like most mercury salts, it is highly toxic and now it is seldom used, except by a few artists.

circadian rhythm The wake-sleep cycle associated with various physiological changes, due to diurnal variations in intensity of light from day to night, therefore roughly a 24-hour cycle.

circumcision Surgical excision of the prepuce of the penis. This has been a common custom since Neolithic times. It probably originated in male initiation rites or coming-of-age ceremonies. It became a cultural fixture in the Jewish religion, in which male children are circumcised on the 8th day, and in Islam, in which it is done in later childhood. It is widespread among others of no particular religious affiliation, often because circumcised fathers want their sons to look as they do. It is said to be desirable in the interest of sexual hygiene, but there is little convincing evidence for its efficacy in this regard. Modern pediatric practice does not encourage circumcision because sexual hygiene can be maintained with an intact prepuce. See also FEMALE GENITAL MUTILATION.

cirrhosis of the liver Fibrotic degenerative changes in the liver associated with certain virus diseases (hepatitis B and C), occupational exposures, and metabolic disorders, including those attributed to chronic ALCOHOL DEPENDENCE.

Citizens Advice Bureau A municipal organization chiefly in the United Kingdom, Australia, and New Zealand, staffed by paid professionals trained in such fields as social work and/or by untrained or partially trained volunteers who provide counseling on miscellaneous social, economic, legal, and housing problems, referral services, etc.

civil liberty One of the fundamental principles of open, free societies, written into constitutions of many nations, civil liberty is the right of citizens to go about their lawful business without intrusive interference by law enforcement officials or other authorities. This liberty can legally be infringed when it exposes others to harm, as can happen with free movement of persons who have dangerous contagious diseases.

civil rights In countries that have victimized certain groups in society, this means emancipation, elimination of segregation, equity, and equality of access to the services and institutions of society. See also HUMAN RIGHTS.

civilization A stage of social development identified by formation of organized communities, permanent settlements, with oral or written records and history, traditions, religious faiths, laws, shared values, customs, beliefs, and artistic achievements. Other features include specialized occupations, commerce, reliance on trade, and multiple societal sectors, including health care, educational, defense and security services. The process of civilization alters naturally occurring ecosystems. Consequently, there are complex relationships between civilization and disease. Advanced civilizations reduce or control many communicable diseases, but often there is a rising prevalence of other public health problems, including nutritional imbalance associated with sedentary occupations and labor-saving technologies, traffic-related injury and premature death, and social, emotional, and some forms of mental disorders.

clade A group of organisms that have evolved from a common ancestor.

claim A legally sustainable request or demand for a service, or payment for a service, usually one covered by some form of collective insurance, for which a claim form is usually required.

class An identifiable group that can be distinguished from a larger whole. Sometimes, as with

SOCIAL CLASS, the criteria used to distinguish a group are contentious, but usually, as with an OCCUPATIONAL CLASSIFICATION, the criteria are unequivocal, or almost so.

classification Assignment to predesignated classes on the basis of perceived characteristics that are shared in common by all members of the class; a means of arranging a heterogeneous group of persons or things. Classifications aim to be comprehensive, systematic, simple, and useful. Many scientists and philosophers have aimed for order in their scholarly field by arranging, classifying, and naming the entities they deal with, from galaxies and planets to viruses. It is a challenge in the biological and medical sciences because expanding knowledge necessitates frequent revisions of an original apparently simple classification system.

classification of disease Arrangement of diseases into groups according to an orderly logical system, usually based on diagnostic categories, organ or system affected, or underlying pathological process. Early attempts to establish such a classification evolved from the BILLS OF MORTALITY, the writings of the English physician Thomas Sydenham (1624–1689), and the clinical and pathological NOSOLOGY of the Scottish physician William Cullen (1710–1790) to a combination based on a hierarchy of identifiable causes, including trauma, infections, cancer, conditions affecting various body systems, etc., developed by the English medical statistician William Farr (1807–1883) and his Swiss colleague Marc d'Espine (1803–1860). This was the precursor of the numerical taxonomy of the BERTILLON CLASSIFICATION, which was adopted by the International Statistical Institute in 1893. Successive revisions at approximately 10-year intervals since then have incorporated refinements based on growth of knowledge and understanding that led to the increased number of rubrics and modified chapters of the INTERNATIONAL CLASSIFICATION OF DISEASES (ICD).

clean air acts Legislation enacted in the United Kingdom, United States, and other countries after environmental air pollution became a pervasive urban problem and its adverse effects on human health (and its economic effects, e.g., on public buildings) could no longer be tolerated. In the United Kingdom, legislation was prompted by the LONDON SMOG disaster of 1952, which caused several thousand deaths; in the United States, the cumulative effect of several persistent problems, such as LOS ANGELES SMOG, led to political pressure for legislative action.

clean energy Energy generated from sources other than combustion of fuel that produces polluting substances. Hydrogen fuel, which combusts to produce water, is one form of clean energy. Others include solar, wind, and tidal power.

clean water acts Legislation enacted by national and state or provincial governments in many industrial nations, with supporting regulations and ordinances setting out ways in which public water supplies are or should be rendered safe for drinking and defining requirements for routine regular testing to ensure that drinking water remains safe.

clearance 1. Formal approval for a service or procedure. 2. The physiological process by which metabolic and many toxic products are removed from the circulation by the liver or kidneys.

clearinghouse An office or agency that collects data and distributes information on designated aspects of national or regional affairs such as health statistics.

climate By implication and usage, this means the long-term seasonally prevailing trends in atmospheric environmental conditions, rather than short-term fluctuations, which are called "weather." HIPPOCRATES described the relationship of climate to health in *Airs, Waters, Places* (4th century BCE). Modern epidemiology and environmental health have identified respiratory and other diseases that are influenced positively or negatively by climatic conditions.

climate change A long-term shift from the usual or expected climate and weather pattern. In the late 20th century, prevailing weather patterns everywhere were changing, with a trend toward global warming, and other trends, including climatic instability, more frequent extremes of hot and cold weather, and more severe catastrophic weather events, such as heat waves and floods. The change has been studied by climate scientists and others in many nations under the auspices of the INTERGOVERNMENTAL PANEL ON CLIMATE CHANGE (IPCC). The IPCC has published periodic reports since the late 1980s. The Report for 2001 contained evidence that recent changes are at least partly, perhaps mainly, the result of human activity, especially the GREENHOUSE EFFECT of fossil fuel combustion. Natural factors influencing climate change include cyclical fluctuations in solar flare activity, impedance of solar radiation by atmospheric dust, precession of the earth's axis, and tectonic plate movements that alter the flow of ocean currents. Climate change has important implications for public health, including increasing distribution and abundance of insect vectors, and deaths, injuries, and social disruptions due to weather-related disasters, such as severe heat waves, hurricanes, severe rain storms, floods, and mud slides attributable to climate change. See also GLOBAL CLIMATE CHANGE.

climate models Estimates or predictions of future climates, usually presented as a set of SCENARIOS in the form of graphs showing the range of predicted temperatures and color-coded maps displaying predicted precipitation and sometimes related features such as vegetation cover and distribution of insect vectors. Climate models display data derived from mathematical models that demonstrate variations in temperature, precipitation, etc., under the range of conditions expected to occur with varying levels of greenhouse gas accumulation and temperature change, impedance of solar radiation, and many other variables. There are wide margins of error, but all modeling methods yield results with a high degree of consistency, and all indicate that the earth has entered a period of warming trends and climatic instability.

climatic zone A geographically defined region in all parts of which the climate is similar.

cline A graded series of characteristics, observed in species from microbes to mankind. The characteristics of the human cline include varying skin pigmentation, facial bone structure, etc.

clinic Etymologically, "clinical" from the Greek *klinikos*, means bedridden, but in modern usage the word "clinic" refers to a setting in which physicians or other health professionals attend to sick (and healthy) people who are not confined to bed. The setting may be within or appended to a hospital, a free-standing institution with a full range of diagnostic and therapeutic facilities, a corner store, a modest one- or two-room structure with a waiting area and a treatment area, or, in a low-income country, war zone, or refugee community, a hut, tent, or meeting point under a tree in the open air.

clinical data set The information about a patient, comprising medical history, physical examination, laboratory and radiological findings, records of treatment regimens, progress, etc.

clinical decision analysis Logical consideration of available treatment options, possible outcomes, and the desirability of each possible outcome. See DECISION ANALYSIS.

clinical ecology A variety of alternative or fringe medical practice that originated in the late 20th century, based on belief in MULTIPLE CHEMICAL SENSITIVITIES as the underlying cause of several intractable ailments such as CHRONIC FATIGUE SYNDROME.

clinical epidemiology Use of epidemiological methods in a clinical setting with patients as the subjects of study. Examples include some CASE CONTROL STUDIES, CLINICAL DECISION ANALYSIS, and CLINICAL TRIALS. Except in COHORT STUDIES, there is seldom a denominator for calculating rates, i.e., a "population at risk." Instead, most inferences from clinical epidemiology are derived from comparisons of population groups, preferably similar in as many respects as possible other than exposure to the factor under investigation. Clinical epidemiologists prefer valid diagnoses in small finite populations rather than broad diagnostic categories or the syndromic approach often used in epidemiological studies of large populations and prefer to use BAYESIAN INFERENCES for analysis.

clinical practice guidelines Patient care protocols, preferably evidence based, that have been established by experts and may be required for accreditation, reimbursement of expenses, etc., by administrators, for example of a HEALTH MAINTENANCE ORGANIZATION.

clinical preventive medicine A method of medical practice that concentrates on opportunistic case-finding, presymptomatic SCREENING, HEALTH RISK APPRAISAL, and strategic and tactical interventions, such as IMMUNIZATION programs, health-promotion strategies such as smoking cessation programs and dietary and exercise regimens, all aimed at promoting good health and preventing disease, and on detecting and correcting departures from good health before these cause irreversible harm. It may be combined with a HEALTH PROMOTION program at the community level. See PREVENTIVE SERVICES TASK FORCE.

clinical preventive services guidelines A summary of current understanding of the efficacy of interventions intended to promote good health and/or prevent disease and injury, set out in the *Clinician's Handbook of Preventive Services* as part of an initiative of the US OFFICE OF DISEASE PREVENTION AND HEALTH PROMOTION known as "Put Prevention into Practice." The work of the PREVENTIVE SERVICES TASK FORCE is now directed by the Agency for Healthcare Research and Quality; details are available at http://odphp.osophs.dhhs.gov/pubs/guidecps/.

clinical trial An EXPERIMENT in which the efficacy and/or safety of preventive, diagnostic, or therapeutic drugs, devices, etc., are studied, usually by giving carefully recorded quantities to each of two or more groups of patients or healthy people who have preferably been randomly allocated to these groups. In a PHASE I CLINICAL TRIAL the aim is to determine the mode of action and safety of a medication. In a PHASE II CLINICAL TRIAL, efficacy of a trial medication is compared to that of a placebo or previously existing medication in a small number of patients who are randomly allocated to receive the test medication or placebo or previously existing medication. A PHASE III CLINICAL TRIAL is a larger trial or trials, often in several clinics or hospitals (multicenter trial) aimed at complete assessment of safety and efficacy.

clinician A physician or other health professional person who treats patients.

clinimetrics The domain of clinical science concerned with rating scales and methods of measuring aspects of physiological and pathological processes. The term was coined by the American epidemiologist Alvan Feinstein (1929–2001).

clone An organism produced by asexual reproduction of cells derived from a previous generation and not from fusion of GAMETES to form a ZYGOTE. Advances in biology have enabled cloning of mammals, such as sheep, pigs, etc. Theoretically, it is possible to clone humans, but there are profound ethical and philosophical objections to this.

clonorchiasis Infection with the Chinese liver fluke *Clonorchis sinensis*, which passes an earlier phase of its life cycle in fish and infects humans who eat inadequately cooked fish.

closed population A population that gains no new members and loses members only to death. It is usually a population of known size.

cluster A collection of events such as new cases of an uncommon or rare disease that occur so closely together in space and/or time as to arouse suspicion that this is not a chance occurrence but has a cause that should be investigated. Epidemiologists and statisticians seek to distinguish between a chance cluster and an epidemic, for instance clusters of uncommon or rare childhood malignancies that may be associated with environmental contamination by carcinogenic chemicals or radioactive waste products from nuclear power plants.

cluster analysis A set of mathematical and statistical procedures that are used to calculate the probability that a presumed cluster of cases is an epidemic, not a random event. The analysis is usually combined with clinical and environmental observations, perhaps aided by experience and intuition to arrive at a decision whether the cluster is an epidemic or a series of random events. It may be a difficult judgment call to distinguish a series of random events from a cluster of events with an identifiable cause.

cluster sampling The use of random sampling methods to select clusters, for example of districts, counties, or households, from a UNIVERSE of all districts, counties, or households that are available for study.

coagulation 1. The process by which bleeding is arrested as a result of physical and biological changes in the composition of circulating blood, with production of insoluble fibrin from fibrinogen, mediated by prothrombin and calcium ions. 2. Aggregation and molecular changes in suspended protein particles as in clotting of milk under the influence of bacterial fermentation.

coal A FOSSIL FUEL, coal is the end product of fossilization of dead vegetable matter. Hard black ANTHRACITE occurs in strata dating back several hundred million years and is mined mostly at depths that have been subjected to pressure of overlying strata and have been compressed, hardened, and dehydrated. Softer brown coal often occurs nearer ground level. Peat is the same material but is younger and not yet fossilized. Coke is coal that has been heated to extract coal gas. The efficiency of these carbon-based fuels is related to their density. Coal was the fuel of the industrial revolution and the underlying cause of many public health problems. Inhaled coal dust causes BLACK LUNG, combustion of coal produces emissions containing toxic ingredients, notably CARBON MONOXIDE, SULFUR DIOXIDE (contaminating sulfur compounds), POLYAROMATIC HYDROCARBONS, including BENZO-α-PYRENE and smaller amounts of LEAD, MERCURY, CADMIUM, and sometimes other toxic substances. The emissions are responsible for considerable SMOG. The sulfur dioxide contaminant in coal smoke combines with water vapor, rain, and fog in ACID PRECIPITATION to cause chronic bronchitis, which is a major public health problem in many coal-burning regions.

coal dust Particles of coal, including atmospheric suspended particles, some of which are small enough to be inhaled (i.e., 10 microns or less) and thus capable of causing BLACK LUNG.

coal gas A fuel produced by distilling coal at high temperatures to extract its gaseous content, consisting of carbon monoxide, hydrogen, and methane in varying concentrations, depending on the quality of coal used to produce it. Coal gas was used widely as a domestic fuel, but it was dangerous, mainly because of the risk of carbon monoxide poisoning, a popular mode of suicide. It has been mostly superseded by NATURAL GAS, i.e. gaseous hydrocarbons, mainly methane.

coal mining One of the principal forms of underground mining, particularly hazardous because coal often occurs in friable strata or seams that collapse under pressure, causing cave-ins that crush trapped workers. Suspended coal dust is flammable, sometimes explosively so, as is methane (known to miners as FIREDAMP). Coal mine disasters are widespread and perennial problems.

coal smoke Emissions from combusted coal, a mixture of several toxic gaseous components and solid particulate matter. Its components include sulfur dioxide, carbonized particles, oily aerosols, and trace amounts of toxic metals such as lead and mercury. Emissions from combusted coal cause air pollution, which has chronic adverse effects on health, and occasional episodes of severe SMOG, with acute effects including an upsurge of deaths from respiratory and cardiac failure, as in Donora, Pennsylvania, in 1948, and London, England, in 1952.

coal tar A sticky black viscous liquid that sometimes occurs naturally or is produced by heating coal. It is used to seal dust on road surfaces, roofing, etc. It and the fumes it emanates when heated contain carcinogens, such as BENZO-α-PYRENE.

coal worker's pneumoconiosis Syn: anthracosis. The common dust disease of coal miners, also called BLACK LUNG, often combined with silicosis if the coal seams are mixed with rock that has to be removed by blasting. In the past, this was very common in all coal mining communities. Its prevalence has been reduced by improved methods of clearing coal dust from the air in mines.

cobalamine The active protein ingredient of vitamin B_{12}. This is essential for rapid cell division, as in production of red blood corpuscles, so deficiency causes pernicious anemia. It occurs only in foods of animal origin, that is, meat, eggs, and milk, so VEGANS can become cobalamine deficient.

Cobalt (Co) A white metallic element combined with iron to make hardened cutting tools and to strengthen magnets. Cobalt is an essential mineral, required for certain enzyme systems, but excessive intake causes cardiomyopathy and interferes with thyroxin production.

cocaine An alkaloid derived from coca leaves, native to the Andes region of South America, where it was a pre-Columbian folk remedy and mood modifying agent. It is the basis for useful local anesthetic agents, but cocaine is a strong central nervous system stimulant and narcotic with mood-modifying qualities. In the early and middle 20th century, it was fashionable among the urban intelligentsia to sniff cocaine, but from about the 1960s, its powerful addictive properties made it a widely used illicit drug, produced in industrial quantities and shipped by criminal gangs to local suppliers and pushers of illicit drug use elsewhere in the world. It is used in several forms, including inhaled powder, combusted smoked cocaine, and, most dangerous, intravenous injection. Sharing needles is part of the culture of intravenous cocaine use, and this has been a major vehicle for transmission of HIV, hepatitis B, and other blood-borne diseases. However, cocaine is much less addictive than nicotine, and despite the association with crime, prostitution, and social degradation, many former addicts are able to break the habit and resume normal life without apparent permanent harm.

coccidioidomycosis An infectious mycotic (fungus) infection of the lungs, occurring mainly in arid desert regions such as Mexico and the southwestern United States. It is relatively uncommon, indolent, debilitating, sometimes subclinical, and a possible, although unlikely, agent in biological warfare.

coccus (Plural: cocci) General name for several genera of spherical bacteria. Those that form clumps include staphylococci, and those that form chains include streptococci.

Cochrane, Archibald Leman (1909–1988) British physician and epidemiologist best known for his work on evaluation of drug treatment for tuberculosis by using randomized controlled trials. In fact, his work on critical evaluation of clinical medicine in studies of observer variation, and on the efficacy, efficiency, and effectiveness of all aspects of health care covered a much wider range than randomized controlled trials.

Cochrane collaboration A network of clinical epidemiologists and others in many countries that collects and distributes results of studies of all varieties of health care interventions, to encourage EVIDENCE-BASED MEDICINE. It emphasizes SYSTEMATIC REVIEWS and META-ANALYSES dealing with therapeutic interventions and publishes the findings on its Web site (http://www.cochrane.org.) and in print journals. The name commemorates the British epidemiologist A. L. (Archie) Cochrane.

Cochrane review group A group of clinicians and others who purposefully gather information about specified clinical problems by conducting CLINICAL TRIALS, META-ANALYSES, and other studies of trials, then disseminating the findings, usually by immediate electronic communication on a WEB SITE. See http://www.cochrane.org.

cockroach Various species of a hardy common household insect pest, regarded as verminous, associated with unclean dilapidated conditions. Despite the dislike they evoke, cockroaches have never been unequivocally identified as vectors of any specific disease, although they play a role in mechanical transmission of some intestinal infections. The health risks from cockroaches may be little, if any, greater than those from insecticides, fumigants, and other heavy-handed but usually unsuccessful endeavors to eradicate them. Cockroaches are an evolutionary success, having survived unchanged through all the environmental climatic changes of the past 100 million years and may still infest the earth after humans become extinct.

code 1. A numerical and/or alphabetical system for organizing and classifying information and data. 2. A formal statement of acceptable ways for members of a defined professional group to behave, i.e., a CODE OF CONDUCT. 3. A method of encrypting to conceal information.

code of conduct A formal statement agreed to by constituent members of an organization that sets out what they may do and must not do, often specifying sanctions for noncompliance. See also ETHICS. An example is the code of conduct for the ethical practice of public health that has been developed by the American Public Health Association. This can be seen at http://www.apha.org/codeofethics/ethics.htm.

codependency A situation in which two or more individuals or groups are mutually dependent and supportive. The relationship may be inherently unhealthy, e.g., when a family member provides a supply of alcohol to a parent or spouse who is an alcoholic.

coding The process of sorting entities such as disease diagnoses into categories and assigning a predesignated number or other identifying symbol to each.

codon The group of three bases found in amino acids, the basic building blocks of chromosomes.

coefficient Strictly speaking, a multiplier; in statistics, a modifier of a numerical entity.

coercive power See POLICE POWER.

coffee A drink brewed from pulverized or finely ground coffee beans according to one of several methods that have become stylized, even ritualized, in the settings where coffee drinking is part of the culture. The mystique of coffee consumption comes from behavior associated with the way it is brewed, the social setting, and the quest for a brew that tastes as pleasing as the aroma promises. The CAFFEINE alkaloid is a stimulant, but decaffeinated coffee provides the pleasures of the social setting and aroma for those apprehensive about the alleged adverse cardiovascular and other effects of coffee. Epidemiological studies provide equivocal evidence of statistically significant associations between coffee drinking, cancer of the bladder, and coronary heart disease, but few serious coffee drinkers have changed their habits in response.

cognitive dissonance Disconnect between the evidence of a person's senses and what the person believes, or between a person's beliefs and what that person says and does, often arising after an action that is inconsistent with beliefs and leading to rationalization, sometimes to changing beliefs or taking corrective action.

cognitive domain In the taxonomy of educational theory, this is the set of intellectual processes responsible for assembling and recalling facts, arranging them in logical order, and deriving a rational conclusion from their synthesis and analysis.

coherence In the logical assembly of evidence, coherence is the quality of evidence that fits most neatly with other facts and existing theories about the situation under investigation. It is an important criterion but must be factored into the totality with caution because occasionally a discordant observation is the first solid evidence leading to REFUTATION of an established belief.

cohort The population group born in a particular period, generally a year or a decade, i.e., a birth cohort. By extension, any defined group that is followed up over time, e.g., in order to discern the incidence and outcome of conditions such as cancer in relation to prior exposures.

cohort study A method of epidemiological study that begins with a hypothesis about the relationship between exposure to specified risks and the occurrence of eventual outcomes, conducted by following up over a long period a group of persons with varying levels of exposure, to determine the outcome in relation to initial and perhaps ongoing exposure after a defined period, usually measured in years or even decades. This method is superior to CASE CONTROL STUDY because it is less susceptible to several kinds of BIAS and CONFOUNDING and can yield more precise estimates of risks. It has provided some of the best available, sometimes the only good evidence, on causal relationships of environmental, occupational, and behavioral risks of coronary heart disease and many varieties of cancer, often in studies of large populations followed up for many years or decades. Examples include the FRAMINGHAM STUDY, studies of the Japanese atomic bomb survivors, and the 50-year study of the smoking habits of British doctors from 1951 to 2001 initiated by the British epidemiologists Richard Doll (1912–2005) and Austin Bradford Hill (1897–1991). It is sometimes possible to use an existing data set collected in the past about a population to investigate current health status in relation to specified past experiences, such as low birth weight, exposure to toxic substances, or diagnostic radiation. That approach is called a historical cohort study. Like other observational studies, cohort studies sometimes lead to serendipitous discoveries, but they are costly and time consuming and require dedicated professional teams to collaborate for long periods, so they are not lightly undertaken. See also PROSPECTIVE STUDY.

co-infection Occurrence of infection in combination with another disease, usually but not necessarily always another infection.

coke 1. The residue of coal that has been distilled to extract coal gas, a porous, brittle solid fuel that burns with relatively fewer emission products than does coal, either in an industrial coke oven or as a domestic fuel. 2. A slang term, now seldom used, for cocaine.

cold chain A method of protecting heat-labile sera, vaccines, antibiotics, and other biological preparations against exposure to high environmental temperatures in hot and tropical countries by preserving them in refrigerated containers until immediately before they are to be given to people in the target population. This is an essential feature of vaccination campaigns in hot regions, especially the tropics. The same methods and procedures operate in reverse to take specimens to regional laboratories.

coliform count A bacteriological test for water quality, using simple culture methods to test for contamination with coliform organisms and other common bacterial contaminants that can cause fecal-oral communicable diseases. A high coliform count is a suspicious sign of the presence of other pathogens, including viruses such as hepatitis A, transmitted by the fecal oral route.

coliform organisms The family of Enterobacteriaceae, Gram-negative motile rod-shaped bacteria, several of which inhabit the gut of many mammals, including humans, without apparent ill effects. However, several coliform organisms do cause diarrhea, and one, *ESCHERICHIA COLI* 0157:H7, causes severe bloody diarrhea and dangerous systemic upsets, including inflammatory renal disease. Some coliform organisms are enterotoxigenic and cause diseases such as TRAVELER'S DIARRHEA, which is often due to *E. coli* organisms. Others are enteroinvasive and cause more severe inflammatory disease with bloody diarrhea. Systemic infection can cause osteomyelitis and septic arthritis.

colinearity Very high correlation between variables.

collagen diseases A group of chronic diseases characterized by aberrant overgrowth of connective tissue. SILICOSIS and ASBESTOSIS are forms of collagen disease.

collective bargaining The process of negotiation between a labor union and management of the industry to which the union members belong. Usually the issues of wages and pensions preoccupy collective bargainers, but other benefits and risks may be at stake. Health risks, compensation, and payment for work-related injury and illness sometimes dominate the bargaining process.

colonization In microbiology, the process a microorganism goes through when it settles on or in a culture medium or host species where it can reproduce or grow and develop.

colonoscopy Visual examination of the mucosal surface of the colon using a flexible fiberoptic telescope introduced rectally.

colorectal cancer A common and frequently fatal cancer with genetic and environmental (dietary) determinants. Genetic tests can detect predisposition, screening for occult blood in the feces may reveal it in the early stages, and its presence is confirmed by colonoscopy and biopsy.

colostrum The precursor of breast milk that is secreted by the female breast from shortly before until some days after childbirth. It is a low-viscosity fluid rich in antibodies and rather lower in fat and carbohydrate content than breast milk.

combustion Conversion of energy stored in a fuel into heat and other combustion products. Most commonly used fuels are carbon based, and the term is sometimes restricted to this usage.

combustion chamber The chamber in a furnace where fuel is ignited and burned; in an incinerator, the place where waste products are consumed.

combustion products The material produced when carbon fuels are burned to yield energy, usually comprising emissions and ash or other residue; the emissions often contain toxic or noxious substances, including polyaromatic hydrocarbons, oxides of carbon, nitrogen, sulfur, etc., that were present as components or contaminants of the fuel.

comfort zone The range of temperature and humidity within which people generally feel at ease and without need of aids to heating or cooling. By analogy, the psychological sense of well-being experienced when in the company of others, whether at work or in social or recreational pursuits.

commensal Literally, eating together. Referring to microorganisms, those that live in or on the body without harm to themselves or their host; some commensal organisms fulfill an essential function by manufacturing substances that their host requires, such as vitamin K, one form of which is synthesized in the gut and is essential to blood clotting.

comminution Fragmentation or breaking into many parts. A term used to describe fractured bones that have broken into many fragments that is also applicable to a community or to a health care system that is fragmented by overspecialization and poor communication.

Commissioner of Health A term used in some jurisdictions, mainly US states, for the chief executive officer of a local or state public health service. This individual is usually, but not always, a physician with specialist qualifications, i.e., board certification in preventive medicine.

Commission on Macroeconomics and Health A WHO-sponsored commission that investigated and made recommendations in 2001 focusing on the relationship between health improvement and economic development. Its recommendations led to the establishment of the global fund to fight AIDS, tuberculosis, and malaria. It also considered the effect of globalized economics on the health status of people in low- and middle-income nations and on the importance of poverty reduction for economic growth and social betterment. See http://www.cmhealth.org/ for details.

Commission on Professional and Hospital Activities A nonprofit American organization founded in Ann Arbor, Michigan, in 1955, to conduct evaluations of the quality of hospital care, using statistical analyses of aspects of patient care, such as length of hospital stay, investigations and treatment regimens, and outcomes of care. Its best known analytic method is the PROFESSIONAL ACTIVITY STUDY, which was conducted in hospitals in the United States, Canada, and several other countries for more than 40 years until being supplanted by computer-based record systems and was one of the standards used to establish CLINICAL PRACTICE GUIDELINES.

common cold Syn: coryza. A very common and highly contagious upper respiratory infection caused by one of several types of viruses (coronaviruses, rhinoviruses) or by mycoplasma or chlamydia. Most people, especially children and young adults, get several colds every year because immunity is short-lived and the ubiquity of common cold viruses as well as viral mutations make infection and reinfection frequent occurrences. Because of the time lost from work due to common colds, they are a major public health problem.

common law The body of law that has become established as a feature of society in the English speaking world, based on longstanding moral values, traditions, and customs. Although there may be no explicit statement of what actually constitutes common law in a nation, it is accepted and acknowledged by judges, lawyers, and the general public. It differs from CASE LAW, which is established by legal precedent, and statute law, which is defined by explicit legislation.

common vehicle A source or potential source of infection that is common to many people, such as contaminated water or food or air laden with pathogenic organisms. Blood and blood products contaminated with HIV, hepatitis B, or other blood-borne pathogens are another example. This mode of transmission characteristically can be responsible for very high attack rates among those who are susceptible to varieties of communicable disease transmitted by common vehicles.

commune A group of people living together in a mutually supportive way; in modern usage, often a group adhering to an alternative or unconventional life style. Such groups sometimes have unconventional approaches to health and health care.

communicable disease Syn: infectious disease, contagious disease. A disease caused by a specific pathogenic agent or its toxic products, arising as a consequence of transmission to a susceptible host of the agent or its toxic products by or from an infected person, animal, or other reservoir. Transmission may be direct person to person; indirect via contaminated food, water, domestic utensils, clothing, etc.; via an insect or animal vector; or directly from the inanimate environment. The words "communicable" and "infectious" are used interchangeably, but the word "contagious" implies direct contact and usually a disease that is more infectious and more serious.

communicable disease control The public health and/or personal preventive measures used to identify the cause, source, and mode of spread of a communicable disease, and the measures adopted to prevent or limit the spread and mitigate or prevent the consequences of infection. The aim is to identify and delineate outbreaks by SURVEILLANCE, to destroy the pathogenic organism or its capacity to invade a human host and cause disease. This can be accomplished by isolating infectious cases, quarantining contacts, disinfecting or erecting a barrier against sources of infection, treating infectious cases to render them noninfectious, and vaccinating or immunizing persons and populations to protect them against infection with specific pathogens.

communication The process by which knowledge, ideas, beliefs, techniques, and methods are transmitted among individuals by word of mouth, printed media, electronic means, etc.

communication network The population of individuals, ranging in size and complexity from a neighborhood to a nation, who are in touch with one another by word of mouth, or other means such as electronic communication. Many people have multiple communication networks of family members, colleagues from work, social, religious, and sporting activities, etc. In the age of the Internet, some communication networks are quite literally worldwide.

communication skills Capacity to speak intelligibly and with clarity, to write and read well, and, just as important, to be a good listener. An essential skill for public health specialists.

community A group of people, e.g., a neighborhood, village, or municipal or rural region or a social group with a unifying common interest or trait, loosely organized into a recognizable unit; a vague but useful term. There is often a sense of belonging, mutual self-interest, and perhaps activism that may lead to collective community action on issues and problems of concern. Elected or otherwise identifiable community leader(s) may represent, advocate on behalf of, and decide issues of importance to the community when it interacts with other groups or persons.

Community-Campus Partnerships for Health A nonprofit organization founded in 1996 to promote population health through community-based research, in-service learning, community service, and other partnership strategies with public health specialists in universities, colleges, and local health departments. See http://www.futurehealth.ucsf.edu/ccph.html.

community care Care of health and social needs that takes place outside of, often away from, and often unconnected with institutionally based care.

community development The process of solving the environmental, economic, social, and public health problems of a community. This is often achieved by teamwork in a multisectoral approach that can also enhance the cohesiveness, self-motivation, vitality, and viability of a community. This has worked well in many settings in low- and middle-income nations. See also HUMAN DEVELOPMENT.

community diagnosis A term coined by the British public health scientist J. N. (Jerry) Morris (b. 1911) to describe the summarized health and social statistics of a defined community, whether it be a nation or a social group within the nation.

community health Although often equated with PUBLIC HEALTH, this term has a more precise meaning when used by specialists in HEALTH PROMOTION and education to describe the desired outcome of their professional activities, i.e., a community in which there are no pervasive health problems, unsatisfactory housing, systemic poverty, unemployment, or other social pathology.

community health center A set of offices for interviews, physical examinations, laboratory tests, and ambulatory treatment used by physicians, nurses, social workers, etc., collectively referred to as community health workers, who attempt to meet the medical, other health-related, and social needs of the people in a community. Users of a community health center may be defined by their enrollment as patients or clients, or they may simply drop in to use the center when the need arises. A crucial requirement for professional staff is teamwork, effective communication among all, collaboration, and avoidance of actions that can impair or erode professional relationships.

community leader An individual identified by community members, perhaps elected by them, who influences them and is recognized by them as their spokesperson and/or advocate. Health promotion programs work best if community leaders are mobilized and active partners.

community medicine The study of health and disease in a community that is considered as an entity, and the provision and evaluation of the health services of that community. One of several terms that came into vogue because of dissatisfaction with the alleged political or emotional associations of the traditional term PUBLIC HEALTH and alternatives such as SOCIAL MEDICINE. In some countries, notably Australia, the term is equated with general or family medical practice, and for this reason it fell from favor among specialists academically trained in community medicine.

community oriented primary care (COPC) A strategic approach to primary health care based on an inventory of health care needs and systematic, coordinated management of identified health problems by members of a primary health care team comprising physicians, nurses, and other health professionals.

Community Preventive Services Guidelines A summary of what is known about the efficacy of population-based interventions intended to prevent or control public health problems, developed by the PREVENTIVE SERVICES TASK FORCE of the US CENTERS FOR DISEASE CONTROL AND PREVENTION, using the same approach as the CLINICAL PREVENTIVE SERVICES GUIDELINES. See http://www.thecommunityguide.org for more information on the effectiveness of interventions that can be applied by public health agencies and others.

community resources The range of economic assets, physical facilities, buildings, plant and equipment, and the human resources, that is, the community health workers who work in and from these physical facilities and are available to meet community health and social needs.

compaction system A method of disposing of garbage and industrial waste that involves compression of the waste matter into as small a volume as possible, using a compactor, a device that applies pressure to loosely stacked or packed material to force it into a smaller volume. Often this involves extrusion of liquid content, which can include a source of infection or toxic effluent that endangers health if it enters aquifers or is widely dispersed in the environment.

comparison group The group with which study subjects are compared, a control group. A vague term that is preferably avoided.

competencies, public health See PUBLIC HEALTH COMPETENCIES.

competing risk An event that removes a study subject from experiencing the outcome that is under investigation. For instance, in a study of smoking in relation to lung cancer, death of coronary heart disease or in a traffic crash is a competing risk.

complement A heat-sensitive ingredient of serum comprising some 20 or more proteins that either has some properties of antibody or is a vehicle for antibody.

complement fixation tests A general name for serological tests that "fix" or inactivate serum complement. The WASSERMAN REACTION for syphilis is an example.

complementary and alternative medicine A general term for a wide range of health care systems and processes outside the range of conventional or orthodox allopathic medicine. These include OSTEOPATHY, CHIROPRACTIC, herbal medicine, hypnotherapy, FAITH HEALING, and many others. Some popular herbal and other remedies used in these systems have been integral to traditional medicine for centuries, and these have been studied, evaluated, their active ingredients identified and refined, and in some cases patented by pharmaceutical corporations.

completed fertility rate The cumulative fertility rate in a cohort of women who have passed the end of their reproductive life, i.e., the total number of births per 1,000 to women aged 49 years and older in a specified population.

complexity theory A conceptual framework that departs from the REDUCTIONISM of scientific thinking by acknowledging that some of the most pressing and difficult problems facing humans early in the 21st century cannot be tackled, let alone solved, by adopting a conventional approach. Problems associated with increasing urbanization, global environmental change, prevention of violent armed conflicts, and the multiple pathological conditions of individuals and populations in an aging society are examples that fall within the realm of complexity theory. These and other complex problems transcend the boundaries of traditional scientific disciplines and can best be approached rationally by a team comprising scientists and technicians from many fields or by persons who are professionally trained in multiple disciplines. See also TRANSDISCIPLINARITY.

compliance Abiding by the advice or instructions of a health professional. Many behavioral scientists prefer to allude to ADHERENCE and suggest that "compliance" is a pejorative word, implying coercion.

compost Decomposed or decomposing stable organic matter such as vegetable kitchen waste, garden residue, that is in the advanced stages of the degradation and destruction of its structure from its original live form. Compost is used to enrich soil for agriculture, etc. It can harbor pathogens such as spores of tetanus and botulism.

composting toilet A toilet capable of converting human feces into compost that can be used as fertilizer. To be effective and esthetically acceptable fecal odors must be minimized and the residue must be reasonably dry, free of fecal pathogens, and safe to handle. This is accomplished by decomposition that relies on actinomycetes, molds, and aerobic bacteria that can be refreshed occasionally

with small quantities of vegetable waste. A composting toilet does not require a water supply or connection to reticulated sewerage or a septic tank. In arid regions or those not connected to a sewerage service, it is a useful alternative method. For more information, see http://www .compostingtoilet.org/.

computed axial tomography The first of the modern diagnostic imaging techniques, computed axial tomography (CAT) scanning uses serial radiographs to generate a sequence of images resembling slices through the body to reveal its inner normal and diseased features. See also NUCLEAR MAGNETIC RESONANCE IMAGING (NMRI).

concentrate (n.) Matter that has been reduced in bulk by a process called concentration; a liquid that has been treated, e.g., by heat or osmosis, to produce a strong solution; a mineral ore from which as much as possible of the extraneous matter has been removed mechanically or by preliminary smelting, leaving a residue known as "tailings."

conceptual framework A statement of theoretical principles to guide logical and systematic development of a research design, a specific policy, or an approach to problem solving. It is sometimes called a statement of principles, and is widely used in social and behavioral sciences.

concordance Agreement, harmony, being of like mind, thus pairs or other groups of people of identical phenotype, e.g., identical twins.

condemned premises A residential or public building that has been declared unfit for human use or occupancy on the basis of health and/or safety criteria after official inspection. Local public health authorities usually are responsible for deciding whether premises should be condemned, and in most jurisdictions they have an obligation to specify the reason. This may be inadequacy of facilities for preparing and cooking meals, unsanitary toilets, overcrowding, lack of ventilation, a combination of factors, or fire hazard, which may be a decision made by the fire marshal, often in collaboration with public health authorities.

condom A contraceptive sheath that fits over the erect penis and prevents ejaculated semen from reaching the uterus and fertilizing the ovum. Thus, it is a BARRIER CONTRACEPTIVE. It is also a protective measure against sexually transmitted diseases. Condoms have a long history dating back to the Romans. In the past they were fashioned from sheep's intestines, canvas, oilskin, and various other materials, few of which could have helped to enhance the pleasure of sexual congress and many of which were not very effective. Today condoms are made of fine latex or plastic, which is an effective barrier to spermatozoa and the pathogens responsible for most sexually transmitted diseases yet does not excessively deaden the senses; some are textured and even flavored. See also FEMALE CONDOM.

confidence interval The range within which the true value of a variable such as a mean, proportion, or rate lies, with a probability that can be calculated using statistical methods. The end points of the confidence interval are the confidence limits. Confidence intervals indicate how precisely the results of an analysis based on a particular population sample approach the true value of proportions, rates, etc., in that sample.

confidentiality The process of and obligation to keep a transaction, documents, etc., private and secret, i.e., confidential; the right to withhold information, e.g.. medical information, from others.

conflict of interest The situation that arises when the objectivity and impartiality of a person's decision making are compromised by the prospect of perceived benefit or harm that the person could or might experience as a consequence of that decision. Conflicts of interest present a frequent, even pervasive, problem in some aspects of modern medical practice and public health, for instance when prospects of commercial gain compromise the objectivity of clinical trials of innovative pharmaceutical preparations. Ethics committees require that conflicts of interest be declared, but merely declaring a conflict of interest does not make the conflict disappear or absolve anyone from the duty to conduct all public affairs impartially.

confounding Distortion of an apparent effect by the operation on that effect of factors whose individual effects cannot be separated. There are several varieties. 1. A situation in which the effects of two or more processes such as the influence on outcome of causal and noncausal factors are not or cannot be separated. Distortion of the apparent effect of an exposure on risk brought about by the association with other factors that can influence the outcome. 2. A relationship between the effects of two or more causal factors that it is logically impossible to dissect into the effect of any one factor. 3. A situation in which a measure of the effect of an exposure on risk is distorted by the association of exposure with other factor(s) that influence the outcome. Confounding is often a troublesome problem in observational CASE CONTROL STUDIES and nonrandomized CLINICAL TRIALS because it is difficult to identify all possible confounding variables.

congenital anomaly An abnormal condition present at or before birth, although not always detected (e.g., congenital blindness, deafness). It is usually attributable to genetic or chromosomal abnormality, sometimes attributable to an infection (e.g., the rubella virus) or an environmental toxin. However, the cause of most birth defects remains unknown. See also BIRTH DEFECT.

conjunctivitis Inflammation of the mucosal epithelium of the eyes, caused by infection, chemical irritants, or ultraviolet or infrared radiation.

consanguinity A close blood (genetic) relationship that can have adverse implications, such as occurrence of birth defects, but may be beneficial if desirable genetic traits are enhanced.

consensus conference A meeting, often a committee, of a group of experts whose aim is to review all available evidence on an issue or problem of concern, for instance the most effective way to treat cancers of specific site and type, and, using CONSENSUS DEVELOPMENT, to reach agreement that can be set out in a formal statement such as a screening or a treatment protocol. The method is used frequently in the United Kingdom and the European Union and by the US National Institutes of Health.

consensus development A process of achieving agreement among members of a group of experts about issues or problems for which a range of possible solutions exists. Two common procedures for this are the CONSENSUS CONFERENCE and the DELPHI METHOD.

CONSORT An acronym meaning consolidated standards for reporting of trials, an initiative of the International Committee of Medical Journal Editors to ensure consistency and quality of the conduct of clinical trials by requiring conformity to a predetermined protocol, consistent use of methods, procedures, participant assignment, masking (blinding) procedures, data analysis, etc. Details and the consort statement are at http://www.consort-statement.org/.

constant An entity often designated n, or k, that remains the same under all circumstances, such as the speed of light and other forms of electromagnetic radiation.

construct (n.) A term used in behavioral sciences to describe a conceptual framework or theory, often called a social construct, based on observations, empirically verifiable facts or events.

construct validity The extent to which an experiment, laboratory test, or set of measurements conforms to or correlates with the underlying theoretical concepts in the field of scholarly activity to which the work in question belongs. See also VALIDITY.

consultation A formal review by expert(s), by definition specialist(s) in the relevant discipline(s) of the status of a patient, a preventive or therapeutic service, or a program. In UK usage, a term for a referral from one doctor to another, usually a specialist, who is called a consultant. A request for expert advice is usually explicit.

Consumer Product Safety Commission The US federal agency responsible for assessing the safety of products such as domestic appliances purveyed on the American market. For details, programs, activities, see http://www.cpsc.gov/.

contact A way that infection is transmitted, describing both the mode and the person from whom the infection is transmitted. Direct contact means transmission from an infected to a susceptible host; indirect contact is transmission via FOMITES or a VECTOR; a primary contact is a person in direct contact with someone harboring an infectious disease; a secondary contact is a person in contact with a primary contact.

contact dermatitis Inflammatory disease of the skin, often chronic, caused by skin contact with an irritant agent encountered in the workplace or the home. Homemakers are frequent victims, affected by exposure to household cleaning agents and other toxic agents.

contact tracing The method of epidemic investigation that is concerned with locating the source of an infection, such as a SEXUALLY TRANSMITTED DISEASE. It uses whatever means are most suitable in the circumstances, often painstaking field work known as SHOE-LEATHER EPIDEMIOLOGY. The most challenging aspect of this work, requiring considerable patience and tact, is tracing contacts of sexually transmitted diseases, usually done by public health nurses.

contagion Transmission of infection by direct contact. In common usage and in public health, "contagious" implies a condition that is highly infectious and usually severe, although one of the most contagious diseases, the common cold, is seldom severe. "Contagion" can be stigmatizing when it is emotionally associated with a distasteful disease, such as leprosy, or with what used to be called venereal diseases, so "contagion" can imply a condition that is unclean or immoral. In *De Contagione* (1546) Girolamo Fracastorius (1484–1553) identified three modes of contagion: direct contact, droplet spread, and via contaminated clothing,

domestic utensils, etc. Other modes of spread are by COMMON VEHICLE spread in infected or contaminated water, food, or air, and vector-borne transmission, but the etymology of contagion, from the Latin *con* (together) *tangere* (to touch) implies intimate contact, so purists prefer to restrict use of the word to communicable diseases transmitted by direct person-to-person contact.

containment The process of preventing the spread of a transmissible infectious disease by limiting the movements of cases and close contacts ("voluntary quarantine") or, as in the smallpox eradication campaign, by vaccinating all contacts of every diagnosed case, which prevented transmission of smallpox from cases to contacts. This tactical approach to smallpox control, suggested by the American epidemiologist Donald Soper (1894–1977) in 1949, was successfully used in the WHO smallpox eradication campaign. Another form of containment is "ring prophylaxis," in which transmission of an epidemic infectious disease spread by person-to-person contact, such as severe acute respiratory syndrome (SARS) or acute influenza A, is halted by prophylactic antiviral treatment of cases and immediate contacts.

contaminant An impurity or undesirable substance that occurs as an ingredient of a useful gaseous, liquid, or solid substance.

contamination 1. The presence of an infectious or noxious agent such as a toxic chemical on or in the body, clothing, utensils, food, water, etc. The presence of matter that is offensive but not infectious is described as POLLUTION rather than contamination. 2. In epidemiology, the situation that arises when a population being studied for one condition possesses characteristics of another, different condition.

contempt of court A serious misdemeanor punishable by fine or imprisonment for disrespect of a directive issued by the presiding official in a court of law, usually a judge. In public health law, it is an effective sanction that can be invoked when, for instance, a factory's management defies an order to cease and desist from polluting the environment.

content analysis The systematic quantitative and qualitative examination of information gathered by pictorial and verbal methods in order to assess a situation such as the prevailing social values of a community.

content validity In the terminology of survey methods, content validity is the extent to which the test items, e.g., questions, opinion statements offered to participants in a survey, are representative of the domain or topic that is the target of the survey.

contingency table A table that arranges sets of data in columns and rows so that relationships between the sets can be studied by means of suitable statistical tests, e.g., the chi-square test.

continuing professional education The term describing a range of designated educational activities that members of health professions such as medicine and nursing are expected and in many jurisdictions required to undertake in order to maintain professional competence. In many specialties, including preventive medicine, this is a requirement for maintaining certification in the specialty.

contraception A general term for methods to prevent pregnancy. BARRIER CONTRACEPTIVES impose an impervious material, usually a condom or cervical diaphragm, between the ejaculate containing the sperm and the uterus and fallopian tubes through which the ovum must pass. Chemical methods use spermicidal jelly or foam, intrauterine devices maintain a constant irritant action on the epithelial surface of the uterus that prevents the fertilized ovum from implanting; hormonal methods, such as the oral contraceptive pill, inhibit ovulation; the RHYTHM METHOD relies on the fact that during the menstrual cycle there is a so-called safe period during which there is only a low probability of the sperm surviving long enough to fertilize the ovum; abstinence relies on not having sexual intercourse. The rhythm method is unreliable, and abstinence is unrealistic. See also BIRTH CONTROL and FAMILY PLANNING.

contraceptive An agent that prevents conception. This may be a mechanical barrier, i.e., a condom, cervical cap, or diaphragm; vaginal foam or jelly (usually spermicidal); intrauterine device; or contraceptive pill.

contraceptive implant Silicone rods trade named Norplant containing progesterone, implanted subcutaneously in a group of six with timed release so progesterone enters the bloodstream continuously for a period of as long as 5 years, providing effective contraception during this period. This is a valuable contraceptive method for nonliterate women in low-income countries.

contraceptive pill Syn: the pill. A compound comprising the steroid hormones estrogen and progesterone, or progesterone alone, which acts by inhibiting ovulation, that has been licensed for use in the United States and most other nations since 1960, after preliminary trials in Puerto Rico. Some variations include the MORNING-AFTER (plan B) PILL and contraceptive implants.

contract A legally binding agreement between parties, customarily a written document that has been signed by the parties to the agreement, and preferably witnessed.

control 1. (n. and v.) Procedures or methods used in a program aimed at achieving a particular goal, such as infection control, pest control. 2. (n. and adj.) Person or persons whose characteristics are used for comparison purposes with a person or persons being studied, as in a case control study or a clinical trial 3. (v.) To regulate, adjust. This word is frequently used, sometimes overused, in many aspects of public health and epidemiology. Its meaning is usually clear from the context.

controlled substance A medication, usually a pharmaceutical preparation, that is subject to strict regulation of prescribing and is not available to the general public in over-the-counter sales.

conurbation An aggregation of urban regions in which several cities are contiguous with one another without intervening rural regions.

convection Carriage of heat energy by movement of a current of water or air.

convenience food A general term for prepared, prepackaged food items, e.g., dehydrated soup packets, cold meat cuts, potted spreads and salads, tinned fruit, ice cream, etc. They are often hygienically prepared in a factory, and by law in many jurisdictions they are required to list all ingredients, including food additives, preservatives, and sometimes calorific content. Their nutritional value varies but is generally good to adequate. See also FAST FOOD, JUNK FOOD.

convenience sample Syn: grab sample. A sample, usually of people, that has been collected by expedient means, such as that they happen to be available for study, not by using a random sampling method. Inferences and conclusions from analysis of data collected in a convenience sample have no scientific validity because there is no way to ensure that the sample is unbiased.

convention 1. A formal gathering of people such as members of professional organizations or people who have a shared concern about a set of issues such as the health of the population. Also a formal statement about matters of importance produced at such a gathering by those assembled, e.g., the United Nations Convention on Human Rights, which drafted the Universal Declaration on Human Rights. 2. A mutually agreed or commonly accepted mode of behavior, dress, speech, etc., from which deviance usually evokes disapproval and occasionally stronger sanctions, such as denial of access to services otherwise available.

coping strategy A system that individuals or groups have worked out to deal with a social and/or emotional situation that would otherwise be intolerable. An example is a woman married to a man who is violently abusive and has chronic alcoholism who may deal with the situation by ensuring that he always has a supply of alcohol readily available.

copper A soft, red metal that conducts electricity; copper, in alloys with tin to make brass and bronze, was one of the first metals used in early civilizations. It is an essential trace element in several enzyme systems and has many compounds of commercial and industrial importance, e.g., copper sulfate is a wood preservative, a fungicide, and used in electroplating. An autosomal recessive disorder of copper metabolism causes hepatolenticular degeneration, a neuropsychiatric condition with involuntary movements and mental deterioration.

copyright The legal protection conferred on inventions, creative works, intellectual property, etc., by official government agencies in many nations when an individual, group, organization, corporation, etc., declares the right to ownership of the copyright article. The legal protection is accompanied by the right to claim royalties when the copyright article is used by others. This can become contentious, for instance when an organization claims ownership of a naturally occurring article, such as an animal resulting from selective breeding (a laboratory strain of cancer-prone mice) or a human gene associated with proneness to breast cancer. The morality and ethics of copyright for commercial gain of discoveries that benefit all humanity have been debated by philosophers and theologians, although the World Trade Organization has ruled that copyright of such discoveries is permissible. Others, including some governments, assert that no one can "own" living organisms or genetic material; they are parts of the global commons.

cordon sanitaire The defensive "barrier," such as isolation procedures, around a focus of infection. This procedure was extensively used in the late 19th and early 20th centuries in attempts to control dangerous epidemics, such as the global pandemic of influenza in 1919. Its failure in that instance contributed to its fall from favor and replacement by more rigorous CONTAINMENT methods based on better understanding of the epidemiology and characteristics of the epidemic agent, host, and environment.

core competencies A term that refers to a list of aspects of competence required by public health professionals, developed by the COUNCIL ON LINKAGES BETWEEN ACADEMIA AND PUBLIC HEALTH in collaboration with individuals and agencies in many academic and practice-based settings. The core competencies include quantitative skills, i.e., ability to compile, analyze, and interpret data about health status and disease distribution; clinical skills, i.e., ability to recognize, diagnose, and assess diseases of public health importance and other community public health problems; policy development to meet perceived needs; managerial and administrative skills, i.e., ability to direct team members, delegate tasks, provide leadership and/or work harmoniously in a team; environmental know-how, i.e., ability to recognize and deal with hazards in public places and private facilities; and familiarity with laws and regulations regarding health. Although it is not included in lists of core functions, a very important requirement for those who work in public health is political savvy. The list was collated and coordinated with the work of task forces on essential public health services and functions. Details and commentary are available at http://www.trainingfinder.org/competencies.htm.

core functions of public health The essential features of the work of specialists in public health. The 1988 Report of the US Institute of Medicine on the *Future of Public Health* categorized core functions under three headings: Assessment, Policy Development, and Assurance. Assessment is the obligation to monitor health status and community needs routinely, regularly, and systematically. Policy development requires comprehensive plans, strategies, and tactics based on available knowledge and responsive to community needs. Assurance is a guarantee that high-priority personal and community health services will be provided for all by qualified organizations and staff under public, private, or mixed public/private auspices. For details and discussion, see http://www.health.gov/phfunctions/activiti.htm.

core values The most fundamental and immutable set of beliefs and attitudes governing behavior of individuals and groups. These are the foundation of BIOETHICS and must be taken into account in health promotion programs, e.g., in aspects relating to human reproduction. See also VALUES.

cornea The specialized translucent epithelial tissue at the front of the eye through which light passes to the lens and retina. Perfect transparency of the cornea is essential to good vision.

coronary heart disease A frequent condition in affluent, well-nourished nations, increasingly also in middle-income nations, often the largest single cause of death for men past middle age. It affects women almost equally but usually a decade or more later in life than men. The fact that it causes so many premature deaths makes it one of the most common public health problems in the world. It is due to atheroma of the coronary arteries, which is related to multiple risk factors, the most important of which are cigarette smoking, hypertension, physical inactivity, high serum cholesterol (related to dietary intake of cholesterol, saturated fats, and trans fatty acids), diabetes, and several other risk factors. Genetic factors can also influence the risk and prognosis of coronary heart disease. See also ISCHEMIC HEART DISEASE.

coroner The public official who presides at an inquiry into the circumstances of death that is otherwise unexplained and similar events that warrant investigation by an inquest. In the United Kingdom and some other jurisdictions, deaths of certain causes that may be related to occupation, e.g., bladder cancer or lead poisoning, are automatically referred to the coroner. In the United States, the medical examiner fulfills much the same functions.

corporation A legal entity that exists in its own right and is distinct from the individuals who comprise it. Varieties in the health field include profit-making, not-for-profit, and professional corpora tions, including some professional associations that have incorporated as legal entities.

correctional facility An American term for a prison, intended to convey the idea of active rehabilitation aimed to prevent or at least to reduce the risk of recidivism. Unfortunately, the social environment sometimes provides a setting for transmission of HIV, hepatitis, and other diseases transmitted in body fluids.

correctional services The services provided by law-enforcement agencies that have several interfaces with health services, e.g., in relation to domestic violence, child abuse, illicit drug use by prison inmates, HIV/AIDS, and other sexually transmitted diseases that are a high risk for inmates. The word "correctional" implies that the services aspire to correct or control the cause or reason the law was violated, but the reality often falls short of this aspiration, e.g., because the service is understaffed with qualified personnel and/or overwhelmed by numbers needing the expert attention required to rehabilitate and prevent recidivism.

correlation The extent to which variables change in unison.

correlation coefficient A statistical measure of the degree of relationship between two variables.

It is represented by the symbol r and in practice it usually refers to a linear relationship that in theory can vary from +1 when there is perfect correlation to -1 when the two variables are inversely related.

cosmetics Preparations intended to beautify those who use them, including innumerable kinds of pigments and powders for skin and lips, etc.; chemicals to alter the color and texture of hair, and usually marketed in the same venues; perfumes, lotions, salves, etc.; and the equipment to apply them to the relevant parts of the body. Cosmetics are as old as, perhaps older than, civilization. Some contain toxic chemicals, so they are actually or potentially harmful, and one function of the FOOD AND DRUG ADMINISTRATION (FDA) and its counterparts in other nations is to evaluate the safety of cosmetics.

cost The value of resources invested in a service, including CAPITAL COST of buildings, equipment, etc., operating cost of upkeep, maintenance, wages and salaries, dressings, medications, etc., each separately itemized in the budget that records where the money comes from and where it goes. Economists, accountants, and auditors distinguish several aspects, including direct, FIXED, INDIRECT, marginal, OPPORTUNITY, unit, and variable costs.

cost-benefit analysis Calculation or estimation of monetary and other costs, social costs such as time lost from work, years of active life lost to disability and premature death, and an estimate of the financial benefits attributable to the activities of a health service. All are expressed as far as possible in monetary terms. The benefits include ability to engage in work and valued familial and social activities, and estimates of added years of active productive life. Value judgments and approximations are inevitable parts of many cost-benefit analyses.

cost-effectiveness Estimation of expenditure and "returns" on this expenditure as health gains, compared with what might have been achieved by using available funds in another way.

cost-effectiveness analysis A variant of COST-BENEFIT ANALYSIS that seeks to identify the least costly way to meet a specified objective. It may be conducted by comparing costs and outcomes in systems that have applied different modalities, or as an abstract exercise using economic and other modeling techniques. It is a measure of the monetary or other costs of an intervention, a service, or an action in relation to its effectiveness in terms of benefits achieved. Public health departments use cost-effectiveness analysis to guide decisions about RESOURCE ALLOCATION.

cost-efficiency The extent to which an action or system is cost-effective.

cost of living index Syn: retail price index. A calculation conducted periodically, usually every month or annually, that compares current costs for specified goods and services, viz. basic staple items such as food, fuel, housing, transportation, with the costs of these items at a baseline, e.g., average costs of the same items in the previous year. The figures for the cost of living index usually are derived from an ongoing government survey. See also INFLATION.

cost-utility analysis A variation of COST-EFFEC TIVENESS ANALYSIS in which the UTILITY of an action or a system is estimated. Utility means the merits, or value, of a specified state of health, such as a health state on the continuum from full functional status to total dependency on others.

cot death (crib death) See SUDDEN INFANT DEATH SYNDROME (SIDS).

cotinine A detoxification product of the metabolism of nicotine that is rapidly excreted by the kidneys. Urinary cotinine concentration can be used to detect recent exposure to tobacco smoke.

cotton dust Suspended atmospheric cotton particles, often mixed with other airborne particles, that induce wheezing and coughing due to an allergic/toxic reaction in the respiratory tract, a precursor or symptom of BYSSINOSIS.

Council for International Organizations of Medical Sciences (CIOMS) A nongovernmental organization affiliated with the World Health Organization, cosponsored by many national and international professional organizations, colleges, academies, etc. CIOMS has sponsored and/or conducted much work on definition of guidelines for ethical conduct in medical practice and research, classification systems, information collection, storage and retrieval, etc. The publications of CIOMS and reports on its activities can be seen at http://www.cioms.ch/.

Council on Education for Public Health (CEPH) An independent nonprofit agency established in 1974, recognized by the US Department of Education, that is responsible for policies, priorities, criteria, and standards for education in public health, and for accreditation of schools of public health and certain educational programs in public health in medical schools and community colleges. Its corporate members are the American Public Health Association and the Association of Schools of Public Health. See http://www.ceph.org.

Council on Linkages Between Academia and Public Health A US professional organization comprising leaders of national associations, colleges, and academies concerned with public health practice, teaching, and research. Its mission is to improve public health education and practice by fostering, coordinating, and monitoring links between academia and the public health and health care communities, developing and advancing innovative strategies to build and strengthen public health infrastructure, and creating processes for continuing professional education. See http://www.phf.org/link.htm.

counseling services A range of services intended mainly for persons who are experiencing stress, e.g., parents and school children and school leavers requiring advice and suggestions about educational and occupational choices, emotional and social support after an unexpected death of a loved one, loss of home and possessions in a disaster. In public health, counseling on risk reduction, avoidance of substance abuse, and mental health are important aspects. Counseling is preferably provided by a professional trained counselor. See also GUIDANCE COUNSELOR.

counterfactual A statement or concept offered as a hypothesis that, although known to be false, can be used in a logical system called counterfactual reasoning, to derive demonstrable truths. It is a useful addition to the range of methods of epidemiological analysis and reasoning in public health policy decisions. When examining the causes and costs of specific diseases, it is useful to have comparisons with hypothetical alternatives, such as an "ideal," rather than an actual frequency distribution of blood pressure or serum cholesterol levels in the population. For example, in considering the costs of tobacco-related diseases, a counterfactual comparison can be made using the hypothetical case in which tobacco use has ceased altogether.

Countrywide Integrated Noncommunicable Disease Intervention (CINDI) An initiative of the European Region of WHO that is modeled on the Finnish North Karelia project, in which active programs of health-behavior change, dietary interventions, traffic injury prevention, and the like, have been implemented to reduce the incidence and prevalence of preventable diseases and disabilities. See http://www.euro.who.int/eprise/main/WHO/Progs/CINDI/Home for details. An equivalent system was introduced in Latin American countries by the Pan American Health Organization, Conjunto de Acciones para la Reduccion de las Enfermedades Notransmissibles (CARMEN). This has been active since the mid-1990s. Comparable national programs have been established in Mauritius and Pakistan.

courtesy staff A designation for medical staff members who have official privileges to admit and treat patients but in most cases use a hospital's facilities only occasionally.

covariate A variable that occurs with another variable of interest and may be a confounding variable, or an effect modifier.

coverage 1. The extent to which the health services provided for or available to the population of a country or region meet the potential or perceived needs of the people. 2.The extent to which a population is protected against a communicable disease by appropriate vaccination or other preventive regimen. 3. As applied to insurance, the extent of financial protection afforded by an insurance program. 4. The proportion of a population that benefits from a particular health care service, e.g., obstetrics, that is theoretically available to all.

cowpox A virus disease of cattle, producing vesicles containing the virus antigen, which provokes antibody formation in humans that effectively immunizes them against SMALLPOX. Smallpox vaccine is manufactured from the serum exudate produced by cowpox lesions.

coxsackievirus A family of more than 20 viruses that cause several kinds of inflammatory changes, including hand-foot-and-mouth disease, aseptic meningitis, and an influenza-like illness. They are named for a city in New York state where the first of this family was isolated.

crack cocaine A derivative of cocaine that either alone or mixed with baking soda can be smoked. Inhalation of crack cocaine produces a more powerful and immediate effect than injection or inhalation of cocaine powder in the form of snuff. It is a highly addictive and dangerous form of cocaine use that can induce cardiac arrhythmia and sudden death.

credentials The official documentary record of training and qualifications that is a prerequisite of employment in a health facility such as a hospital.

cresol An organic chemical in which one or more hydroxyl groups in the benzene ring are substituted with isomers to form a volatile liquid that is used as an industrial disinfectant and in the manufacture of dyes, plastics, and antioxidants. It is toxic and irritant, absorbed through the skin, and can cause death from asphyxiation or neurological, renal, and hepatic damage.

Creutzfeldt-Jakob disease A fatal degenerative brain disease caused by PRIONS, proteinaceous particles that enter the body in contaminated human tissue, such as transplanted cornea or human growth hormone prepared from extracts of human pituitary gland, and probably also from ingested prions of animal origin, such as nerve tissue in meat from beef cattle infected with the prion that causes BOVINE SPONGIFORM ENCEPHALOPATHY (BSE). In humans this causes VARIANT CREUTZFELDT-JAKOB DISEASE (vCJD). The eponym commemorates the two German neuropsychiatrists who identified and described the disease, Hans Creutzfeldt (1885–1964) and Alfons Jakob (1884–1931). Further information is available at several Web sites, including that of the World Health Organization (http://www.who.int/mediacentre/factsheets/fs180/en/) and the CJD Surveillance Unit at the University of Edinburgh (http://www.cjd.ed.ac.uk/), which maintains a cumulative incidence record of newly reported cases worldwide.

crisis intervention The emergency or "first aid" management of medical, social, psychological problems that usually declare their presence by causing an emergency requiring immediate action. The intervention may be the opportunity to begin longer-term management and amelioration of the underlying problem that precipitated the crisis.

criterion (Plural: criteria) A standard by which something is judged.

critical appraisal Systematic evaluation of a process, service, research design, etc., consisting of a detailed scrutiny and logical analysis of all phases of the process with the aim of ensuring that it conforms to acceptable standards, or, if it does not, identifying the shortcomings of the service, process, research design, and procedures.

critical care The level of medical and nursing care, including close surveillance and monitoring of vital signs, fluid and electrolyte balance, etc., provided for seriously ill and injured patients and those in the immediate postoperative period.

critical path analysis A systematic study of all phases in the conduct of a program or the operation of a service. This begins with complete description of each phase and examination of the extent to which each phase conforms to ideal standards, and continues with a study of the interactions of phases, searching for evidence of effective interlocking of each part with others. The aim is to maximize the efficiency of the system.

critical population size The minimum number of people required to sustain indefinitely an infectious pathogen, i.e., large enough to ensure that there is a specified probability of infectious agents encountering susceptible hosts. The specified probability varies with the nature of the infectious agent, its route of transmission, environmental conditions, and other factors that can all be observed, measured, counted, and included in the complex stochastic processes that are part of the mathematical theory of epidemics.

cross-cultural study A scientific study that compares variables such as determinants of health, among people from differing cultures or ethnic groups. This approach has been a popular way to study associations of disease, notably coronary heart disease, with factors such as differences in diet, occupation, leisure activities, among different cultural communities whether in the same or different countries. An example is the Seven Countries Study of coronary heart disease (see http://www.epi.umn.edu/about/7countries/results.shtm).

cross-infection An infection that is transmitted from one person to others in an institution such as a workplace or school. When it occurs in a hospital or other health care facility, it is classified as one form of NOSOCOMIAL INFECTION.

crossover design A research design sometimes used in clinical trials, in which the study and comparison regimens are switched after observing the effects on the study group, in order to determine whether the PLACEBO effect has influenced the outcome.

cross-sectional study A study that examines the relationship of health to other variables of interest at a particular time without regard for past conditions; thus a PREVALENCE study.

crowd behavior An ancient observation is that groups of people, crowds, and mobs behave in qualitatively and quantitatively different ways from the individuals that comprise them, often less rationally and in a more extreme and sometimes violent manner. There is a mutually reinforcing character to crowd behavior that can be exploited by demagogues and *agents provocateurs* with harmful consequences both for members of crowds, as when mob hysteria causes vulnerable persons to be injured, even trampled to death, and for others caught up in events, such as riots and episodes of soccer hooliganism and the like. Exploiting crowd behavior for desirable ends such as conduct beneficial to health seems usually to be less easily achieved.

crude death rate Syn: crude mortality rate. The frequency of death in a specified population during a specified period. It is calculated by dividing the number of deaths in the period by the estimated person-time at risk of dying during this period, usually a calendar year. The midperiod population

is a convenient approximation. It is called the "crude" death rate because no adjustment is made to allow for age composition of the population or for other conditions or circumstances. Thus, comparisons of crude death rates in different populations have limited value and must be interpreted with caution.

cryptococcosis A mycotic infection of the dermis, predominantly seen in tropical regions.

cryptosporidiosis A protozoan infection of domestic and wild animals that can infect humans. It causes inflammation of the gastrointestinal and respiratory tracts. The protozoa are excreted in the feces of infected animals and pass to humans if the animals inhabit the catchment area of a reservoir and the water is inadequately filtered before people drink it (the organism is relatively resistant to chlorination). In this way, about 400,000 people were infected in Wisconsin in 1993. It is usually a mild disease but can be serious, even fatal, in immunocompromised persons.

crystal meth The popular name for illicitly manufactured methamphetamine, an easily produced substance that is widely used by certain underground and counterculture groups, mainly young people and increasingly in rural and urban youth in the United States and elsewhere. It is a member of the AMPHETAMINE group, highly addictive, and suspected of causing permanent damage to the higher centers of the cerebral cortex.

Culex pipiens A common culicine mosquito along the eastern seaboard of the United States and Canada, and a vector for several diseases, including WEST NILE VIRUS.

cult A belief system that unquestioningly accepts a set of values, rituals, symbols without regard for unverifiable assertions that may be part of the belief system. It may be characterized by norms and values and sometimes by related ways of living and behaving that deviate from the accepted norms and values of the rest of the community. Cults, including some religious SECTS, sometimes have beliefs and behaviors that expose them to health risks different from those in the general population. Some are "health conscious," e.g., are nonsmokers, abstainers from alcohol, or vegetarians, regularly participate in exercise, and have significantly better health indicators than the general population. Some cults have health-harming beliefs, e.g., rejection of conventional health care systems and preventive regimens, including recommendations about infant and child immunizations.

cultural anthropology See ANTHROPOLOGY.

cultural barriers Impediments to communication between mainstream culture and members of a societal subgroup that is culturally distinct in significant ways can have implications for health. At a simple and obvious level, communication is impaired if the subgroup has language differences. Other important cultural barriers are imposed by major differences in values relating to marital customs, the role and status of girls and women, permitted and proscribed foods, standards of personal hygiene, etc.

cultural relativism The process of decision making that projects onto a person or a population the norms and values of the decision maker when the decision is being made about a person or population from a different culture or ethnic group. It has been used in ethical decision making, where it is criticized as infringement of autonomy of the person or group affected by the decision.

cultural sensitivity The ability to recognize, understand, and react appropriately to behaviors of persons who belong to a cultural or ethnic group that differs substantially from one's own.

culture 1. A nutrient medium on or in which microorganisms can be grown. 2. A set of beliefs, traditions, customs, values, and religious, artistic, and intellectual qualities that are common to a loosely defined group of people, such as citizens of a country or members of an ethnic community.

culture-specific disorders Conditions uniquely associated with a certain culture include unusual behavioral disorders, such as "amok," which occurs among Malays, with a period of quiet, solitary brooding followed by an outburst of violently destructive, sometimes homicidal, conduct. Chinese men can experience an acute hysterical state called "koro," in which they believe their penis is shrinking and will disappear into the abdomen. In Haiti and Jamaica, a form of BLACK MAGIC called "voodoo" is associated with evil spells that induce debility and death. FEMALE GENITAL MUTILATION, originally a tribal custom in northeast Africa, often causes difficult childbirth and chronic vulval and urinary infections. A culture-specific disorder in the United States is the high mortality and injury rate associated with easy access to and frequent use of firearms in INTERPERSONAL VIOLENCE.

cumulative frequency distribution The distribution of variables displayed visually. With Gaussian (normally) distributed variables, this is a characteristically S-shaped curve.

cumulative incidence rate The proportion of a specified group who experience the onset of a condition during a specified period, usually a calendar year. The specified period may be longer, as in cumulative lifetime incidence rate.

cumulative trauma disorders A collective name for a group of conditions associated with frequently repeated minor injury or musculotendinous strain. Examples include work-related back pain, REPETITIVE STRAIN DISORDER, tennis elbow, BEAT KNEE, etc.

curie A measure of radioactivity, in which 1 curie $=3.7 \times 10^{10}$ atomic disintegrations per second. The unit honors the memory of the Polish chemist and nuclear physicist Marie Curie (1867–1934). The curie has been superseded by the SI unit the BECQUEREL.

curve fitting An attempt to discern underlying mathematical order in the distribution of a variable by plotting it graphically with the hope or expectation that the display will conform to a recognizable mathematical formula, e.g., a normal or log-normal distribution.

custodial care Patient care provided in a secure institution, i.e., with restricted right of egress. This is used mainly to care for people with serious mental disorders who are unable to care for themselves and/or are at risk of harming others. Custodial care may be short term or long term. Long-term custodial care in mental hospitals often raises concerns about protection from risks such as transmission of fecal-oral infections by persons whose mental disorder involves absence or loss of capacity to maintain personal hygiene.

custody Legally recognized responsibility for and authority over others, e.g., child custody as designated in a divorce settlement, incarceration of alleged and convicted criminals in prison.

custom Habitual or usual way of behaving. Customs are the time-honored habits, ways of life, and modes of social intercourse of a community or cultural or ethnic group that often have implications for health. For instance, it was a polite custom in Western society throughout most of the 20th century to offer a cigarette when introduced to strangers.

customs The agency in virtually all nations responsible for screening possessions of persons who enter the country or import goods. This agency is primarily a tax-gathering arm of government, but it has important health-related functions in excluding illicit drugs and hazardous products and, in collaboration with public health authorities, applying and enforcing control measures against human, animal, and plant diseases.

CUSUM An acronym for cumulative sum, referring to the sum of a series of measurements. This is used to demonstrate a change in trend or direction of a series of measurements over time. To calculate the CUSUM, a reference figure such as the expected average measurement is selected, then, as each new measurement becomes available, the reference figure is subtracted from it, and a cumulative total is produced by adding each successive difference.

cut point An arbitrarily chosen value in an ordered sequence, such as the level of systolic and diastolic blood pressure, that is used to designate sections of the entire sequence, such as the level at which blood pressure is designated as high or abnormal and in need of treatment.

cyanosis Bluish discoloration of the skin caused by deficiency of oxygen and accumulation in the blood of reduced hemoglobin.

cybernetics The study of electronic communication, feedback, and control mechanisms.

cyclamate An artificial noncalorific sweetening agent.

cyclical trend A regularly recurring pattern, e.g., of seasonal fluctuation in prevalence of insect vectors or respiratory infections in primary school children.

cyclopropane Syn: trimethylene. An anesthetic gas, cyclopropane is explosive and a liver toxin.

cyclosporin An immunosuppressant, given to patients undergoing organ transplants.

cysticercosis Infection with the pork tapeworm, *Taenia solium*, specifically the somatic stage of the infection in which cysts of the larval worms lodge in tissues and organs, commonly in muscles and subcutaneous tissues but sometimes in vital organs, such as the brain, where they can cause serious symptoms, such as epileptiform seizures.

cystic fibrosis A disease inherited as a recessive genetic condition expressed when offspring inherit the gene on chromosome 7 from both parents. The disease causes malfunction of intestinal and pancreatic secretory glands and sticky mucous secretions in the bronchial tubes, leading to repeated respiratory infections, bronchiectasis, and life expectancy usually limited to 2 to 3 decades, despite treatment with detergent inhalant spray, antibiotics, etc. Counseling of parents carrying the gene, and possibly genetic engineering, offer prospects for prevention. A common intervention when both parents are known to carry the gene is prenatal chromosome determination and elective termination of pregnancy.

cytochromes Pigmented heme-containing proteins that occur in the mitochondria of organisms that use aerobic respiration. They are essential for most energy generation in the body.

cytogenetics The aspects of the science of genetics based on the study of cells, especially their microscopic chromosomal structure.

cytology The science devoted to the properties of cells, which are studied by microscopy, culture, and other means.

cytomegalovirus A type of host-specific herpes virus that causes serious ocular and pulmonary disease in immunocompromised persons.

cytosine A complex organic compound that is an important component of RNA and DNA

D

dairy A place to milk cows, store milk, and often process milk into butter, cheese, and other dairy products. In size and complexity, it varies from a simple lean-to shed for the family cow to a large mechanized barn where many cows are milked using mechanical milking machines in a setting akin to a factory production line and from which milk is transported in tankers. In all dairies and especially in those that serve many people, the milk can become a vehicle for fecal-oral and other pathogens, so cleanliness, scrupulous hygiene, and freedom from infection of dairy workers are essential. Inspection of dairies and dairy workers is an important function of SANITARIANS.

damp In the mining industry, "damp" (from German *dampf*, steam) means smoke, fumes, or gas. Thus, for instance, FIREDAMP is the methane gas that causes explosions in coal mines.

damper A flanged plate that partially opens or closes to vary the flow of air into the combustion chamber of a furnace, controlling the rate of combustion and modifying the emission products. In general, combustion is more complete and emissions less when the air flow is greatest.

dander Dandruff, i.e., skin flakes mixed with mites, fungus particles, etc., occurring on domestic animals such as horses, dogs, and cats. Cat and horse dandruff are frequent causes of asthma and other allergic reactions in sensitive humans, especially children.

dapsone A sulfone compound used mainly to treat leprosy. It is also used to treat *Pneumocystis carinii* infections that complicate HIV/AIDS and other conditions, including malaria, systemic lupus erythematosus, and actinomycosis infections.

Darwin, Charles (1809–1882) The British naturalist who transformed biology and concepts of the place of humans in nature. In 1831 to 1835 he sailed on HMS *Beagle* on a voyage to chart parts of the coasts of South America, the Galapagos Islands, and Australasia. He collected many biological and paleontological specimens, and in 1859, after reflecting on his observations and conclusions, he published in *The Origin of Species* a theory of EVOLUTION that revolutionized the biological sciences, making him one of the most influential scientists who ever lived. Among much else, Darwin's theory explains the evolution of antibiotic-resistant pathogenic microorganisms.

Darwinian fitness, selection See EVOLUTION and FITNESS.

data (Plural of datum, a fact) A set of facts or items of information, usually quantitative.

data bank A source of data, such as the accumulated records of clients or patients who have attended a clinic during a specified period.

data base An organized set of data, often a set that has been partially processed and is available for more detailed analysis.

data dictionary, directory A set of tabulated information about the contents of a data base.

data dredging An unkind description of the conduct of a desperate or dishonest investigator who attempts to demonstrate a "significant" result by using a sequence of statistical tests that were not in the original research protocol. This conduct has been summed up in the remark: "If you torture the data enough, they'll confess to anything!" Not to be confused with DATA MINING.

data integration The process of combining data bases from several sources to eliminate redundancy and achieve a broader view.

data management The method of recording, organizing, and storing information, for instance, handwritten or typed on alphabetically arranged charts, or direct keyboard entry into a computer. Electronic scanning can be used to achieve a "paperless office," but this has the disadvantage that files may be accidentally or deliberately corrupted (a problem that applies also to data protection). See also MEDICAL RECORD.

data mining Systematic, purposeful analysis of large files of raw data or an already analyzed data base using MULTIVARIATE ANALYSIS, with the expectation that useful information, e.g., on relationships between outcomes and their possible causes, will come to light. An example is the discovery by this means of occupational exposure risks of rare malignancies.

data protection Procedures adopted to ensure that the CONFIDENTIALITY of sensitive personal information is maintained. Examples include secure record storage systems (filing cabinets that are locked at all times and accessible only with a key held by authorized persons) and encryption of computer-stored files to ensure that they are accessible only to authorized persons who possess the access code. Data protection DIRECTIVES in the European Union have established an elaborate system to preserve confidentiality, sometimes at the cost of destroying or denying access to information or potentially important findings that it would be in the public interest to obtain and use. Other problems arise because computer-based secrecy has challenged a whole underground industry of computer hackers to break the code, and this they do embarrassingly often.

data set An alternative name for a data base.

date rape drugs These are drugs that dull consciousness and/or reduce inhibitions, thus making it easier for a man to overcome a woman's resistance to sexual advances. Three drugs have been mainly used for this purpose. They are gamma hydroxybutyric acid (GHB), Rohypnol (flunitrazepam), and ketamine (ketamine hydrochloride). They are tasteless and dissolve readily in alcoholic drinks. See http://www.4woman.gov/faq/rohypnol.htm for details.

day care A system for providing shelter and supervision of infants, toddlers, and preschool children whose parent(s) have no one else with whom to leave them while at work or otherwise occupied. Some jurisdictions provide day care at public expense or it is subsidized; in others, the parent(s) must pay for it in full. The quality varies, as do the benefits, such as early socialization and the risks of harm to children from such causes as CROSS-INFECTION.

day hospital A hospital, or a designated portion of a hospital, where people receive care during part or all of the day and go home at the end of the day. The care may be medical, surgical, psychiatric, supportive-social, or any combination of these. A day hospital is not the same as an OUTPATIENT or AMBULATORY CARE department of a hospital because it is specialized, not episodic, usually one-time-only, although sometimes provided on a recurring basis.

DBCP See DIBROMOCHLOROPROPANE.

DDT (dichloro-diphenyl-trichloroethane) Synthesized in 1874, DDT was discovered to be an insecticide in 1939 by the Swiss chemist Paul Müller (1899–1965), thus winning him the Nobel Prize. It was used successfully to treat lice-infested populations in Europe toward the end of World War II, aborting threatened epidemics of typhus. In the 1950s and early 1960s, it was successfully used in a WHO-coordinated plan to eliminate malaria-carrying mosquitoes in many regions where malaria had previously been endemic. However, mosquitoes soon became DDT resistant. Moreover, DDT is not biodegradable, kills many birds, is stored in fatty tissue, is excreted in breast milk, and bioconcentrates at higher levels of terrestrial and marine food chains. In humans, it is hepatotoxic and neurotoxic and possibly genotoxic and carcinogenic. It was banned as an insecticide in the United States and most of Europe in the early 1970s, but is still widely used in low-income nations.

deadly nightshade The common garden plant *Atropa belladonna*, the flowers of which contain hyoscine and scopolamine, two drugs that in overdoses cause flushing, dilated pupils, rapid heart rate, hallucinations, coma, and death. The name *belladonna* (beautiful maiden) derives from the flushed face and dilated pupils caused by ingesting the flowers. Medicinally, both drugs are used as antispasmodics, in preoperative medication, etc.

deafness Hearing impairment, which has many preventable causes, including antenatal rubella; middle-ear infection in childhood; damage to the cochlea, the organ of hearing, by exposure to excessive noise in industry; loud music; discharge of firearms, etc. Deafness has many other causes, include prenatal injury; nerve damage due to drugs, e.g., streptomycin; and impacted wax in the external auditory canal. It is a serious and often underappreciated impairment.

death Cessation of cardiovascular, respiratory, and neurological activity for a sufficient period to cause irreversible pathological deterioration of vital organs. The traditional definition of death—irreversible cessation of circulatory, respiratory, and neurological functions—has become less valid since the development of LIFE SUPPORT SYSTEMS and devices to ventilate lungs and artificially stimulate contractions of heart muscle. Individual organs and body systems can "die," but life ceases only when a person experiences BRAIN DEATH, after which organs may be harvested.

death certificate A VITAL RECORD, signed by a licensed physician or other designated official, containing personal identifying information (name, birth date, sex, place of residence, and death) and specifying the CAUSE OF DEATH. The cause of death is recorded with the immediate or direct cause stated first, followed by ANTECEDENT CAUSE(S) OF DEATH, i.e., condition(s) leading up to the immediate cause, and finally the UNDERLYING CAUSE OF DEATH, which is the one coded with the ICD NUMBER and entered in vital statistical tables of causes of death. Other significant conditions are also recorded. In many jurisdictions, death certificates include further details, such as occupation, Social Security or insurance number, birthplace, and, for RECORD LINKAGE purposes, the deceased person's father's name and/or mother's maiden name. Copies of death certificates are required for legal purposes by next of kin, and by civil authorities, pension fund administrators, etc., to close the accounts of those who had been getting pensions or other benefits. In many countries, death certificates are permanently stored in their original paper form or on microfiche and are available for study by authorized persons, including public health research workers.

death rate Syn: mortality rate. The frequency with which death occurs among a designated population during a designated period, usually a calendar year. Conceptually, this is the number of deaths divided by the amount of PERSON-TIME at risk of death within the designated period. In practice, it is calculated by counting the number of deaths in the period, customarily a calendar year, divided by the midyear population, and, to produce a whole number rather than a fraction, multiplying by 1,000. This yields the CRUDE DEATH RATE. For comparison with other times and places, the death rate is standardized. (See STANDARDIZATION.) Death rates are published in statistical reports tabulated in several ways, e.g., by age group, sex, cause, geographical distribution, occupation.

death registration The formal procedure of recording and notifying death has been a statutory legal requirement in most organized jurisdictions for more than 100 years. The details are contained in the DEATH CERTIFICATE. This is a legal document, as well as the source of tabulated data on causes of death. In developing countries, registration usually begins on a trial basis in one or more defined districts and extends to the rest of the country as resources expand to permit this.

decibel A measure of sound intensity (loudness). Because decibels are measured on a logarithmic scale, each decibel unit represents a tenfold increase in sound intensity. The threshold of hearing is 0 dB; normal conversation is 60 dB; a food blender 3 feet away is 90 dB; a diesel truck 30 feet away is 100 dB; a power mower 3 feet away is 107 dB; amplified rock music 6 feet away is 120 dB; a jet aircraft engine 100 feet away is 130 dB. Sound intensity above about 120 dB can permanently damage hearing.

decision analysis A system of logic that uses elements of GAME THEORY and OPERATIONAL RESEARCH to identify and quantify all available choices and their outcomes at each stage in designing a plan for preventive or therapeutic interventions. Each of the choices and probabilities of the outcomes of each choice can be visually presented in a DECISION TREE. The relative value of each outcome can be expressed as a UTILITY or quality-of-life measurement.

decision theory A specialized branch of logic that provides a conceptual framework and formal rules for decision making. One of the pioneers in this discipline was the British mathematician Charles Lutwidge Dodgson (1832–1898), better known by his pseudonym Lewis Carroll, author of *Alice's Adventures in Wonderland* and other works that playfully illustrate the rules of formal logic.

decision tree A diagrammatic presentation of the sequence of decisions (choices) available at each stage in management of problems in which the outcome of each decision presents two or more further alternatives and therefore requires further decisions.

decomposition Decay of organic waste matter, a natural process facilitated by the presence of aerobic bacteria. It is the usual mode by which organic matter is decomposed in soil and in many sewage disposal systems; anaerobic decomposition caused by the action of anaerobic bacteria often produces foul and noxious odors. This occasionally happens when organic matter decays in the depths of freshwater lakes and can lead to eruptions of poisonous gas, such as methane.

decompression syndrome Syn: caisson disease, the BENDS. The response to a sudden decrease in ambient air pressure, as when the high-pressure environment required to counteract the effect of water pressure on a fragile submerged vessel is suddenly reduced, or when an aircraft climbs suddenly to high altitude. Release of dissolved gases (oxygen, nitrogen, carbon dioxide) from blood and other body fluids, even synovial fluid in joints, bursts capillaries, arterioles, and venules and produces multiple air emboli. The condition is acutely painful and can be fatal. It requires emergency treatment in a decompression chamber, where air pressure is gradually restored over a period of hours to normal atmospheric pressure. The condition is both depth- and time-dependent, so scuba divers who immerse for long periods in relatively shallow water may be vulnerable.

deductive reasoning A method of reasoned argument in which a conclusion or inference must logically follow from observed facts in combination with related axioms, premises, or principles. This is the underlying method of Sherlock Holmes and many other fictional detectives. Another phrase for this is "particularizing from the general." See also INDUCTION.

dedusting The process used to remove suspended particles from air, using a water spray or passing air through an electronic filter, which causes charged particles to aggregate. In industrial and mining operations, this process is sometimes used as a way to reduce the risk of exposure to harmful inhaled dusts, such as silica, but on its own it is not very effective.

DEET (N,N-diethyl-3-methylbenzamide) Formerly called N,N-diethyl-toluamide. DEET is an insect repellent, i.e., a chemical that insects such as mosquitoes and ticks avoid. Exposure to high concentrations of DEET can cause cerebral seizures, so it is advisable not to use it as an insect repellent to protect small children.

defensive medicine The method of practice by physicians fearful of litigation against them because they have failed to detect a condition or failed to treat a condition adequately. This often leads to excessive use of diagnostic tests, and/or costly and potentially dangerous overtreatment. Defensive medicine is deplored by good physicians and abhorred by administrators of medical insurance programs because it drives costs to excessive heights.

defibrillator A device that sends a strong electric charge to the myocardium, thus stimulating conduction tissue, and capable, under favorable circumstances, of restoring regular sinus rhythm to a heart that has gone into ventricular tachycardia or fibrillation, or has ceased beating. See also CARDIOPULMONARY RESUSCITATION (CPR).

deficiency disease A disease caused by a dietary deficiency of protein or an essential mineral or vitamin. The many varieties include iron deficiency anemia, IODINE DEFICIENCY DISORDERS (IDD) associated with dwarfism and mental retardation, vitamin A deficiency associated with BLINDNESS caused by XEROPHTHALMIA, and vitamin B deficiency associated with BERIBERI.

defoliant An herbicide that selectively kills plants with broad leaves, used in conifer forests to eliminate so-called weed trees that compete for nutriment. Several varieties are widely used as domestic and agricultural weed killers. They are artificially manufactured plant hormones. Some contain DIOXINS as contaminants and thus may be an occupational hazard for agricultural workers.

degrees of freedom A term used in STATISTICS to describe the number of independent comparisons that can be made between the variables in a study.

deinstitutionalization The transition from institutional (custodial) to community-based care of mental disorders, which was facilitated by development of psychoactive drugs and modern office-based psychotherapeutic methods. It was perceived as a progressive trend because custodial care often had punitive elements, and was said to be cheaper than custodial care. As a bureaucratic process, it was sometimes heartless. Not all of the people with chronic mental disorders who had previously lived in mental hospitals and other long-stay institutions were identified and effectively treated by community-based psychiatric services after they had been ejected from the institutions that sheltered them. An unintended consequence has been the emergence of a new public health problem: a sharp increase in the prevalence of homeless mentally ill people. Enlightened psychiatrists and mental health administrators have avoided this problem by establishing a THERAPEUTIC COMMUNITY. See also LONG-TERM CARE.

Delaney clause A legislative addition to the US Food, Drug and Cosmetics Act, proposed by Representative J. J. Delaney in 1958, prohibiting the use of food additives that are known to be carcinogenic. The European Union and other nations have similar protective legislation. The Delaney clause has frequently been subjected to political pressure, usually to relax standards, for instance, about use of agricultural pesticides and food additives. For a recent impartial report, see http://www4.nationalacademies.org/news.nsf/isbn/POD 375.

deletion syndromes Any of several inherited diseases attributable to loss of a chromosomal segment. Most such syndromes are associated with gross physical and often mental deficiency.

delinquency A word often used by law enforcement officials to describe antisocial adolescent behavior ranging from vandalism to violent crime. Delinquency has a public health dimension because of the risks of substance abuse, sexually transmitted disease, the coexistence of mental and emotional disorders, etc. Often it can be prevented, and successful intervention is possible for common precursor situations, such as parental alcohol and drug abuse and domestic violence.

delivery room Syn: labor room, labor ward. The room in a hospital or birthing center where the neonate is delivered. A term not usually applied when delivery is by cesarean section, an operative procedure that is conducted in the operating room of a hospital.

delphi method Circulation to a selected panel of experts of repeated sequences of questions, each subsequent sequence being refined or composed in light of responses to the preceding round. The aim is to arrive at a limited number of workable alternative solutions to the problem or problems that have been considered by the members of the panel. Ideally, the identities of panel members are unknown to each other so as to reduce the possible effects of biases and to avoid the risk that one person's ideas and opinions may dominate those of other members of the panel. The term derives from the oracle of Delphi in ancient Greece, who reputedly could make prophesies and offer wise words about the right course of action in many situations.

delusion A false belief that is not changed by reasoned argument. Delusions are a feature of some serious mental disorders, notably paranoia and schizophrenia. See also HALLUCINATION.

demand A term used in economics to describe willingness or ability to pay for goods or services. In the terminology of health economics, it means desire for or willingness to seek health care.

deme A group of persons or animals who are studied in their natural habitat or ecosystem. From Greek *deme*, a township or natural division that circumscribes a population from others.

dementia A neuropsychiatric disorder in which memory and intellectual functions are lost. The possible causes include pathological changes in the brain, such as those that occur in ALZHEIMER'S DISEASE, senile dementia, cerebrovascular disease, drug or alcohol addiction, and environmental toxins. The many varieties of dementia and Alzheimer's disease in particular are common enough to constitute a major public health problem, and in contemporary Western populations with small families and increasing numbers of elderly people with no close kin, a difficult economic and social problem. The term senile dementia is loosely used, but precise diagnosis is important because effective interventions vary and are dependent upon the underlying cause. No effective treatment of Alzheimer's disease or generalized cerebrovascular disease is available, but dementia caused by some toxins or by severe hypothyroidism respond to specific therapy.

demographic and health survey A method of assessing family status and health conditions in low- and middle-income nations by questionnaire or interview survey of representative samples of households, focusing on variables relating to reproductive health, infant and child illness and death, use of immunizations, dietary supplements, and other pertinent information about health and access to and use of health care services. Typically, the data are derived from a representative sample of at least several thousand and obtained by means of standardized interview schedules. Information about methods is at http://www.measure dhs.com/aboutsurveys/dhs_surveys.cfm.

demographic transition The change in long-term trends in fertility and mortality from high rates to low, accompanied by a change in the age composition of a population as birth rates and death rates both decline, following roughly in parallel a decline in infant and child mortality rates. The result is a decrease in the proportion of children and young adults and an increase in the proportion of older persons in the population, i.e., AGING OF THE POPULATION. See POPULATION PYRAMID.

demographic trap The situation that arises in a country or region when the population exceeds the CARRYING CAPACITY of its local ecosystem, there is nowhere for the people to go, and the economy produces insufficient goods or services to exchange for food and other essentials. The consequences include famine requiring food aid, migration out of the affected region, epidemics, and violent armed conflict. All these happened in some low-income countries in Africa in the late 20th century and in some Pacific islands early in the 21st century. This situation was predicted by the British clergyman and amateur scientist Thomas Robert Malthus (1766–1834) in his essay on the *Principle of Population* (1798).

demography The scientific study of populations that focuses on their size, distribution, age structure, fertility, marital patterns, migrations, mortality, and the social, cultural, economic, and other determinants of variations in any or all of these features. Demography has interfaces and features in common with vital statistics, epidemiology, sociology, and economics and is one of the essential basic sciences of public health.

demonstration project A health program, service, facility, or professional staffing structure, or a combination of these, usually publicly funded, often large, established and evaluated to determine whether it constitutes an improvement on previous ways of achieving the desired outcomes.

dengue fever A tropical and subtropical virus infection transmitted by Culex mosquitoes, such as *Aedes aegypti* and *Aedes albopictus*, with symptoms of high fever and severe muscle pains (thus the name breakbone fever). The hemorrhagic variety is very serious, resembling YELLOW FEVER. Dengue is not transmissible directly from person to person but only via mosquito bites. It is endemic in many tropical regions, in urban as well as rural communities. There is no specific treatment, but the disease usually runs its course and confers a type-specific immunity.

denominator The lower part of a fraction used to calculate a rate, ratio, or proportion. The population, or population-experience (as in person-time, passenger-distance, etc.), at risk of experiencing an event of interest.

densitometer An instrument that measures the degree of opacity of a translucent gaseous or liquid medium, e.g., the degree of opacity of urban haze due to air pollution.

dental (chairside) assistant A person who assists a DENTIST. Formerly this was often a young woman or adolescent girl who was trained on the job by the dentist. Formal training is available in technical colleges. The occupational risks may include mercury poisoning from mixing the amalgam used to fill teeth and radiation exposure from dental x-ray machines.

dental caries See CARIES.

dental hygiene Systematic, frequent (preferably after every meal) cleaning of teeth with a toothbrush, removal of detritus between the teeth by dental flossing, and massaging the gums. Most adults can do this themselves, but it can be done more thoroughly by a DENTAL HYGIENIST.

dental hygienist A trained person, licensed after formal assessment at the end of training, who is skilled in removal of tartar from dental enamel ("scaling"), flossing, topical application of fluoride paste, and education on oral hygiene.

dental sealant An inert, stable, and long-lasting plastic compound used by dentists to close small fissures in dental enamel and thereby prevent or retard the occurrence of dental caries.

dentist A person who is professionally trained and licensed to prevent and treat diseases of the teeth, gums, and adjacent tissues, notably dental caries, malocclusion, periodontal disease, gingivitis, oral cancer, and dental or oral manifestations of systemic disease.

dentistry The specialized care of the teeth and adnexa. Restorative dentistry focuses on repairing decayed (carious) teeth and often includes regular sessions conducted by a dental hygienist. Orthodontics is devoted to correcting the alignment and position of teeth that are not aligned in a manner that permits efficient mastication and/or improperly positioned. Preventive dentistry is a specialty of public health, as well as dentistry, that emphasizes ways to preserve and protect dental health, using such methods as population-based FLUORIDATION of drinking water and personal care and dental health education by a DENTAL HYGIENIST.

deontological ethics Syn: duty-based ethics. An approach to ethical reasoning and decision making based on the moral theory that certain aspects of conduct must be adhered to, regardless of possible consequences, because they are integral to inviolable beliefs about what is right and wrong. The emphasis tends to be mainly on eschewing what is wrong, e.g., it is wrong to take human life, rather than abiding by the belief that it is a moral duty to do what is right or good.

deoxyribonucleic acid (DNA) The nucleic acid compound of adenine, guanine, cytosine, and thymine that is the genetic structure of chromosomes and occurs in body cells in the characteristic DOUBLE HELIX shape first identified by the British molecular biologist Francis Crick (1916–2004) and his American postdoctoral graduate student James Watson (b. 1928), assisted by the British x-ray crystallographer Rosalind Franklin (1920–1958), the New Zealand physicist Maurice Wilkins (1916–2004), and the American chemist Linus Pauling (1901–1994). Crick, Watson, and Wilkins received the Nobel prize for this work in 1962.

Department of Health and Human Services (DHHS) The US government department responsible for all civilian federal health services. It includes some large, well-known, important agencies and centers, e.g., the Centers for Disease Control and Prevention, National Institutes of Health, Food and Drug Administration, Indian Health Service, and a number of others. For details, organization, and activities, see http://www.dhhs.gov.

Department of Health, Education and Welfare (DHEW) The precursor of the Department of Health and Human Services, which underwent an administrative reorganization when a separate federal Department of Education was established.

Department of Health, Social Services and Public Safety (DHSSPS) The UK government department responsible for administering the British National Health Service, the affiliated social services, and public health and health protection services. The Department of Health and the Department of Social Services were separate ministries for some years but in 1999 were amalgamated and broadened to include public health and health protection services. For details and current information, see http://www.dhsspsni.gov.uk/.

dependency The status of a person who is unable to live an independent existence because of age (infancy, childhood, frail elderly); chronic or acute illness, injury or infirmity; or disability caused by impairment.

dependency ratio The ratio of dependent persons (infants, children, frail elderly, and the infirm) to the others in the population who support them, either directly or by collective social security.

dependent variable In statistics, a variable the value of which is affected by other variable(s).

depleted uranium Uranium residue from which radioactive components have been wholly or mostly excluded during the use of this metallic element in the nuclear industry. Depleted uranium is used in weapons, for instance, in armor-piercing shells. There is equivocal anecdotal and epidemiological evidence that exposure of combat troops and noncombatants to depleted uranium has adverse effects on health, including increased risk of malignant disease.

deposition 1. The process by which particles of a substance settle on a surface, e.g., the epithelial surface of the upper respiratory tract. 2. Testimony given under oath, e.g., as at an inquest.

depression 1. An emotional disorder associated with persistent gloomy mood; sadness; guilt feelings; unhappiness; loss of interest in family, friends, and work; preference for being alone; feeling of worthlessness; crying fits; and other symptoms, such as sleep disturbances, psychomotor agitation, or fits of crying, loss of appetite, and loss of energy. It can be a prolonged condition lasting months or years, a recurrent disorder, which may be familial and is sometimes called BIPOLAR DISORDER, or a sudden disease of acute onset leading to profound depression with the belief that life is not worth living—a very dangerous condition because it frequently leads to suicide. Depression is a common and often unrecognized public health problem. 2. A prolonged period of severely reduced economic activity. In the early 1930s, a particularly severe period, known as the Great Depression, afflicted all industrial and many agricultural nations worldwide.

deprivation In public health, this term usually applies to the status of children who are deprived of food, shelter, adequate clothing, or other necessities of life, such as protective immunizations against common infectious diseases; deprivation renders them vulnerable in many ways that child protection agencies aim to control. Deprivation can occur to anyone, adult as well as child. It is also common among REFUGEES and DISPLACED PERSONS or populations. The word applies also to emotional deprivation, which can be an underlying determinant of personality disorders.

dermal exposure The skin, the largest organ of the human body, is the protective shield against many physical, chemical, and biological agents that would otherwise cause harm. However, it is not impervious to all possible environmental insults. Physical agents, e.g., heat, cold, ionized radiation, can all harm the skin. Many chemicals are toxic, even corrosive. Biological agents include some that induce toxic or allergic reactions in or on the skin, such as poison ivy, and some pathogenic organisms gain entry to the body through the skin. All these can be classified as dermal exposure.

dermatitis Inflammation of the skin. This can be acute, subacute, or chronic and has many possible causes, including pathogenic organisms, physical and chemical irritants, allergic reactions, psychological stress, and atopic eczema. Dermatitis is a common occupational disease.

dermatology The medical specialty concerned with the study, diagnosis, and treatment of diseases of the skin.

dermatophytosis Fungus infection of the skin. Several common varieties of this often stubbornly persistent infection are tinea pedis (ATHLETE'S FOOT) and tinea capitis (RINGWORM), a fungal infection often acquired from domestic pets. Ringworm can also infect the trunk, groin, and perianal region. A less common variety affects the fingernails, causing chronic paronychia.

DES See DIETHYLSTILBESTROL.

desalination Extraction or removal of dissolved salts from sea water. Available methods include distillation, osmotic processes using ion-exchange resins, and reverse electrophoresis. All methods are energy intensive, but in some regions, e.g., the Middle East, solar energy is used. Distillation yields sterile water; the other methods do not necessarily remove all pathogens.

desensitization 1. A method of treatment for hypersensitivity to allergens that consists of steadily increasing doses of the allergen aimed at inducing formation of blocking antibodies. 2. A method of treating alcoholism and substance abuse that relies on conditioned reflexes.

designated driver An automobile driver who has been selected in advance before a party or social outing during which intoxicants will be served, who remains sober to drive inebriated friends home afterward; a means to avoid traffic crashes due to IMPAIRED DRIVING.

designer drug A mood-modifying pharmaceutical preparation specifically intended for social use, e.g., ECSTASY, an illegal derivative of amphetamine that induces euphoria and hallucinations and has dangerous adverse effects on the cardiovascular system and can cause sudden death.

determinant A definable entity that causes, is associated with, or induces a health outcome. It may be a factor or combination of factors that can be classified as inherited or acquired. The latter, lumped together as environmental determinants, include biological, behavioral, social, economic, cultural, and other factors. Any combination of these may be determinants of health.

determinism The philosophical belief that everything in life is predetermined or that there is a predestined cause-effect relationship for everything that happens. Adherents to this belief system sometimes disdain or eschew preventive or therapeutic interventions because of the notion that fate, rather than science, determines what will happen to them.

deterrent fee In a fee-for-service health care system, a deterrent fee is one that inhibits contact between someone seeking health care and the source of its provision. It is intended as a form of economic rationing system, but it can act as a barrier between persons who need health care and the service or agency that could provide this care.

detoxification Elimination or drastic reduction of a toxic dose of a substance, such as alcohol or a narcotic drug, usually relying on a combination of a specific antidote and metabolic action of the body. This may take some time and is best done under medical observation in a "detox center" or specially established clinic.

detritus 1. The heaviest component of solids in sewage sludge, usually comprising mainly inorganic matter. 2. Amorphous body tissues, e.g., atheromatous arterial deposits.

developed country In the language of international affairs, including INTERNATIONAL HEALTH, this is a country whose citizens have on average a sufficient income to enjoy the good things of life and usually have access to a wide range of publicly provided and private services in the health, education, social welfare, housing, transport, commercial and industrial sectors, as well as state-supported defense and security services. See also INCOME LEVELS and WORLD BANK CLASSIFICATION.

developing country A country that is lacking in the services and facilities enjoyed by people in developed countries, such as personally owned automobiles and homes with water-carried sewage disposal systems. Use of this term is resented by people in nonindustrialized nations with a low per capita income and a long history with rich traditions, such as India and China. Because of this, the term LOW-INCOME COUNTRY may be preferable, but in reality no catch-all phrase adequately summarizes national socioeconomic status. Other terms are "the South," a term used by the German statesman Willy Brandt (1913–1992), and third world. See also INCOME LEVELS, WORLD BANK CLASSIFICATION.

development 1. In biology, the processes of growth, formation of adult tissues and organs, etc., leading to accomplishment of maturity. 2. As in the phrase child development, the process by which latent capabilities emerge or are brought out. 3. In economics and international affairs, increase in per capita income, goods and services, etc., associated with trade, commerce, and industrialization, generally leading to improved quality of life, as measured by the HUMAN DEVELOPMENT INDEX, a process allegedly accelerated by GLOBALIZATION.

development grant Funds disbursed by an international agency, or by a national or regional government, and/or material and/or human resources in lieu of cash, in order to establish and/or enhance needed human services such as health care, education, etc.

developmentally handicapped A general term to describe children who fail to achieve their expected intellectual milestones with or without associated physical disabilities. This term is sometimes preferred because it has fewer pejorative overtones than mental retardation. "Developmentally impaired" would be a preferable term.

deviance 1. In mathematics, a set of values that deviate from another sequence or set without specifying the direction or magnitude. 2. In the health sector, the word often describes sexual behavior that deviates from accepted norms and values and is deprecated by most people in the society or culture. But norms and values can change. Homosexuality was regarded as deviant in Western industrial nations until about the middle of the 20th century and then in most progressive Western societies it began to be accepted as a normal, although relatively uncommon, variation of human sexuality. In some cultures homosexuality is still considered abhorrent, disgusting, and even a capital crime. Pedophilia is considered deviant in Western industrial nations, but child marriage is acceptable in some cultures. In short, "deviance" is often an emotionally loaded, as well as a culture-specific, term. The public health sector and the law enforcement sector have varying reactions and responses that are influenced by societal norms and often by the values of individual professional workers.

devolution The political process by which authority and responsibility for management of public affairs, including health services, shifts from central government agencies and departments to local or regional equivalents, conferring greater autonomy on citizens at the grassroots level.

dewatering 1. Extraction of sufficient liquid content from sewage sludge to render it useful as fertilizer by means of a mechanical spreader. 2. Application of methods to dry out waterlogged ground to permit construction of foundations for high-rise buildings.

dew point The temperature at which moisture (dew) begins to appear on a solid surface when the temperature of this surface is falling and there is water vapor in the atmosphere.

diabetes A metabolic and systemic disease in which carbohydrate metabolism is disrupted by an insufficient supply of INSULIN to meet the body's metabolic needs. Type 1, or insulin-dependent diabetes, formerly called juvenile diabetes, is caused by destruction of insulin producing pancreatic cells, probably an autoimmune disorder that may often be viral in origin (e.g., associated with the mumps virus). Type 2, or non-insulin-dependent diabetes, is due to relative insufficiency of insulin, i.e., carbohydrate intake exceeding the capacity of the pancreas to produce insulin, often associated with obesity. Both types have implications for preventive medicine, in presymptomatic screening, and in efficient control to minimize the incidence of such dangerous consequences as diabetic ketosis, insulin coma, and complications, e.g., renal and retinal damage and coronary heart disease.

diagnosis The intellectual process of determining the nature of disease or injury and the "disease label" that is the end product of this process. This "label" may be a precisely defined disorder that has been identified by a battery of tests, a probability statement based on what is most likely among several possibilities, an opinion based on pattern recognition, or mere guesswork, a shot in the dark. Usually applied to individuals, the word is also used in the context of COMMUNITY DIAGNOSIS, in which the health problems of a community are identified, defined, and categorized.

diagnosis-related groups (DRGs) The term used by hospital and medical insurance carriers in the United States and some other countries to classify patients according to the nature and level of intensity of the medical care that they require and that is eligible for insurance coverage. Although the concept is useful to insurance carriers and other third-party payers, it tends to constrain clinical decisions relating to the cost of care within boundaries that do not necessarily allow for exceptional cases.

Diagnostic and Statistical Manual of Mental Disorders (DSM) The manual developed and published by the American Psychiatric Association, containing the list of diagnoses of psychiatric illnesses and the criteria that should be used to arrive at each specified diagnosis. The 4th edition of this manual (DSM-IV) was published in 1994, and a revised version (DSM-IV-TR) was released in 2000. It has been criticized because it may have too many rather arbitrary and artificially narrow categories and because it assigns "disease labels" to conditions that many social scientists and other experts outside the field of psychiatry regard as normal behavioral variations. For example, the sorrow accompanying bereavement is given the label "depression" (implying that it requires psychiatric treatment) if it continues for more than 2 months. For details, see http://www.appi.org/book.cfm?id=2025.

dialectic The method of reasoning that proceeds by question and answer and logical argument, famously illustrated by the dialogues of Socrates (470–399 BCE) as recorded by Plato (c. 428–347 BCE). Teaching of epidemiology and other public health sciences can be conducted by dialectic.

dialysis Separation of crystalline (usually inorganic) chemicals from colloid (usually organic) compounds, using a semipermeable membrane, which allows passage of low molecular weight compounds and blocks or filters the heavier compounds. The process is widely used in chemistry. It is used in medical practice in renal dialysis to treat patients with renal failure.

diapause Retarded or suspended development of an insect, a phase akin to hibernation, in which an insect (and pathogens it carries) can survive for prolonged periods when the environment is too cold or too dry to sustain the next developmental stage. See also OVERWINTERING.

diaphragm 1. The muscles at the lower end of the thorax in air-breathing vertebrates that, when they contract, act like a piston to suck air into the lungs. 2. The cervical diaphragm is the barrier method of contraception that acts by preventing passage of spermatozoa to the uterus.

diarrhea Passage of frequent loose, watery stools, often associated with the presence of pathogens responsible for the condition. Diarrhea is a symptom, not a diagnosis. The cause must always be sought. The condition ranges from mildly annoying to acutely life threatening when it is accompanied by severe fluid and electrolyte loss, especially in infants and children, among whom it causes 3 to 4 million deaths annually, despite ORAL REHYDRATION THERAPY (ORT).

diatomaceous earth Syn: kieselguhr. A form of clay containing a high content of calcified or fossilized organisms, including mainly diatoms. It is widely used industrially as an abrasive (which can cause pneumoconiosis), a filtering agent, and an absorbent vehicle for explosives, such as nitroglycerin, i.e., dynamite.

dibenzo[a,h]anthracene One of the emission products of incompletely combusted carbon fuels that is a known animal and probable human carcinogen. It may also be an endocrine function modulator that interferes with androgen receptivity.

dibromochloropropane (DBCP) A liquid pesticide that was used from the 1950s as a soil fumigant to control plant nematodes. In the early 1970s, it was found to be hepatotoxic, an animal carcinogen, and, most significantly, to produce male infertility and sterility by causing gross deformities and malfunction of spermatozoa. Its use is prohibited in the United States and the European Union.

3-3'-dichlorobenzidine One of the aromatic amine dyes, it is a known animal carcinogen and a suspected human bladder carcinogen on the basis of its structural similarity to benzidine.

dichloromethane One of the halogenated industrial solvents; occupational exposure to the fumes of this substance causes angina and myocardial damage.

dieldrin Halogenated organochlorine pesticide that bioaccumulates in the food chain of birds, causing reproductive failure. It is also an animal teratogen and is no longer used. See BIOACCUMULATION.

diesel fuel emissions Combusted diesel fuel often contains a high content of particulate matter, as well as noxious and toxic fumes, including several known and probable human carcinogens, irritant aldehydes, heavy metal contaminants (lead, mercury), and sulfur. Diesel-powered vehicles are a major source of fine particulate matter in urban outdoor air. Stagnant air in densely populated urban areas with many buses and heavy transports may be so loaded with toxic emissions as to present a real danger to health.

diesel oil Petroleum fuel used in heavy traction engines for trucks and buses, often incompletely combusted and a source of emission products that are an important component of urban SMOG.

diet The composition of food intake, often that for a person or a specified group over a specified period, e.g., the daily diet, or dietary intake. There are many specialized diets, some based on religious beliefs, others composed to ameliorate, cure, or prevent specific diseases. Examples include salt-free, gluten-free, and phenylalanine-free diets for hypertension, celiac disease, and phenylketonuria, respectively. Many patients with diabetes follow strict dietary guidelines to limit calorific intake. Many variations of low-calorie diets are popular in upper-income countries where obesity is prevalent. Jews and Moslems have religious beliefs that proscribe pork; orthodox Jews adhere to even more rigorous requirements. Many Hindus and a few Christian sects have a VEGETARIAN diet. In lay language, "dieting" usually means reducing calorie intake to lose weight. See also RECOMMENDED DIETARY ALLOWANCE (RDA).

dietary fiber Cellulose and other indigestible material of vegetable origin that adds bulk to the stools, and enhances the progress of digested material in the gastrointestinal tract. It is believed to be a desirable dietary ingredient, and some epidemiological evidence suggests it protects against diarrhea and some chronic gastrointestinal diseases, so it is a beneficial dietary component.

dietary guidelines A statement of the desirable composition and amount (weight, volume) of food and drink for persons of specified age, sex, occupation, etc. Such a statement of dietary guidelines may be vague and generalized or detailed and precise, the latter being more common, for instance, in RECOMMENDED DIETARY ALLOWANCES (RDAs) for persons with metabolic disorders such as diabetes

mellitus, celiac disease, etc. Many developed nations publish and periodically revise sets of dietary guidelines. See, for example, http://www.health.gov/dietaryguidelines/.

dietetics The science and techniques of composing and supervising diets, usually for people with special needs, such as those who have diabetes, are obese, have metabolic disorders, or have other conditions for which a dietary regimen is important.

diethylstilbestrol (DES) A synthetic estrogen compound with hormonal properties and actions similar to those of naturally occurring (physiologically produced) estrogen. It was used from the 1940s to the early 1970s to treat gynecological conditions, including threatened miscarriage and menopausal symptoms. Unfortunately, it is a mutagen and a carcinogen. Its use in early pregnancy led to the occurrence in offspring of many cases of genital dysplasia and a high incidence of otherwise rare and histologically unusual vaginal cancers in late adolescence and early adult life.

dietitian A health professional who specializes in composing and supervising diets, especially for people with metabolic disorders and many kinds of disease requiring special food intake.

differentials A term used by demographers and vital statisticians to describe the observed rate differences in health experience of specified segments of the population.

diffusion In sociology, the process by which new ideas, rumors, fashions, etc., are communicated and spread in a community, often facilitated by word of mouth as well as via the media.

digester A tank in which solid or semisolid sewage sludge undergoes organic decomposition in the process of settling.

digit preference The tendency when recording measurements on a scale such as the height of the mercury column in a sphygmomanometer to "round off" the reading to the nearest multiple of 10, for example, so an actual reading of blood pressure of 136/72 is recorded as 140/70.

digitalis The active alkaloid ingredient of the garden plant foxglove, *Digitalis purpurea*, the traditional folk remedy for heart disease that was used from medieval times or earlier to treat disorders of the pulse and heart beat. The British physician William Withering (1741–1799) was responsible for the promotion of digitalis from folk to orthodox medicine. Refined and less toxic pharmaceuticals, e.g., digoxin, are prepared from digitalis, or synthetically manufactured.

digitizer A device for converting nominal or numerical data to the binary digit system.

diisocyanates Toxic chemical fumes, principally toluene diisocyanate, produced in manufacture of polyurethane plastics; these substances cause acute respiratory distress. Repeated exposure causes chronic emphysema.

dimercapropanol Syn: BAL (British antilewisite). Under the name British antilewisite, this compound was originally developed as an antidote to the poison gas Lewisite, a form of mustard gas. It was found to be an effective treatment for heavy metal poisoning with lead and mercury compounds, and is still occasionally used as an antidote to poisoning with lead and mercury.

1,1-dimethylhydrazine A substance used as rocket fuel, in the manufacture of antioxidant rubber compounds, in pesticides, and for other purposes. It is a possible human carcinogen. Exposure can cause liver damage, but usually recovery is complete if exposure ceases.

dioxins A family of organochlorine compounds. The most well-studied and most toxic member is 2,3,7,8-tetrachlorodibenzo-*p*-dioxin (2,3,7,8-TCDD), which occurs in trace amounts in some combustion products and in other compounds that have (or had) many industrial uses, notably the phenoxy herbicides, and AGENT ORANGE, in particular. Dioxins cause a disfiguring skin eruption, CHLORACNE, and are carcinogenic and possibly mutagenic.

diphtheria An acute bacterial disease that primarily affects the upper respiratory tract, causing obstruction of the airway. The causal organism, the diphtheria bacillus (*Corynebacterium diphtheriae*), also produces a toxin that causes paralysis of respiratory and peripheral muscles and myocarditis. Until the development of diphtheria vaccines and antisera, there were frequent deadly epidemics, and it was a common cause of death in childhood. It can be prevented by mass immunization of vulnerable infants and children and illustrates the principles of HERD IMMUNITY in that epidemic transmission usually ceases when about 60% to 70% of the susceptible population has been immunized.

diphyllobothriasis The intestinal infection caused by the fish tapeworm, acquired by eating inadequately cooked freshwater lake fish.

diploid A cell having two sets of chromosomes, i.e., in the process of cell division.

dipstick An absorbent strip of paper impregnated with a chemical reagent that changes color on exposure to a specific substance, e.g., acetone, sugar in urine.

directive An administrative order that may have the force of law, i.e., failure to comply may be punished by fines, imprisonment, or other severe sanction.

disability Reduced capacity of a person to perform usual functions, usually the consequence of an IMPAIRMENT, such as impaired mobility or intellectual impairment. May cause HANDICAP.

disability-adjusted life years (DALYs) A population-based measure of the BURDEN OF DISEASE and injury expressed in terms of hypothetical healthy life years that are lost as a result of specified diseases and injuries. DALYs display the difference between a country's life expectancy and either the maximum life expectancy empirically found, which currently is in Japan, or an arbitrary standard of 80 years for males and 82.5 years for females. DALYs comprise lifetimes lost completely because of death and healthy life years "lost" from onsets of nonfatal diseases and injuries, weighted to equivalent years completely lost (e.g., 2 years in a state half as bad as death has a "disability weight" of 0.5). Lost years of healthy life are calculated from a reference life table, usually with life expectancy of 80 years for males and 82.5 years for females. Estimates of DALYs attributable to various causes are derived from many sources, including consolidated mortality and morbidity statistics, health survey data, epidemiological studies, other health indicators, such as health-related census records, expert judgment, and modeling studies aimed at ensuring consistency. DALYs use a "disability weight" multiplied by chronological age to reflect the burden of disability, and yield estimates that accord greater value to fit than to disabled persons and to those in middle years of life than to youthful or elderly people. A methodological weakness of calculating DALYs is inadequate evidence to estimate the impacts of each major specific cause of chronic disability. Another weakness is that the concept of DALYs assumes a continuum from good health to disease, disability, and death that is not universally accepted, especially by representatives of the community of long-term disabled persons. Nevertheless, DALYs are useful in health policy making and in setting priorities. A discussion of the significance and a description of methods used in calculating DALYs can be found at http://www.worldbank.org/html/extdr/hnp/hddflash/workp/wp_00068.html.

disability-free life expectancy An estimate of the number of years a person can expect to live before impairment(s) limit(s) ability to perform usual activities. It is calculated in the same way as LIFE EXPECTANCY, with an adjustment using "disability weight," as with DALYs.

disaster A naturally occurring or manmade event that disrupts the environment and human or animal habitats, causes widespread distress, and often loss of life and usual occupations. Disasters may be sudden, acute, unexpected, unanticipated, short-term or long-term, or slowly developing, insidious, with progressively increasing severity. Examples include floods, droughts, earthquakes, forest fires, and the destruction of life and property accompanying violent armed conflicts. MASS CASUALTIES occur with several varieties of natural and with many manmade disasters.

disaster management Syn: disaster relief. The organized efforts of society to cope with disasters, usually administered by a national or regional agency: by the Federal Emergency Management Agency (FEMA) in the United States and comparable agencies in other countries. Disaster management is a collaborative effort by medical, public health, law enforcement, defense, public administration, and communication sectors of society. Major disasters, such as massive earthquakes, large hurricanes, famines, and the Indian Ocean tsunami of December 2004, require international aid, provided by UN agencies, nongovernmental organization, and voluntary groups. First aid, triage, emergency shelter, provision of food and potable water, vector control, public health services including vaccinations, and reuniting family members are among the high-priority activities in disaster management. Details on management are available at several Web sites, including http://www.fema.gov/ and http://www.unhabitat.org/programmes/rdmu/. Some varieties of natural disasters and many manmade disasters are theoretically preventable.

discharge 1. Formal release of a patient from a hospital, an event that is documented officially for medical, administrative, legal, and financial reasons, and generates a record that can be used to compile hospital discharge statistics. 2. The fluid exudate from a wound, ulcer, or other lesion that allows the escape of body fluids. 3. Release of emissions or factory waste products into the environment, often causing contamination of air, water, or ground with toxic substances.

discharge planning Organized efforts by medical, nursing, social support, and other personnel to ensure that persons discharged from the hospital receive effective care on re-entering the community.

discounting An adjustment to cost estimates to allow for the fact that future monetary units

(dollars, pounds, Euros, etc.) will have a different value from those at present, usually a smaller value because of the effects of inflation. Discounting applies an interest rate equivalent to the rate of inflation to produce estimates of future values at specified future times.

discount rate The specific numerical calculation that is applied to arrive at an estimate of the future value of monetary units.

discriminant analysis A statistical method used to separate two or more sets of data that are initially mixed together.

discrimination The process of making distinctions among a mixed group of people, usually with the implication that some prejudice is applied in making these distinctions. It has often been accompanied by some form of SEGREGATION and victimization.

disease Literally, dis-ease, the opposite of ease or comfort, a general word descriptive of any departure from good health. Best applied to a physiological and/or psychological departure from normal function, as contrasted with ILLNESS, which is the subjective state of the diseased person. A disease is a conceptual entity defined by clinical, pathological, and epidemiological criteria that enable it to be studied systematically.

disease control The method(s) and procedure(s) used to prevent and/or treat disease. This is the main business of public health practice. Preventive methods are classified as primary, secondary, and tertiary PREVENTION. In practice, control of communicable diseases relies on surveillance, notification of cases of contagious and other communicable diseases, specific control measures such as isolation and application of measures such as chemoprophylaxis, vector control for vectorborne diseases, and many other specific and general control methods. Other methods of control are used to reduce the effects of injury, cancer, heart disease, and harmful behaviors, such as use of aggression and domestic violence, excessive alcohol consumption, and cigarette smoking.

disease register A documentary account of persons with specified disease(s). This may be a listing of patients attending a clinic or hospital arranged in diagnostic categories, e.g., patients with epilepsy, congenital heart disease, or drug dependency. However, the term is usually applied to a population-based, disease-specific register, or REGISTRY, that records information about all persons in a specified diagnostic category in a defined jurisdiction, e.g., a CANCER REGISTRY.

disease taxonomy A taxonomy is an orderly system of nomenclature that abides by set rules and procedures. Disease taxonomies vary in their adherence to this principle. Some aspects, such as the chapters in the International Classification of Diseases, follow an anatomical or body-system orientation, and others are based on etiology and pathogenesis.

disinfectant A chemical solution or substance that can be applied to contaminated sites, such as toilets, hospital floors, and, in the case of some disinfectants, to skin surfaces, in order to kill pathogens, preferably without harm to other living things, including humans and domestic pets.

disinfection The process of treating an area (e.g., of skin surface) or an environment to rid it of pathogenic organisms by applying a DISINFECTANT.

disinfestation Use of chemical agents to eliminate infestation of the body with external parasites such as *Sarcoptes scabiei*, the pathogen responsible for SCABIES.

disinsection, disinsectization Treatment of an environment, such as a warehouse or a goods container, with an insecticide or other substance (e.g., a poisonous gas) to rid it of insect pests.

disparities in health Syn: inequalities. Differing levels of health indicators, such as life expectancy and infant and perinatal mortality rates, that are observed among segments of a population, discernible in the size of the HEALTH GAP between the highest and the lowest segment of the population, that often correlate with economic indicators, educational level, employment, and housing conditions. Disparities in health were recognized as a challenge to public health systems and services by the English medical statistician WILLIAM FARR. They have provided incentives for initiatives aimed at improving living conditions and health status for deprived communities, such as ethnic minority groups in upper-income countries, and for international nongovernmental organizations in low-income countries.

dispensary A place that provides pharmaceutical preparations, drugs, dressings, and medications for those who need them, located often in a hospital or clinic, or more often a free-standing drug store, shop, or agency. Also the name given to the book in which the composition of medications is recorded.

displaced persons People who have been obliged by war, natural disaster, political persecution, ethnic cleansing, or other cause, to relinquish their usual home and habitat, and seek refuge elsewhere within their own country, i.e., INTERNALLY DISPLACED PERSONS in the terminology of the United Nations. The same people are designated REFUGEES when they cross the frontier into another country. The intergovernmental organization that deals with displaced persons is the International Organization for Migration (IOM), and the United Nations High Commissioner for Refugees (UNHCR) manages the care of refugees. Many nongovernmental organizations also participate in provision of aid to both displaced persons and refugees.

distal cause A cause that underlies or is remote from the more obvious direct cause of a departure from good health. For example, atmospheric contamination with ozone-destroying substances, such as CHLOROFLUOROCARBON compounds, is a distal cause of skin cancer due to increased ultraviolet radiation flux.

distal risk factor A behavioral or environmental factor that has a remote or indirect causal influence on a specific disease outcome. Many etiological factors in chronic diseases fall into this category. This does not mean a relationship that is remote in time, or one that has a long latency period, but one that acts indirectly by way of its influence on the chain of causation. An example is the presence in the atmosphere of ozone-destroying substances, such as freon gas from air conditioning equipment leading to attenuation of the ozone layer, higher levels of biologically active ultraviolet solar radiation, and consequently greater risk of skin cancer and cataract. Thus, the use of ozone-destroying substances is a distal risk factor for skin cancer and cataract.

distance education A set of educational methods that can be used to teach people who are remote from their teacher(s). Formerly this relied on correspondence courses, in which written or printed lessons, projects, problems, and examination questions were distributed to students by mail. Today the entire process, known as distance learning, usually operates via the Internet or by radio or television links.

distribution-free method A method of statistical analysis that does not depend on the mathematical form of the underlying distribution that is being analyzed.

distributive justice A term used in BIOETHICS to describe equitable, even-handed distribution of goods and services, and impartial decisions, in contrast to prejudicial decisions. Distributive justice is the aim of an egalitarian society and may involve initiatives such as AFFIRMATIVE ACTION that "level the playing field" or right past wrongs by providing preferential services for disadvantaged population subgroups. Because this is not impartial, it is sometimes perceived as unjust and therefore presents new ethical problems.

diuretic A pharmaceutical preparation used to treat fluid retention by promoting renal excretion of electrolytes and the fluid in which they are dissolved.

diving injuries The principal occupational injury risk for commercial divers is BAROTRAUMA. Recreational divers using compressed air tanks are also at risk of barotrauma. Other common injuries include spinal cord injuries, not uncommonly quadriplegia, caused by crush injury to the cervical spine following a dive into shallow water, and lacerations from reef shellfish, coral, etc.

Dix, Dorothea (1802–1887) An American social activist and reformer, best known for her advocacy of humane treatment for persons with mental illness.

DMF Abbreviation for decayed, missing, filled teeth, a term used mainly in dental epidemiology as an indicator of dental health level in a population.

DNA See DEOXYRIBONUCLEIC ACID.

DNA typing Each individual has a unique sequence of DNA that is the basis for individuality. An individual's sequence of DNA codes is identified by the POLYMERASE CHAIN REACTION to magnify the amount of DNA available for analysis. DNA typing has great utility in forensic medicine.

Doctors Without Borders See MÉDECINS SANS FRONTIÈRES (MSF).

domestic violence A general term for violence directed against children in a family, i.e., CHILD ABUSE; against a spouse or partner; against a dependent older person, i.e., ELDER ABUSE; or against some other household member.

dominance A position of ascendancy or influence over another. In biology, a species that is dominant over another that occupies the same ecosystem. In genetics, the expression of alleles in the phenotype in contrast to the failure of alleles to be expressed, in which case they are recessive. See RECESSIVE TRAIT.

Donora A city near Pittsburgh in Pennsylvania that in 1948 was the setting for a severe SMOG episode that caused many respiratory deaths due to exacerbation of chronic respiratory disease. The Donora disaster provided impetus to clean air legislation in the United States.

do not resuscitate (DNR) A medical request issued by a doctor and/or patient or next of kin that, in the event of cardiac and/or respiratory arrest, no resuscitation measures should be conducted, but the patient should be allowed to die in comfort without heroic intervention.

dose The quantity of a drug, ionizing radiation, etc., administered to a person for therapeutic purposes. The word is used colloquially to describe an episode of illness, as in "a dose of flu."

dose-response relationship The relationship of observed outcomes in a patient or population to the quantity of medication or level of exposure to an environmental health determinant. For instance, a linear dose-response relationship reflects a direct increase in risk as exposure increases. The dose-response relationship has central importance in toxicology and environmental health. The cumulative dose, as well as the size of an individual dose, may be important, for instance, in exposure to trace amounts of carcinogens, such as those in tobacco.

dosimeter An instrument for measuring the quantity of an agent (e.g., ionizing radiation) or drug or other substance to which persons or a population are or may be exposed.

double-blind study A RANDOMIZED CONTROLLED TRIAL in which the allocation of study subjects to receive or not receive the regimen being tested is concealed from both the subjects and from the investigator(s) conducting the trial. The aim is to reduce the effects of BIAS, such as the PLACEBO effect and the HALO EFFECT, as well as selection bias and observer bias. Some people consider the use of the word "blind" offensive in this context, and to respect their sensibility the term "double-masked study" is proposed as an alternative.

double helix The architectural shape of paired DNA strands in the nucleus of cells in the process of cell division.

doubling time The average time it takes for a population to double in size. A population with a high proportion of young people in the reproductive age group, a high birth rate, and a high completed family size, has a brief doubling time. Kenya, with a doubling time of about 20 years, is an example of a nation with a very brief doubling time. In several western European nations, e.g., France, Italy, Sweden, the population is not increasing—the doubling time is infinite.

douche A jet of water or a watery solution directed at part of the body (as in a shower). The term is usually applied to a vaginal douche, used (usually ineffectively) to wash out the vagina after sexual intercourse as a contraceptive method or as a feminine hygiene practice.

doula Also daula. A word derived from Greek δουλη, meaning "experienced woman," specifically a woman who is capable of assisting normal childbirth. In obstetrics and medical anthropology, a doula is a laywoman who assists normal childbirth in a birthing center, or a traditional village midwife, who is sometimes a traditional healer. A doula often also advises on aspects of infant care, feeding, etc.

Down syndrome Syn: trisomy 21 syndrome. An inborn defect in which the affected person has an extra chromosome 21, a condition of unknown origin that apparently starts at conception and may be associated with a defect in male or female chromosomes. The physical stigmata (formerly called "mongolism") affect facial appearance, stature, and the limbs, including the hands, and intellectual development is retarded to varying degrees. Affected children may have other problems, such as congenital heart disease, increased risk of leukemia, and amyloid brain plaques resembling those of Alzheimer's disease. The eponym for the condition commemorates the British physician John L. H. Down (1828–1896), who provided the first detailed clinical description.

downward mobility A sociological term for progression from a higher to an inferior position in the socioeconomic scale, e.g., from an original professional or managerial status to an unskilled working class status. Downward mobility is associated with chronic mental and personality disorders, alcoholism, and substance abuse. It also commonly happens to displaced persons and refugees who become immigrants to countries where their qualifications are not recognized. Downward mobility characteristically is associated with poor health outcomes.

DPT, DPTP Initial letters of the combined vaccines for diphtheria-pertussis-tetanus and diphtheria-pertussis-tetanus-poliomyelitis, recommended for immunizing infants against these diseases. See VACCINE-PREVENTABLE DISEASE, usually given in coordination with the MMR VACCINE.

dracunculiasis Syn: Guinea worm disease. Infection with a nematode worm, *Dracunculus medinensis*, that has a life cycle in which the larval stage is passed in minute freshwater Crustacea (*Copepoda*, or water fleas). These infect humans when they drink water containing the water fleas. The disease was formerly common in West Africa, Yemen, and India. It is yielding to efforts to eradicate it but is still endemic in about a dozen countries in Sub-Saharan Africa.

drain 1. A channel, conduit, or gutter that carries wastewater or sewage from its place of origin. An open drain such as those commonly found in many low-income countries can be a source of infection if children play in it or people drink water from it. 2. In surgery, a tube or packing to release pressure of accumulated fluid, sometimes a potential source of nosocomial or hospital-acquired cross-infection.

drainage A network of drains, as in a reticulated sewage disposal system. Also used to describe the CATCHMENT AREA of a water reservoir.

Dr Foster A Web site that provides access to information about all aspects of health care in the United Kingdom, including descriptions of diseases and their appropriate treatment, health care services, and contact details for general practitioners and consultants (specialists) arranged by locality, etc. The site is accessible to the general public and health professions. See http://www.drfoster.co.uk.

drift Movement of water, air, people, or things, generally in a particular direction. See GENETIC DRIFT and SOCIAL MOBILITY.

drinking water Syn: potable water. Water that is safe and fit for drinking without risk of disease caused by pathogens or chemical contaminants. Water is essential to life. The required daily intake varies with environmental conditions and physiological demands. On average, an adult weighing 70 kg has a minimum daily requirement of 2.5 liters, more if fluid loss is increased by sweating in hot conditions or hard physical work.

droplet A small drop of fluid such as mucous secretion, technically a drop just visible to the naked eye, that can remain airborne briefly and may be projected for distances up to 1 to 2 meters by sneezing, even by talking. It is a common source of person-to-person spread of pathogenic organisms.

droplet nuclei Particles from 1 to 5 microns in size that are the desiccated residue of liquid aerosol drops or droplets emitted in coughing, sneezing, or speaking, comprising dehydrated mucous secretions that usually contain viable microorganisms, including pathogens. Some disease agents, notably *Mycobacterium tuberculosis*, can survive for long periods in droplet nuclei and cause disease when they eventually invade a susceptible host.

dropout Someone who leaves or defaults from a setting where they have been observed, e.g., a dropout from the educational system, a dropout from an epidemiological or social study.

drug A substance, such as a chemical compound, that is used for medicinal purposes. The word applies to all such substances, but popular usage may imply that it modifies the mood and/or emotional state of the person who takes it. Drugs can be classified as PRESCRIPTION DRUGS, which are prescribed by a physician; PROPRIETARY drugs, which carry a trademark; GENERIC DRUGS, often marketed under their pharmaceutical names; OVER-THE-COUNTER DRUGS, which can be purchased by the general public in a pharmacy or shop; and ILLICIT DRUGS, which are mainly addictive narcotics or mood-modifying substances that are prohibited by law.

drug abuse, addiction The term used to describe inappropriate and usually compulsive and irrational use of prescribed or over-the-counter medication and (more commonly) to describe the use of illicit addictive drugs.

drug dependence The condition of people unable to function without resort to a drug or drugs, whether licit or illicit, to which they have become pharmacologically addicted or habituated. Drug dependence may be physical (pharmacological) or psychological and may be associated with tolerance of larger doses than normally tolerated.

Drug Enforcement Administration (DEA) The US government agency that aims to control the problems associated with drug dependency and addiction. The name of the agency implies a coercive and punitive approach, and its methods are mainly based on the premise that these are criminal activities, rather than illnesses requiring treatment and prevention. The DEA devotes very little of its budget or professional expertise to medical, social, and public health aspects, including prevention and treatment of drug abuse. See http://www.usdoj.gov/dea/.

drug sensitivity A term usually applied to unusual susceptibility to the action of a drug or to an atypical, idiosyncratic, or adverse reaction. Because it is imprecise, the term is preferably avoided.

dump A place where solid waste is deposited, with the implication that no environmental protection measures are employed.

dumping The act of disposing of waste—solid waste on land, liquid waste, such as bunker oil, at sea—with the implicit assumption that this is done irresponsibly.

dunnage Material used to secure a cargo in a ship's hold or on the deck, or the contents of a cargo container. Scraps of wood and cardboard are commonly used, and are often the vehicle that carries unwanted passengers such as larvae of insect vectors or pathogenic organisms. Ensuring that dunnage is free from this risk is seldom part of the precautions that exporters and importers take against introduction to new ecosystems of quarantinable or other diseases of plants, animals, and humans.

dust Fine particles of solid matter. There are many varieties, some naturally occurring, such as fine particles of earth that are blown about by the wind in the process of soil erosion, and many varieties of industrial origin, most of which have adverse effects on health.

dust mites Tiny arthropods, invisible to the naked eye, that live indoors on carpets, mattresses, bedding, etc. Individuals can become sensitized to house dust mite fecal allergens, and this may be a cause of increased episodes of asthma.

duty An obligation to act, perform a function; also the function itself. The obligation may be identified as part of a job description or a moral responsibility. See also FIDUCIARY RESPONSIBILITY.

dyes A large, miscellaneous group of substances that change the color of cloth or other material when they are immersed in the substance or it is applied to the surface. Some occur naturally, e.g., indigo, which was greatly prized in antiquity for this property. German organic chemists developed many ANILINE dyes in the late 19th and early 20th century, and these became the basis for large and powerful chemical corporations. Other valuable products, including antibiotics and explosives, were developed from the same organic chemical bases.

dynamic population A population that is changing in composition, e.g., age distribution.

dysentery Bloody diarrhea, either chronic and intermittent or continuous, caused by chronic inflammatory or infective disease of the intestinal tract. The numerous causes include infection with bacteria, amebae, or intestinal parasites.

dysfunction Departure from normal physiological and or psychological function.

dysgenic (adj) An agent that has adverse effects on genes or chromosomes, e.g., ionizing radiation, many industrial chemicals.

dyslexia A common learning disorder of children that sometimes persists into adult life, characterized by inadequate ability to recognize words or individual letters in words, and, when copying these down, to make mistakes in transcription. It can be dangerous when workers fail to read or misread and therefore misunderstand warning labels on toxic products.

E

ear protectors Devices to protect the organs of hearing, i.e., eardrums, auditory ossicles, and cochlea from loud NOISE, e.g., due to machinery, gunfire. The simplest ear protectors consist of ear plugs that fit in the external auditory canals. Larger devices resembling headphones fit over the head and effectively insulate against very loud noise, e.g., from nearby jet aircraft engines.

early detection A phrase describing prompt identification of incipient or early disease and, by implication, intervention to arrest, treat, and cure it in a timely manner; and the early detection of environmental, social, and behavioral hazards to health. Methods of early detection include questionnaires, interviews, physical examinations, SCREENING tests, procedures and equipment for environmental monitoring, e.g., of drinking water, indoor air quality, ionizing radiation levels. Early detection is an important role of primary care physicians, who can use many opportunities that arise in the course of incidental and continuing care of patients to conduct simple screening tests for early evidence of serious conditions, such as cardiovascular disease, diabetes, and cancer.

early warning system In public health, methods and procedures used in SURVEILLANCE to detect, as soon as possible, any departure from normal that may indicate an impending public health emergency, such as an epidemic. Early warning systems focus mainly on communicable diseases, e.g., epidemic influenza, which can declare its presence by an otherwise unexplained sudden increase in sickness absences from work and deaths from pneumonia. Epidemiological surveillance is the main defense against new and EMERGING PATHOGENS. Early warning systems also employ environmental monitoring, e.g., of the distribution and abundance of insect vectors, detection of trace amounts of environmental toxins, and abnormally high levels of ionizing radiation.

Earth Charter A statement of principles considered essential for sustainable development drafted by environmentalists and endorsed by many agencies and some local governments in various parts of the world, setting out what were considered to be realistic goals for consumption of resources and disposal of waste in ways that are considered sustainable. Details and the text of the Charter can be seen at http://www.earthcharter.org/.

earthquake A natural DISASTER caused by tectonic plate movement. Earthquakes vary greatly in frequency, duration, and character, and in intensity, which is measured on the logarithmic RICHTER SCALE. Regions where tectonic plate movement is greatest are most earthquake prone. Some earthquake-prone regions also have active volcanoes. Earthquakes and some volcanic eruptions can lead to great loss of life when people are crushed by falling masonry or drowned in tsunamis, and can be followed by epidemics, e.g., due to contaminated water supplies and other health-related sequelae associated with destruction and severe damage to infrastructure. Like all natural disasters, earthquakes require RAPID EPIDEMIOLOGICAL ASSESSMENT and considerable deployment of public health services.

Earth Summit Syn: Rio Summit. The United Nations conference on sustainable development in Rio de Janeiro in 1992, at which most of the world's political leaders acknowledged that the future of the human race required measures to achieve a balance between environmental sustainability and economic development. There was little agreement about ways to achieve this balance. The relationship of public health to sustainable development was not discussed. See also JOHANNESBURG SUMMIT, KYOTO PROTOCOL, and WORLD SUMMIT ON SUSTAINABLE DEVELOPMENT.

eastern equine encephalitis One of several ARBOVIRUS diseases spread by Culex mosquitoes in North America; it is primarily a disease of birds, but both horses and humans can be affected.

Ebola fever A severe viral hemorrhagic fever that occurs in occasional and mostly localized epidemics in central Africa. It causes high fever and multiple hemorrhages from mucosae, including in the eyes, nose, mouth, and gastrointestinal tract. It has a very high case fatality rate, ranging from 50% to 90%. It is caused by a filovirus that is presumably transmitted to humans from wild animals or their meat or skins because epidemics have been associated with killing and eating "bush meat," i.e., locally available monkeys and rodents. See also EBOLA-MARBURG VIRUS DISEASES and the Web site listed there for further information.

Ebola-Marburg virus diseases Acute tropical hemorrhagic fevers with a high case fatality rate, caused by related but antigenically distinct viruses in the filovirus group. Some members of this group of diseases may be zoonotic infections of rodents or monkeys, but the host species of others, including the usual central African form of

Ebola disease, is not known. A summary of the current status is available at http://www.cdc.gov/ncidod/dvrd/spb/mnpages/dispages/ebola.htm.

echinococcosis See HYDATID DISEASE.

eclampsia Syn: toxemia of pregnancy. An acute life-threatening disease occurring usually late in pregnancy, characterized by severe hypertension, fluid retention, renal failure, convulsions, etc. If detected early and given appropriate treatment, it can be reversed. Without early and aggressive treatment, it can be life threatening.

E. coli See *ESCHERICHIA COLI.*

ecological fallacy Syn: aggregation bias, ecological bias. An error of logical inference arising from confusion of data at different levels of organization. An example is "particularizing from the general" by assuming that a particular individual faces the same risk of dying from coronary heart disease as the whole population in the "risk category" to which the individual belongs. It can arise in studies of exposures and outcomes in groups, rather than individuals, when probabilities based on groups are particularized to persons.

ecological footprint The dimensions and composition of the ecosystem(s) required to sustain a population, or a particular part of it, such as a hospital, a factory, a holiday resort complex, a jet passenger aircraft. The term is applied mainly to large urban populations to draw attention to their required input of resources and output of waste products, which almost always exceed those available within their political boundaries by a wide margin.

ecological niche The habitat to which a species is, or can become, adapted. Colonization, mass migration, and globalized trade and commerce have led to transport of many species from their original habitat to other places. For example, *Aedes albopictus*, the Asian tiger mosquito, was imported to southern Europe and to the southern United States as larvae in pools of water in car tires imported for retreading. This robust mosquito easily withstands cold winter weather. It found a favorable ecological niche in its new environment and has proliferated widely. It is a vector for dengue and viral encephalitis, and became a local disease vector in its adopted habitat.

ecological study An investigation in which population groups, rather than individuals, are the unit of study, usually aimed at identifying and explaining association between the groups and their environments. As a research method, ecological study is fraught with difficult problems, notably the inability to allow for the effects of CONFOUNDING variables. See also ECOLOGICAL FALLACY.

ecology The scientific study of interrelationships among all the organisms that occupy a habitat, and between all these organisms and their environment, i.e., the ECOSYSTEM. Ecologists often study discrete, specified ecosystems, such as a freshwater lake, transition zones between savannah and desert, or coral reefs, seeking to identify stressors, determinants of stability, etc. The word was coined by the German zoologist Ernst Haeckel (1834–1919).

econometrics The branch of economics concerned with collating and analyzing economic data.

economic index The term "index" is used by economists in several contexts, most commonly in the expressions COST OF LIVING INDEX and INFLATION INDEX, which both reflect the declining value of monetary units over time.

economics The branch of scholarly activity concerned with the production, consumption, and transfer of goods, services, and wealth, and with the allocation of finite resources. Economics has many specialties including, MACROECONOMICS, MICROECONOMICS, and HEALTH ECONOMICS.

economy class syndrome Peripheral venous thrombosis that can be a consequence, especially for middle-aged and elderly passengers, of sitting more or less immobile in long-haul jet aircraft, particularly but not only in the cramped economy class seats. Inability to move about causes venous stasis, which encourages thrombosis. Occasional fatalities occur from this condition.

ecosystem An identifiable entity in which the resident living organisms interact with one another and with their inanimate environment in such a manner that the flow of energy among all remains approximately constant and in balance. Ecosystems range in size from the entire biosphere to a drop of pond water, comprising all the living organisms and nonliving components that interact in the system. The term was coined by the British biologist A. G. Tansley (1871–1955).

ecosystem distress syndrome The situation that arises when the balanced equilibrium of an ecosystem is disrupted by a failure or disruption of an essential link or links in its chain of being. This can happen as a consequence of human-induced pollution of a water source, introduction of alien species, a change in prevailing temperature range or other environmental conditions, or many possible combinations of these variables.

Although there may be no adverse effects on human health, there are sometimes indirect health consequences. An example with beneficial effects on human health is draining swamps, which destroys an aquatic ecosystem but, by eliminating mosquito breeding sites, reduces the risk of mosquito-borne diseases such as malaria. An example with adverse health effects is the ecosystem distress in an industrial zone, such as that in which a mining and smelting operation or a petrochemical plant has polluted the environment, killed the vegetation, destroyed wildlife habitat, and exposed human residents to toxic substances such as lead, mercury, and organic compounds such as dioxins and PCBs.

Ecstasy Syn: MDMA. The popular name for a powerful derivative of METHAMPHETAMINE, easily made in clandestine laboratories, taken in pill form, and used to induce a state of euphoria ("high"), mainly by young people in group settings, such as nightclub rave parties. It causes altered states of consciousness, hallucinations, and side effects including tachycardia, hypertension, and acute heart failure, and its use may be followed by rebound depression and paranoia. It is addictive. See also CRYSTAL METH.

ectropion A condition of outward deviation of the eyelids, associated with advanced aging and loss of elasticity of the skin that prevents the eyes from closing efficiently so the conjunctivae and corneas become inflamed and easily infected. Untreated ectropion endangers eyesight.

eczema An inflammatory condition of the skin associated with redness, scaling, itching, and perhaps serous or purulent exudation that may be localized or generalized and has many possible causes, including allergies, occupational irritants, and impaired immune responses.

edema Accumulation of fluid in the tissues, as a result of venous obstruction or fluid-electrolyte imbalance, e.g., in renal failure, impaired peripheral circulation as in cardiac decompensation, etc.

EDTA See ETHYLENE DIAMINE TETRA ACETIC ACID.

education The process of receiving or giving systematic instruction, and transfer of knowledge, ideas, concepts, methods, techniques between a teacher or educator and a learner or student. Education is an integral component of many aspects of public health practice. Public health nurses educate pregnant women and new mothers about prenatal and postnatal care. Health promotion and health education are essential features of health maintenance, used in smoking cessation programs, cardiovascular fitness regimens, dental hygiene, and dietary regimens, and are provided by television and print media, as well as by family physicians, public health professionals, dentists, and other health professionals.

educational objectives Specific statements about expectations at the end of an educational course or program, usually expressed in relation to three domains. The cognitive domain is the knowledge acquired; the affective domain is the set of emotions or values changed by the program or course; and the psychomotor domain is the set of new skills and behavior patterns acquired as a result of the course or program. These objectives are assessed in many ways during health professional training programs and in other settings, such as KAP surveys, that are an integral feature of family planning programs, especially in low-income countries. See also KAP.

education and training for public health A phrase encompassing all aspects of preparation for a professional role and responsibility in public health practice. The content, methods, and results depend on the profession. In the case of public health nurses and physicians, it includes extensive professional education in classroom and practical sessions interspersed with in-service training.

effective dose The smallest quantity of a pathogenic agent or concentration of a substance that is capable of producing a measurable outcome, such as occurrence of disease or relief of symptoms. Applied to ionizing radiation such as x-rays, it is an exposure level adequate for diagnostic purposes but insufficient to have harmful consequences. When long-term followup studies revealed adverse effects of even small exposures to diagnostic x-rays, this dose was revised downward. In toxicology, ED50 is the dose that has a measurable effect on 50% of subjects. Compare LD50.

effective population size The average number of people in the population who (a) contribute genes to the next generation or (b) are required to sustain a communicable disease agent in the population indefinitely, as herd immunity declines or new susceptible members are added to the population at a rate balancing or exceeding the numbers becoming immune after infection.

effective stack height The height of a factory chimney stack considered adequate for dispersal of emissions into the atmosphere that in combination with convection currents and prevailing winds is believed adequate to dilute toxic emissions to safe levels. The critical word is "adequate": emissions can remain harmful to people, other living things, and the fabric of buildings, no matter how diluted and dispersed by air movement.

effectiveness As used in clinical epidemiology, this is a measure of the extent to which a medical intervention, such as preventive immunization, dietary regimen, or surgical procedure, does what it is supposed to do. It can be assessed in quantitative terms, for instance, when weight reduction is a measure of the effectiveness of dietary intervention.

effect modifier A factor that modifies the action of a causal factor. For example, age modifies the effect for many conditions, and immunization status modifies the action of pathogenic organisms as causal factors in specific communicable diseases. See also CONFOUNDING.

efficacy The capacity to produce an effect. In clinical epidemiology, the extent to which an intervention produces a beneficial result under ideal circumstances. In health care services, the benefit or utility to an individual of a preventive or therapeutic regimen or service or a disease-control program.

efficiency 1. The end results achieved in relation to expenditure of money, resources, effort, and time that have been aimed at achieving these results. This is a measure of the economy or resource costs in relation to the output or end results of an intervention. 2. In statistics, efficiency is the precision with which a study design or a test can estimate a parameter of interest. In HEALTH ECONOMICS, several categories of efficiency are recognized, including: ALLOCATIVE EFFICIENCY, concerned with resource allocation; PRODUCTIVE EFFICIENCY, concerned with identifying the best way to produce desired health outcomes, and TECHNICAL EFFICIENCY, concerned with the suitability and quality of equipment, facilities, etc.

effluent This word is used (often with pejorative associations) to describe all forms of matter that flow out from a source: the outflow of storm or waste water, sewage, industrial pollutants, gaseous emission products from a factory or furnace, and the products of radioactive decay.

effluent guidelines, regulations Discharge of household waste water, sewage, and many specific industrial toxic by-products into rivers, lakes, and the sea is unregulated in some jurisdictions, subject to voluntary guidelines in some and to regulations of varying rigor and enforceability in others. Problems and disputes arise in many circumstances, for instance, when standards vary in different jurisdictions sharing riparian rights to

the same waterway, as was the case with the Rhine and Danube rivers in Europe until international agreements and European Union directives addressed the issue. A similar set of problems and issues was addressed by the International Joint Commission that deals with the North American Great Lakes. Gaseous effluent guidelines are often included in CLEAN AIR ACTS.

effluent sampling Procedures aimed at assessing the composition of industrial effluents. These procedures may specify sampling methods, or sampling may be haphazard. They are usually the responsibility of local health and environmental agencies, who may or may not have the authority to order corrective action when effluent discharges are found to be harmful.

egg count Syn: cyst count. Microscopic examination of feces for presence and number of eggs and cysts of intestinal parasites, including helminths, protozoa, and encysted bacteria.

egg products Eggs are a staple dietary item and have numerous uses and varieties of culinary preparation and presentation. Most are safe and nutritionally beneficial. Eggs occasionally carry pathogens, such as certain *Salmonella* species, and they have a high cholesterol content, but many dietitians believe the benefits of egg products outweigh possible hazards from the high cholesterol level, although not, of course, the risk of contaminating pathogens.

Ehrlich, Paul (1854–1915) German organic chemist whose work on dyes led him into studies of suitable stains to identify bacteria and thus to searching for drugs to treat bacterial infections, especially syphilis. In collaboration with others at the Koch Institute, in Berlin, he developed the arsenical compound salvarsan, the so-called MAGIC BULLET, which killed the treponema of syphilis without killing the patient. He received the Nobel Prize for Physiology or Medicine in 1908 for this work.

ekistics The study of human settlements with particular reference to how they adapt and evolve in changing circumstances, how they function, and the cultural, social, occupational, and economic interactions of the people in a settlement. The word was coined by the visionary Greek architect and urban planner Constantinos A. Doxiadis (1913–1975) and first used by him in lectures delivered in 1942.

elder abuse Physical or psychological assault or aggression directed against elderly people, whether by a family member, in the form of DOMESTIC VIOLENCE or other maltreatment, or by strangers, such as a street gang of teenagers.

eldercare A set of services that include both formal and informal arrangements for home and community-based care of elderly people, including friendly visits, provision of hot meals, home nursing care, etc., usually paid for by a combination of public funds and charitable donations.

electrolyte An ion or compound derived from an element, such as sodium, potassium, or carbon, that when dissolved or suspended in a liquid medium transmits an electric current and is deposited on the positive or negative electrode, depending on whether the electrolyte is negatively or positively charged. Electrolytes are normally in biochemical balance in serum and other body fluids. An essential feature of intensive care is maintenance of electrolyte balance.

electromagnetic field (EMF) The zone around an electrical power source in which instruments can detect ELECTROMAGNETIC RADIATION. This has two components: electric power measured by voltage and magnetic radiation produced by the current.. Electromagnetic fields that may harm health possibly include those generated by mobile or cellular telephones. Electric field strength (volts/meter) depends on the voltage independent of current size. Magnetic field strength (amps/meter) reflects the amount of current passing through a conductor, independent of voltage, and is produced by moving electric charges. A 50 to 60 Hz electrical and magnetic field moves along a live domestic electric power cable, but the strength diminishes with distance from the source. Common building materials shield against electric, but not against magnetic, fields. Both components have biological effects at extremely high levels not experienced by the general population. Power frequency magnetic fields from high-voltage electric power lines, transformers, etc., have been found in epidemiological studies to be associated with an increased risk of cancer, especially leukemia and possibly brain cancer in occupationally exposed adults and residentially exposed children. The mechanism is unknown. See also EXTREMELY LOW FREQUENCY (ELF) ELECTROMAGNETIC RADIATION.

electromagnetic radiation Waves of energy that travel through space at the speed of light, possessing properties of waves (radiation) and particles (photons, neutrons, etc.). There are several interrelated but distinct and different components of the same phenomenon, each with varying effects on health and physiological function according to its wavelength. The shortest wavelength cosmic and gamma waves and ultraviolet radiation are mutagenic and carcinogenic. Life as we know it is possible on earth only because the earth's mag-

netic fields and the ozone layer in the ionosphere filter out most of the harmful radiation before it penetrates to the biosphere. Longer wavelength electromagnetic radiation has zero, minimal, or equivocal human health effects that are the subject of considerable research interest. See also IONIZING RADIATION.

electromagnetic spectrum The range of frequencies and wavelengths of electromagnetic radiation. These extend from very short wavelength highly penetrating cosmic and gamma rays, through ultraviolet, visible light and infrared, to longer wavelength radio waves. Cosmic and gamma rays have wavelengths in the range of 10^{-17} to 10^{-11} meters; x-rays, 10^{-10} to 10^{-8} meters; ultraviolet light, 230–400 nm (UV-A: 320–400 nm, UV-B: 200–320 nm, UV-C: 230–290 nm); visible light, 740–390 nm; infrared radiation, 10^{-5} to 10^{-3} to meters; and radiofrequency waves, 10^{-2} to 10^5 meters.

electromyography The instrumental measurement of the minute electrical charges generated during muscle contraction and relaxation. Electrocardiography is a specialized variety of this.

electron microscopy Use of beams of electrons to visualize very small objects. Electron beams have wavelengths of 0.04 nanometers (nm) and can reach a resolving power of 0.2 to 0.5 nm. Scanning electron microscopes produce a three-dimensional perspective image, although the resolving power is somewhat less than that of transmission electron microscopes.

electrophoresis Migration of electrically charged particles in a colloidal solution toward the electrode with the opposite charge. This is the underlying process in the SOUTHERN BLOT and similar diagnostic test procedures.

electrostatic precipitation A useful, although rather costly, method of removing suspended atmospheric particles is to filter air through a grill with positively and negatively charged plates, to which suspended particles are attracted and on which most of them are deposited.

elimination 1. In physiology, excretion of waste metabolic products, such as hydrogen ions, urea, and carbon dioxide in expired air. 2. The control of a previously prevalent communicable disease by reducing case transmission to a predetermined low level, although not necessarily to zero. The aim is to achieve a situation where the infecting agent cannot sustain itself in the population or, as with leprosy, with an elimination threshold of less than 1 case per 10,000 population, until the disease no longer presents a major public health problem. In 1991, WHO defined this threshold for tuberculosis as attainment of a prevalence rate of active cases below one case per million. Elimination differs from ERADICATION OF DISEASE in offering the potential for the disease to return if the host-agent-environment conditions change in favor of the agent. This approach has worked well in the regional elimination of poliomyelitis and measles in many industrial nations.

ELISA See ENZYME-LINKED IMMUNOSORBENT ASSAY.

El Niño A warm sea current originating in the western Pacific equatorial region that flows east from the Indonesian archipelago, across the Pacific Ocean, then south along the coast of Ecuador and Peru. The location where the current reaches South America periodically fluctuates in relation to other climatic changes that profoundly affect weather conditions over much of the world quite remote from South America. An El Niño southern oscillation (ENSO) is correlated with heat waves and droughts in the heartland of North America and Australia and with anomalous weather and precipitation in Europe, Africa, and Asia. El Niño oscillations do not cause these widespread climatic changes; they are merely one of the observed effects of more fundamental processes that affect the global climate. Similar changes in the Caribbean Sea, Gulf Stream, and other Atlantic Ocean currents influence the frequency and strength of violent climatic events, notably HURRICANES in Central and North America. The health impacts associated with ENSOs include increased incidence and prevalence of vector-borne and other diseases affecting tropical and temperate zones worldwide. CHOLERA entered South America in 1990 during an ENSO, causing more than half a million cases.

elutriation The process of separating solid particles of varying size and density by straining or sieving them, or allowing them to settle at differing rates when they are suspended in fluid. The process is used both to reduce or remove altogether the suspended particulate matter in emission products of combustion, and to separate solids from liquids in a sewerage system or industrial waste disposal system.

embargo 1. A barrier to the passage or transmission of goods that is usually legally enforceable. This is used, for instance, to prevent importing of infectious, toxic, or otherwise harmful goods. 2. Time-limited restriction on release of information that often depends on an honor system.

embryo The earliest developmental stages of a fertilized ovum at which cellular differentiation begins. After the 8th week of gestation, the human embryo is described as a fetus and has recognizable limbs, functioning heart, etc.

emergency In public health, a situation that threatens life, personal, and population health and safety, human settlements, habitat, generally associated with environmental change from equilibrium to an unbalanced state. It is usually sudden in onset but may develop gradually. Examples include floods, hurricanes, earthquakes, droughts, and manmade situations, such as violent armed conflict, that require intervention to restore stability. See also DISASTER.

emergency measures organization (EMO) A system or agency that many nations have in some form to coordinate and administer responses by relevant services and sectors of society whenever emergency situations arise. The sectors directly involved include public health and therapeutic health care services, communications, law enforcement, fire services, local and regional administrative services, and the hospitality industry that can provide accommodation for people displaced from their homes. See also FEDERAL EMERGENCY MANAGEMENT AGENCY (FEMA).

emergency medicine The medical specialty concerned with the immediate care and management of life-threatening illness and injury. In practice, most emergency medicine specialists devote most of their time and energy to dealing with conditions that are not serious, let alone life threatening. The ability to recognize dangerous contagious diseases is a required skill in emergency medicine because the index case may present as an emergency.

emergent, emerging infections A term used to describe newly identified diseases. More than 30 such diseases have been identified since 1970, demonstrating that the ecological relationship of humans and pathogenic organisms continues to evolve. Recently emerged infections include HIV/AIDS, Legionnaires disease, Lyme disease, several varieties of tropical viral hemorrhagic fevers, hantavirus pulmonary syndrome, severe acute respiratory syndrome (SARS), and avian influenza. See http://www.cdc.gov/ncidod/eid/index.htm for current information.

emerging pathogens A descriptive term for a miscellaneous group of more than 30 pathogens that have been identified since approximately 1970. Most are responsible for life-threatening, communicable diseases, most of which have occurred, and in some cases declared themselves for the first time, in epidemic form. They include the pathogens responsible for Legionnaires disease, HIV/AIDS, Ebola-Marburg virus disease, hantavirus, Lyme disease, *Helicobacter pylori*, new varieties of hepatitis virus, several tropical hemorrhagic fever viruses, the viruses responsible for SARS, and avian influenza.

emetic A pharmaceutical compound or substance that induces vomiting. Emetics have a mixed history in folk medicine, in lay methods of emergency treatment, in formerly fashionable therapeutic regimens, and as a feature of bulimia. They have a place in emergency management of episodes of poisoning but must be used with knowledge of the appropriate emetic to use with specific types of poison. For instance, saline is a popular emetic, but it makes barbiturate overdose worse because saline promotes solution of barbiturates; and in corrosive poisoning, emetics may aggravate the damage and even cause rupture of the mucosal lining of the esophagus or stomach.

emission guidelines, limits, standards The US Environmental Protection Agency and its counterparts in other jurisdictions have compiled and published lengthy lists of allowable amounts of toxic and otherwise harmful emission products. See, for instance, http://www.epa.gov.

emission products, emissions The products of combustion. The extent to which combustion generates pollutants is measured in these emissions. Carbon-based fuels are the most commonly used, and the principal emissions are oxides of carbon, especially carbon dioxide. Most carbon fuels produce other emission products, including oxides of nitrogen, and more toxic emissions from trace amounts of sulfur, lead, mercury, and other elements that are contaminants of the complex compounds that make up carbon-based fuels. The phrase also applies to emission products of nuclear fuels.

emotional distress A term used in legal circumstances, e.g., in TORTS, to describe damage of a nonphysical or pathological nature for which people may seek to claim compensation.

emphysema A CHRONIC OBSTRUCTIVE PULMONARY DISEASE (COPD) with destruction of the architecture of alveolar walls, formation of bubble-like spaces, loss of elasticity of lung tissue, progressively increasing dyspnea, and right-sided heart failure. It occurs in chronic or recurrent bronchitis or other inflammatory disease and is often attributable to lifelong CIGARETTE SMOKING or to a PNEUMOCONIOSIS such as silicosis.

empirical (adj) Syn: rule of thumb. Based on past experience and observation of how well that experience worked. Until the advent of EVIDENCE-BASED MEDICINE, clinical practice was largely empirical.

empiricism The method of thinking and practice based on experience and observation, rather than on a particular underlying theory. This has been the dominant method of discovery and advances in medicine and other observational sciences. Many theories of disease causation and approaches to rational therapeutic regimens are based ultimately on empiricism. Empiricism is also the name of a school of philosophical thought.

employment insurance A politically palatable name for UNEMPLOYMENT INSURANCE, i.e., payment of a subsistence allowance to wage and salary earners who have lost their jobs, in a time-limited period during which they are seeking new employment.

emporiatrics Syn: TRAVEL MEDICINE. The branch of medical specialization concerned with diseases associated with travel and travelers. "Travel medicine" is a preferable name for this field.

empowerment The process of conferring decision-making capacity upon those who previously had been unable to decide matters for themselves or had limited ability to do so. Examples include recognition of and reaction to the needs of handicapped people, and actions to elevate the status of women and to enhance reproductive freedom. Conferring autonomy and devolving power to indigenous colonized people is another important application of this process. Community empowerment is an integral component of many health-promotion programs and of AIDS control programs.

empty calories A term sometimes used to describe calories derived from consumption of sugar, starch, and other carbohydrate foodstuffs that contain neither vitamins nor minerals, i.e., they have no nutritional value other than provision of energy.

emulsifier An agent that promotes the suspension of a liquid substance in a liquid medium.

enabling factors A set of social, cultural, behavioral, economic, political, or other conditions that may facilitate or impede the interaction of antecedent causes with the occurrence of a disease or other health-related phenomenon. For example, poverty, overcrowding, and poor nutrition are enabling factors for the invasion and progression of the tubercle bacillus; access to family planning and contraceptive counseling without impediment is an enabling factor for good maternal and infant health.

enamel The hard, shiny white calcium compound comprising the outermost layer on the crown of teeth. It is hard enough to cut or grind most foodstuffs into fragments during mastication. The formation of caries-resistant enamel uses enzymes that require trace amounts of fluoride, which is therefore an essential trace element. See also CARIES.

encephalopathy, spongiform See TRANSMISSIBLE SPONGIFORM ENCEPHALOPATHY.

endangered species An animal or plant species that has been so reduced in distribution and/or abundance as to be at risk or extinction because its gene pool has declined to a level where propagation of healthy offspring is unlikely to occur. Endangered species are useful as an early warning signal of ECOSYSTEM DISTRESS.

endemic (adj) Refers to the constant presence in a population of a condition such as a communicable disease. A HOLOENDEMIC disease is one that affects a high proportion of children, leading to relative resistance to reinfection in adult life, so the incidence of new cases and prevalence of existing cases are lower among adults than children; an example is malaria in many tropical regions. A HYPERENDEMIC disease is constantly present at a high rate of occurrence (prevalence) among persons in all age groups.

endobiotic An endogenous substance that produces a toxic metabolite when it is metabolized.

endocrine disorders A wide range of conditions associated with malfunction of endocrine glands including absent, insufficient, and excessive production of hormones. Several have characteristic clinical features, sometimes associated with a distinct physical appearance. Causes include surplus or deficient production of hormone, associated with environment or diet, or with an inflammatory or neoplastic lesion of the affected endocrine organ. Sometimes hormonal dysfunctions interact, for instance, when pituitary dysfunction affects the function of the thyroid, suprarenals, and gonads. Public health relevance of endocrine disorders arises in several ways, for instance, in control of iodine deficiency disorders and in screening for diabetes.

endocrine disruptors Syn: endocrine modulators. A group of compounds with actions that mimic, inhibit, or modulate the effects of naturally occurring endogenously produced hormones, such as estrogen, progesterone, thyroxin, androgen, etc. They include artificial estrogens, such as DIETHYLSTILBESTROL, DDT, dioxins, PCBs, Kepone, some polyaromatic hydrocarbons, and several other industrially or therapeutically important chemicals or their toxic by-products.

endocrine system The word "system" is applicable to the interacting endocrine glands, including the pituitary, thyroid, suprarenal, and testes or ovaries, all of which influence and are affected by the secretions of the others. The endocrine system also includes the pineal, parathyroid, and pancreas glands, which do not interact and influence each other's functions in quite the same way. All have in common the fact that they produce HORMONES essential to normal bodily functions.

endocrinology The study of the endocrine glands, their actions, interactions, and the HORMONES that the endocrine glands produce.

end-of-life care See PALLIATIVE CARE.

endogamy Syn: inbreeding. Selection of a sexual partners, i.e., marriage, from within a relatively small and restricted gene pool, often a defined, often close-knit ethnic group, as in the caste system of India and also among the members of a cultural minority, such as an immigrant community.

endogenous (adj) Produced or originating within an organism.

endometriosis A chronic condition in which tissue that microscopically resembles endometrial tissue proliferates in the pelvis outside the uterus, causing painful intercourse, irregular menstrual periods, and usually impaired fertility.

endometrium The lining of the uterus that undergoes periodic changes, i.e., hypertrophy and increased vascularity during the menstrual cycle in preparation to receive a fertilized ovum. When a fertilized ovum is not implanted, the outermost endometrial layer is shed during menstruation.

endorphins Naturally occurring peptides and polypeptides secreted by brain tissue and probably by other organs with qualities resembling those of hormones. These compounds are produced when pain and some other forms of acute stress occur and have calming and pain-alleviating properties. Some athletes and persons with anorexia nervosa seem to become "addicted" to the psychogenic effects of endorphins, leading them to engage in compulsive excess physical activity.

endotoxin A toxin that is released only when the organism dies, i.e., not excreted by living organisms. Most endotoxins are produced by bacterial cells.

end stage disease Disease that has reached an irreversible stage, a term most often applied to advanced renal disease but equally applicable to disease of the liver, lungs, etc.

energy The force generated by combustion, e.g., of calories during metabolism, or carbon-based fuels in a furnace or power plant, and by radioactive nuclear transformation. Several sources and types of energy include kinetic, thermal, nuclear, etc.

enriched uranium Uranium that has been refined to increase the proportion of highly radioactive isotopes contained in it so it can be used to manufacture nuclear weapons. See also DEPLETED URANIUM.

ENSO See EL NIÑO.

enteric disease Disease of the gastrointestinal, i.e., enteric system, usually infections or inflammation, e.g., ESCHERICHIA COLI, Shigella, and SALMONELLA infection of the gastrointestinal tract.

enteric fever An obsolete name for TYPHOID fever.

enterobiasis Infection with pinworms, Enterobius vermicularis, a common childhood condition.

enterotoxin A toxic metabolic product of certain bacteria, notably staphylococci, that acts on the epithelial cells of the gastrointestinal tract, causing spasmodic contraction and sometimes acute inflammatory reactions, shock, and/or hemorrhage. Many enterotoxins are tasteless and odorless, and some, including staphylococcal enterotoxin, are heat stable. Clinically, they commonly reveal their presence by inducing explosive bouts of vomiting and diarrhea, an acute illness that has many names (la turista, Montezuma's revenge, Delhi belly, Gippy tummy, and other names unfit for publication).

enterovirus A general name for poliovirus and picornavirus transmitted by the fecal-oral route and as a rule residing in the gastrointestinal tract, although some cause diseases primarily affecting the central nervous system. The diseases due to these include poliomyelitis and aseptic or viral meningitis.

entitlement Money, goods, or services provided for persons or families by reason of their status, such as invalid or old age pensioner, or an obligation of a present or former employer.

entropion A condition in which scarring or contracture of the tissues of the eyelids causes an inward distortion, preventing complete closure of the eyelids, conjunctival inflammation, and inadequate lubrication of the cornea. It is a common complication of TRACHOMA, and unless prevented by antibiotics or treated surgically, it causes blindness.

environment The setting and conditions in which events occur. The total of all influences on life and health apart from genes, comprising the physical world and the economic, social, behavioral, cultural, as well as physical conditions and factors that are determinants of health and well-being.

Environment Agency The agency of the British government responsible for setting standards and monitoring environmental quality. Its activities are described and brief reports on relevant topics appear at http://www.environment-agency.gov.uk/.

environmental engineering Applications of engineering science and technology to the improvement of environmental conditions or amelioration of environmental pollution. These include measures to control pollution of air, water, soil, abatement of nuisances, etc.

environmental epidemiology The use of epidemiological methods to study the effects of exposure to environmental determinants of health. The International Society for Environmental Epidemiology (ISEE) defines these determinants as any or all of the physical, chemical, biological, social, economic, cultural, and behavioral factors that affect health. Interactions of genetic and environmental factors are also included. This definition is almost identical to the definition of EPIDEMIOLOGY without the qualification "environmental." Environmental epidemiology further specifies its domain with examples such as health effects of urbanization; built environments; agricultural development; energy production and combustion; pollution of air, water, soil, and food by toxic chemicals; ecosystem disruption; human-animal interactions; and much else.

environmental health The branch of public health science and practice concerned with the whole range of environmental determinants of health, i.e., the physical, chemical, biological, social and behavioral factors in the environment that influence health and disease occurrence, and with diseases of environmental and occupational origin, such as ASBESTOSIS, smog-related BRONCHITIS, occupationally related cancers, LEAD POISONING, and RADIATION SICKNESS, as in CHERNOBYL. A large component of environmental health is OCCUPATIONAL HEALTH/MEDICINE, which is a specialized field of public health science and practice that often involves clinical work.

environmental health criteria documents A set of official publications produced by the WORLD HEALTH ORGANIZATION and the INTERNATIONAL AGENCY FOR RESEARCH ON CANCER, and by national agencies including the US NATIONAL INSTITUTE FOR OCCUPATIONAL SAFETY AND HEALTH, specifying safe and unsafe levels of exposure to environmental agents that can cause disease. The criteria are set by a combination of laboratory, clinical, and epidemiological observations and periodically revised. See http://www.who.int/ipcs/publications/ehc/en/.

environmental hypersensitivity A rather ill-defined "new" disease that some authorities believe does not exist, with symptoms that include headaches, skin rashes, breathlessness, nausea, and vomiting, said to be caused by exposure to any or all of a range of environmental factors that are associated with modern urban living. Some people with it have symptoms similar to those associated with the SICK BUILDING SYNDROME.

environmental impact assessment A set of toxicological tests and epidemiological procedures that can be used to determine post hoc whether the presence of an industry has had adverse environmental effects or to estimate before an industry is established what its effects on the environment are likely to be.

environmental justice The concept of equity in risk management that aims to ensure that communities near potentially polluting industrial sites are not more exposed to environmental health risks than are more affluent communities further removed from the source of pollution.

environmental laws, regulations Most nations, and often smaller administrative jurisdictions within nations, have enacted laws and promulgated supporting enforceable regulations aimed at preventing and mitigating the impact of industrial pollution and toxic contamination on human habitat, and sometimes to protect wildlife sanctuaries. Laws and regulations are better than nothing but seldom provide adequate control of transborder and global environmental toxins. They rarely provide any protection against environmental harm that is merely esthetically unpleasant, such as unsightly advertising billboards, open-cut mining and quarrying operations, offensively loud noise, etc.

environmental pollution A term that covers all forms of contamination of the environment by domestic and industrial substances that can cause harm.

Environmental Protection Agency (EPA) The US government department that is responsible for assessing and managing environmental risks to human health. The EPA is expected to measure, monitor, and make recommendations about amelioration of environmental health hazards. Its activities are sometimes impaired by political intervention, for instance under some administrations that have rescinded existing safeguards. For details of programs, etc., see http://www.epa.gov.

environmental refugee A refugee or internally displaced person whose movement has been enforced by loss or severe disruption of usual habitat as a consequence of a natural disaster, such as flood, volcanic eruption, drought, or extensive forest fires.

environmental sciences The sciences concerned with the environment, which include geography, meteorology, physics, chemistry, biology, ecology, toxicology, epidemiology, and often others, including social and behavioral sciences when the impact of these on environments is considered.

environmental terrorism A terrorist attack aimed at deliberate destruction of the environment or at an ecosystem. Crop destruction has been used in military strategy since antiquity, but attacks by terrorists are comparatively recent. Examples include deliberately set forest fires and destruction of hydroelectric dams and oil installations. All have obvious implications for public health.

environmental tobacco smoke A specific form of indoor air pollution due to the presence of tobacco smoke, especially SIDESTREAM SMOKE, which contains several known carcinogens and many other toxicants.

environmental toxicology The scientific study of toxic substances that can contaminate air, water, soil, and food. This science focuses mainly on acute toxicity but is concerned also with long-term and intergenerational effects, although the economic incentive to market new products usually leads to environmental release of new chemicals before sufficient time has elapsed to permit adequate testing for adverse long-term and intergenerational effects. The Food and Drug Administration (FDA) and its counterparts in the European Union and some other countries became more diligent about testing for long-term and intergenerational effects after the problems with DIETHYLSTILBESTROL (DES), but many of the regulations have since been relaxed under pressure from the pharmaceutical and chemical industries.

enzyme-linked immunosorbent assay (ELISA) A rapid, reliable, relatively cheap biochemical test for specific normal and abnormal molecular constituents of blood and other body fluids. This test can be used to detect just about any antigen and antibody, e.g., HIV antigen.

enzymes Compounds that catalyze a biochemical process, e.g., assimilation, absorption of food in which many enzymes are involved, secreted by salivary, gastric, and intestinal glands. Enzymes are essential for most biochemical processes. Their deficiency or malfunction causes many diseases.

eosinophilia The presence in peripheral blood of abnormally large numbers of eosinophilic white blood corpuscles, which is associated with allergic and immunological disorders.

epichlorohydrin A colorless toxic liquid used to make epoxy resins, adhesives, plasticizers, pharmaceuticals, textile chemicals, etc. It is absorbed through cutaneous and mucosal surfaces and by inhalation. It is an acute toxin and a known animal and suspected human carcinogen.

epidemic The occurrence in a community or specified population of deaths or cases of a condition in numbers greater than usual expectation for a given period of time. The word comes from the Greek *epi* (upon) and *demos* (people). The word originally applied to outbreaks of contagious disease, but broadened in the 20th century to include conditions of noninfectious origin, such as traffic crashes, coronary heart disease, cigarette smoking, imitative (copycat) suicide, and other behavioral health problems. The meaning of "usual expectation" varies widely. Thus, the reappearance of a single case of a contagious disease such as diphtheria or typhoid in a community from which it had been eliminated would be grounds for initiating full epidemic precautions. The occurrence of a CLUSTER of cases of a rare condition, such as an uncommon variety of cancer, also requires investigation to determine whether it is a chance event or an actual or incipient epidemic. The existence of an epidemic may be self-evident or be revealed only by diligent surveillance of available information from all relevant sources. An example of the latter was the occurrence of excess deaths from pneumonia among members of the American Legion who had all attended a convention in Philadelphia but many of whom fell ill and died after returning home. Investigation of this epidemic led to the discovery of LE-GIONNAIRES DISEASE. Epidemics of cancer in which the responsible agent was revealed only after surveillance and epidemiological study include lung cancer caused by cigarette smoking, hemangiosarcoma in vinyl chloride workers, and genital dysplasia and cancer in the daughters of women who took DIETHYLSTILBESTROL (DES) during pregnancy.

epidemic curve The diagrammatic representation of the course of an epidemic, which varies according to the nature and cause of the epidemic. For instance, a food-borne epidemic caused by contamination of a food item in a particular meal has an explosive onset, in which many people are affected simultaneously, then a rapid reduction

and cessation; an epidemic that spreads from person to person from an initial INDEX CASE has a slower onset and more protracted course, dying down slowly as the number of susceptible persons declines.

Epidemic Intelligence Service (EIS) A service and training program initiated in 1951 at the US Public Health Service Communicable Diseases Center (now the Centers for Disease Control and Prevention) under the direction of Alexander Langmuir (1910–1993). The original aim of the EIS was to investigate the epidemiology of communicable disease outbreaks with unusual features, large and life-threatening epidemics, and epidemics of unidentified conditions. The EIS has an illustrious history of important discoveries that have clarified many previously mysterious disease outbreaks in the United States and elsewhere in the world. By early in the 21st century, the EIS Officer Training Program had trained almost 3,000 epidemiologists and stimulated development of similar programs in several other countries. For further information, see http://www.cdc.gov/eis/.

epidemic investigation A set of procedures to identify the cause, i.e., responsible agent, affected persons, circumstances and mode of spread, and other relevant factors involved in propagating an epidemic, especially one with unusual features and one that is not self-limiting and presents a significant threat to public health. Investigation may require deployment of personnel and resources to identify the INDEX CASE, ask questions about exposure of both cases and noncases in the affected community, conduct microbiological tests, etc. In epidemics affecting large numbers and in dangerous life-threatening epidemics, especially with exotic and unfamiliar pathogens, this may be a fast or a protracted process, but it may be accelerated by RAPID EPIDEMIOLOGICAL ASSESSMENT.

epidemic theory The branch of mathematics concerned with fitting statistical models to the empirically observed facts about incidence of communicable and other diseases, including data on all quantifiable determinants, behavior of infectious agents, environmental conditions, and host resistance. The aim is to develop models that can be used in planning effective epidemic control programs, as well as predict conditions and circumstance in which epidemics can be expected.

epidemic threshold According to epidemic theory, the number and/or density (proximity) of susceptible persons required for an epidemic to occur. The MASS ACTION PRINCIPLE defines the epidemic threshold as the reciprocal of the INFECTION TRANSMISSION PARAMETER.

epidemiological transition theory A theory postulated by the Egyptian demographer Abdel Omran (b. 1925) in 1971 that visualizes several phases in the interactions of human populations with infectious disease agents. These include the "age of pestilence and famine," the "age of receding pandemics," and the "age of degenerative and manmade diseases," three generalizations based on the history of epidemics in Western civilization during the past 1,000 years. While the theory more or less fits the observed facts in Western nations over much of this period, anomalies appear when observations from other parts of the world and a longer time period are included. A rapid transition occurred in some low-income countries and regions, with enlightened policies on empowerment of women and on family planning, notably in Sri Lanka, the Maldives, and Kerala state in India.

epidemiologist A specialist in epidemiology. This may be a physician, nurse, medical scientist, microbiologist, veterinarian, statistician, or member of any of several other professions.

epidemiology A word first used in English in 1873 by J. P. Parkin to describe the science that deals with epidemics. A related word, *epidemiologia*, had been used in Spanish for about 100 years at that time. Epidemiology was one of three powerful scientific methods deployed against the oppressive public health problems of 19th century industrial Britain, Europe, and the United States (the others were bacteriology and physical sciences). Epidemiology burgeoned as an increasingly rigorous science based on observation, inference, and experiment around the middle of the 20th century, with development of methods, notably CASE CONTROL and COHORT STUDIES to investigate noncommunicable diseases such as coronary heart disease and cancer and RANDOMIZED CONTROLLED TRIALS to evaluate therapeutic and preventive regimens aimed at control of these conditions. The definition developed by an internationally representative expert group for the *Dictionary of Epidemiology* (1983) is "the study of the distribution and determinants of health-related states or events in specified populations and the application of this study to control of health problems."

epigenesis Certain sites, called epigenetic sites, on the DNA molecule are capable of inducing or suppressing gene expression. Some of these sites are prone to alterations that are expressed as genetic defects or malformations, such as congenital heart defects.

episode An event that usually has a well-defined beginning or onset, recognizable features and duration, and identifiable termination. In the health sector, the word is often used in relation to an episode of illness or a specific phase during the course of an illness.

epistemology The study of the basic foundations for knowledge, including scientific knowledge, and the ways this is augmented and modified by new discoveries.

epizootic An epidemic in an animal population, often with the implication that it can also affect human populations.

epoxy compounds These useful compounds include industrial solvents and resins and are the base for powerful adhesives. Many are toxic by inhalation or absorption through the skin, causing a variety of reactions, including dermatitis and asthma.

Epstein-Barr virus The herpesvirus that causes infectious mononucleosis and Burkitt's lymphoma (nasopharyngeal cancer) and is associated with several other malignant conditions, including some cases of leukemia and non-Hodgkin lymphoma. It was one of the first viruses identified as an agent or cause of cancer. It is named for the British microbiologists Michael Epstein (b. 1921) and Yvonne Barr (b. 1932).

equal protection A fundamental principle of common law and a constitutional right in the United States and many other nations is that all citizens, regardless of other distinguishing characteristics, have a right to the same level of protection from harms and from unlawful actions by others. This resembles the ethical principle of equity, impartiality, or distributive justice.

equipoise A condition of uncertainty about the possible benefits or harms of a preventive or therapeutic regimen. In public health and in preventive and clinical medical practice, this is usually an indication for a RANDOMIZED CONTROLLED TRIAL.

equity Fairness, evenhandedness, impartiality in dealing with others; an important concept in BIOETHICS, especially in relation to human rights. Achieving equity of access to health care services, regardless of social, ethnic, and cultural status, has become a high-priority health policy issue for all UN health-related agencies, including WHO, UNICEF, UNAIDS, and the World Bank. See also AFFIRMATIVE ACTION and SOCIAL JUSTICE.

eradication of disease Ending all transmission of an infectious disease agent by bringing about the extermination of the disease agent. This was achieved worldwide for SMALLPOX by a policy of SURVEILLANCE and CONTAINMENT, made possible by the fact that vaccination of a smallpox contact before the disease declares itself clinically will prevent that contact from getting the disease; because the smallpox virus has no other host than humans, it dies if it cannot infect new cases to perpetuate itself. Similar methods of eradication have worked regionally for DRACUNCULIASIS, MEASLES, and POLIOMYELITIS but would not work for communicable diseases that have different agent-host relationships, such as alternative animal hosts.

erectile dysfunction disorder Inability to achieve or maintain an erection of sufficient strength and duration to perform sexual intercourse. The causes may be psychogenic, neurological, endocrine, or vascular. Common causes in previously potent men include systemic disease, such as diabetes and/or arteriosclerosis. The advertising of drugs such as Viagra has led many men to seek treatment and thus to considerable increase in estimates of the prevalence, now believed to be 30% to 50% of men older than 50 years, increasing with age. See also IMPOTENCE.

erethism A condition of nervous irritability associated with various stimulants, including MERCURY POISONING.

ergonomics The science and technology of relationships between workers and their working environment that deal with aspects conducive to enhancing comfort and efficiency and reducing work-related physical and psychological harm. Ergonomics seeks to fit machines to the workers who use them, e.g., ensuring that fatigue is minimized among operators of keyboards and computer screens, and that small-framed women can operate heavy machines designed for men.

ergot A fungus disease of rye and corn. If humans ingest grain or flour infected with ergot, they can experience a dramatic psychotic disturbance and peripheral vascular disease with excruciating pains in the gut and extremities, called St. Anthony's Fire; the condition was relatively common in medieval Europe.

ergotamine An amine alkaloid derived from the toxin of ergot that in small controlled doses is a therapeutically useful vasoconstricting agent used routinely in the third stage of labor to control postpartum hemorrhage, and used in clinical medicine to treat migraine.

ergotism A condition, known as St. Anthony's Fire in medieval Europe when consumption of infected flour was a common occurrence, that causes acutely painful ischemic muscle cramps. These are due to ingestion of the toxin produced by a fungus that infects wheat, rye, and other grains used to make flour for bread. In addition to the severe pain, ergot causes bizarre hallucinations resembling those caused by LSD. Episodes of ergotism occasionally occur in modern times, as in the Soviet Union during the famines of the 1920s and in France in the early 1950s.

error A false or mistaken result or belief. RANDOM ERROR is the portion of variation in results or measurements attributable to chance factors. SYSTEMATIC ERROR is usually the consequence of a defective measuring instrument or technique, and often can be detected and corrected by recourse to CALIBRATION, SAMPLING, or STANDARDIZATION.

error, type I See ALPHA ERROR.

error, type II See BETA ERROR.

error, type III A term used to describe the situation when an investigator uses unsuitable research methods to address a problem, leading to the outcome of finding "the right answer to the wrong question." A common form of this is to use methods that detect interindividual differences, when the problem requires methods that can detect differences between population groups, or vice versa.

errors of logical reasoning Any of several common flaws in logic fit this description. They include false inferences and conclusions, such as the ECOLOGICAL FALLACY or TYPE III ERROR, i.e., use of unsuitable or the wrong kind of statistical tests. The history of medicine offers many examples, including discredited theories of disease causation that led to harmful therapies, such as excision of most of the colon for the nonexistent disease called auto-intoxication, based on the premise that the digested contents of the large intestine poisoned the system.

erysipelas An acute, sometimes recurrent streptococcal infection of the skin with raised, red, indurated inflammatory patches on the face and body.

erythema nodosum An inflammatory-allergic streptococcal skin infection that sometimes occurs as a feature of RHEUMATIC FEVER.

erythroblastosis fetalis A severe form of RHESUS FACTOR incompatibility that causes fetal destruction and death late in pregnancy.

erythrocytes Syn: red blood corpuscles. The oxygen-carrying cells in mammalian blood. They are disc-shaped cells with a flattened or slightly depressed center and no nucleus. The pigmented hemoglobin they contain imparts the red color to blood.

erythromycin A broad-spectrum antibiotic that can be used systemically or topically to treat many diseases that do not respond to other antibiotics. It is a bacteriostatic agent rather than a bacteriocidal one, is less inclined than other antibiotics to promote resistant strains of organisms, and is less toxic than most other antibiotics.

Escherichia coli 1. A ubiquitous family of Enterobacteriaceae, Gram-negative, nonmotile rods whose natural habitat is the gastrointestinal tract of humans and many animals. They are usually not pathogens, but some strains occasionally cause enteritis, urinary tract infections, cystitis, and peritonitis. One specific strain, *E. COLI* O157:H7, associated with drinking water contaminated by fecal material and with eating underdone meat or meat products, causes a dangerous, hemorrhagic diarrhea, often leading to renal damage and other complications.2. A ubiquitous COLIFORM ORGANISM that is a common cause of (usually) low-grade infection of the gastrointestinal tract and can also infect other systems, e.g., the urinary tract. Some types of E. coli can cause very serious infections.

***Escherichia coli* O157:H7 infection** A potentially fatal infection that causes acute gastroenteritis with bloody diarrhea and generalized systemic disease, sometimes including renal failure. This may be primarily a zoonotic infection, often transmitted to humans in contaminated water supplies. The contamination may have animal more often than human sources, for example, when manure from a FEED LOT pollutes an aquifer that is a source of drinking water.

esophageal cancer A frequently fatal cancer associated with exposure to certain dietary and other environmental factors, including carcinogens in tobacco (pipe and cigar smokers are especially prone to this cancer), and to regional variations in dietary components. For example, it occurs in Iran and in parts of China in association with high dietary intake of NITROSAMINES.

essential amino acids More than 20 amino acids have been identified as essential to human life, including the four that are the basic building blocks of the DNA molecule: adenine, thymine, cytosine, and guanine.

essential drugs and medicines A simplified pharmacopeia of life-saving drugs compiled for WHO, required to treat and prevent the commonly occurring life-threatening diseases and aimed mainly toward low-income countries. See http://www.who.int/medicines/rationale.shtml.

essential public health services A set of services provided by public health agencies that are considered to be required for health protection and disease prevention. A WHO-sponsored delphi study in 1995–1997 arrived at a consensus among internationally recognized public health experts that some public health functions are essential everywhere, so services to provide these are required in all nations. These functions include disease monitoring and surveillance; environmental protection; health promotion; communicable disease control; health legislation; occupational health services; specific health services for children and other vulnerable groups; and the management, administration, and evaluation of public health services. The essential functions are:

1. Monitor health status to identify community health problems.
2. Diagnose and investigate community health problems and hazards.
3. Inform, educate, and empower people about health issues.
4. Mobilize community partnerships to identify and solve health problems.
5. Develop policies and plans to support personal and community health efforts.
6. Enforce laws and regulations that protect health and safety.
7. Connect people and the services they need.
8. Assure a competent workforce for personal and community health.
9. Evaluate effectiveness, accessibility, and quality of personal and community health services.
10. Conduct research to gain new insights and seek innovative solutions.

At its plenary session in 2000, the Pan American Health Organization added two more to make a total of 12 essential public health functions: namely,

11. Management capacity to organize public health systems and services.
12. Reducing the impact of disasters and emergencies on health.

See http://www.lachsr.org/en/thesaurus/00000228.htm. See also CORE FUNCTIONS OF PUBLIC HEALTH.

estradiol The female sex estrogen hormone responsible for sexual maturation, i.e., growth of the breasts, broadening of the female pelvis, maturation of the ovaries, and monthly ovulation in accord with the timing of the biological clock.

estrogens Female sex hormone, a group of steroid hormones of which the most important is estradiol, which is responsible for the growth and essential functions of the female genital tract, including the preparation of the uterus for implanting of the fertilized ovum. See also PROGESTERONE. Estrogen production declines at the time of the menopause, and this is said to be responsible for menopausal symptoms, such as hot flashes.

ethane A gaseous aliphatic compound that usually occurs with methane in NATURAL GAS.

ethanol C_2H_5OH, the simplest alcohol, the active ingredient of all alcoholic drinks. This is a colorless, volatile flammable liquid, produced by fermentation of grains, fruits, etc. Taken in moderation, it is a mild stimulant and sedative, reduces inhibitions, can be addictive and habit forming; in excess quantity, it is a cumulative poison that causes, or is associated with, liver, peripheral nerve, and brain damage.

ethers A group of alkyl compounds. The best known is diethyl oxide $(C_2H_5)O_2$, a volatile solvent that was used for more than 100 years from the middle of the 19th century as an anesthetic agent.

ethical relativism The form of ethical reasoning in which the values of a particular group are assumed to apply to another group with quite different values and beliefs. Ethical relativism is flawed by failure to take into account these differences. See also CULTURAL RELATIVISM.

ethical review Formal review by a properly constituted group such as an INSTITUTIONAL REVIEW BOARD (or its equivalent in other countries). It is mandatory that all publicly funded research involving human subjects (participants), research involving human tissues or laboratory animals, and some other kinds of research comply with ethical requirements. These are specified in guidelines, such as those of the National Institutes of Health, and in codes of conduct and guidelines prepared by professional organizations, such as the American Public Health Association.

ethics The branch of philosophy dealing with distinctions between right and wrong, with the moral consequences of human actions. Aristotle identified many virtues that are components of the good life or of the ethical person, in *Ethics* (4th century BCE). Some of Aristotle's virtues, including truthfulness, integrity, compassion, are the basis for one approach to applications of ethics in the health sector. Other approaches include principle-based ethics, based on the four principles respect for autonomy, beneficence, nonmaleficence, and equity or justice; and duty-based ethics or deontology, which means behaving according to tenets defined by beliefs, usually in a particular religious faith. See also BIOETHICS and VIRTUE-BASED ETHICS.

ethnic cleansing A euphemism for attacks on and violent destruction and driving out of their habitat of a group of people who are ethnically distinct from their aggressors. It may involve violent armed assaults, murder of whole households, mass rape of girls and women, by military or paramilitary forces or by gangs of armed thugs. The end results include internal displacement and flight across international frontiers of surviving members of the targeted group, often preceded by large-scale loss of life and followed by the public health problems of REFUGEES.

ethnic group A community or group of people with distinctive social, cultural, and behavioral characteristics that distinguish them from others in the same or different country or society. Members of an ethnic group share the same language, have similar ways of life and a common history, preserve traditions and customs from one generation to the next, identify themselves as members of that ethnic group, and often have a common genetic heritage. In countries where the population includes high proportions of immigrants from earlier generations, members of an ethnic group are sometimes identified by a hyphenated name (Armenian-Americans, Ukrainian-Canadians, Italian-Australians, etc). Ethnic groups sometimes display epidemiological patterns of disease that differ from prevailing patterns of others in the same country, which may relate to their genetic heritage, lifestyle, dietary factors, or a combination of these.

ethnicity A term for the ethnic group to which people belong. Usually it refers to group identity based on culture, religion, traditions, and customs. In some contexts, it is a "politically correct" term equivalent to the word "race," which may have pejorative associations.

ethnography The scientific study of customs, habits, and behavior of specified groups of people, usually applied to tribes or clans of people in non-literate societies.

ethnomedicine Medical practice focused on the health behavior and problems of ethnic groups.

ethology An old meaning of this word was the study of ethics, but its modern meaning is the study of animal behavior.

ethylene diamine tetra acetic acid (EDTA) A CHELATING AGENT, a molecule that reacts with toxic metals, such as lead and mercury, to form stable, soluble, nontoxic, and more readily excreted compounds. It was formerly used as an antidote to poisoning with these heavy metals.

ethylene dibromide An industrial chemical used in pesticides and as a scavenger to remove impurities in petroleum fuels. It is a renal and hepatic poison and a suspected human carcinogen and can cause oligospermia and therefore impaired male fertility.

ethylene oxide A colorless gas used in the manufacture of the popular antifreeze ethylene glycol. It is a respiratory and mucous membrane irritant. It is mutagenic: exposure during early pregnancy can induce miscarriage, and it is a probable human carcinogen.

EU Acronym for the European Union.

eugenics A word coined in 1883 by the British biologist Francis Galton (1822–1911) meaning good breeding. Galton believed that marital unions between people of what he regarded as "excellent genetic stock" could be expected to produce offspring with the same or similar qualities. From then until the 1920s, eugenics was a prominent feature of public health theory, and textbooks such as Rosenau's *Preventive Medicine and Hygiene* (1913) contained extensive and detailed chapters on the practice of eugenics, with discussions about "sterilizing the unfit." The practice and the theory were soon discredited by demonstration of its failure as an approach to better population health, the taint of elitism, and its use by the Nazi regime in Germany. However, it was practiced until the 1970s in Sweden and in Alberta, Canada, until the 1960s.

euphenics A word coined by the American biologist Joshua Lederberg (b. 1925) to describe the environmental amelioration of harmful genetic defects, for instance, the dietary management of phenylketonuria.

European Public Health Association An organization with members drawn from the nations of the European Union (EU). It has a journal, the *European Journal of Public Health*, advises the European Parliament on health issues, and advocates on behalf of its members and the people of Europe. It is a coalition of national public health associations of member states of the EU. For information, see http://www.eupha.org.

euthanasia Literally, a gentle, easy death. In modern usage, the means of achieving a gentle and easy death, with an implied suggestion that this can be facilitated by medical means.

eutrophication Enrichment of nitrogen and phosphate nutriments in an aquatic ecosystem, e.g., by sewage disposal in lake water. In deep lakes, eutrophication can happen in subsurface layers, leading to oxygen lack in deeper waters, death of fish or other marine life because of this, and formation of toxic algal blooms that may make the water smell and taste unpleasant so that it is unfit for drinking and irrigation. In extreme cases, eutrophication causes sudden upheaval of deep waters that release lethal amounts of anaerobically generated toxic gases, such as methane.

evaluation Efforts aimed at determining as systematically and objectively as possible the effectiveness and impact of health-related (and other) activities in relation to objectives and taking into account the resources and facilities that have been deployed in the activities being evaluated. There are many ways of attempting this task, none fully satisfactory. One approach is to evaluate the resources and facilities, another is to examine how these work in practice, and a third is to assess outcomes, preferably in relation to inputs. Some methods attempt to employ all three approaches together. An important reason for evaluating health services and systems is to answer questions about costs in relation to benefits.

event horizon The most distant point or period of time at which it is possible to discern the effects attributable to a specific cause. A concept that is useful in environmental health when effects may be separated from their causes by many decades.

event node Syn: decision node. The point in a DE-CISION TREE at which alternative choices arise and a decision must be made as to which choice to take.

evidence The assembled information and facts on which rational, logical decisions are based in the diverse forums of human discourse, including courts of law, and in the practice of EVIDENCE-BASED MEDICINE among many others.

evidence-based decision making Logical, consistent use of the best available evidence from proven basic scientific sources, preferably augmented as necessary by facts from current verified peer-reviewed research, to inform policy decisions and routine practice. This approach to decision making ought to apply to all aspects of life, for instance, decisions in courts of law, as well as in biomedical science, medical practice, and public health. The evidence used in decision making should be systematically collected, assessed, and applied, bearing in mind the HIERARCHY OF EVIDENCE when considering its quality, validity, and relevance. In considering evidence, the standards of proof vary and are often passionately debated. Direct observation and precise measurement are regarded as solid evidence that can provide firm proof in many circumstances. On the other hand, epidemiological evidence is mainly circumstantial, thus giving opponents of public health measures based on epidemiological evidence many opportunities to refute it. Lawyers representing the tobacco industry, for instance, have often been successful in refuting epidemiological evidence, although in recent years they have found it increasingly difficult to deny the weight of accumulated evidence that tobacco is harmful. See also HILL'S CRITERIA and LOGIC.

evidence-based medicine Consistent use of best available evidence, preferably from current peer-reviewed sources in electronic and print media, to inform decisions about optimum patient management; decisions should consider the needs and preferences of individual patients. This evidence comes from many sources, especially reports from the COCHRANE COLLABORATION.

evidence-based public health Application of best available evidence in setting public health policies and priorities. The evidence comes from official vital and health statistics and from peer-reviewed publications in EPIDEMIOLOGY, SOCIOLOGY, ECONOMICS, and other relevant disciplines. Evidence-based public health is an approach that makes informed, explicit use of validated studies to arrive at judicious decisions on public health policies and best practices.

evil eye A manifestation of BLACK MAGIC, in which a person believed to have supernatural powers casts a spell over others who, by the power of suggestion, fall ill and sometimes even die.

evolution The process of change with successive generations, by which microorganisms, plants, animals, and humans adapt to changing environmental influences by undergoing anatomical and physiological modifications. These influences change slowly over time that is better measured on a geological, than a human lifetime, scale. The existence of evolution as a fundamental biological process is denied by believers in the literal truth of the story of creation as told in the book of Genesis, who uphold a theory called creationism, but the unassailable observational evidence for the reality of evolution includes the occurrence of antibiotic-resistant microorganisms. This fundamental biological concept must be used to inform many decisions in medical and public health practice, for instance, regarding best methods of management of environmental pests and infections due to antibiotic-resistant pathogenic organisms.

exanthem (Plural: exanthemata) A skin rash. The term applies to any and all varieties of skin rash but is mostly used in describing the infectious exanthemata, i.e., infectious diseases causing a skin rash, formerly common in childhood, e.g., measles, rubella, chickenpox, scarlet fever.

exclusionary rule in medical law This is the principle that illegally obtained evidence is not admissible in a court of law. It is important when, for instance, proof of corporate culpability for environmental pollution depends on incriminating documents obtained without authorization by a WHISTLE-BLOWER.

excreta The waste products of metabolism and the residue of digested food intake. In humans and other mammals, soluble chemical waste products are excreted mainly in the urine. Solid waste, including the products of bacterial action in the gut, is excreted in feces. Carbon dioxide and excess water vapor are excreted by the lungs in expired air.

excretion rate The rate at which substances are excreted from the body, often after metabolic transformation. This rate varies considerably. Some toxic substances are stored in body tissues and very slowly excreted, e.g., fat-soluble pesticides are stored in fat, lead is stored in bone.

exercise Muscular activity that requires energy expenditure, using inspired oxygen to transform and metabolize carbohydrates. AEROBICS or AEROBIC EXERCISE maximizes this process. Calisthenic exercise increases the mobility and agility of limbs and trunk.

exhaust gases A general term for gases that are released by combustion of fuel and decomposition of organic matter and are often toxic. Almost all exhaust gases are produced by carbon-based fuels, so they consist of oxides of carbon, often also oxides of other ingredients, e.g., nitrogen, sulfur, as well as contaminants or additives to petroleum fuels. These are the principal ingredient of urban SMOG and environmental pollution. See also OFF-GASSING.

exit problem A term used by family physicians to describe a problem mentioned seemingly as an afterthought by patients just as they are going out the door. This may in fact be the real reason for the encounter but could not be mentioned until the patient plucked up enough courage to mention it, half-hoping the physician would dismiss it. Public health administrators encounter exit problems, too, under similar circumstances, and these may be serious and important.

exogamy Mating between people from altogether different gene pools.

exotoxin A toxin secreted or excreted by a pathogenic microorganism that harms health by disrupting or inhibiting essential physiological functions. An example is the exotoxin produced by the diphtheria bacillus that has an inhibitory effect on the conduction tissues of the heart.

Expanded Programme on Immunization (EPI) As practiced by WHO and UNICEF, usually in collaboration with national agencies, this is a systematic program of immunization against communicable diseases of infants and children that in the preimmunization period had high incidence and high morbidity and mortality rates. The diseases against which immunizations are given usually include diphtheria, pertussis, tetanus, poliomyelitis, measles, and hepatitis B; and sometimes rubella and mumps.

expectation of life Syn: life expectancy. The average number of years an individual of given age can be expected to live if current mortality rates continue to apply. This is a hypothetical statistical abstraction, calculated on the basis of existing age-specific mortality rates.

expected years of life lost A measure of the impact of premature deaths due to disease or injury on national statistics. This measure calculates separately for each specific cause the number of years of life lost before reaching normal life expectancy and adds the results to arrive at a global figure comparable to the BURDEN OF DISEASE.

experiment A scientific study in which the investigator deliberately alters some of the conditions of whatever is being observed in order to study the effects of making the alteration(s).

experimental epidemiology As used by early 20th century epidemiologists, this term meant the observation of how infections spread in populations of experimental animals such as rats or guinea pigs. In the 1970s, the term was used for randomized trials, but this usage is preferably avoided.

experimental error As commonly used, this term means error introduced by faulty instruments, contaminating ingredients in reagents, etc., rather than error due to human failings, such as OBSERVER ERROR.

experimental study As customarily used, this term applies to experiments on human subjects, e.g., randomized controlled trials, for which ethical approval is mandatory.

expert witness A person with particular knowledge, skill, experience in a defined or specified field, generally recognized by peers in that domain of human affairs, who is called upon to testify in a court case in the capacity of an acknowledged authority on the subject.

exponential growth Strictly speaking, this means a rate of growth that abides by an exponential distribution. As loosely used in demography, it often means a growth rate greater than increments that follow an arithmetical progression. The actual growth rate in the middle years of the 20th century population surge was described by demographers as hyperexponential.

exposure 1. In communicable disease control, contact with a source of a disease agent that leads to transmission of the agent to a new host. 2. In environmental hazard control, the amount of a disease agent such as a toxic substance to which person(s) have been exposed and that may lead to disease or clinical signs, but not necessarily the same as DOSE, which is the amount that actually acts on the body. 3. In noncommunicable disease control, "exposure" refers to any influence on health outcomes, including social influences on behavior such as adoption of cigarette smoking, or the process by which an agent or a factor such as high blood pressure influences health. Exposure to an agent can have beneficial, i.e., protective, rather than adverse, consequences.

exposure assessment The process of determining whether exposure to an environmental agent has adverse effects on health. Ideally, this assessment is conducted by means of epidemiological and/or toxicological studies, and, depending on the nature of the exposure, it may be necessary for these to be long-term studies. For instance, exposure to low-level ionizing radiation may not have harmful consequences for decades and exposure to endocrine disrupters might not exert effects until the next generation. Establishing cause-effect relationships becomes extremely difficult in situations such as these.

exposure limit The measured amount of an environmental agent that, if exceeded, is harmful to health, usually expressed as MAXIMUM ALLOWABLE CONCENTRATION (MAC).

extended family A multigenerational group of people related by blood and marriage, often comprising an identifiable head (a patriarch or matriarch), their offspring and spouses, and the children of this second generation; often there are additional relations, cousins, second cousins, etc., all of whom recognize their kinship and possess a high degree of family solidarity. Extended families were the norm in pastoral and agrarian societies but have often broken down into NUCLEAR FAMILIES (two generations, i.e., marital partners and their children) in industrial societies, where there is usually higher geographical mobility. Extended families transmit traditions about infant and child care, provide mutual support, and can offer a health-sustaining environment to all who belong to them, although sometimes they perpetuate customs that are harmful to health.

extinction 1. In biology, the complete disappearance of a species by extermination of breeding stock, which happens as a consequence of loss of habitat, excessive predation, inability to adapt to altered conditions in the supporting environment and ecosystem—almost always the result of human activity. In the early 21st century, species extinction is occurring at an unprecedented rate with unpredictable consequences. 2. In environmental science, the property of ionizing radiation that declines and ceases naturally or as a result of artificial impedance.

extremely low frequency (ELF) electromagnetic radiation The long wavelength radiation emitted by electrical appliances and high-voltage power lines, that, it has been suggested, may have ill-defined adverse biological and human health effects.

extrinsic allergic alveolitis, pneumonitis An inflammatory disease of allergic origin affecting the bronchioles, alveoli, and interstitial lung tissue. It can occur after repeated exposure to many varieties of organic dusts. Two forms of it are FARMER'S LUNG and SILO-FILLER'S DISEASE.

extrinsic incubation period The period required for development in the nonhuman host of the life stage of parasites that pass portions of their life cycle in humans and portions in other species. The term is most often applied to the portion of the malaria parasite's life cycle that is passed in the definitive host, i.e., the female mosquito.

eye injuries Occupational or recreational injuries of the eyes and adnexa are extremely common, but because the bony orbit protects the eyes, these injuries are not often a serious threat to eyesight. Nonetheless, all must be treated seriously. Common injuries include corneal and conjunctival foreign bodies and corneal lacerations. Penetrating injuries are much more serious and often cause permanently impaired vision.

eye strain A common, although rather ill-defined, condition associated with work involving use of the eyes for intense close work, such as proofreading, detailed budgetary preparation, and also prolonged working with computer monitors.

F

fabrication of data The invention or falsification of observations or results of experiments. This is a very serious form of SCIENTIFIC MISCONDUCT or FRAUD that is a criminal act occasionally perpetrated by overly eager, dishonest, or corrupt scientists.

face validity The apparent relationship of findings or observations to the topic that is under investigation or observation ("on the face of it"). See also VALIDITY.

facies The facial appearance and/or expression. The word is used in the context of the facial appearance or expression typical of specific diseases, such as the protuberant staring eyes and anxious expression often associated with hyperthyroidism.

facilitator An individual who leads and acts as a catalyst in discussions, eases or encourages an activity. In international or multicultural conferences and in adversarial situations such as disputes between labor and management, a facilitator ideally is someone who understands and can interpret to each party the point of view of the other parties, and can present the facts impartially while seeking reconciliation and consensus development.

factitious As applied to health, this describes a state or condition such as physical blemishes that could be the consequence of illness or injury but is under the subject's voluntary control. Thus, a factitious injury is a deliberate, usually self-inflicted injury. A factitious disorder resembles MALINGERING in some respects, but it may be a symptom of serious mental disorder or of the condition known as MUNCHAUSEN SYNDROME, in which often bizarre symptoms and physical signs are fabricated.

factor From Latin *facere*, to do, to make. Literally a maker, a person who performs a designated function in an organization. In common public health and epidemiological usage, the word describes a specific agent, event, or process that brings about a change in health status or initiates a specific outcome. Sometimes the word is used loosely as a synonym for a causal agent when the correct term is usually DETERMINANT or RISK FACTOR. See also PROTECTIVE FACTOR.

factor analysis Statistical methods and procedures for seeking patterns of interrelationships among many variables by grouping those that correlate, using analysis of correlations among sets of variables, such as the scoring systems for rating scales used in surveys.

Factor VIII A specific protein ingredient in blood that promotes clotting. It is absent or deficient in hemophilia, so concentrated preparations of Factor VIII are used to prevent bleeding and treat the exacerbations that hemophiliac patients experience. This was a vehicle for transmission of HIV and hepatitis C infection to large numbers of children and adults with hemophilia in the early 1980s, before this transmission route was identified and HIV screening tests were developed.

factory A place where workers are engaged in making something. The legal definition under the UK Factories Acts has varied since the first Act of 1803. Currently, it is a place where 10 or more workers are employed, using machinery. Factories Acts in the United Kingdom and similar legislation in other countries aim mainly to ensure that working conditions are safe, noxious and toxic processes are under control, and environments are unharmed. Violations are common and difficult to control.

factory farming Highly intensive rearing of livestock, such as pigs, heifers, turkeys, and chickens, relying on fortified feeds rather than grazing or free-range foraging for food, with emphasis on adding bulk to meat to enhance its price when it is marketed. Factory farming becomes an economic imperative as the need for food increases in an affluent world with exploding urban populations, but it has been associated with several serious disease outbreaks, including localized but dangerous epidemics of *E. COLI* O157:H7 infection attributable to contamination of aquifers and wells by large quantities of animal manure, and possibly with mad cow disease, i.e., BOVINE SPONGIFORM ENCEPHALOPATHY, due to use of contaminated feeds (with subsequent human cases of VARIANT CREUTZFELDT-JAKOB DISEASE). See also FEED LOTS.

facultative Descriptive of organisms that can adapt to other ways of surviving than that which is usual for them. Thus, a facultative anaerobe is an aerobic organism that can also live and perhaps reproduce in anaerobic conditions.

Faculty of Public Health The organization for physician specialists in public health in the United Kingdom. It is a specialist faculty of the Royal Colleges of Physicians of the United Kingdom. It sets the standards for specialists in the discipline, conducts examinations for entry to the specialty, and is also the academic professional association for physician specialists in public health. This organization has had several name changes. It began as the Faculty of Community Medicine in 1980, then became the Faculty of Public Health Medicine, and in 2002, changed its name again to the Faculty

of Public Health. See http://www.fph.ac.uk for details.

fads and fashions Responses of populations or defined groups to collective influences from opinion leaders or peer pressure. These responses may be irrational but can profoundly alter ways people behave, dress, eat, fall ill, and are treated for their diseases. Examples include women's shoes, which fashion dictates must look "attractive," despite evidence of structural and functional harm they may do to the feet, diets that rely on starvation or bizarre ingredients, and, in the 19th century, tight corsets that constricted women's waists, sometimes deforming and even crippling them. Harmful fads and fashions in medical care have included bloodletting, purging, colonic irrigation, irradiation for acne and other complaints, and psychosurgery. Some currently popular drug treatments may fall into the category of harmful, but only time will tell.

failed state A nation or comparable administrative jurisdiction in which essential infrastructure, including health services, law enforcement, and other necessities for collective and personal health and safety, has broken down because of lawlessness and anarchy. A sharp rise in all or most indicators of population ill health and premature death occurs in failed states.

failure rate The proportion of unsuccessful procedures, examinations, etc., in a series.

failure to thrive The condition of infants and small children who do not achieve developmental milestones within the range expected for their age. It can be an indicator of nutritional deficit, or of developmental abnormalities, some of which are difficult to detect or identify in infancy, and/or of chronic diseases of infancy and childhood, such as cardiorespiratory or gastrointestinal disorders.

fair employment practices See AFFIRMATIVE ACTION.

faith-based programs and services These are programs and services organized, administered, and usually staffed by members of a particular denomination of a religious faith. Educational programs, services, and support for the indigent and the needy have long been provided by many Christian denominations, Jewish temples, and Moslem mosques, and by Hindus and Buddhists. Hospitals evolved from, and some remain institutions staffed by members of, religious orders. The concept became controversial in the United States in 2001, when the administration encouraged faith-based agencies in the health and social services sectors to assume responsibilities for services that had traditionally been secular, although the US Constitution explicitly separates church and state. This policy shift caused concern because some faith-based agencies might proselytize and may not provide needed services, such as advice on contraception or other aspects of human reproduction of which their faith disapproves.

faith healing A form of alternative or unconventional medicine that functions on the belief that illness can be arrested and even cured by faith alone, such as by prayer or the intercession of a supernatural power. CHRISTIAN SCIENCE is a form of faith healing.

Fallopian tubes The duct through which the ovum passes on its way from the ovary to the uterus, where it implants if fertilization has occurred. The operation of TUBAL LIGATION consists of excision of a small segment and tying off the cut ends to prevent passage of ova, thus sterilizing a previously fertile woman. The name commemorates the Italian pathologist and anatomist Gabriele Fallopio, or Fallopius (1523–1562).

fallout Descent to the earth's surface of suspended atmospheric particles. The term is used mainly in the context of RADIOACTIVE FALLOUT from nuclear explosions and accidents (see CHERNOBYL). It applies also to emissions of combusted carbon-based fuel, which can include toxic ingredients, such as trace amounts of lead, mercury, and other metals, polyaromatic hydrocarbons, and other fine particulate matter. Worldwide, the fallout of trace amounts of lead and mercury in emissions from coal-fired power generators and furnace factories produces prodigious quantities measuring in the range of many tonnes per annum per 100 hectares.

fallout zone The region affected by fallout. This obviously is influenced by the direction and strength of prevailing winds, which often create an elliptical zone, called a PLUME, downwind from the source of the emissions.

false memory syndrome A controversial condition in which it is claimed that an impressionable person is encouraged by a therapist to "remember" events that never happened. "Recovered memories" often involve accounts of sexual abuse that is said to have taken place in infancy or early childhood. It is difficult to establish the truth in these cases, but careers of some physicians, nurses, and school teachers have been blighted by unprovable accusations of sexual abuse that are based on such recovered memories.

false negative A negative test result occurring in a person who actually has the disease or possesses the attribute for which the test is done. If this occurs in testing for potentially lethal conditions such as cancer, the consequences of declaring persons healthy when they are not can be very serious. Rates of false-negative and false-positive test results are indicators, respectively, of the SENSITIVITY and SPECIFICITY of SCREENING TESTS.

false positive A positive test result in a person who actually does not have the condition for which the test is being done. This can have serious consequences when, on the basis of screening test findings, people are wrongly diagnosed and further investigated or treated for such conditions as cancer, leading to unnecessary risks, sometimes including radiotherapy or major surgery; in addition, the individuals experience needless anxiety about the implications of having such a disease.

falsifiability A principle on which the advance of science is based, that relies on the process of finding evidence that a scientific finding, belief, or theory is false. It is elucidated in the writings of the Austrian (later British) philosopher Karl Popper (1902–1994). The process of REFUTATION is an important way in which science advances, when previously accepted "truths" are shown by observation, experiment, and logical analysis to be untrue.

family 1. A group of two or more persons united by genetic heritage or adoptive or marital ties or the common law equivalent, who may or may not live together in the same household but who often share the same family name and usually function in mutually supportive ways (although many varieties of dysfunctional families occur). A family is an established entity in law and religion. Structural variations include NUCLEAR FAMILY, EXTENDED FAMILY, and SINGLE-PARENT FAMILY. Sociologists and psychologists have identified functional variations, such as autocratic, democratic, and autonomous decision making about church going, children's schools, contact with health care services, and uptake of vaccinations, that help to determine the health status of children. 2. In biology and TAXONOMY, a family is a division of an ORDER.

family contact disease Illness that occurs among family members who acquire a disease of occupational origin, such as ASBESTOSIS or BERYLLIOSIS, as a result of exposure to the causal agent (asbestos fibers, beryllium dust, etc.) that is brought home on the exposed worker's clothing. Infants and small children are vulnerable to family contact diseases of occupational origin.

family court A court of law that seeks to resolve disputes between family members, often involving domestic violence, spouse abuse, etc., therefore frequently involving health issues.

family health A term used to describe the concept of health status of the family unit as a whole, i.e., parent(s) and child(ren) considered collectively. Use of the term in this way recognizes that dynamic psychological and physical interaction of family members can influence the physical, mental, and emotional health status of all, either beneficially or harmfully. In a dysfunctional family, psychodynamic transactions induce disruption, hostility, and malicious acts, rather than mutual love and support.

family medicine, family practice Syn: general practice. The branch of medical practice that has evolved from general practice, that is now recognized as an important specialty focusing on the continuing care of the entire family, with emphasis on disease prevention and health promotion, as well as treatment of incidental and chronic disease.

family physician Syn: general practitioner. A specialist in family medicine.

family planning A term applied both to individual initiatives and to community-wide approaches to spacing of births by restricting excessive numbers of pregnancies through the use of education about reproductive health and instruction on effective contraceptive methods. See also BIRTH CONTROL and CONTRACEPTION.

family planning association An organization dedicated to aspects of human reproduction, especially to educating girls and women about human fertility and ways to control it. Such organizations exist at every level, from international to local, in most literate societies. They derive inspiration from founders of the family planning movement such as MARIE STOPES in Britain and MARGARET SANGER in the United States, and leadership, educational material, etc., from national organizations in countries where they are legally permitted to function. Their educational activities and their capacity to provide contraceptive supplies are impeded, sometimes aggressively, by some religious leaders and fanatics in some nations.

family study In-depth examination by social worker(s), psychologist(s), etc., of the way a family functions, usually preliminary to intervention aimed at correcting unhealthy or abnormal situations.

family therapy Intervention by a trained social worker or other qualified health professional who works with the family as a social unit, seeking the best way to ensure healthy interactions among family members.

family violence See DOMESTIC VIOLENCE.

famine Extreme scarcity of accessible food supplies of the population of a country or region over an extended period, leading to hunger, malnutrition, starvation of those affected with deaths due to this among the most vulnerable members of the population, weanling children, and those who have pre-existing diseases, such as chronic infections. Many famines occur because of inequitable distribution rather than overall shortages of available food. Famine is a DISASTER requiring intervention and often external food aid.

farmer's lung An allergic-inflammatory pneumonitis that occurs as an occupational disease of agricultural workers, attributable to inhalation of dust from moldy hay, containing spores of any or all of several varieties of fungus species.

Farr's laws WILLIAM FARR demonstrated that epidemics decline at a mathematically predictable rate, using empirical observations of a smallpox epidemic to confirm this. He later formulated several other mathematical equations and laws that apply to epidemics, e.g., that prevalence of a disease can be calculated from the mathematical product of incidence and the average duration.

Farr, William (1807–1883) A British physician who became the first Compiler of Abstracts in the Office of the Registrar General of England and Wales, where he worked for more than 40 years, studying, analyzing, and reporting on all that could be learned from the annual records of deaths. He established the analysis of vital statistics as an essential tool in public health services.

fascioliasis Liver fluke (*Fasciola hepatica*) disease, which is ZOONOSIS of sheep and cattle in South America, the Middle East, and parts of Asia with humans as occasional hosts. In humans it causes symptoms affecting the liver and biliary tract, such as colicky pains and jaundice.

fasciolopsiasis An intestinal trematode infection of pigs and humans with *Fasciolopsis buski*, transmitted by the fecal-oral route, endemic in southeast Asia, e.g., rural regions of Thailand.

fast breeder reactor A NUCLEAR REACTOR that uses fast-moving neutrons to convert uranium to plutonium and by nuclear fission creates more fuel than it uses. An important use of a fast breeder reactor is to manufacture plutonium for military purposes, rather than to generate electric power. It creates large quantities of radioactive waste with a very long half-life, and if the reactor releases radiation into the environment because of accident or inadequate protection against leakage, it can contaminate large areas for prolonged periods—centuries, rather than decades.

fast food Prepackaged, sometimes partly or fully cooked food that can be purchased in supermarkets for home consumption with minimal preparation. The same term describes foods that are cooked or reheated and served in franchised outlets in many countries. Available varieties include hamburger, fish fillets, chicken, pizza, and french fries, with token amounts of vegetables and liberal use of condiments. The environment of many fast food outlets and the fact that staff are often poorly trained prompt public health authorities to monitor them to ensure that they do not become a nidus for food-borne diseases. Fast food is often nutritionally adequate but has a high content of carbohydrate and fat (including TRANS FATS), so people whose diet consists largely of fast foods can become obese. See also JUNK FOODS.

fasting Abstinence from food. This can be voluntary or involuntary, total, partial, periodic, episodic, or prolonged (as in hunger strike). The motive may be concern about body weight, part of religious observance, as it is for Moslems during the month of Ramadan, or a requirement for certain biochemical tests, such as fasting blood sugar estimation.

fatality rate A term often used loosely and incorrectly by the media to describe the number of deaths observed in a designated group of people, such as the victims of a natural disaster in which the deaths occur simultaneously or close together in time. It is seldom a rate in the true sense of the word because there may be no clearly defined denominator or time dimension, and for this reason use of the term fatality rate (rather than fatality ratio) should be discouraged. Contrast the precise term CASE FATALITY RATE.

fatherhood The status of a male who is identified as a parent, with obligations, e.g., taking part in child rearing, and rights, e.g., to state-provided paternity benefits, accompanying this.

fatigue 1. Exhaustion, associated with overwork, long working hours, strenuous physical work, demanding intellectual work. A condition predisposing to work-related injury. 2. Muscle fatigue, associated with excessive and/or repetitive activity of particular muscle groups. 3. Metal fatigue, a physical change in the molecular structure of metal, associated with increased fragility.

fatty acids The general term for monobasic carboxylic acids that are ingredients of fats and oils that include acetic acid and formic acid among others, and long-chain compounds such as oleic, palmitic, and other fatty acids.

fatty liver A condition associated with excessive intake of alcohol in which the liver is enlarged, soft, but functionally intact. It may be a precursor of hepatic cirrhosis.

favism An acute toxic reaction to ingestion of fava beans or exposure to the pollen of the bean plant caused by a genetically determined aberration of glucose metabolism, causing headache, fever, convulsions. It occurs mainly in regions where the beans are grown, e.g., Mediterranean countries.

feasibility study An investigation, usually on a modest scale, aimed at finding out whether it would be practicable to carry out a more formal, larger-scale research project.

fecundity The capability of producing live-born offspring. This can be assessed only in retrospect, as there is no consistently reliable and valid way of testing for potential fecundity.

Federal Emergency Management Agency (FEMA) The US government agency, now part of the Department of Homeland Security, that organizes and administers plans to cope with natural and manmade disasters involving loss of life, loss of habitat, and destruction of essential infrastructure. FEMA coordinates with local agencies, including security, law enforcement, local and regional administrative services, hospital and public health services, the media, transport, and communications. Most nations have comparable systems. Concern about terrorism in the early 21st century has led to enhanced attention to the work of this agency in the United States and similar reactions in the United Kingdom, European Union, and many other nations. See http://www.fema.gov/.

feebleminded An obsolete (and derogatory) term for mental retardation, the condition now often described as "intellectually challenged" or "intellectually impaired."

feedback A signal that indicates how a system is functioning and enables some adjustment or control procedures to be applied. Where this process is under continuous control, a feedback loop is established. The system may be mechanical, biological, or human.

feed lots Land set aside for supplementary feeding of animals, typically close to transshipping and slaughtering facilities, often on the outskirts of a city. Because the animals produce large quantities of manure, public health concerns often arise, e.g., potential contamination of water supplies. The cattle in feed lots receive fortified feeds that may be a vehicle for transmission of pathogenic organisms, such as the prion of BOVINE SPONGIFORM ENCEPHALOPATHY.

fee-for-service system A payment method used in many nations, especially for general or family medical practice and in other personal health services, such as dentistry, in which patients (or their medical insurance carriers) pay a designated fee for each item of service that they receive from their physician. Fee-for-service payment systems have the advantage of personalizing health care, but the disadvantage that the fee may be a deterrent that inhibits people who need care from obtaining it in a timely manner. In low-income nations and nations with inadequate provision for comprehensive medical insurance coverage, out-of-pocket fee-for-service expenses exacerbate poverty. See also CAPITATION, which is a contrasting payment system.

female circumcision See FEMALE GENITAL MUTILATION.

female condom A BARRIER CONTRACEPTIVE employing a latex pouch that fits into the vagina, completely shielding the vaginal epithelium from contact with the penis, and vice versa, thereby reducing considerably the risk of sexually transmitted diseases, such as HIV/AIDS and genital herpes, as well as the possibility of pregnancy.

female genital mutilation An ancient tribal custom that persists in parts of Africa (Somalia, Kenya, Sudan, Egypt, etc.) and the Middle East (Yemen) that is believed by those who practice it to ensure purity and chastity of women. At its least traumatic, the procedure involves no more than an incision in the prepuce of the clitoris, and this is an initiation rite among some educated urbanized tribal groups in Kenya. The most radical operation (usually done on small girls by rural village midwives) amputates the clitoris, excises the labia minora, and sutures the raw tissue remaining, leaving a small hole for the passage of menstrual blood. Sexual intercourse for these women is painful, childbirth is hazardous, and postnatal fistulas, genitourinary infection, and offensive vaginal discharge lead to chronic ill health. This radical form of mutilation has been exported with migrants to industrial nations in Europe and North America and, although illegal there and in most countries from where the women originally came, it is still practiced clandestinely.

female labor force Working women identified in labor statistics as receiving wages or salary for their work, in contrast to unpaid women who often work harder and longer hours as homemakers, caring for husbands, children, dependent elderly relations, etc.

female-male gap A demographic term for the numerical or percentage difference between the numbers of males and females in each age group in the population. Unless distorted by selective abortion of female fetuses and/or female infanticide, the female-male gap at birth is about 5 to 6 per 100, i.e., there are about 105 to 106 male births for every 100 female births. A demographic profile in which there are 110 or more boys aged 5 to 9 years, or 10 to 14 years, per 100 girls is an indication of selective factors, such as abortion of female fetuses and/or female infanticide. The same term is used to describe other sex differences, e.g., in literacy levels, health status indicators.

fermentation chamber, tower A silo fitted with horizontal shelves on which macerated solid waste is deposited, aerated, and encouraged to undergo fermentation through the action of an agent such as yeast, while undergoing agitation. Fermentation of decaying organic matter produces methane, which can be used for domestic or commercial purposes.

fertility The production of live offspring, excluding stillbirths, fetal deaths, and miscarriages.

fertility drug The lay term for hormones such as progesterone and pituitary extract, used to enhance the prospect of ovulation and successful implantation of a fertilized ovum. Their use is sometimes complicated by multiple pregnancies, i.e., simultaneous release of several ova, and fertilization of all. Pregnancies with seven or more fetuses have been reported with associated high rates of fetal loss, premature births, and very low birth weight infants. One approach to this has been to "cull" surplus fetuses, which has raised difficult moral and ethical issues.

fertility rate Loosely, the rate at which live infants are added to the population of women in the reproductive age range. The term is preferably avoided. See GENERAL FERTILITY RATE.

fertility ratio A seldom-used measure of the fertility of a population that is calculated by using females in the reproductive age groups, i.e., 15 to 49 years, as the denominator and the number of girls younger than 15 years in the same population as the numerator.

fertilization Fusion of male (sperm) and female (ovum) sex cells (gametes) to produce a single cell that develops into an embryo, fetus, infant, and eventually into an adult.

fertilizers Classes of compounds used in agriculture, horticulture, etc., to promote growth of food crops. Most fertilizers are nitrogen-rich compounds, and some are also rich in phosphate and potassium compounds. Some contain trace elements such as zinc and molybdenum to correct soil deficiency. Natural fertilizers include many kinds of manure, human excreta, guano, some forms of which may contain high concentrations of pathogenic organisms, cysts of intestinal parasites, etc. Artificial (chemical) fertilizers mostly alter soil chemistry when used for prolonged periods, and rainfall runoff from fertilized fields can disrupt freshwater ecosystems.

fetal alcohol syndrome A developmental fetal defect due to maternal alcohol consumption that causes toxic damage to fetal embryonic cells, producing mental retardation and, in severe forms, growth retardation, small cranial size, and a characteristic facial appearance. It occurs in 25% to 50% of offspring of mothers who consume excessive quantities of alcohol during pregnancy. To avoid this condition, women are advised to avoid alcohol altogether from the beginning of pregnancy.

fetal death Syn: STILLBIRTH. Death that occurs before complete expulsion from the uterus of a fetus or the product of conception at any time during the pregnancy after the gestational stage when the fetus is normally considered to be viable. This is variously defined as after the 20th or the 28th week of gestation.

fetus A developing embryo that has reached the stage of organ development, i.e., 8 weeks or more after conception.

fiberglass Very fine filaments of silica glass used primarily as a replacement for asbestos as an insulating material because it was believed to be biologically inert, without the dangerous adverse effects of asbestos. However, inhaled fiberglass particles can cause pulmonary fibrosis. Molded fiberglass is used in boat-building, etc., and its carriage in a volatile solvent and "fixer" exposes workers to hazards, notably damage to the cornea unless protective goggles are used.

fiberoptics Bundles of fine glass tubes are used to transmit light, i.e., electromagnetic radiation, along cables that have a very high capacity and low impedance of signal strength, making this an extremely efficient means of transmission that is widely used in computing and telephony. These are also used in flexible endoscopes for cystoscopy, gastroscopy, bronchoscopy, etc.

fibroid A common benign tumor of the uterus, usually consisting of smooth muscle and fibrous cells. It usually occurs late in a woman's reproductive life or after the menopause but can disrupt pregnancy and labor if large fibroids arise earlier in reproductive life.

fibromyalgia Syn: polymyalgia rheumatica. A condition causing chronic muscle pain, primarily affecting the upper limbs, back, and shoulders and affecting women several times more frequently than men. The persistent pain responds sluggishly to analgesics, often causes insomnia, and may lead to depression.

fiduciary responsibility The legal duty to act in a position of trust for the benefit of others. For example, physicians have a fiduciary responsibility to act for the benefit of their patients. Elected and appointed officials in a public health department have a fiduciary responsibility to act for the benefit of the people in the community the department serves. This fiduciary responsibility includes the duty of elected officials and their delegates to ensure the provision of adequate staff, facilities, and funds for the performance of essential public health functions.

field This word has several scientific meanings, each of which is usually clear from the context: 1. A theme or topic of specialization; 2. A community or region selected for epidemiological or social scientific study; 3. All that is visible through the eyepiece of a microscope; 4. The range of concepts embraced by a particular science.

field study A research project conducted outside a university, health department, etc., generally with study subjects who live in the community or "field" that has been selected for study.

fieldwork Scientific study or routine investigation that is conducted in a setting away from the office, clinic, department, etc., where the scientist or professional worker is usually based.

fight-or-flight reaction Throughout the animal kingdom, an instinctive response to aggression or threat from members of the same or another species is either to resist (fight) or run away (flight). In humans this instinctive reaction is often partly or wholly suppressed, but the release of adrenalin, the hormonal reaction that is part of it, persists. This may be an etiological factor in hypertension. See also SYMPATHETIC NERVOUS SYSTEM.

filaria A genus of thread-like parasitic worms prevalent mainly in tropical regions. The adult worms live in the mesentery, connective tissue, and lymphatic vessels, where their obstructive and inflammatory effects cause swelling called elephantiasis. The larval worms are transmitted by mosquitoes, in which early developmental stages are completed before the almost adult worms infect new hosts when infected mosquitoes partake of a blood meal. The life cycle was worked out by the British physician and naturalist Patrick Manson (1844–1922) and was a model for the elucidation of other mosquito-borne infections, notably malaria.

filariasis Infection with any of several varieties of filaria, nematode worms in the *Filarioidea* family. These are transmitted to humans in the larval stage by mosquito bites. Both culicine and anopheline mosquitoes can transmit filarial worms.

filoviruses A family of anatomically distinct viruses characterized by filamentous structure, which include several that cause extremely dangerous and highly contagious hemorrhagic fevers. They include the viruses responsible for Ebola virus disease, Lassa fever, and Marburg disease.

filter A method or device for separating ("filtering") solid from liquid ingredients in a suspension composed of a mixture of liquids and suspended solid particles. The word is also used to describe the process of sorting people according to predetermined criteria, such as presence of communicable diseases, although this is preferably called SCREENING.

filth diseases A term coined by the British social administrator Charles Murchison (1830–1879) in 1858 and widely used by the public health reformers of 19th century England to describe a class of diseases associated with the unhygienic conditions that prevailed in the urban slums of the early industrial period. The filth diseases included all the departures from health associated with poor personal hygiene, lack of adequate sanitation, presence of vermin such as rats and cockroaches, poverty, and overcrowding, for instance several children obliged to sleep in the same bed, which enhanced the risk of cross-infection with serious respiratory diseases such as tuberculosis. These diseases include respiratory and gastrointestinal infections, diseases spread by ticks, lice, and fleas. The term is obsolete and pejorative, but the conditions described by the term still occur among some poor and underprivileged people even in rich industrial nations.

filtration An important stage of reservoir WATER TREATMENT in which water is led over filtration beds of coarse gravel on which algae grow profusely, then through progressively finer sand before entering the reticulated water supply. The gravel and sand are mechanical filters; the algae are biological filters.

financial index See ECONOMIC INDEX.

fine suspended particulate matter (FSP) Atmospheric dust or solid particulates in emission products of combustion with an aerodynamic diameter of 2.5 microns or less (also known as PM_{25}) that remain suspended in the atmosphere. Particles of less than 2.5 mm ($PM_{2.5}$) can penetrate to the alveoli and contribute to pneumoconiosis or chronic respiratory disease.

firearms A collective name for handguns, rifles, shotguns, and similar potentially lethal weapons that in most civilized jurisdictions are required to be registered with law enforcement authorities and with access restricted to demonstrably responsible users for defined purposes.

firedamp An archaic term for METHANE that forms an explosive mixture with air in coal mines.

firefighting 1. The occupation that is equal in importance to policing in maintenance of public safety. Firefighters are at high risk of occupational death and injury and some risk of chronic respiratory disease from smoke inhalation. 2. (*jargon*) The ad hoc treatment of the consequences of exposure to a health hazard that would be better controlled by eliminating or reducing the health hazard, rather than waiting for it to cause adverse effects. An example is treatment of individual cases of a childhood infectious disease preventable by immunization, rather than immunizing all susceptible children in the population to prevent the disease from occurring in the first place.

first aid A set of mostly simple measures to provide immediate emergency treatment of painful injury or life-threatening cardiac or respiratory crises. In an ideal world, everyone would be able to clear an airway, position unconscious persons to maintain a clear airway, stop severe bleeding, and immobilize fractures. It is a requirement in many jurisdictions for a specified proportion of staff in an organization to be trained in first aid. Some first aid measures, e.g., reduction of dislocated shoulder, splinting limb fractures, have ancient origins. Others, such as CARDIOPULMONARY RESUSCITATION (CPR) and the HEIMLICH MANEUVER for obstructed airway, are modern innovations.

fiscal year The 12-month period selected for accounting purposes at which an annual balance sheet is prepared and subjected to rigorous auditing and scrutiny by all interested parties. The fiscal year may be the same as a calendar year, but often another cutoff date is selected; for instance March 31 or April 30 marks the end of the government fiscal year in some nations.

fission 1. The mechanism by which the nucleus of a cell divides to form two cells where previously there was only one. 2. Nuclear fission, division of an atom into two, usually with release of energy in the form of ionizing radiation and charged particles.

fitness 1. Physical fitness is a set of attributes that include ability to engage in strenuous exercise or hard physical work without becoming distressed by breathlessness and rapid heart action, a state achieved or attained by a regimen of regular, frequent exercises. 2. Genetic fitness is a measure of the reproductive success (relative survival) of a particular phenotype or population group.

fixed assets Syn: tangible assets. Real property, equipment, etc., for which a value is assessed or assigned in balance sheets when a budget is compiled.

fixed costs The component of costs in the balance sheets or financial statements, e.g., of a health department, that remain unchanged over a defined, relatively long period; fixed costs include overhead—costs of lighting, indoor climate control, rental of buildings and equipment, and core staff—although these may be separately itemized in budgets and balance sheets.

flame retardant A chemical compound used to impregnate fabrics in order to render them fire resistant. One group of such substances, POLYBROMINATED BIPHENYLS (PBBs), acquired notoriety when it accidentally contaminated cattle feed and caused an epidemic of bizarre wasting disease in 1973. Several hundred people, including pregnant women, consumed contaminated dairy products, and many developed a complex persistent neurological and generalized disease. A related flame retardant containing polybrominated diphenyl ethers is widely used in electronic equipment.

flashcard A card that indicates alternative response categories for participants in a survey when they are asked to reply to questions that have a finite, limited number of possible responses.

flaviviruses A family of viruses that includes many arboviruses and the virus of hepatitis C.

flavonoids A family of phenolic compounds that include many natural plant pigments.

fleas Small wingless arthropods that are parasitic on birds, domestic pests, animals, and humans and include important disease vectors, notably PLAGUE, transmitted between rats and to humans by the rat flea, *Xenopsylla cheopis*. They derive nourishment from the host's blood, which they drink through mouth parts adapted for piercing skin and sucking blood.

Flexner Report A report prepared for the Carnegie Corporation in 1910 by the American educator Abraham Flexner (1866–1939) that identified serious deficiencies in medical education and recommended changes, including organized programs of basic medical sciences and clinical instruction. The Flexner Report had a profound and permanent influence on medical education throughout the world.

flies The insect order of *Diptera*, winged insects that typically feed on fluids, including blood and decayed organic matter. They include houseflies, blackflies, botflies, and many others that are either serious pests or disease carriers or vectors.

flocculation From Latin *floccus*, a flock of sheep. Aggregation of suspended particles in a fluid medium into a loose mass resembling tufts of wool, a process that occurs in some chemical reactions, in the flocculation tanks of sewage treatment plants, and, by adding alum, in reservoir water that can become potable if suspended particles are filtered out or settle to the bottom, which is easier after flocculation than before.

flood Overflowing of large amounts of water onto land that is normally not submerged. This can result from rivers bursting their banks after heavy rainstorms, tidal surges accompanying severe storms, collapse of a reservoir or dam, obstruction of river flow by ice buildup in the spring thaw, landslides, etc. A flood is often a sudden catastrophic event that has significant health consequences, including loss of homes and habitat, displacement of large numbers of people, contamination of water supplies by sewage from inactivated sewage treatment works, toxic chemicals escaping from waste dumps, etc., in short, a major public health emergency. For example, hurricane Katrina in 2005 caused flooding of much of the city of New Orleans because of a combination of storm surges and breaches in the protective levees, with the loss of several hundred lives, many billion dollars in damages, widespread environmental pollution, and destruction of essential public health infrastructure.

flood plain A region of flat land beside a river bed, made up of sediment deposited in previous floods. Flood plain land is usually very fertile because sediment is rich in nutriment, and this encourages people to settle there. But it is likely to flood again when the river is running with higher water than usual after heavy rains or during the spring thaw. Such land should never be used for sewage treatment plants, toxic waste dumps, or high-density housing purposes. Flood plains are unsuitable settings on which to build large cities, but for geopolitical and economic reasons many cities do exist on flood plains.

flow chart A diagram in which the stages in a process are set out in boxes connected by arrows to show the connections between the stages.

flu See INFLUENZA.

flue A chimney or smoke duct to convey emissions from combusted fuel to the outside world.

fluke A type of trematode flatworm, generally parasitic, for example, the liver fluke, *Fasciola hepatica*, that primarily infects sheep and occasionally people. The worms that cause SCHISTOSOMIASIS are trematodes or flukes, and these are the cause of major public health problems in several parts of Africa and Asia.

fluorescein A dye that dissolves in alkaline solutions to produce green fluorescence. Its medical uses include staining specimens in order to visualize bacteria microscopically and staining the conjunctival sac in order to visualize foreign bodies.

fluoridation The planned, systematic addition to reservoir drinking-water supplies of carefully measured amounts of sodium fluoride, to achieve a level of 0.7 to 1.2 parts per million. This level has been shown by many large-scale epidemiological studies to provide a fluoride intake adequate to enable formation and renewal of dental enamel, thereby greatly reducing the risk of dental caries, but this concentration is not so large as to cause FLUOROSIS.

fluoride pollution An environmental hazard of emissions from aluminum smelter stacks that can cause FLUOROSIS among exposed populations living downwind in the fallout zone from the plume.

fluorocarbons A group of stable organic compounds formerly widely used industrially as solvents, refrigerants, and aerosol propellants because of their supposed inert quality but then found to react with and destroy stratospheric ozone and thus are now subject to an embargo.

fluoroscope A diagnostic instrument that directs a beam of x-rays through the body so as to cast an image on a fluorescent screen. This was widely used in the 1930s to 1950s, e.g., to determine at weekly examinations whether sufficient air had been injected into an artificial pneumothorax (used

to treat tuberculosis by collapsing the affected lung); the consequence was later onset of cancers. e.g., of the breast, attributable to repeated small doses of ionizing radiation. The use of fluoroscopes in shoe stores in the 1930s to the 1950s was abandoned for the same reason.

fluorosis A condition of dental enamel and bones that results from excessive intake of fluoride, manifested by unsightly mottling of dental enamel and increased bone density, sometimes with deformity if the condition has been very severe at the time of growth spurts.

fly ash Large solid particles that are contained in emissions from fuel combusted in a furnace and emitted with the smoke plume unless trapped by a dust separator or BAFFLE CHAMBER.

focus group A group of people selected because of their interest or special knowledge of an issue or problem, who are brought together by invitation from a community leader, such as a public health official who seeks their views on alternative courses of action that might be taken to deal with a problem or issue of concern. Focus groups are widely used by political leaders and are sometimes used by social science and other public health research workers to help clarify the most suitable way to study a problem. Findings or results of focus group analysis are readily influenced by selection biases of several kinds, so they should always be viewed with cautious skepticism.

fog A thick mist of water vapor suspended in the atmosphere; cumulus clouds have the same composition, and one form of fog is cumulus clouds at ground level, but more often fog is caused by condensation of water vapor at the earth's surface as the temperature changes to a level that encourages condensation. Fog is a hazard in many coastal regions. Fog may aggravate respiratory disease, but aerosol medication is used in a "therapeutic fog," for instance, to treat asthma. See also SMOG.

folic acid A water-soluble vitamin in the vitamin B group that plays an essential role in purine metabolism and in the formation of red blood cells. Folic acid deficiency leads to anemia. A high intake of folic acid before and during pregnancy protects against the occurrence of neural tube defects (spina bifida) in the offspring.

folklore Beliefs passed on from one generation to the next, often throughout many centuries, especially in preliterate cultures, that include many ideas about FOLK MEDICINE. Pharmacological research has shown that some aspects of folk medicine and healing are effective, but it is difficult to discern whether they originated by chance or by application of empirical observations that may have been made in the first place many centuries or even millennia ago.

folk medicine Remedies, usually for common ailments, usually comprising herbs or substances plentifully available that have been believed and/or found by experience to be effective treatment for people with common symptoms such as "rheumaticky" pains, shortness of breath, and menstrual irregularities. Some folk medicines work because they contain pharmacologically active ingredients, some by the power of suggestion. Many are culture specific.

folkways A term from cultural anthropology meaning customs that have become firmly established and transmitted throughout many generations and are characteristic of the society.

follicle-stimulating hormone A hormone produced by the pituitary gland that stimulates the growth and maturation of ovarian follicles and the growth of oocytes and also stimulates formation of spermatozoa in the testes.

followup study An assessment that focuses on persons who have previously been the subjects of research, clinical investigation, or therapeutic intervention. Followup studies include COHORT STUDIES, in which study subjects are reassessed at specified intervals, and surveillance by cancer registries and clinics from which 5- and 10-year survival rates for treatment of cancer at various sites are derived.

fomites Plural of fomes, from Latin *fomes, fomitis*, tinder. Articles such as utensils, clothing, children's toys that, by becoming contaminated with pathogenic organisms, can transmit disease.

food Natural or artificially modified substances that are edible, containing any or all of the basic nutritional substances, i.e., carbohydrates, proteins, and fats, and sometimes essential minerals and vitamins, that when consumed and digested are metabolized and converted into energy.

food additive A substance or agent intentionally added to food, generally to commercially processed food. Additives include preservatives, coloring agents, and mineral or vitamin supplements.

food allergy An adverse reaction to ingested food that contains allergens or toxins. A true food allergy is induced by ingestion of a protein or peptide to which the person is hypersensitive or allergic, and can vary from an acute, life-threatening anaphylactic reaction to a mild urticaria. Some so-called food allergies have a different basis: they are really toxic reactions to specific chemicals, such as monosodium glutamate.

Food and Agriculture Organization (FAO) The United Nations agency based in Rome that was established after World War II and has grown into the largest UN agency. Its mandate is to improve human nutrition everywhere, enhance agricultural productivity, monitor food supplies, intervene when food stocks are depleted, and, if possible, take necessary corrective action to limit unsustainable practices such as overfishing when a species is endangered. It works closely with related UN agencies, notably the WORLD FOOD PROGRAMME, which provides food aid at times of scarcity and FAMINE. See http://www.fao.org for details of current activities.

Food and Drug Administration (FDA) The agency in the US Department of Health and Human Services that oversees the safety and efficacy of medicinal drugs, monitors food safety and purity, and reviews the safety of related products, such as biological preparations, cosmetics, and proprietary preparations, and the safety of food for animals, as well as for humans. It liaises with state agencies, public interest groups, the food industry, and the pharmaceutical industry. It has an advisory and policy-forming role for the US government and is sometimes accused of yielding to the influence of the pharmaceutical and food industries, rather than giving priority to the public interest. The FDA has wide-ranging roles and functions, described in detail at http://www.fda.gov.

food bank A charitable community social service that collects surplus food from restaurants, hotels, grocery stores, etc., accepts donations from private citizens, and distributes food to needy persons. Food banks supplement the often inadequate social safety net in some affluent nations, where large gaps exist between those who have and those who lack adequate resources to feed themselves and their children. Because much of the food is donated surplus supplies, it does not necessarily provide well-balanced dietary intake, especially for children, but at least it helps to prevent frank starvation.

food-borne disease A class of diseases attributable to the contamination of food by disease agents, such as a pathogenic organisms and their toxins. These diseases include many kinds of gastroenteric infections, ranging from mild diarrhea to severe life-threatening diarrhea and vomiting with fluid and electrolyte loss caused by conditions including salmonella, shigella, and staphylococcal gastroenteritis, typhoid, botulism, and more, as well as diseases caused by toxic chemicals of other than biological origin. Some food-borne diseases can also be WATER-BORNE DISEASES, e.g., *Salmonella* infections and CHOLERA. Foods that are especially vulnerable to food-borne disease include prepared dishes containing milk and eggs, cold meat and meat products that can become culture media for *Staphylococcus aureus*, and salads that have not been adequately cleansed of contaminants that contain or convey pathogens.

food chain The natural biological transmission of nutriment or energy by ingestion and digestion from one species to others, beginning with single-celled phytoplankton in marine food chains, and moving through progressively larger marine species, all the way to the largest predators. Land-based food chains begin with soil bacteria that nourish plant species, which rely on chlorophyll to metabolize carbon-based proteins and sugars, and these plants nourish herbivorous animals, which in turn provide nourishment (protein, carbohydrate, fat, minerals, vitamins) for carnivores and omnivores, including humans. Green plants are in fact the primary setting for transfer of energy, ultimately originating from solar radiation, into forms that can be used by all other species that feed on plants or on those creatures that feed on plants.

food groups A rather loose and imprecise way to classify foods according to their composition, i.e., principally comprising carbohydrates, fats, proteins, or rich in a specific mineral or vitamin. For example, citrus fruits might be classified as members of a food group rich in vitamin C. Rather than serving a scientific purpose, food groups are a reminder of the virtue of dietary diversity.

food handlers This designation describes the large, heterogeneous occupational group engaged in every phase of the food industry, from primary production through processing to distribution, preparation, cooking, and serving food. High standards of personal hygiene and freedom from contagious diseases are prerequisites for employment as food handlers, especially at the distal (consumer's) end of the system, i.e., preparation, cooking, and serving food in restaurants and cafeterias. This occupational group includes many part-time and temporary workers who are often poorly trained and may be disease carriers.

food irradiation A method to prevent or retard deterioration of food caused by fungus infection or bacterial decomposition, by exposing it to a short burst of ionized radiation, such as may be produced in a nuclear power plant. This is a highly effective method of food preservation, but it is regarded with suspicion by many consumers because of a mis-taken belief that the food continues to emit harmful ionizing radiation long after it has been treated.

food poisoning A general term for contamination of food by agents of disease. Contaminants that cause food poisoning fall into several groups: 1. Infection with pathogenic organisms (see FOOD-BORNE DISEASE); 2. Bacterial food poisoning, caused by effects of bacteria on epithelium of the gastrointestinal tract or bacterial toxins (e.g., STAPHYLOCOCCAL ENTEROTOXIN); 3. Chemical food poisoning, caused by accidental or deliberate contamination of food by chemical poisons, e.g., toxic pesticides in feed grain, the Spanish cooking oil disaster; and 4. Poisons of plant or animal origin, including poisonous fungi, CIGUATERA FISH POISONING.

food policy An aspect of public policy focusing on efforts to achieve equitable distribution of food and a healthy balanced diet, especially for children. Nations have established food policies formally or informally in several ways. One way was the British food rationing program during World War II, which established an equitable food distribution system to ensure adequate intake of protein, fat, carbohydrate, vitamins, and minerals for all children, as well as for the general population. One result of this was a conspicuous improvement in indicators of healthy child development. In peacetime, many nations have made recommendations about desirable food intake, and from time to time international agencies such as the World Health Organization issue statements, for instance on RECOMMENDED DIETARY ALLOWANCES (RDA), and advisory notices about dietary habits that contribute to the risk of obesity, diabetes, and coronary heart disease.

food preservation Treatment to prevent spoilage of food by bacterial decomposition. There are several ancient and some modern methods. Some foods can be sun-dried to reduce water content or immersed in brine ("salted"). Another method, used with fruit, is immersion in sugar (syrup) or conversion to jam or jelly. Canned (tinned) food is hermetically sealed after killing bacteria, usually with heat. Irradiation kills bacteria without altering the appearance or taste.

food rationing In times of scarcity, such as interruption of supply lines in wartime conditions or severe natural disasters, rationing is a way to ensure that all members of the population get a fair share of available food supplies. An interesting side effect of wartime rationing in the United Kingdom and some European nations was that, for the first time, economically deprived segments of the population, and especially their infants and children, received enough food for healthy growth and development, leading to a generation born during the deprived Depression years of the 1930s and nourished on wartime and postwar rations that was taller and fitter than their parents.

food safety Policies, strategies, and tactics sanctioned by laws and regulations, monitored and enforced by national, state, provincial, and/or local public health authorities, aimed at ensuring that all aspects of production, distribution, marketing, and preparation of food are safe, free from contamination by harmful toxins, disease agents, etc. Food safety is an important component of routine public health protection in all organized societies, although food standards vary.

food security Measures adopted to ensure a safe regular food supply from producer to consumer. This is a concern of civil defense authorities and others. In many nations, a senior cabinet minister oversees arrangements to ensure food security.

food stamps A public assistance program for the needy in the United States and some other nations that provides coupons in lieu of cash to be exchanged for designated food items at participating grocery stores and supermarkets.

food standards A set of criteria that have been determined by experts in relevant scientific and technical disciplines, including microbiology, biochemistry, nutrition, and dietetics, stating the acceptable qualities for all commonly marketed foodstuffs, for example specifying content of minerals, preservatives, conditions of storage, shelf life, safe levels of food additives, and the like. One routine task in public health services, usually at a national level, is the monitoring and surveillance of food standards.

Food Standards Agency The British government agency that sets and monitors standards on food quality and nutritional requirements and provides information for health professionals and the general public. Its Web site, http://www.food.gov .uk, provides links to many specific details about food and nutrition and current information, for instance, about commercial foods that have been approved or withdrawn from the market.

forced expiratory volume (FEV) A physiological measurement of "forced vital capacity" using a simple instrument to measure the volume of air expelled from the lungs on complete exhalation. It is measured by FEV_1, the maximum volume of air the person can exhale in 1 second.

force of morbidity A theoretical measure of the number of new cases of a condition that occur at a point in time or per unit of population-time, e.g., in person-time (person-years) at risk.

force of mortality A theoretical measure of the number of deaths of a condition that occur at a point in time or per unit of population-time, such as person-years at risk.

forecasting An essential feature of rational planning in all human activities, including all in the health sector, is a systematic method of anticipating and preparing for the future. This may be done in several ways. The simplest is to extrapolate observed demographic, vital statistical, and epidemiological trends from the past through the present and on, as far as feasible, into the future. This works well enough for some situations but not for others, and it fails to take account of unpredictable events, such as new medical discoveries, the appearance of a new and deadly disease such as HIV/AIDS, natural or manmade disasters, or major changes in the body politic, such as the collapse of the Soviet Union. For these and other reasons, it is desirable to develop imaginative alternative SCENARIOS and also to attempt to shape the future by VISIONING. Forecasting is essential, despite the discouraging observation that forecasts that were made in the past have so often been proven wrong by unfolding events.

foreign body An unwanted object that is inhaled, ingested, or lodges in a part of the body, such as the conjunctival sac, where it can cause pain, distress, inflammation, etc.

forensic medicine The specialized branch of medicine concerned with investigation of deaths and injuries due mainly to other than natural causes, i.e., accidental or intentional violence or deliberate infliction of harm on self or others. Its predominant science is forensic pathology, but other sciences, including toxicology, forensic anthropology, and aspects of physics, chemistry, meteorology, and many other scholarly fields, are often relevant.

formaldehyde A toxic, flammable, irritant gas. In a strong solution in water, it is called FORMALIN, which is widely used as a preservative of tissues and cadavers. Formaldehyde is a carcinogen, and occupational exposure to formalin or formaldehyde is a known cancer risk.

formalin A 40% solution of FORMALDEHYDE in water that is used, among other things, as an embalming fluid and to preserve pathological specimens. It is an animal carcinogen.

formula feeding Infant feeding by means of substitutes for human breast milk that are made up according to a formula that mimics as closely as possible the composition of breast milk. In many developing countries, the use of unsafe water to prepare the formula and dilution of the formula because it costs more than the family budget allows can have disastrous consequences, revealed in many studies sponsored by UNICEF and the WHO. Manufacturers of infant formulas reluctantly accepted an international convention on advertising and promotion of infant formula but continue to promote their products in ways that many consider to be unethical.

formulary A collection of specific drugs and prescriptions for therapeutic remedies, such as the officially approved and printed books published by national agencies, hospitals, etc.

fortified food Food that has been modified to increase the content or concentration of specific ingredients, generally protein and sometimes carbohydrates, vitamins, or minerals.

fossil fuel A generic name for carbon-based fuels derived from carboniferous compounds that are recovered from strata deposited during an earlier era of the earth's existence. COAL in its various forms is a fossil fuel; petroleum oil is a fossil fuel, too, but some geologists and paleontologists believe that the origin of petroleum is different, i.e., a mixture of dead organic matter and naturally occurring compounds.

foster care Care of infants and/or children by someone other than parents or legal guardians, usually with the implied assumption that this is done under the authority of an official public agency, such as child protection services.

foundations These are organizations from which funds are available to support causes, including medical and scientific research. Some derive funds wholly or partly from government sources, others from gifts and/or bequests, and a few encourage additional support in the form of charitable donations from members of the general public. Several foundations have long played a prominent role in the advance of medical science and experimental or demonstration projects, such as community clinics. These include the Rockefeller Foundation, the Ford Foundation, the Milbank Memorial Fund, the Nuffield Trust, the Commonwealth Fund, the Bill & Melinda Gates Foundation, the Wolfson Foundation, and many others. Many activities of foundations in low- and middle-income nations, such as provision and evaluation of family planning services, often resemble the activities of nongovernmental organizations.

founder effect In population genetics, the principle that when a small sample of a large population establishes itself as a new isolated genetic entity, its gene pool contains only a fraction of the genetic diversity of the original larger population from which the sample came.

foundling An abandoned infant who is "found" in a church or on the doorstep of a rich person's home, having been left there by a desperate woman unable or unwilling to care for it. In the 19th century and earlier, foundlings were common enough to justify special hospitals and orphanages to care for them. The practice of indigent mothers abandoning newborn infants still occurs rather frequently in India, Pakistan, and other low-income countries and occasionally in wealthy countries, including the United States and Canada. There is not necessarily a penalty for ABANDONMENT in such circumstances.

foundry workers Workers in a factory that prepares iron, steel, and other metallic castings from molten metal. The work is hard, very hot, and usually dusty and noisy. The specific occupational hazards include infrared radiation-related cataracts, deafness from exposure to loud noise, and, in some situations, pneumoconiosis.

fourfold table Syn: 2×2 table. A table comprising two columns and two rows allowing direct comparison of two sets of data.

foxglove This herb, *Digitalis purpurea*, was known to folk healers for many centuries as a useful remedy for disorders of the heart. Its active ingredient, digitalis (from which digoxin is prepared), was first isolated early in the 20th century.

Fracastorius The Italian monk Girolamo Castor, known as Fracastorius (1478–1553), worked out several ways infection can be transmitted. He described direct person-to-person transmission in the mock heroic poem *Syphilis Sive Morbis Gallicus* (1530), which gave us the name of syphilis, and in *De Contagione* (1546) described DROPLET spread and spread by FOMITES. Thus, he brought about a paradigm shift in the understanding of ways diseases could be caused, spread, and controlled.

fraction Two numerical quantities wherein one is divisible in whole or in part by the other. Fractions are the basis for other expressions, including RATES, RATIOS, and PROPORTIONS.

fragile X syndrome A genetic disorder associated with mental retardation due to a mutation at one end of the X chromosome. It is the most common genetic cause of male mental retardation.

frail elderly A term used to describe elderly people who for the most part need help to complete daily living tasks and sometimes need medical care and social support in order to function independently in the community.

framework A material or abstract structure that is the basis for a more complete entity. Thus, the foundations and supporting beams are the framework for a building; the skeleton is the framework for vertebrates, including humans; and the preamble and themes for successive clauses are the framework for a constitution, such as that of the World Health Organization, a treaty among nations, or legislation enacted by the elected officials of a democratic government.

Framework Convention on Tobacco Control (FCTC) A document presented to and approved by the delegates at the World Health Assembly in 2003 that sets out the measures required by national governments and international trade agreements to limit the worldwide public health problem of tobacco consumption. The convention limits advertising and the sale of tobacco to children and has several restrictions on trade in tobacco products. It came into force in February 2005. By March 2005, 102 nations had signed the Framework Convention, and 57 had ratified it. For details and current status, see http://www.who.int/tobacco/framework/en/.

Framingham Study A series of long-term cohort epidemiological and biomedical investigations that have been conducted with volunteers from the population of Framingham, Massachusetts, since 1948, primarily to investigate RISK FACTORS of coronary heart disease. The Framingham Studies established the importance of behavioral risk factors, such as lack of exercise, cigarette smoking, and physiological and metabolic factors, such as high blood pressure, elevated serum lipids, and non-insulin-dependent diabetes. Many important findings have emerged from this series of investigations. See http://www.nhlbi.nih.gov/about/framingham/ for details.

Frank, Johann Peter A German physician (1745–1821) trained in Heidelberg and Strasburg, professor of medicine at Göttingen, Pavia, and the Allgemeines Krankenhaus in Vienna, he wrote a nine-volume treatise *System Einer Vollständigen Medizinischen Polizey (A Complete System of Medical Policy*, 1779–1827). This described the basic principles of personal hygiene and public sanitation that would protect the health of the populace. Frank emphasized the importance of laws and regulations in protecting and improving population health.

fraud Deception or misrepresentation in which the true situation is deliberately withheld or perhaps is not known, as when there is FABRICATION (or invention) OF DATA, or, more often, when the facts are falsified with intent to deceive. There are many ways this can happen, all of them crimes that require exposure and appropriate corrective action. In public health, fraud may occur in the conduct of research work in any of the sciences on which protection of health depends, or in any of several ways that dishonest, corrupt, or incompetent public health officials may betray their trust, e.g., failure to carry out routine safety tests on food, milk, or water.

freedom of choice The situation that ideally exists in liberal democracies when all people can decide for themselves how to conduct their lives, as long as they abide by the law and do not harm others. The phrase often has a special meaning in relation to the REPRODUCTIVE RIGHTS of women who can choose whether or not to become and remain pregnant.

freedom of information See ACCESS TO INFORMATION.

freon The trade name for FLUOROCARBON compounds used as refrigerants that destroy ozone in the upper atmosphere. By international agreement, they are being phased out of production, but a flourishing black market has persisted, especially in freon for air conditioners in cars, where the risk of escape into the atmosphere is considerable.

frequency An imprecise general term that is used to describe the occurrence of conditions, in particular diagnostic categories when it is not feasible to distinguish incidence and prevalence.

friendly societies A collective name for a large number of insurance programs to help cover the costs of medical care, prescribed drugs, and partial support of inpatient hospital care, operated by national service clubs and the like, in the United Kingdom, European nations, Australia, and New Zealand before these nations had comprehensive tax-supported health care insurance systems.

friendly visitor A person who regularly contacts infirm, elderly, or other housebound people to attend to their needs for shopping, housekeeping, etc., and provide company and conversation. This may be a self-generated voluntary activity or part of a formal program organized and perhaps financially subsidized by a local health and social services department. See also BUDDY SYSTEM.

fringe benefits Nonmonetary rewards additional to salaries that are provided for professional staff and others in many organizations. Benefits may include contributions to retirement income and payment of part or all of employees' health insurance. Some nations require that benefits be wholly or partly portable, i.e., they follow a beneficiary from one post to another in a different organization. In other nations, including the United States, there is no legal obligation for portability of fringe benefits, which can have serious implications for medical and hospital insurance benefits.

fringe medicine Varieties of alternative or unorthodox health care that are "on the fringe" of acceptability because they lack scientific credibility, are tainted with charlatanism or quackery, or imply other dubious practices. Examples beyond the range of science include aromatherapy, color therapy, reflexology, and many other practices of unproven benefit.

frostbite Thermal injury resulting from exposure to a cold environment. To conserve heat for vital organs, peripheral blood vessels contract under the influence of extreme cold, causing blood flow to become so sluggish that clotting occurs, leading to peripheral ischemic damage, ranging from localized necrosis to gangrene of the extremities.

FTE See FULL-TIME EQUIVALENT.

full-time equivalent (FTE) An expression used in compiling statistics on staffing structure in which allowance is made for the presence of part-time workers. When preparing and auditing the budgets of health departments and hospitals, the number of hours per week and eligibility or otherwise for fringe benefits are important considerations.

fume, fumes Volatile matter produced by combustion, generally a mixture of aerosols, gases, and solid particles, as in many varieties of smoke from combusted biomass fuels. Fumes are often toxic and/or an asphyxiant when inhaled. Fumes produced by molten metals remain suspended in the atmosphere long enough to be an occupational hazard of smelting. See METAL FUME FEVER.

fumigant A substance used in fumigation, e.g., to rid a building of pests. Common fumigants are sulfur dioxide, ammonia, and naphtha. Many fumigants are toxic to humans, and those who work with them must wear respirators.

fumigation The process of applying or injecting pesticide fumes into a closed space with the aim of disinfecting it or ridding the space of pests such as insects or rats.

function 1. In mathematics, the relationship of two or more variables, often expressed in symbols as well as or instead of numbers. 2. In organizations, the specific task(s) of designated person(s). 3. In

physiology and medicine, the way a body system or an organ is working, which can be assessed by means of suitable tests.

functional analysis A rigorous evaluation of the responsibilities, activities, and actions of designated divisions, sections, and individual persons in an organization.

functional illiteracy A state in which a person has some ability to read and perhaps to write, such as ability to sign a document, but is unable to comprehend the information in the document.

fungal infection Infections that usually affect vulnerable moist places on epithelial surfaces, such as flexures, the inside of the mouth and vagina. They include candida or thrush, paronychia, and athlete's foot. In immunocompromised persons, e.g., persons with AIDS and those undergoing chemotherapy, fungal infections can be systemic and lethal, e.g., when meninges are infected with aspergillosis.

fungicide An agent, usually chemical, that kills or inhibits reproduction of fungus.

furans A family of chemicals that are produced when chlorinated hydrocarbons, especially polychlorinated biphenyls (PCBs) are incompletely combusted. They have toxicity similar to PCBs and related compounds that cause chloracne.

furnace 1. In industry, a specially constructed combustion chamber in which fuel such as coal is burned with supplementary oxygen to achieve high temperatures capable of melting ores and making high-grade alloys. The fumes are often irritant or toxic, and the emissions may be a source of severe air pollution. 2. In dwellings, a furnace supplies central heating, using coal, oil, coal gas, or natural gas. It can be an occasional cause of fires, explosions, or gas poisoning.

fusion In cytology, the intimate mixing of genetic material from two cells. In physics, mixing of two or more elements, as in smelting of ores; also, the joining together of nuclei in nuclear fusion.

futile care Health care that can have no beneficial outcome but merely prolongs needlessly, and often at considerable expense in money and resource allocation, the process of dying and the duration of suffering for both patient and caregivers.

fuzzy logic Literally, imprecisely defined, vague, or confused logic. A branch of logical reasoning in which propositions may not be either true or false but contain varying degrees of truth. This is applied in machine intelligence.

G

Gaia hypothesis An ancient concept stated in modern scientific language in 1968 by the British biophysicist James Lovelock (b. 1919). The biosphere is an entity with living and nonliving components that interact to shape the evolution of the planet as an integrated ecosystem. Healthy interaction of the components is required for the integrity and survival of this global ecosystem. Similar ideas are part of the belief system of some so-called primitive or animistic cultures and occur in ancient myths and legends. Lovelock advanced empirical supporting evidence for the Gaia hypothesis. In Greek myths, Gaia was the daughter of Chaos and the mother of Uranus. The concept of SUSTAINABLE DEVELOPMENT implicitly acknowledges the Gaia hypothesis.

Galton, Francis (1822–1911) British biologist, one of the founders of GENETICS, author of *Hereditary Genius* (1869), which analyzed the physical and intellectual characteristics of successive generations of several hundred prominent British families. He coined the expression "regression to the mean" to describe the tendency for successive generations to show less extreme qualities than their progenitors. Galton's mathematical approach laid the foundations for the modern science of BIOSTATISTICS, refined by his pupil Karl Pearson and others.

gambling A form of RISK-TAKING BEHAVIOR that reflects a widespread human denial of the laws of chance and is manifest in all common variations of games of chance played for money, based on a throw of the dice, toss of a coin, distribution of playing cards shuffled and dealt to players, or prediction that one horse will run faster than the others around a track. It can become an addictive or compulsive behavior and a health problem, reducing families to penury. Criminals, charities, and governments capitalize on the urge to gamble and reap large financial rewards by ensuring that the odds always favor them. Bayesian statistics is a byproduct of gambling.

gamete A specialized female or male sex cell, containing half the number of chromosomes that occur in a somatic cell, and fusing with its counterpart at FERTILIZATION to produce a zygote that has the normal number of diploid chromosomes and develops into a fetus, an embryo, an infant, and eventually an adult.

game theory A branch of mathematical logic described in *The Theory of Games and Economic Behavior* (1944) by the Hungarian-American mathematician John von Neumann (1903–1957) and the German-American mathematician Oskar Morgenstern (1902–1977). Game theory calculates the likelihood of each of a range of possible reactions of a hypothetical adversary to a set of specific acts or strategies. Game theory has many applications, in systems analysis, some aspects of psychotherapy, and in resolving conflicts, such as industrial disputes.

gamma globulin A large protein molecule comprising at least five distinct classes of protein components called IMMUNOGLOBULINS, involved in immune reactions, designated IgG, IgA, IgM, IgD, and IgE. Many, if not all, possess the capacity to react with and bind or inactivate specific antigens. It is collected from human serum and injected as a method of boosting passive immunity to certain infections, notably measles and hepatitis A, that could otherwise cause serious illness when no other treatment or preventive methods are available.

gamma hydroxybutyric acid (GHB) A colorless, tasteless powder or pill that dissolves readily in water or alcohol. It is licensed for use to treat narcolepsy, but it is more notorious as a DATE RAPE DRUG because it induces clouded consciousness, reduces or blocks memory of events that occur while under its influence, is a muscle relaxant, and can be manufactured in a home laboratory.

gamma radiation Ionizing radiation in the range 10^{-14} to 10^{-10} meters wavelength; very high-energy, penetrating, biologically active, ionizing radiation, emitted by radioactive substances and during very high-speed collisions between nonradioactive subatomic particles. Gamma radiation is teratogenic, mutagenic, and carcinogenic.

gangs Social groups, usually of adolescents and young adults, often single-sex groups, that may form, dissolve, and form again with changed membership. They provide mutual emotional and social support for their members, may operate on the fringes of or entirely outside the accepted norms and customs of society, may defy authority figures and engage in criminal behavior. Their relevance to personal and community health includes promotion of risky or harmful behavior, such as promiscuous sexual conduct, alcohol and other substance abuse, and assaults on nongang members, girls and women, elderly people, and ethnic or other minorities. Public health authorities sometimes succeed in directing the energy of gangs to desirable social purposes, such as clearing derelict industrial sites or delivering groceries to housebound infirm people.

Gantt chart A scheduling technique developed by the American engineer Henry L. Gantt (1861–1919) showing graphically each of the activities of all members of an organization arranged by days and duration of tasks, but usually not showing interconnections among activities. The method of PROGRAM EVALUATION AND REVIEW TECHNIQUES (PERT) is superior in this respect.

gap The disparities or inequalities in status among defined subgroups of the population. One widening gap is the disparity in health status, strongly correlated with income, education, housing conditions, values, and behavior between the highest and the lowest socioeconomic classes in a nation or subsections of the nation. Another health gap often exists between certain ethnic groups and the mainstream society in which they are embedded.

garbage Syn: trash. Solid domestic waste, comprising organic matter, such as vegetable residue and food scraps, often mixed with containers, wrapping, etc., in which the food was supplied.

garbage disposal methods In urban and suburban communities, collection and disposal of domestic and industrial waste is an important service, usually provided by local government agencies. In affluent communities, the quantity is prodigious, amounting to many tonnes per person per annum. Methods of disposal include LANDFILL, incineration, dumping at sea, and separation into components that can be recycled, composted, or recovered and reused, and other components not amenable to any of these more environmentally friendly approaches.

gas The physical state of matter with the property of indefinite expansion in which atoms and molecules are widely separated, loosely distributed, and move randomly at high speed. Many gases have great importance in health and public health, beginning with the gases that comprise the atmosphere: oxygen, nitrogen, carbon dioxide, and trace amounts of others. Several gases are widely used as fuels and/or occur as products of industry, notably coal gas, natural gas, propane, methane, and petroleum gas. Some of these gases and many others that are used in or occur as by-products of industrial processes are toxic, asphyxiant, or biologically active in some other way. Several gases emitted as combustion products of carbon-based fuels are important atmospheric pollutants that are the ingredients of SMOG. Several gases are used as anesthetic agents. See also COAL GAS, NATURAL GAS, SEWAGE GAS, and SOUR GAS.

gas barrier A device or air flow that can divert the flow of gases in a controlled solid waste site.

gas chromatography A method of analysis in which a specimen is vaporized and introduced into a stream of carrier gas, usually helium, where it is conducted through a chromatograph column and separated into constituent parts that travel at specific rates and are detected as they emerge in a characteristic time sequence. This permits both qualitative and qualitative analysis of components. Compare paper ELECTROPHORESIS, which analyzes substances by volatilizing them and passing them through a porous inert filter using an inert carrier gas such as argon. Markers for components are traces left at a particular position on the filter when an electric current is passed through it.

gaserator A special high-temperature incineration chamber that is used to dispose of dead animal carcasses, condemned foodstuffs, and other potentially harmful material that would leave a residue if combusted in an ordinary incinerator.

gas exchange The physiological, biochemical, and biophysical processes whereby oxygen is absorbed and carbon dioxide is released by hemoglobin molecules in the alveoli in the lungs.

gasification The industrial process of converting solid fuel to gaseous form.

gasoline Syn: petrol. Refined distillate of petroleum, a volatile liquid that is the fuel for internal combustion engines. The exhaust emissions from gasoline combustion often contain ingredients harmful to health, notably lead-ethyl additives and carbon-based atmospheric pollutants. Gasoline fumes, sometimes inhaled as an intoxicant, are dangerously toxic.

gas sampler An instrument that measures the concentration of specific gases such as carbon monoxide in the ambient air of the enclosed space of an indoor sports arena.

gas scrubber A device to remove solid particulate matter from the emissions in a furnace stack, usually consisting of high-pressure fine water jets. These also reduce emissions of some soluble gases and fumes, e.g., toxic sulfur compounds, but not lead or mercury emissions.

gastroenteritis An inflammatory reaction of the gastrointestinal tract that causes vomiting and/or diarrhea. It is usually caused by invading pathogenic organisms or their toxins, sometimes by chemical contaminants in ingested food. Some forms of gastroenteritis are infectious and can be transmitted by droplet spread from person to person, but most are caused by infected food handlers and/or fecal contamination of ingested food, i.e., by the fecal-oral route. Fastidious hand-washing by food handlers is the most important preventive measure.

gastroenterology The medical specialty concerned with diseases of the gastrointestinal tract and related organs, especially the liver, pancreas, and spleen.

gatekeeper A word used to describe a receptionist in a clinic, a health worker who exercises a TRIAGE function, or an official who stands between persons requiring a health service and those who are able to provide this service. In this latter sense, the word has an unflattering and sometimes rather threatening connotation.

gateway An agency, service, or individual that is the means of ingress to the health care system. Gateway services and agencies include community clinics, general practitioners, family physicians, nursing services, pharmacies, public health professionals, support groups, etc.

gateway drug A readily available mood-modifying drug or substance that is legal, such as alcohol, tobacco, volatile glue, or an illegal but not rigorously policed substance, such as marijuana, that is believed to render people more susceptible than they might otherwise be to use more dangerous illicit and more addictive substances. The concept of gateway drugs posits that they are at one end of a continuum of substances and frequently lead to use and abuse of more dangerous HARD DRUGS. There is little or no convincing evidence to support this concept.

gauss The unit of measurement of a magnetic field, now superseded by the SI units webers per square meter and teslas. The name commemorates the German physicist Karl Friedrich Gauss (1777–1855).

Gaussian curve, distribution See NORMAL DISTRIBUTION.

gay An adjective meaning cheerful or carefree that acquired an association with loose morals and sexual licentiousness in the 19th century, and in approximately the 1940s came into use among members of the homosexual community to describe male homosexuality. In this context, it has no pejorative connotation.

gay and lesbian movement In an increasingly tolerant society that upholds human rights, one segment of society that was long marginalized and victimized was the minority group comprising male and female homosexuals. In the last 2 to 3 decades of the 20th century, this group became increasingly assertive, and the gay and lesbian movement that was established in many countries has since won many concessions that have led toward recognition and equity.

Geiger counter An instrument that measures radioactivity in atomic and subatomic particles, named for the German physicist Hans Geiger (1882–1945), who developed it while working with the New Zealand physicist Ernest Rutherford (1871–1937) in Manchester, United Kingdom.

gender In grammar, the designation of a noun as masculine, feminine, or neuter. Now the word is used to designate the sex of individuals and groups. This usage probably originated as a genteel euphemism for the sex of individuals or groups. It has evolved into a broad concept that designates not only sex but also the sexual orientation and sometimes the cultural context of persons and groups. In this sense, "gender" is a social construct.

gender bias A preference for persons of a particular sex (which it has become politically correct to describe as their "gender") in hiring, promotion. To some extent gender bias is built into the English language, which often uses masculine nouns and pronouns to embrace all humankind. Gender bias generally favors males in senior management and the leading professions, restricting females to subservient lower-rank positions and certain professions, such as nursing and school teaching. Initiatives driven by a renewed sense of social justice and the political imperative of AFFIRMATIVE ACTION have aimed to "level the playing field" so classes of aspiring entrants to some professions, including medicine and law, sometimes now have a majority of women.

gender gap The discrepancy between male and female numbers either in demographics or in various trades and professions. Since the development of ultrasound techniques for prenatal sex determination, the preference for male children in some countries and easy access to abortion have led to a serious distortion of the natural FEMALE/MALE RATIO of liveborn infants, creating a new variety of gender gap that could have serious social consequences when these birth cohorts reach marriage age.

gender identity The psychological sense of the self as masculine or feminine. This is not always the same as gonadal sex. A few individuals who are genetically members of one sex feel and act as though they are members the other sex.

gene A hereditary unit that occupies a particular position (locus) on a chromosome. Genes pass from parents to offspring with coded information contained in segments of DNA sequences on chromosomes, and these DNA sequences determine many aspects of an individual's makeup. The collective name for an organism's genes is the genotype, and the individual organism is the phenotype. Genes are structural, involved in composition of organs, tissues, etc., or regulatory, for instance, directing hormones, enzyme systems, etc. The DNA sequence that makes up individual genes is responsible for the codes for specific characteristics, such as blood group, hair and eye color, usually in combination with other genes. The complex DNA structure of genes helps to explain why and how they can undergo mutation, and it has become the basis for molecular level studies of evolutionary biology.

genealogy The study and recording of family lineage that involves tracing ancestry back for as many generations as possible. This is of interest to all seeking to explore their roots and a feature of the belief system of members of the MORMON denomination, who believe they can aid the salvation of their identifiable ancestors' souls by retroactively baptizing them into the Mormon faith. For this reason, the Mormons maintain comprehensive genealogical records at their world headquarters in Salt Lake City, Utah, which can be used to trace an individual's ancestry and by research workers studying the inheritance patterns of diseases, such as cancer.

gene-environment interaction Syn: nature-nurture. This is defined as the varying effects of an environmental factor on disease outcome for individuals with different genotypes. Many aspects of health and disease result from the interplay of inherent characteristics and environmental influences. The inherent, mainly genetic determinants influence susceptibility and resistance to invading pathogens, including those causing major communicable diseases, such as smallpox, plague, influenza, and to physical environmental factors, such as solar radiation or exposure to tobacco smoke. The innumerable environmental influences include physical, biological, social, and cultural factors to which individuals react in multiple ways that may be associated with, while not necessarily explaining, the occurrence of many diseases.

gene expression The extent to which genotypes are manifest in an individual's phenotype, or in the occurrence of specific genetic traits.

gene pool The total genetic information possessed by the reproductively active population.

general adaptation syndrome A theory of disease etiology proposed in the late 1940s by the Austrian-Canadian endocrinologist Hans Selye (1907–1982) to explain the pathogenesis of many common diseases, including hypertension, peptic ulcer, asthma, and cancer, that may be attributable to short-term or long-term bodily reactions to stress. The theory proposes three stages of pathophysiological response: 1. Initial alarm reaction, the first response to physical or emotional threat, i.e., the FIGHT-OR-FLIGHT REACTION, characterized by accelerated heart rate and respiration, muscle tension, sweating, and anxiety; 2. Resistance stage, in which the alarm reaction is sustained, even indefinitely, or coping mechanisms are developed; 3. Exhaustion stage, in which physiological responses are overwhelmed, causing physical and/or psychological symptoms, including hypertension, anxiety states, depression, substance use and abuse, and insomnia.

general circulation model (GCM) A complex theoretical construct incorporating mathematical models, empirical observations of fluctuations of winds and ocean currents, and algorithms, aimed at predicting future trends in climates over large regions or the world as a whole. The variables include topographical features, wind direction and ocean current movements, and temperature readings. GCMs have become an important feature of CLIMATE MODELS and forecasts since the 1990s, when concerns began to mount about the physical, biological, economic, social, and health implications of global climate change.

general fertility rate A measure of the fertility of a population using the annual number of live births as the numerator and the number of women in the reproductive age group (15–44 or 15–45 years) as the denominator.

generalization The aspect of logic that deals with formation of generalizable rules and theorems. It can and often does lead to false conclusions when loose generalizations are based on incomplete or faulty evidence, deliberately ignoring evidence that refutes the generalization, as in racist theories about character or flaws in logical reasoning.

generally regarded as safe (GRAS) A designation by the FOOD AND DRUG ADMINISTRATION of many commonly used chemicals, including pharmaceuticals, cosmetics, food additives, industrial chemicals, etc., that have been tested and found safe. In routine daily use, empirical observation has confirmed their safety. These substances are listed by the FDA with this designation.

general practice Syn: family practice. The branch of medical practice that is concerned with the first contact and usually continuing care of unselected persons in the population, previously undifferentiated as regards their age, sex, medical condition, social background, occupation, etc. The general practitioner who encounters such persons as patients is usually their first point of contact with the health care system. General practice offers scope for the opportunistic early detection of important serious diseases, including hypertension, diabetes, and cancer, which may be more cost-effective than screening programs for these conditions.

General Register Office The British government agency responsible for collecting, collating, analyzing, and disseminating statistics on vital events, births, marriages and common law unions, divorces and separations, and deaths. It was originally an agency of the government of England and Wales, established in 1842 in response to an Act of Parliament, and WILLIAM FARR was the first compiler of abstracts. Its activities and the vital statistics it produces are accessible at http://www.gro.gov.uk/gro/content.

generation This word has several meanings: 1. The process of creating; 2. All the offspring born to pairs of parents in a specified period, thus loosely speaking, a COHORT; 3. The average time that elapses between the procreation of one generation and that of its offspring. This ill-defined period has varied over historical time according to changes in marital customs, spacing of children, and average age at marriage or at first conception. In the 20th century, it varied from about 20 to 22 years to 25 to 28 years in the industrial nations.

generation effect The variation in physical fitness and health status that can be observed between birth cohorts born in successive decades, caused mainly by the different environmental, dietary, and other factors and determinants to which each cohort is exposed from conception onward.

generation gap Differences in values, behavior, lifestyle, and often economic, educational, and employment opportunities and prospects between one generation of a family and the next or between different age cohorts in the population. Differences in growth and development and in physical and mental health status often accompany other age cohort differences.

generation time In communicable disease epidemiology, the time interval between invasion of a host by an infectious pathogen and the stage of maximum infectivity of the host, i.e., when the host is excreting pathogens at maximum number, volume, or rate. See also MASS ACTION PRINCIPLE.

generic drug A pharmaceutical preparation that is marketed under its pharmacological name, rather than a trade name copyrighted by a commercial manufacturer. Generic drugs are usually not subject to patent, are generally considerably cheaper than PROPRIETARY DRUGS, and often are as efficacious, sometimes more so.

gene therapy Treatment of inherited disorders by modifying the genetic material in germ cells of prospective parents. Until recently, this therapeutic approach was of theoretical interest only, but progress in human genomics has increased the feasibility of intervention to correct genetically determined diseases. However, as of 2005 almost all experimental attempts to prevent the birth of offspring with inherited conditions such as hemophilia, cystic fibrosis, and other serious diseases had been unsuccessful.

genetic code The sequence of nucleotide triplets (CODONS) of DNA and RNA that specify the sequence of amino acids for protein synthesis and thereby determine aspects of inheritance and of growth and development of organs, tissues, and individuals. Molecular genetic techniques permit the genetic code or "genetic fingerprint" to be precisely identified. The genetic code makes each human being unique and different from every other person. Genes are made up of base pairs of nucleotides, adenine, guanine, thymine, and cytosine; in humans there are about 25,000 genes and 3×10^9 base pairs, so when conception occurs and equal numbers of chromosomes and genes from each parent contribute to the genetic makeup of the offspring, the probability that two individuals will have identical genetic makeup is less than 1 in 30 trillion, a fact that is used in DNA testing for forensic purposes.

genetic counseling The method and process of analyzing and discussing the risks that a marital pair may produce genetically defective offspring, based on what is known and can be learned about family history and heritable conditions. The length of human generations, uncertainties about inheritance of many traits, and the random occurrence of mutations that can cause conditions such as cystic fibrosis and hemophilia make genetic counseling less predictable than the outcome of breeding experiments with roses or racehorses. The extent to which findings from the HUMAN GENOME PROJECT and advances in GENETIC ENGINEERING can be applied in medical and public health practice remains uncertain.

genetic disorders A large class of conditions that includes single-gene disorders, inborn errors of metabolism, chromosomal abnormalities, etc. Many can now be identified by genetic screening and some, e.g., PHENYLKETONURIA, can be treated by appropriate intervention.

genetic drift The random variation in gene frequency that occurs from one generation to another and that over many generations can lead to changes in distribution of phenotypes in the population as a whole if some gene frequencies are associated with greater REPRODUCTIVE FITNESS than are others.

genetic engineering A set of techniques and procedures that are used to alter the genetic composition of a species. Genetic engineering has been applied mainly to plants, domestic animals, and insects and used commercially to enhance the nutritional value of feed crops, poultry, and pigs. An important application is in the development of genetically modified insect vectors so that they cannot act as host species for pathogens or cannot reproduce efficiently. As yet, genetic engineering has not been applied to any extent in humans, but the possibility that it might be has led to debates by theologians, bioethicists, geneticists, and politicians about the potential dangers and uncertain benefits of interfering with the human genome in this way, despite the considerable potential benefit for individual families afflicted by lethal gene defects, such as cystic fibrosis and Huntington's disease.

genetic epidemiology The branch of epidemiology dealing with the distribution, determinants, and control of diseases in groups of people related by blood ties and with inherited causes of disease in population groups. The function of genetic epidemiology is to investigate genetic factors in disease causation and control. It relates to MOLECULAR EPIDEMIOLOGY and has made rapid progress since the development of molecular biology and the HUMAN GENOME PROJECT.

geneticist A scientist, e.g., a biologist or a clinician, who specializes in genetics. Recent discoveries in genetics have led to a considerable increase in the numbers of geneticists in research and practice, and to evolution of specialization in aspects including molecular genetics, genetic counseling, and genetic engineering.

genetic linkage The fact that some of the characteristics associated with genes that are fairly close to each other on a chromosome tend to be inherited together so that characteristics associated with these genes rather often occur together in the offspring.

genetic marker A genetically determined characteristic that is usually readily identifiable by direct observation.

genetic polymorphism The maintenance of proportions of genetic subtypes in a large interbreeding population. This is an important determinant of diversity of a large population.

genetics The scientific study of heredity and inheritable diseases. This includes Mendelian genetics, the study of inheritance patterns of dominant and recessive characteristics, single-gene disorders, population genetics and genetic epidemiology, the study of effects of genetic determinants and factors on disease distribution in populations, and molecular genetics, which is studies at the interface of molecular biology and genetics. Genetic engineering and the HUMAN GENOME PROJECT are applications of molecular genetics.

genetic shift An abrupt transition in a genetically determined characteristic that is presumably due to a mutation. This happens with some pathogenic microorganisms, such as the influenza virus, and explains the origin of some antibiotic-resistant strains of pathogenic bacteria. Evolutionary biologists have gathered evidence that genetic shift probably accounts for some evolutionary changes that differentiate earlier forms of higher organisms studied by paleontologists from their contemporary counterparts.

Geneva Conventions International agreements signed by most of the world's nations in 1864 and revised and expanded in 1949 that established rules for combatants in violent armed conflicts, treatment of prisoners of war, civilians, and the social fabric of occupied countries. These include explicit prohibition of certain kinds of weapons and rules that all nations originally agreed to honor regarding medical personnel, treatment of prisoners of war, and maintenance of essential services, including restoration of public health infrastructure and treatment of civilians in occupied territories. Sadly, combatant nations often flout these conventions, although they complain vociferously if any of their citizens or combatants are alleged to have been victims of violations by their adversaries. See http://www.genevaconventions.org/ for a reference guide.

genital examination Medical examination of the genitalia. Often this is an emotionally delicate matter, especially for women and girls when the examining physician is a man, and in some cultures, as well as in the most permissive, increasingly the presence of a chaperon is mandatory. In the armed forces, the procedure, colloquially known as "short arms inspection," has been used for about 100 years as a way to screen for venereal or sexually transmitted diseases, although its efficacy for this purpose is doubtful.

genital herpes A sexually transmitted disease, caused by herpesvirus type 2 or other types of herpesvirus, that causes ulceration and inflammation of the skin and mucosal surfaces of the genital tract. It is highly contagious, indolent, and often resistant to treatment, but it resolves well if antiviral treatment begins early. It has occurred in near-epidemic form among promiscuous adolescents and young adults in several large urban centers in the United States and Europe.

genital mutilation Surgical modification of the external genitalia. This ancient custom has been practiced in various forms on members of both sexes in many cultures since Neolithic times. Male genital mutilation has been a tribal custom in many cultures since prehistoric times. It usually consists of CIRCUMCISION, excision of the prepuce, which may be done in infancy, early childhood, or around the time of adolescence as an initiation rite. It is an essential feature of the religious customs of Jews and Moslems. In some cultures, such as certain tribes of Australian Aborigines, other forms of male genital mutilation have been practiced, e.g., subincision, which consists of incising the urethra, so urine and ejaculated sperm emerge from the junction of the scrotum and the base of the penis. FEMALE GENITAL MUTILATION is also an ancient practice that appears to have developed, perhaps several millennia ago, in northeast Africa as a tribal custom aimed to ensure the purity and chastity of girls.

genocide The extermination, usually by brutal armed aggression, of members of an ethnic group. Human history offers many examples: massacres of Armenians by Turks in 1915, Stalin's collective farm policies in the Ukraine in the early 1930s, the Nazi extermination of Jews and Gypsies in parts of Europe that they controlled in 1938–1944, and, in more recent history, the ETHNIC CLEANSING policies of the Serbs in the former Yugoslavia in 1992–1994, the massacre of Tutsis by the Hutus in Rwanda in 1994, and the destruction of rural subsistence farming communities in Darfur, western Sudan, by government-supported nomadic tribesmen since 2004.

genogram A diagram showing family relationships over three or more generations used in studies of genealogy, e.g., to show the occurrence of disorders of genetic origin.

genome All of the genes carried by an individual member of every species of living creature. See also HUMAN GENOME PROJECT.

genomics The study of the genome, closely related to genetics and molecular biology. It began with studies to map the positions and the sequence of individual genes in chromosomes, and with attempts to identify the functions of as many genes as feasible, including in particular those that are or seem to be essential for normal healthy development and metabolic functions and those that appear to be associated with occurrence of abnormalities of many kinds. Its main achievement is the HUMAN GENOME PROJECT, which is hoped eventually to make possible the control and perhaps the prevention of many inherited and other genetic disorders.

genotype The genetic composition of an individual, as distinct from physical appearance.

gentrification The social and economic transformation of INNER CITY slums into expensive housing for affluent professional people by architectural improvements, modernizing and improving kitchens and bathrooms, etc. Generally regarded as a desirable form of URBAN RENEWAL, the process can have adverse consequences for former occupants whose social networks are disrupted and who may be left homeless or forced to relocate to accommodation that is distant from their workplace, requiring costly and time-consuming commuting.

genuine progress indicator (GPI) A composite measure of economic well-being. The GPI includes economic contributions of the family and the community and of the natural habitat and conventionally measured economic production. It considers more than 20 social and environmental factors and differentiates between economic transactions that add to well-being and those that diminish it, integrating these so the benefits of economic activity can be weighed against costs. Per capita gross domestic product (GDP) in the United States more than doubled from 1950 to 1999, but while the per capita GPI increased in 1950–1969, it declined by 45% in1970–1999. The GPI reveals that much which economists consider economic growth measured by GDP is really fixing problems caused by earlier errors and social decay from the past, borrowing resources from the future, or shifting functions from the community and household realm to the monetized economy. The GPI suggests that the costs of the economic trajectory of the United States and similar nations have begun to outweigh the benefits. The GPI adjusts for factors such as income distribution, adds the value of household and volunteer work, and subtracts the costs of crime and pollution. Because the GDP and the GPI are both measured in monetary terms, they can be compared. GPI provides a more valid economic indicator than does gross national product (GNP) for studies of population health. For further details, see http://www.redefiningprogress.org/projects/gpi/.

geocoding A method of classifying personal data according to the place of residence, using precise indicators such as postal or zip codes. This is a useful device for many epidemiological studies and for purposes such as SOCIAL MARKETING.

geographical pathology The aspect of pathology that deals with the geographical distribution of specific pathological conditions. It resembles and may be the same as descriptive epidemiology or may be a more anecdotal aspect of the work of pathologists.

geographic information system (GIS) An information system based on digitally constructed maps, sometimes using GEOCODING as one element of the data base. Satellite imaging and remote sensing have greatly expanded the scope of GISs, for instance, by making it possible to identify changes in composition of vegetation and amounts of precipitation in tropical regions that relate to changes in the distribution and abundance of insect vectors, such as mosquitoes and blackflies. An important application is in GEOMATICS, which is used for many purposes, including assessment of time trends in geographical distribution of diseases such as malaria. For an introduction and details, see http://www.gis.com/.

geography The scholarly activity concerned with the configuration and topography of the world and the distribution and abundance of humans and plant and animal life on earth. Geography is an ancient discipline that flowered in the era of exploration from about 500 BCE to 1900 of our era. The original concern with charting the world has given way to detailed study of natural resources, land use, distribution of population, and interfaces of geography with demography, economics, and politics. Its public health relevance is mainly through some aspects of descriptive epidemiology (medical geography or geographical pathology) and economic and sometimes political geography.

geomatics The collection, processing, storage, and analysis of geographic information. A new and important application is sequentially generated computer maps to show regional and temporal trends and variations, e.g., in vegetation cover, and incidence and/or prevalence of conditions in various sectors of society, including the health sector.

geometric mean See MEASURES OF CENTRAL TENDENCY.

geothermal power Energy derived from the earth's volcanic interior, for instance, from hot springs, geysers, or heat energy in subsurface strata. In theory this is a virtually inexhaustible source of energy because the heat is derived from the pressure of overlying strata. In practice, it is difficult to extract and use. Iceland is a model of how it can be done: geothermal power supplies the nation's needs for heating domestic and public buildings, but similar methods are not always feasible. As a source of energy, geothermal power has a great advantage in being nonpolluting.

geriatrics The medical specialty concerned with the care of the elderly, a loosely defined age range, often with care of infirm and dependent elderly, although preventive geriatrics seeks to anticipate deterioration of organs and prevent organ failure, sometimes by intervening at younger ages, around age 55 to 60 years, and providing health-promotion and disease-prevention regimens that will enhance prospects for independent healthy life at later ages. See also GERONTOLOGY.

German measles A colloquial name for RUBELLA.

germ cell The zygote that is formed by the union of two gametes.

germ theory The theory of disease causation by tiny living creatures was proposed or hinted at by scholars, philosophers, and physicians in antiquity. The theory was confirmed after the invention of the microscope by the Dutch lens-grinder ANTONI VAN LEEUWENHOEK (1632–1723) and the rise of BACTERIOLOGY in the second half of the 19th century under the intellectual leadership of FRIEDRICH GUSTAV JACOB HENLE, ROBERT KOCH, LOUIS PASTEUR, and others.

gerontology The scientific study of the aging process. From the Greek *geront,* meaning old man. Although this science focuses on anatomical, physiological, and pathological phenomena associated with aging, it can begin the study with humans, or organisms, or at any age from conception onward.

gestational age The age of the fetus measured from the date of conception. In the past, it has been estimated from the first day of the last normal menstrual period before the beginning of pregnancy. Ultrasound allows a more precise estimate. It is expressed in completed days or weeks of pregnancy. Variations of gestational age include preterm (less than 37 weeks or 259 days), term (37–42 weeks or 259–293 days), and postterm (42 weeks or 294 days, or more).

gestational diabetes During pregnancy, glycogen metabolism is sometimes temporarily disrupted, leading to glycosuria and other signs of glucose intolerance. This is not true diabetes mellitus, but may be a premonitory manifestation of later onset of diabetes, so preventive medicine includes extra vigilance when women have had glucosuria during pregnancy.

ghetto A circumscribed, usually poor and deprived section of a city. The word originally referred to a district reserved for Jews in 15th-century Venice to segregate them behind walls guarded by sentries to prevent them from "contaminating" the Christian population elsewhere in the city. The word became an international term for similarly segregated localities for Jews in other European cities. The system disappeared in the social transformation of Europe after World War II. The term has survived to describe urban slums and ethnic neighborhoods, e.g., occupied by African American and Hispanic people, in many large US cities and their counterparts in other countries.

giardiasis Infection with the protozoan intestinal parasite *Giardia lamblia* and other members of this family, transmitted person to person or from animals to humans via water, including water collected from catchment areas contaminated by the excreta of infected animals. This can cause diarrhea, colicky abdominal pain, loss of appetite, and general malaise but may be symptomless. It is common in regions with poor sanitation but can occur anywhere. Control requires personal hygiene, enteric isolation of cases, and improved sanitation. It can be treated with metronidazole.

gingivitis Inflammation of the gums, often chronic and accompanied by foul-smelling breath and loosening of teeth in their sockets. It is an indicator of poor oral hygiene and may be a sign of more serious disease, e.g., vitamin C deficiency (scurvy).

Gini coefficient A measure of the degree of dispersion or inequality in a set of values that is used mainly in economic analyses, e.g., in HEALTH ECONOMICS, where it is used to calculate variation or income inequality. It was invented by the Italian economist Corrado Gini (1884–1965). It can be calculated in several ways, e.g., $G = 1 + 1/n - 2/n^2 \check{y} \,[y_1 + 2y_2 + 3y_3 + \ldots + ny_n]$, where $y_1 \ldots y_n$ are individual incomes in diminishing order of size, $\check{y}$ is the mean income, and n is the number of individuals.

ginseng Several varieties of herb that have been widely used for many centuries in Chinese traditional medicine as a tonic and supposed sexual stimulant. It is said to reduce symptoms of fatigue, enhance hormonal activity, and restore or strengthen sexual potency. In experimental studies, it has been found to stimulate corticosteroid and testosterone secretion, raise blood pressure, and elevate mood. It may sometimes be mildly addictive and therefore can be harmful, especially to elderly men with cardiovascular disease.

glanders A disease of horses, donkeys, and mules caused by *Burkholderia* (formerly *Pseudomonas*) *mallei*. It is serologically indistinguishable from the agent of MELIOIDOSIS, which occasionally infects humans, in whom it can cause a fatal bronchopneumonia.

glandular fever See INFECTIOUS MONONUCLEOSIS.

glass ceiling A colloquial term for imperceptible but impenetrable barriers to career advancement, usually impeding the professional advancement of women and members of VISIBLE MINORITIES but applicable to other identifiable individuals on the basis of accent, mode of dress or behavior, social background, etc. The existence of the barrier is seldom acknowledged and may be denied, but facts frequently demonstrate selective discriminatory hiring and/or promotion practices.

glaucoma Elevated pressure of aqueous humor in the eyes, usually a chronic condition caused by faulty drainage, that if untreated can impair circulation of blood in the vessels supplying the optic nerve and so cause restriction of visual fields and eventually blindness. Elevated pressure can be detected by SCREENING TESTS and treated to prevent further visual deterioration. By restricting peripheral visual fields, glaucoma impairs capacity to drive safely on public roads, so in this respect it can become a potential public health problem as well as a personal health problem.

Global Alliance for vaccines and Immunization (GAVI) A multilateral international coalition to promote vaccine development, dissemination, and delivery to populations that need vaccines, especially in low-income countries. The partners and donors include the Bill & Melinda Gates Foundation, the World Bank, WHO, UNICEF, nongovernmental organizations, national governments, research institutes, and manufacturers of vaccines. GAVI has been active in developing new vaccines for meningococcal meningitis, Japanese B encephalitis, and others, and improving vaccines for pertussis, rubella, etc. Details are available at http://www.vaccinealliance.org/.

global budget A system of financing aspects of health care, such as community clinics, in which a lump sum is provided by the health care financing agency or authority, and decisions about the allocation of funds to staff, facilities, etc., are left to the discretion of local staff.

global burden of disease A term that appeared in the World Bank's *World Development Report* in 1993, also called BURDEN OF DISEASE, to describe the loss of healthy years of life in a specified population, usually that of a nation or occasionally a specified group. It is assessed in a population by DISABILITY-ADJUSTED LIFE YEARS (DALYs). The concept gave rise to some important activities and initiatives by the WHO. Further information and links to studies of the global burden of disease are at http://www.who.int/topics/global_burden_of_disease/en/.

global climate change A trend in the physical environment of the planet, sometimes imprecisely called global warming because an increase in average global temperatures that has been observed in recent decades is part of the process. Global climates have changed many times during the earth's long history, under the influence of variations in solar flare activity, the precession of the earth's axis, the impedance of solar radiation by atmospheric dust such as that emitted by massive volcanic eruptions, tectonic plate movement that modifies the direction and force of ocean currents, and other natural processes. The INTERGOVERNMENTAL PANEL ON CLIMATE CHANGE (IPCC) has been studying the phenomenon since 1985. In its reports in 1995 and 2001, it stated that the current trends can be partly attributed to the effects of human activity, especially to the increase in atmospheric burden of GREENHOUSE GASES produced by combustion of carbon-based fuels that permit solar energy to reach the earth's surface but block the escape back to space of radiation reflected from the earth's surface. The main effects, in addition to a long-term warming trend, include increased frequency of climatic extremes and violent weather events, sea level rise, and a range of adverse health effects that include harm due to heat waves and smog, increased frequency of vector-borne diseases, and displacement of populations because of habitat loss. See http://www.ipcc.ch for details.

global commons A term describing aspects of the biosphere held in common by all people and other living things everywhere. The global commons include the atmosphere and its features (climate, weather patterns, and precipitation); the oceans; the world's stocks of biodiversity;, and wilderness regions, of which Antarctica is now the only one uncontested. Nations and private corporations increasingly claim ownership rights over other natural features previously regarded as part of the global commons, such as tropical and boreal rainforests and large river and lake systems, in which several or many nations claim riparian rights.

Global Fund to Fight AIDS, Tuberculosis and Malaria Established in 2001 as a consequence of the UN COMMISSION ON MACROECONOMICS AND HEALTH, bringing together governments, civil society, the private sector, and affected communities in a new funding mechanism for programs to control three priority diseases of great public health importance. As of 2004, US$1.5 billion had been committed to support 154 programs in 93 countries. See http://www.theglobalfund.org/en/.

global governance A system of administrative supervision and decision making above the level of individual nations, intended to cope with problems that transcend national interests. In the mid-20th century, it was partially achieved under United Nations auspices with monetary systems and exchange rates, and through UN agencies, such as the United Nations Development Programme, the Food and Agriculture Organization, the World Health Organization, and the World Bank. Global governance works well in agreements on time zones, measuring units, many currency exchange rates, and international health regulations, but in most respects, many nations, especially the most powerful, put short-term national interests above the interests of the world as a whole.

globalization A process with institutional/social and political/economic dimensions that became a pervasive force for change in the last 2 decades of the 20th century. Social and institutional dimensions include the spread of education, literacy, and scientific and technical expertise, including many aspects beneficial to population and personal health, accelerated by radio, television, and the Internet and by capacity building in low income countries by international and bilateral aid agencies. Economic and political dimensions of globalization have had a mixed impact on social well-being and population health. Often the impact is beneficial, but in some low-income nations, the existing subsistence economies have been harmed and rural migration to periurban slums and shantytowns has been accelerated. The philosophy of economic liberalism encouraged by the World Bank and the World Trade Organization aims to reduce and eventually eliminate national barriers to trade and commerce, with the premise that free markets promote democracy as well as enhanced wealth for all participants. This is manifestly not universally so. In the health sector, globalization encourages mobility of skilled professional workers, many of whom have migrated from poor to rich nations, jeopardizing provision of essential human resources in many places.

global public goods for health Public goods and services are those open to all and provided at public expense or sometimes by a wealthy donor. Examples include defense, fire and police services, roads and parks, and public health and emergency medical services. Global public goods for health are services and measures such as health information systems, international health regulations, and epidemic investigation and control procedures, provided by the World Health Organization, other UN agencies, various nongovernmental organizations, and national agencies such as the Pasteur Institute and the US Centers for Disease Control and Prevention. For details, see http://www.who .int/trade/distance_learning/gpgh/en/.

Global Public Health Intelligence Network A WHO-Canada collaborative network of Internet-based early warning systems for contagious disease outbreaks that uses routine national and regional disease notification systems and also media reports of unusual outbreaks of contagious or other diseases (e.g., chemical poisoning). Information gathered at the main clearinghouse in Ottawa is transmitted to national public health agencies worldwide. This network has become increasingly relevant in the current period of heightened concern about bioterrorism. Its activities are described at http://www.phac-aspc.gc.ca/media/nr-rp/2004/2004_gphin-rmispbk_e.html.

global village A term describing the capacity for all the world's people to communicate virtually instantaneously with one another by electronic means, i.e., by radio, television, and the INTERNET, although the last of these did not exist when the term was coined by the Canadian media scholar and communications theorist Marshall McLuhan (1911–1980).

Glossina See TSETSE FLY.

glove box A sealed container that is opaque to ionized radiation but translucent to optical wave lengths and is used to handle radioactive material, such as isotopes being prepared for medical purposes, using heavy lead-lined gloves that do not transmit ionized radiation. A similar device, although not radiopaque, is used to manipulate preparations of dangerous pathogens and the cultures, or experimental animals, used to investigate them.

glucagon A polypeptide hormone secreted by the islets of Langerhans of the pancreas that elevates blood sugar levels.

glucocorticoids A family of steroid hormones secreted by the adrenal cortex that includes hydrocortisone and others. Their main functions include regulation of metabolism, especially of carbohydrates, and anti-inflammatory, antiallergic action.

glucose The monosaccharide carbohydrate $C_6H_{12}O_6$ that is the main source of energy in the body, produced from glycogen and combusted into water and carbon dioxide.

glucose-6-phosphate dehydrogenase Metabolism of carbohydrates requires the action of this essential enzyme. Hereditary deficiency of the enzyme occurs in some populations, associated with severe hemolytic anemia when triggered by certain dietary ingredients such as fava beans.

glue ear The consequences of recurrent middle-ear infection in small children who have been treated with antibiotics but left with serous effusion into the middle ear, causing deafness.

glue sniffing A dangerous addiction, mainly of adolescents, due to inhalation of volatile vapors of the solvent used to bond the adhesive glue used to assemble model airplanes. The commonly used solvent is toluene, a central nervous system depressant that in small doses causes euphoria. Addicts enhance the effect by placing the solvent in a plastic bag, and as they lose consciousness, they may asphyxiate themselves or die of toluene overdose.

glutamate See MONOSODIUM GLUTAMATE (MSG).

gluten A wheat protein that plays a role in the pathogenesis of celiac disease, which is an inflammatory condition of the gastrointestinal tract. Elimination of gluten from the diet effectively controls celiac disease.

gluten-free diet A diet that avoids flour and other carbohydrates that contain gluten, containing flour from sources other than wheat. This diet is required for treatment of celiac disease.

glycerides Fats and oils composed of esters of glycerol.

glycerol Syn: glycerin. A colorless, sweet, syrupy liquid constituent of fats and oils used in the manufacture of foodstuffs, pharmaceuticals, and explosives. It is nonirritating so is sometimes used in emollient lotions for infants with sensitive skin to alleviate or prevent diaper rash.

glycogen A metabolic product of glucose and starches. Disruption of glycogen metabolism is manifested by diseases associated with deficiency of enzymes involved in glycogen storage, or any of about a dozen other varieties of metabolic upset.

goal A desired condition or state of affairs that is to be achieved within a specified time frame. See also OBJECTIVE and TARGET.

goiter Swelling of the thyroid gland that is usually associated with malfunction, either deficiency or excess, of thyroxin production. Endemic goiter occurs in regions that are geologically deficient in iodine, i.e., where IODINE DEFICIENCY DISEASES are a prominent public health problem, which is treated and eliminated by iodized salt for cooking and condiment use.

goitrogen A substance that tends to lead to formation of goiter, e.g., vegetables such as kale and spinach that block the uptake of dietary iodine.

Goldberger, Joseph (1874–1927) American public health physician who studied PELLAGRA and demonstrated in epidemiological and dietary studies that this disease was caused by a nutritional deficiency, not an infectious organism, as had previously been suggested. His studies included controlled trials of dietary regimens; the trials were excellent in most respects but were done without ethical approval and would not be approved by modern ethics review committees.

gold standard A slang or jargon term for a measurement, test, method, or procedure that is considered to be the best available.

gonad A sex gland (testis in males, ovary in females); appears in pairs. These produce the gametes and also sex hormones, testosterone, progesterone, estrogens, etc. The gonads become active at adolescence, promoting the development of secondary sex characteristics.

gonadotrophic cycle The cyclical fluctuation of hormone production that is one of the bases for the study of CHRONOBIOLOGY. The *how* of cyclical variations that control pubertal changes and menstrual rhythm is well understood, but *why* it happens at pubertal and menopausal age epochs and, in the case of menstruation, with a regular cycle of 28 days, is not clear.

gonadotrophic hormones The hormones, including chorionic gonadotrophin, the follicle-stimulating hormone (FSH), luteinizing hormone, and prolactin produced by the anterior portion of the pituitary, that are responsible for growth and maturation of the gonads at puberty, and in females for the regulation of the menstrual cycle, lactation, and, when hormone production declines, for the onset of menstruation. In males, gonadotrophins are responsible for production of sperm.

gonococcal infection Infection with *Neisseria gonorrhoeae*, a Gram-negative diplococcus that has been widely distributed throughout the world for several hundred years (since the beginning of the period of European colonization) and before that, in Europe, since early in the Common Era. It is primarily a sexually transmitted disease, GONORRHEA, but also infects the conjunctiva and occasionally the synovial membrane of limb joints. The acute infection often evolves into chronic urethritis, salpingitis, pelvic inflammatory disease, etc., which impair fertility. Neonatal gonococcal conjunctivitis, caused by mother-to-infant transmission of infection as the infant passes through the birth canal, can cause blindness, and for many years has been prevented by routine administration of silver nitrate eyedrops immediately after the birth of the infant.

gonorrhea A very common sexually transmitted infection that can be virtually symptomless in women but that causes a painful urethritis in men. For many years after the development of antibiotics, it was well controlled by a single large dose of penicillin, but penicillin-resistant *Neisseria gonorrhoeae* are widely prevalent now, so treatment has become more challenging. Information is available at http://www.niaid.nih.gov/factsheets/stdgon.htm.

good chemical practices A set of guidelines produced by committees of the American Chemical Manufacturers Association, setting out procedures for the use and safe disposal of potentially toxic or hazardous manufactured chemicals such as pesticides. The fact that the industry has sponsored these guidelines demonstrates recognition that many chemicals are potentially or actually harmful to health, but the statements tend toward the platitudinous, and some epidemiologists and other public health workers believe that the industry and the public would be better served by developing safer products. Similar guidelines have been developed in other industries, e.g., good agricultural practices.

goodness of fit The extent to which empirical observations accord with predictions of statistical or other mathematical models.

good Samaritan laws Legislation enacted in some jurisdictions, e.g., states within the United States, to protect health workers and others from legal action for damages if there is an untoward outcome when they go to the aid of critically ill or injured persons outside of a medical setting. Good Samaritan laws also usually specify that there is no duty or obligation of bystanders to render assistance, even if they are professionally qualified to do so.

gossypol An aromatic amine derivative of cotton-seed oil. It is toxic and reduces sperm counts to levels that are usually sufficient to impair fertility. It has been used since the 1920s by the Chinese as a male oral contraceptive. However, clinical trials in China in the 1980s of its safety and relative efficacy have shown that some users experience irreversible sterility, and a small proportion experience toxic nephritis. Its use has been discouraged in Western industrial nations.

gout A metabolic disease associated with disrupted excretion of the purine component of globin metabolism and deposition of uric acid crystals in joints, predominantly occurring in older people. Acute attacks can be prevented or at least ameliorated by a dietary regimen that restricts purine intake. Drug-induced gout can occur as a complication of medication, e.g., with diuretics.

Graafian follicle The cellular fluid-filled sac in a mammalian ovary in which an oocyte develops, matures, and in humans, bursts once a month to release an ovum that passes from the ovary to the uterus through the fallopian tube, and is then ready for fertilization. The name commemorates the Dutch microscopist Reijneer de Graaf (1641–1673), who first described it.

gradient of infection The range of possible host reactions to an invading pathogenic organism, from inapparent subclinical through mild clinical to severe to fulminating and overwhelming generalized fatal bacteriemia (or viremia). Usually, an overwhelming or fulminating infection leads to segregation of the victim, thereby reducing the risk of transmission. On the other hand, mild and subclinical infections that do not incapacitate leave the infected person able to move around and infect others.

grain dust The airborne matter comprising a mixture of pollen, organic particles, and inorganic dust that often evokes an allergic reaction or toxic-allergic reaction, such as alveolitis, as occurs, for instance, in FARMER'S LUNG. This reaction is sometimes called grain fever.

Gram stain A widely used staining technique in bacteriology that was originally invented by the Danish bacteriologist H. Gram (1853–1938). This staining method uses crystal violet, an iodine solution, ethanol, and a counterstain to decolorize. It distinguishes purple-colored Gram-positive from Gram-negative microorganisms that are clarified by the counterstain, thereby separating almost all pathogenic bacteria into these two large families of Gram-positive and Gram-negative organisms.

granuloma inguinale An ulcerating disease that occurs mainly in developing tropical countries, presumably caused by the Gram-negative *Klebsiella donovani*. It produces indolent granulomatous lesions on the genitalia and adnexa. Transmission is mainly, but not exclusively, by sexual contact with an infected person.

graph A visual display of the relationship between two or more variables, commonly two variables with one plotted on the horizontal and the other on the vertical axis.

Graunt, John (1620–1674) A London merchant haberdasher, amateur scientist, and fellow of the newly established Royal Society who made several notable contributions to the natural sciences, Graunt is remembered mainly for his work on the BILLS OF MORTALITY, which he analyzed to show how mortality varied by cause from year to year and differed between the sexes and from rural areas to the city of London. He reported his analyses in *Natural and Political Observations, Mentioned in a Following Index, and Made Upon the Bills of Mortality* (1662) and on this basis is regarded as a founding figure in the science of VITAL STATISTICS.

gravidity The number of pregnancies a woman has experienced, whether completed or ending before term in miscarriage, abortion, or stillbirth. See also PARITY.

gravimetric methods Analyses of liquids such as urine by assessing their specific gravity.

gray (gy) The SI unit for the amount of absorbed radiation dose equal to supplying one JOULE of energy per kilogram. The name honors the British radiobiologist L. H. Gray (1905–1965).

gray literature Unpublished papers and reports, academic dissertations, etc., that by common agreement are of sufficient quality to be reliable, verifiable, and acceptable sources of original observations for citation purposes.

gray market The unconventional, usually non-monetary economy that functions by a barter system or cash payments without documentation for sale tax purposes.

Gray Panthers An advocacy group, whose members are usually all elderly people, to promote the interests, publicize the needs, and seek enhanced services and resources for persons in these age groups and those who care for them.

gray water Water in an aquifer, canal, river, or lake that is so seriously contaminated by domestic wastewater or industrial toxins that it requires decontamination before it is fit to be used even for irrigation. Untreated, it is not potable and cannot be made available for domestic animals to drink. See also WASTEWATER.

green energy Energy that is generated without polluting the environment by adding to the burden of atmospheric greenhouse gases or causing other environmental harm, such as loss of human and wildlife habitat by construction of large hydroelectric dams. Available varieties of green energy include solar and wind power, tidal power, and geothermal energy sources.

greenhouse effect The process that maintains the atmosphere in the biosphere at a relatively even temperature. The phenomenon was described and explained in 1896 by the Swedish astronomer Svante Arrhenius (1859–1927). Short wavelength solar radiation that reaches the earth's surface and warms the biosphere is reflected back into the atmosphere as longer wavelength, but if the atmosphere contains high concentrations of GREENHOUSE GASES that trap the longer wavelength radiation, the biosphere gets warmer. Several greenhouse gases, notably carbon dioxide, methane, and CFCs, are by-products or pollutants produced by combustion of carbon-based fuels. Accumulation of greenhouse gases in increasingly higher concentrations leads to GLOBAL CLIMATE CHANGE or global warming.

greenhouse gases Gases that permit the passage of solar radiation from the sun to the earth's surface but impede the escape back into space of longer wavelength infrared radiation, thus trapping it in the earth's atmosphere. Gases incriminated in this process include carbon dioxide, which is one of the principal ingredients contained in the emissions of combusted carbon based fuels, methane produced by digestion or decomposition of vegetation, oxides of sulfur and nitrogen, and CFCs, which are also ozone-destroying substances.

griseofulvin An antibiotic that is effective against many fungus infections. It can be taken by mouth or applied topically. In the body, it is concentrated in the skin, so it is especially useful to treat fungus infections of the skin, such as ringworm.

grit Coarse particulate matter, generally exceeding 75 microns in size, that settles rapidly from the air in which it is suspended, e.g., as emissions from a coal-burning furnace.

gross domestic product (GDP) A measure of the amount of goods and services produced by a national economy over a specified period, generally a year, calculated by summing the output of all goods and services at market value. The total includes only goods and services that reach the market, are consumed, or are invested. Income arising from investments and possessions outside the nation are not included. See also GENUINE PROGRESS INDICATOR (GPI).

gross fertility rate Also called "general fertility rate," this is the number of live births to women aged 15 to 44 years or 15 to 49 years per 1,000 women in a year.

gross national product (GNP) The gross domestic product (GDP) plus income that accrues from investment and services outside the nation, minus income earned within the nation that is sent abroad.

ground level contamination The amount of contamination measured at low altitude (ground level), e.g., on vegetation, from a polluting substance such as airborne lead or other heavy metal contained in emissions from a furnace.

groundwater Water that flows or is trapped in aquifers and subsurface soil strata.

group dynamics The psychological and social interactions that occur among and between members of a group that may demonstrate cause-effect connections, development of empathy, antipathy, bonding relationships, and the reverse. Groups sometimes take on a "group personality" that is unique and different from that of other groups who undergo similar or identical experiences (as seen, for instance, with successive classes of medical students). This may be the consequence of subtle influences exerted over the group by a leader or leaders.

group leader A person who facilitates interaction among members of a group and others outside the group, recognized by group members and others as the leader or spokesman. The group leader may be chosen by consensus among group members, elected, or appointed by an outside authority. The last of these is unlikely to work well if not accepted by members of the group.

group practice Medical and other health care services provided by a group that often comprises physicians and other health professionals, each of whom specializes to a greater or lesser extent, and within which patients are often referred by the physician who first sees them, to the group member who is best qualified by expertise and experience to deal with the patient's problem. Group practice has the added virtues of permitting time off from work at nights and weekends and pooling of resources and facilities. Many group practices now provide a range of preventive and health promotion services, as well as care of incidental disease and injury.

group therapy A treatment method used mainly in psychotherapy in which group members share information and ideas about their emotional and social problems and in open discussion seek ways to resolve their problems. Groups are led by a trained psychologist or psychiatrist. Small groups (up to 6 or 8) may help to resolve problems, but the process is time consuming, and success is not assured. Staff meetings of public health departments or other professional organizations sometimes have some of the features of group therapy and may help to resolve social and emotional problems, such as interpersonal tensions among staff members.

growth curve A graphical display of the increase of height and weight of individual infants from birth through infancy and childhood, often with a printed template of the normal range against which the observed changes can be compared. These are used by pediatricians and nutritionists to assess development of infants and children. In famines and nutrition surveys in low-income countries, upper arm circumference measurements are often used as an alternative when assessing nutritional status.

growth hormone A hormone produced by the pituitary gland that controls human growth and differentiation. Deficiency of growth hormone causes short stature or, in extreme cases, dwarfism. Growth hormone derived from extracts of human pituitary glands collected at necropsy was used for a few years to treat the condition, but unfortunately was contaminated by the prion that causes CREUTZFELDT-JAKOB DISEASE, with a consequent medical disaster. This has now been superseded by synthetic growth hormone. Excess growth hormone causes gigantism, sometimes with disfiguring features, and is more difficult to detect early and to treat effectively.

growth rate A demographic term for the rate, usually expressed as a percentage, at which the population of a nation or other defined geopolitical region increases or decreases as numbers of births and deaths fluctuate. Immigration and emigration may be factored into the rate. Throughout most of recorded history growth rates have been positive and remain so in nations with high birth rates and high proportions of young people. However, in nations with low birth rates and high proportions of old people, growth rates decline, and in some, such as several Eastern European nations, Russia, and Japan, the growth rate has become negative in recent years. This has important economic and social implications for methods of support for the aged and infirm.

guardian An adult who has legally recognized responsibility for the care and supervision of child(ren) or for adults incapable of caring for themselves.

guest worker Anglicized version of the German *gästarbeiter*, a term used throughout the European Union to describe migratory or transitory laborers, usually from Eastern Europe, Asia Minor (Turkey), or the northern Mediterranean nations. Although they may reside more or less permanently in the nation where they work, they do not have the same rights as citizens and are sometimes victims of exploitation by employers. Generally, their health status is inferior to that of citizens of their host country, and often they have inferior access to health services. Migratory agricultural workers in the United States have similar status and similar health problems.

guidance counselor A professionally trained person, skilled in identifying available options and suggesting to young people the range of potential occupations and career opportunities open to them. The aim is to find the best fit between these and the student's scholastic performance, aptitude, and interests. Guidance counselors may be teachers or other members of staff of a school or higher education setting, or of a large organization that has a diverse workforce. Guidance counselors may have a role in the detection of social and emotional problems among adolescents, although they are not formally trained for this and not appropriately compensated.

guidelines A formal statement about a recommended defined policy, function, or activity. Examples include guidelines for screening procedures, the CLINICAL PREVENTIVE SERVICES GUIDELINES, and for the ethical conduct of practice and research in occupational health, epidemiology, etc., and clinical practice guidelines. There may be sanctions against those who violate the guidelines, but generally guidelines are more loosely structured than codes of conduct and seldom strictly enforced.

Guide to Clinical Preventive Services The report of the US PREVENTIVE SERVICES TASK FORCE, now published in its second edition, describes and comments on a wide range of preventive services that practicing physicians can use, including screening, counseling, and early interventions. One important feature of the *Guide* is its critical evaluation of each service discussed. The text is available at http://odphp.osophs.dhhs.gov/pubs/guidecps/.

Guillain-Barré syndrome An acute disorder of spinal nerve roots, probably immunological in origin, occurring as a complication of other conditions, such as viral infections, characterized by paralysis of peripheral muscles, often ascending from the legs through the trunk to the upper limbs and occasionally extending to respiratory and facial muscles. The condition mostly affects motor nerve roots, but there is often some accompanying sensory loss. Progression may continue for some weeks, followed by a period of stability and usually a slow recovery. It was thought to be an adverse reaction to vaccination, notably anti-influenza vaccine against swine influenza in 1976 in the United States, but reanalysis of the data suggested that the number affected could have occurred by chance, rather than as a consequence of vaccination. The eponym honors the French neurologists Jean Barré (1880–1971) and Georges Guillain (1876–1961). Further information is available at http://www.ninds .nih.gov/disorders/gbs/gbs.htm.

guinea pig A rodent that has been extensively used in experimental studies of vaccines, drugs, etc., to test their safety before they are given to humans. Humans used in medical experiments are often called "human guinea pigs."

Guinea worm See DRACUNCULIASIS.

Gulf War syndrome A condition observed among service personnel who served in the Gulf War in 1991, characterized by fatigue, limb pains, and symptoms resembling some of those associated with POST-TRAUMATIC STRESS DISORDER. Investigations have revealed equivocal evidence that the syndrome may sometimes have been attributable to environmental exposures, e.g., to organophosphate chemical weapons and/or depleted uranium used in armor-piercing shells.

gumma A granulomatous swelling of skin or internal organ, such as the liver, that in the past was a common characteristic of untreated syphilis. Modern antibiotic treatment methods have made this an uncommon or rare sequela.

gun control Procedures and processes required by law to control access to and use of guns, especially handguns, which are subject to rigorous control measures in many nations. In the United States, this is a state responsibility, and standards and procedures vary from attempts to maintain quite rigorous control of access to and use, especially of handguns, to the policies of jurisdictions where it is permissible to carry concealed handguns and even to use them in a preemptive manner when there is a self-perceived threat against a person.

gun lobby A political pressure group that advocates easy access to and ownership of guns, including handguns and (in the United States) assault weapons. The most aggressive and effective such lobby in the United States is the NATIONAL RIFLE ASSOCIATION.

Guthrie test A reliable test for the detection of phenylalanine in the urine, used to screen newborn infants for PHENYLKETONURIA. It was developed by the American microbiologist Robert Guthrie (1916–1995).

Guttman scale A measurement scale devised by the American psychologist Louis Guttman (1916–1987) for grading responses to interviews and self-completed questionnaires in which each possible response category represents an increasingly positive (or negative) expression of the response to the question or statement in that item of the survey.

gynecology The branch of medical and surgical specialization concerned with prevention and treatment of diseases of the female genital organs. The preventive components include pelvic floor exercises aimed at minimizing postnatal gynecological problems, such as uterine prolapse and urinary incontinence, and the Pap smear for early evidence of cancer of the cervix.

H

habit A behavior that has become a customary or regular part of life, often to the extent that it is done without conscious thought or almost automatically, and recognized as a way to render life orderly. Health habits such as hand-washing and covering the nose and mouth when sneezing or coughing are important disease-control activities best acquired in early childhood. Habits may become compulsive, as with gambling or alcohol consumption. See also HABITUATION.

habitat The environment that under ideal conditions is favorable to a species, enabling it to grow, develop, reproduce, and flourish indefinitely. A species does not flourish if the habitat is polluted or depleted of resources needed for it to grow, develop, and reproduce.

habituation Decrease in reactivity to repeated stimulation, as with repetitive sensory input, and doses of sedatives or stimulants, so that larger doses are required to produce the desired effect. In habituation to drugs, alcohol, or other substances, progressively larger doses are necessary to produce the desired effect.

habitus (obsolete) Bodily configuration, especially of adults, sometimes called plethoric (stocky, broad-framed) or asthenic (thin-framed); intermediate types are called sthenic (broad-framed thin) and hyposthenic (thin-framed plump). In the early 20th century, habitus was believed to be associated with temperament and predisposition to certain diseases, but there is little or no good evidence to support generalizations along these lines.

Haddon's model for traffic-related injuries The American physician and founding director of the National Transportation and Safety Commission, William Haddon (1926–1985) analyzed the factors responsible for traffic-related injury. In 1963, he produced a model of three phases (before, during, and after injury occurred), and the human, vehicle-related, and environmental factors that were associated with the injury. He presented these in what became known as Haddon's matrix, shown below.

Haemophilus influenzae A pathogenic organism responsible for acute respiratory infection with a tendency to complications, including otitis media and meningitis, characteristically of infants and children. This happens especially often with *H. influenzae* B infection (Hib), and Hib vaccine is recommended as effective protection against this risk.

hair analysis Two forms of analysis can be conducted on hair. 1. Spectroscopy and chemical analysis can detect certain kinds of metallic poisoning, notably arsenic, as readers of detective fiction know. 2. DNA analysis to identify individuals is possible if roots of hair are available. Both forms may fall within the purview of specialists in FORENSIC MEDICINE. Hair "analysis" is sometimes used in drug screening and is also a feature of several varieties of quackery.

half-life The time in which the concentration of a substance, such as the radioactive content of an element or the body burden of a toxic chemical, is reduced by half.

halfway house Syn: group home. A semisheltered setting, preferably an inconspicuous house in a residential area rather than a place that looks like an institution, in which persons can live and work part time while undergoing treatment or rehabilitation for various forms of mental disorder, on parole after release from prison for committing a criminal offense, during treatment for alcohol or substance misuse, or if for some other reason they need unobtrusive professional supervision.

hallucination The subjective sensation of a sensory input that does not match the objective reality, that is, seeing, hearing, feeling, or smelling something that does not in fact exist. An erroneous visual, auditory, tactile, or olfactory signal received by conscious centers in the brain that record sensations or events that do not exist. The causes include toxic encephalopathy, delirium induced by high fever, and psychiatric disturbances. See also DELUSION.

hallucinogen A substance, e.g., a legal or illicit drug, that gives rise to hallucinations.

halocarbons Syn: halogenated hydrocarbons. A large family of hydrocarbon chemical compounds containing halogens, i.e., fluorine, chlorine, bromine, iodine. These compounds include TRIHALOMETHANES, some of which are weakly carcinogenic, CHLOROFLUOROCARBONS (CFCs) that have been used as refrigerants, solvents, and are stratospheric ozone-destroying substances, polyhalogenated hydrocarbons, etc.

halo effect The way an observer's generally positive perception of an observed individual's personal qualities, and sometimes other emotions such as affection or prejudice, can influence the behavior of the person observed, and thus the observer's judg-

Haddon's model

Haddon's model	Human Factors	Vehicle Factors	Environmental Factors	
			Physical	*Socio-economic*
Pre-injury Phase	Alcohol	Unstable	Poor visibility	Ignorance
Injury Phase	Resistance to injury	Hard, sharp surface material	Flammable	Lack of enforcement
Post-injury Phase	Existing conditions	Rapid deceleration	Emergency medical response	Lack of funding for care and rehab

ment of specific behavioral characteristics and the overall assessment of the observed individual. This works in treatment, too. The manner, attention, and caring attitude of a health care provider can influence the response to therapeutic and other interventions. See also HAWTHORNE EFFECT.

halogens A class of chemicals containing one of the elements fluorine, chlorine, bromine, or iodine. Many are biologically active and are essential components of body fluids, enzyme systems, and the like. At doses higher than trace amounts, they are usually toxic. For example, fluorine is an extremely lethal poison, despite being essential for dental enamel formation.

halothane An anesthetic gas that became popular in the 1950s because it was nonflammable and had fewer adverse effects than did alternatives such as nitrous oxide. Halothane is chemically similar to carbon tetrachloride, is hepatotoxic, and sometimes causes hepatic necrosis.

Hamilton, Alice (1869–1970) A pioneer American occupational disease specialist, renowned for innovative studies of "dangerous trades." She received her medical degree from the University of Michigan in 1893 and worked on occupational diseases in Illinois, at Harvard Medical School, and for the US Bureau of Labor. Her work, summarized in *Industrial Poisons in the United States*, consolidated her reputation as the world's leading industrial toxicologist of her time.

Hammurabi's code Usually called the Code of Hammurabi, this is a set of principles and rules of conduct for physicians and others who serve the people, composed during the reign of the Persian emperor Hammurabi (c. 1800–1900 BCE). This code emphasized the physician's duty to preserve good health. It included rewards for success in this endeavor and drastic punishments, such as amputation of a hand for failure to prevent or cure disease of an important person.

hand-foot-and-mouth syndrome An indolent vesicular eruption affecting infants and debilitated elderly patients, caused by coxsackievirus or enterovirus infection.

handguns Short-barrelled firearms to which access is restricted in most Organization for Economic Cooperation and Development (OECD) nations because of their lethal potential in the hands of the inexperienced, the irresponsible, and criminals. The United States is an exception. The US Constitution is interpreted as conferring on all the right to bear arms. In some states, legislation permits people to carry concealed handguns, and in Florida they may be used preemptively to respond to a perceived threat. The US death rate due to handguns (much higher than in any comparable nation) is demonstrably related to easy access.

handicap Reduced capacity to perform designated tasks or fulfill expected occupational or social roles and functions because of impairment, disability, inadequate training for the task or role, or other circumstances. Applied to children, "handicap" often implies the presence of IMPAIRMENT or other circumstances that hamper normal growth and development or reduce learning abilities. See INTERNATIONAL CLASSIFICATION OF FUNCTIONING, DISABILITY AND HEALTH for the WHO definitions of these terms. A handicap usually imposes disadvantages, such as limited access to desired occupational and social opportunities. Many people with impairment or disability consider that their handicap is at least partly due to society's expectations and the roles that follow from these expectations. See also DISABILITY.

handicap-free life expectancy The average number of years of life a person can be expected to live free of handicap if current patterns of mortality and handicap continue to apply.

hand-washing The practice of disinfecting hands with soap and water is supposedly universal in patient care although not always performed conscientiously. It was recognized to be a necessary step in prevention of infection in the Allegemeines Krankenhaus in Vienna by the Hungarian physician IGNAZ PHILIPP SEMMELWEIS (1818–1865) and the American physician OLIVER WENDELL HOLMES (1809–1894) at the Boston Lying-in Hospital. Each independently concluded on the basis of observation and experiment that hand-washing prevented puerperal sepsis, but both had the same experience of aggressively hostile rejection of their beliefs by fellow professionals.

hantavirus infection A ZOONOSIS primarily affecting wild rodents that causes hemorrhagic fever when the virus invades humans, usually through inhaled aerosolized rodent droppings. It causes several varieties of serious and often fatal hemorrhagic fever, including hantavirus pulmonary syndrome, Korean hemorrhagic fever, epidemic nephropathy, and epidemic hemorrhagic fever. Epidemics occur in parts of East Asia, and sporadic cases occur elsewhere, including North America. See http://www.cdc.gov/ncidod/diseases/hanta/hps/ for details.

haphazard sample A group that is selected without regard for any rigorous method of sampling, without using either a random allocation procedure or a systematic nonrandom sampling method, such as every tenth name in a telephone directory. A haphazard sample is just that, i.e., a selection based on no formal predetermined rules whatever. It cannot be considered an unbiased sample. The "person in the street" approach of television interviewers usually uses haphazard sampling.

haploid number The number of chromosomes in a GAMETE, i.e., half the number in a ZYGOTE.

hapten An organic substance that combines with a protein to form antibody.

harassment Intimidation, bullying, threatening, or coercive behavior, including manner of speech, usually by a superior toward a subordinate, sometimes by colleagues in an organization. See also SEXUAL HARASSMENT.

hard data Data that have been directly observed and recorded, such as objective measurements of biochemical and physiological variables, as contrasted with soft data, such as responses to questions in an interview, about which there may be doubts, e.g., errors of interpretation.

hard drug An addictive drug such as HEROIN or COCAINE, so called because its use is usually illicit, often associated with crime, and users easily become addicted to it. In contrast, "soft" drugs are either legal or less addictive, such as MARIJUANA.

hard liquor An alcoholic beverage with a high alcohol content, generally a distilled or fortified spirit with alcohol content of 30% or more, such as whisky, gin, vodka, rum, or fortified or distilled wine, such as brandy.

hard science A term sometimes applied to physical sciences and aspects of biological sciences where empirical observations and verifiable, frequently replicated experiments have confirmed the facts and established a firm theoretical foundation for them. This is not to say that the scientific truths so established are immutable, as demonstrated by replacement of the Newtonian paradigm in physics with relativity and quantum mechanics.

hardship A situation, circumstance, or condition that is unusually stressful, difficult to tolerate, and causes the person(s) experiencing it an undue burden of distress, pain, or financial difficulties. Hardship in some occupations can justify compensation, such as extra financial recompense (a hardship allowance), and can be a reason for seeking damages in a legal action against the agent responsible for it.

hard water Water containing high concentrations of calcium and/or magnesium that does not readily react with soap to create a lather and leaves a layer of precipitated salts on the lining of boilers and inside kettles. Ecological, but not epidemiological, evidence suggests that populations drinking hard water have lower incidence of cardiovascular disease than do those using soft water.

hardwired A colloquial term for a neural pathway or circuit that is present from infancy and persists throughout normal life, such as sensory and motor connections through the brain, as contrasted with neural pathways that can be modified by development of conditioned reflexes. In electronics, a hardwired circuit is one that is permanently interconnected.

Hardy-Weinberg law The principle enunciated by the British mathematician G. H. Hardy (1877–1947) and the German geneticist Wilhelm Weinberg (1862–1937) according to which gene frequencies and genotype prevalence remain constant in a population of infinite size in the absence of mutations, nonrandom mating, and other selective factors such as migration.

harm A physical, emotional, and/or social or political injury to an individual or group that is suffered or brought about by an agent such as a person, institution, or organization. In law, the word is used to refer to deliberately inflicted injury, but in medicine and public health, it can apply also to injury caused by inadvertent acts.

harmonic mean The sum of reciprocals of all the values in a set divided by the number of values in a set. See MEASURES OF CENTRAL TENDENCY.

hashish An oily alkaloid resin derived from MARIJUANA that contains a high concentration of TETRAHYDROCANNABINOL (THC). It is an active psychotropic substance but is not addictive.

hate crime A violent crime such as murder, assault, mutilation, or a less physically harmful offense such as property damage or desecration of graves that is motivated by unreasoning hatred, frequently based on ethnic or racial differences between the perpetrator(s) and the victim. A special class of hate crime is violent assaults on homosexual men. The perpetrators of hate crimes often are motivated by racial or ethnic prejudice but may be mentally disturbed. The victims may suffer mental and emotional trauma, as well as physical harm.

HAV Hepatitis A vaccine.

Hawthorne effect Any effect on the behavior of individuals and groups due to knowing that they are under observation. Frequently this knowledge promotes behavior that those observed believe the observer(s) expect(s) or hope(s)to see, i.e., the effect is usually beneficial. The name derives from the observations made of workers' behavior at the General Electric plant in Hawthorne, Illinois, and reported by the Australian-born sociologist Elton Mayo (1880–1949) in *Social Problems of an Industrial Civilization* (1949). Later work has shown, however, that the effect is not consistent or predictable. See also, and compare, HALO EFFECT.

hazard The word means "risk" and is the name of a gambling card game. In public health and epidemiology, it is often a synonym for RISK FACTOR, meaning the inherent capability of an agent or a situation to have an adverse effect, that is, a factor or exposure capable of adversely affecting health or causing harm or injury. Health hazards may be behavioral, such as tobacco smoking; physical, such as exposure to toxic chemicals; biological, such as exposure to infectious pathogens; or psychological, inducing stress. See also RISK.

hazard assessment See RISK ASSESSMENT.

hazard identification The methods and procedures that are used to decide whether a hazard actually exists. These methods derive from epidemiology, toxicology, and many other sciences. See also RISK ASSESSMENT.

hazardous air pollutants Air pollutants that are known risks to health. The US Environmental Protection Agency has listed a number of these, including emissions, fumes, or gases containing arsenic, asbestos, benzene, beryllium, mercury, vinyl chloride, and radionuclides. There are, of course, many others, notably lead. The EPA Web site (http://www.epa.gov/trs) lists more than 180 hazardous air pollutants. European Union regulations set generally more rigorous standards than those of the United States regarding exposure to most hazardous air pollutants.

hazardous material A general term for any substance that is hazardous to health, e.g., a toxic chemical, radioactive material, or biological matter containing pathogenic organisms.

hazardous pollutant A hazardous substance such as a toxic chemical that contaminates the environment, i.e., the air, water for drinking or irrigation, soil, or food. Hazardous pollutants such as lead, mercury, and arsenic can occur in furnace emissions, and many kinds of toxic chemicals used in or occurring as by-products of industry can enter water courses (rivers, lakes, aquifers) or leach out of toxic dump sites.

hazardous substance See HAZARDOUS MATERIAL.

hazardous waste disposal Waste matter often contains material actually or potentially harmful to health. The largest category is INDUSTRIAL WASTE, mainly toxic chemical by-products of industrial processes. This is often deposited in lagoons or quarry pits adjacent to industrial sites and is a major component of BROWNFIELDS or INDUSTRIAL WASTE sites. Another important category is HOSPITAL WASTE. This consists of used wound dressings, hypodermic needles and other sharp or cutting items colloquially known as SHARPS, contaminated material of many other kinds, discarded doses of diagnostic or therapeutic medications, etc. Disposal of hospital waste presents problems because incineration is usually regarded as the safest method, but this can produce dioxins and furans when plastic materials are incinerated. In some settings, notably in low-income countries, recourse to incinerators is limited, and hospital waste is dumped where scavengers can salvage and repack items such as syringes, raising other added risks.

hazard rate Syn: force of morbidity, instantaneous incidence rate. A theoretical measure of the risk that a specified event will occur at a particular point in time.

haze Obscured atmosphere due to the presence in the air of opaque gases or suspended aerosol or solid particles that refract and/or reflect light. This may be a normal atmospheric phenomenon due to temperature and humidity changes at or near the earth's surface, but when it occurs in a region containing large human settlements, it can be caused by the presence of trace amounts of sulfur dioxide and/or the effect of solar ultraviolet radiation on oxides of nitrogen contained in automobile exhaust emissions. This is the mechanism for the notorious LOS ANGELES SMOG.

haze coefficient Usually called coefficient of haze (CoH). This is a measure of the atmospheric impedance of light caused by suspended atmospheric particles or aerosols. It can be measured by absorption on a white filter paper of suspended particles when air is passed through the filter paper under a standard pressure or by means of light-scattering optical technology.

HbsAg Hepatitis B surface antigen, a protein substance shed from the surface of hepatitis B virus particles that is the antigen from which hepatitis B vaccine is prepared.

HBV Hepatitis B vaccine.

HDL See high density lipoprotein.

HDL/LDL ratio The ratio of high to low density LIPOPROTEINS. It may be used to assess the risk of coronary heart disease, which is greater when the ratio is low, but the LDL/HDL RATIO is preferred because it produces a number greater than 1 rather than a decimal fraction.

head lice Infestation of the scalp hair with the head louse, *Pediculus capitis*, which is a common condition in school children but can affect people of all ages. It is transmitted by direct contact from one child to another and often affects high proportions of children in one class. It occurs in children from affluent, as well as deprived and overcrowded, homes.

head of household The adult member of the household who is identified as the principal decision maker. This was traditionally the male head, who was often the principal, or only, income earner. In household interview surveys, this individual may be the respondent for the family, although the mother may be a better source of information about children's nutritional intake and health status. In some situations, the head of the household is asked to give informed consent on behalf of all household members, but this is not ethically acceptable for research involving human subjects. In parts of Sub-Saharan Africa, where HIV/AIDS has decimated adult populations, the head of the household may be the oldest of several preadolescent children. Functionally, sociologists identify several varieties of decision making within families or households. Three simple categories are democratic, in which decision making is discussed by all, and all agree to the decision; autocratic, in which the head of the family or household decides for all without discussion; and autonomous, in which each member of the family or household makes decisions independently of the others.

Head Start Program A program that began in the United States under the administration of Lyndon Johnson in the 1960s, aimed at improving the physical and intellectual development of socioeconomically deprived infants and children by evaluating their progress in achieving developmental milestones, implemented by financial support for food and milk supplements in kindergartens, etc. Similar programs have operated for many years in Britain, other European Union nations, and Canada; most began before the American Head Start programs and have been less subject to interruption by funding cuts when the governing party has reduced its support. Evaluations have demonstrated the efficacy of such programs in enhancing development of learning and social skills. For details see http://www2.acf.dhhs.gov/programs/hsb/.

health Derived from an Old English word *hal*, meaning hale, hearty, sound in wind and limb, health has been defined in many ways. The preamble to the constitution of the World Health Organization (1946) defined health as "A state of complete physical, mental and social wellbeing and not merely the absence of disease or infirmity." In 1984, WHO-sponsored discussions about health promotion led to a revised description and definition that condenses to "The extent to which an individual or a group is able to realize aspirations and satisfy needs, and to change or cope with the environment; health is a resource for everyday life, not the objective of living; it is a positive concept, emphasizing social and personal resources as well as physical capabilities." This implies that individuals, families, and communities have some control over many determinants of their health There are several alternative definitions, including the following: 1. A structural, functional, and emotional state that is compatible with effective life as an individual and as a member of family and community groups. This definition is made up of physiological and functional ingredients that can be measured or at least assessed objectively. 2. A sustainable state of equilibrium or harmony between humans and their physical, biological, and social environments that enables them to coexist indefinitely. This does not necessarily imply that the environment or life-supporting ecosystem must remain unchanged; however, its capacity to adapt or adjust to change is not adversely affected by human activities, and changes in aspects of the environment and/or the life-supporting ecosystem do not adversely affect human health. See also HOLISTIC HEALTH, POPULATION HEALTH, and WELLNESS.

health-adjusted life expectancy (HALE) Life expectancy expressed in QUALITY-ADJUSTED LIFE YEARS (QALYs). This is a way to take into account the effect on life expectancy of chronic disease and disability, which as a general rule can be expected to shorten life.

health administration Syn: health care administration, health services administration. The art, science, and techniques of ADMINISTRATION and MANAGEMENT as applied to health or hospital services. Health administration is concerned with human and material resource allocation, assessing and meeting needs for health care, evaluating outcomes of care, and appropriate application of relevant health-related disciplines, such as vital statistics, demography, sociology, and epidemiology. Health administrators may enter the field from professions such as medicine, nursing, accountancy, or business management, and in the past often had little or no formal training. Now it has become almost mandatory to possess professional training and a qualifying degree or diploma, usually graduate education to master's degree level in a university, school of public health, or college of applied technology.

health advocacy The process of educating about and explaining determinants of health, drawing attention to risk factors for disease, injury, and premature death, and encouraging adoption of policies, strategies, tactics, and personal behaviors, such as lifestyle choices that may promote good health. This is done in many ways, including health education in schools, community groups, clubs and associations, and the media, such as television, magazines, newspapers, and, increasingly, the Internet. It may be done one to one or with small groups or a mass audience. Health advocacy is a concern of many health professionals, professional groups, voluntary agencies, public interest groups, lobby groups, and other organizations, including FOUNDATIONS, such as those concerned with heart disease, cancer, antismoking campaigns, prevention of impaired driving, control of toxic wastes, reduction of atmospheric pollution, etc.

health agency A general term for an organization, large or small, governmental or private, that provides some aspect of services concerned with health promotion, protection, treatment, long-term care, or rehabilitation. In some nations, designated nongovernmental health agencies receive benefits such as tax-supported subsidies or waiver of taxation on funds they generate.

Health and Human Services See DEPARTMENT OF HEALTH AND HUMAN SERVICES (DHHS).

Health as a Bridge for Peace A multidimensional policy and planning framework that has WHO sponsorship. Its premise is that low-intensity conflict in developing countries, and some other violent armed conflicts, are interrelated with public health problems, requiring intervention that offers opportunities for peace building. The aims and achievements of this initiative can be seen at http://www.who.int/hac/techguidance/hbp/en/.

health behavior The actions people undertake that influence their health status. These actions are influenced by the combination of understanding, insight, beliefs (VALUES), and practices that define the patterns of actions that influence people's health status, and may promote, preserve, and protect good health, or if aspects of behavior are harmful, such as driving cars at excessive speed, unsafe work practices, or cigarette smoking, may lead to injury, death, or chronic disease.

health belief model A conceptual model of health-related behavioral factors affecting health that was developed by workers in the US Public Health Service in the 1950s. The model emphasizes the role of cognition (understanding) and beliefs (VALUES) and explains how behavioral determinants influence ways individuals behave in matters affecting their health. Evaluations have shown that the model is a less reliable and consistent predictor of health-related behavior than others, notably the PRECEDE-PROCEED MODEL, but it has had some success in control strategies for HIV disease.

health benefit A valued enhancement in functional capacity or quality of life attributable to an intervention in the prior health status of a person or population group.

Healthcare Commission The UK agency that monitors performance in the British National Health Service, produces reports, and advises the general public, health service workers, and the government about many aspects of health and health care, how people can access the services they need, and much else. See http://www.healthcarecommission.org.uk/Homepage/fs/en.

health care delivery system A term used to describe how a national, regional, or local health care system is organized, administered, provided, and paid for, sometimes to a circumscribed system such as that under the auspices of a specific medical and hospital insurance carrier or HEALTH MAINTENANCE ORGANIZATION. Use of the word "delivery" is deprecated by critics who point out that health and health care cannot be "delivered." Health care can be offered or provided, and it may (or may not) be used by those who need or want it.

health care expenditure In national accounting of budget allocations and personal expenditure, money devoted to prevention and care of sickness comprises a substantial component of gross national expenditure. This includes personal health care costs; costs of drugs, dressings, and appliances; costs of hospital and long-term care; costs of personal services provided by physicians, dentists, physiotherapists, and others; costs of local, regional, and national public health services aimed at protecting community health and preventing diseases and injuries; and costs of administration. Collectively, the health sector absorbs about 10% of national expenditure in Organization for Economic Cooperation and Development (OECD) nations, less in low-income nations. There is a wide range, from 6% to 7% in France and the United Kingdom, through 10% in the Nordic nations, to 14% to 15%

in the United States. The allocation among personal costs (out-of-pocket expenses), costs covered by insurers through individual or group health plans, and costs paid directly from public revenues varies more widely. Many health economists believe that one reason health care expenditure is higher in the United States than in other OECD nations is waste and duplication inherent in a system of fragmentary insurance systems, each with its own administrative overhead costs. The US system also leaves more than 40 million people without health insurance coverage. Another reason is the extensive use of costly technology and prescribed medication. The US federal agency overseeing national expenditure on health care is the Centers for Medicare and Medicaid Services, formerly the Health Care Financing Administration (HCFA).

Health Care Financing Administration (HCFA) Now called the Centers for Medicare and Medicaid Services, this is the US government agency responsible for managing and evaluating federal funds applied to cover the costs of medical and hospital care for elderly, infirm, and indigent sick in the United States. See http://www.cms.hhs.gov/ for information.

health care industry A term used mainly in the United States to describe that part of the health sector of society comprising the organized hospital-based and community-oriented health care services for which in many, but by no means all, instances there is financial provision for payment through a medical and hospital insurance plan or through a tax-supported program such as Medicare or Medicaid. The health care industry is an important component of the national economy. In the United States, it absorbs about 14% to 15% of the gross domestic product; in most other rich industrial nations, about 8% to 12%; and in most low-income nations, less than 5%.

health care organization A term used in many countries to mean any of several varieties of organized systems of medical care, including prepaid group medical practices, collective group insurance-covered, fee-per-service medical care, and community clinics organized and run by nonprofit or profit-making organizations. In the United States the term means more or less the same but is usually applied to health maintenance organizations.

health care provider A bureaucratic term to describe a health service worker who encounters a patient or client and deals with one or more aspects of a person's health problem. This may be a physician, nurse, dentist, physiotherapist, social worker, or other professional person. The term could also apply to a radiographer, pharmacist, or others who provide diagnostic or therapeutic services but usually are agents carrying out orders rather than active interveners in the encounter.

health care system The total human and material resources that a nation or community deploys to preserve, protect, and restore health and to minimize suffering caused by disease and injury, and the administrative and organizational arrangements involved in using these. The main components of the system are primary community-oriented personal health care, hospital-based specialized care, and public health services. The "system" can also be said to include self-care and informal care provided by family members and friends.

health center The offices of health professionals who work as a team or in a loose coalition to provide ambulatory medical and related services to a community. The word "health" is often a misnomer, as there may be little emphasis on promoting and protecting health; services are mostly or entirely devoted to medical care and other services for the sick. In such cases, the term "medical center" or clinic would be more accurate, but it is less often used.

health communication The design and delivery of messages and strategies based on consumer research to promote the health of individuals and communities. This is an important way in which expert opinion on every aspect of health is conveyed to those who need it, for instance, advisory messages to the general public about many aspects of health problems. The term also applies to the two-way flow of surveillance information in communicable disease notification, cancer registries, and the like.

health counseling The strategies, methods, and procedures used by physicians, nurses, or other health care workers to explain the nature of health problems and conditions to individuals and groups, as part of the process of dealing with these problems and conditions.

health department The branch of national, regional (i.e., state, provincial, territorial), or local (i.e., municipal, county, city) government concerned with the provision, administration, resource allocation, financing, surveillance, and evaluation of services for health promotion and protection. Health departments are publicly funded and originally focused on public health, but in many nations they have become increasingly involved in financial and administrative aspects of personal health services. Many public health departments provide some aspects of personal health care services, for instance maternal and child care, treatment of sexually transmitted and other infectious diseases, and services for elderly infirm and housebound chronic sick. Many such health departments require malpractice insurance coverage for staff in these services, which is an increasingly costly component of expenses.

health development The initiatives aimed at improving health status and establishing secure personal and community health services in developing or low-income countries. These include education; environmental and housing improvement; provision of sanitary and hygiene facilities; immunization programs; maternal and infant care services; ensuring access to safe water, food, and nutrition; and, in a wider context, improving infrastructure, such as transport and communication.

health disparities Syn: health inequalities, health gap. The difference between the levels of health indicators that are observed in a defined population group and the level that would be expected if this group had the health experience of the segment of the population that ranks highest in health indicators. The observed difference in levels of specific indicators of health status, e.g., LIFE EXPECTANCY and DISABILITY-ADJUSTED LIFE YEARS (DALYS), among different socioeconomic groups or other categories of the population are generally used when assessing these disparities quantitatively.

health economics The specialized branch of economics devoted to the study of costs, benefits, resource allocation, use, inputs, outputs, and outcomes of all forms of health care. One way in which the health sector differs from other sectors of society is that the supply-demand paradigm of the marketplace is not fully applicable because at least some, perhaps most, personal health services and virtually all public health services are necessities, rather than optional expenditures. An important aspect of health economics is analysis of UTILITY, defined as the value of a state of health in quality-of-life terms. However, health economics is inseparable from the POLITICS of health services, and decisions about health economics are often ideologically driven, and therefore are subject to change with the changing fortunes of political parties.

health education The range of learning resources and teaching programs concerned with aspects of health and its preservation and protection. Health education often begins in the family and is a feature of school systems almost everywhere. (See SCHOOL HEALTH SERVICES.) It may begin in kindergarten and continues through primary school, often into secondary education, with emphasis on exercise, diet, care of teeth and skin, discussion of sexually transmitted disease, ways to cope with one's own sexuality and social relationships, teen pregnancy, avoidance of smoking, alcohol and drugs, etc. Health education is provided by school teachers and nurses and sometimes by specially trained educators or physicians. It is also conducted in the community and with subsets of the population, including pregnant women, workers, people about to retire, and the elderly.

health enhancement A term used by specialists in health promotion to describe initiatives and activities aimed at elevating health levels of well and chronically sick individuals and groups to a greater height than they had previously enjoyed. This is achieved by compiling an inventory of health needs, such as regular exercise regimens to enhance physical fitness, social activities to widen acquaintance and friendship networks, and active smoking cessation programs.

health expectancies Summary measures of health that combine life table estimates of survival with estimates of average amounts of time spent in less than perfect health. An example is HEALTH-ADJUSTED LIFE EXPECTANCY (HALE), in which life expectancy is adjusted to allow for average length of time spent at each level of health, a readily comprehended figure that is sometimes politically useful. See also HEALTH GAP INDICATORS (MEASURES).

health fair A community-based, health-promotion program based on demonstrations, displays, and dialogues between professional staff and the public, usually organized as a feature of a county fair or located for a period in a shopping mall. Health fairs may include screening facilities for hypertension, diabetes, glaucoma, cancer, etc. The aims include provision of health-promotion and disease-prevention services at a local community level, achievement of higher levels of "health consciousness," and drawing attention to local health hazards that require correction.

health field concept A conceptual model of determinants of health that was used by the authors of a visionary report, *A New Perspective on the Health of Canadians*, also called the Lalonde Report, released in 1974 in the name of the Minister for Health, Marc Lalonde, and written by public health scientists in the Canadian government department of National Health and Welfare. The health field concept identified human biology, lifestyle, environment, and health care organization as the four principal determinants of health.

Health for All by the Year 2000 The goal of the World Health Organization in the 1980s, often mistaken for a slogan. It was resolved by the World Health Assembly in 1977 that the main social target of governments and of WHO should be attainment by all the world's people by the year 2000 of a level of health that would permit them to lead a socially and economically productive life. This goal would be implemented by ensuring access to essential PRIMARY HEALTH CARE and reduction by finite amounts of the burden of disease, disability, and premature death. The goal was never achieved because of many obstacles, notably lack of political will to implement measures that would achieve it. The onset of the HIV/AIDS pandemic was an important aggravating factor. See also ALMA-ATA DECLARATION.

health gap See HEALTH DISPARITIES.

health gap indicators (measures) Summary measures of population health that estimate the shortfall between the actual health levels of a population and what would be expected in an optimal reference state. The gap is usually measured using DISABILITY-ADJUSTED LIFE YEARS (DALYs) lost or POTENTIAL YEARS OF LIFE LOST (PYLL) usually from specific causes. These have the advantage of facilitating estimates attributable to specified diseases and risk factors but also the disadvantage that the "units of healthy time lost" may have no intrinsic meaning.

health goals Sets of quantitatively expressed health and vital statistics that health planners aspire to achieve by specified target dates. The World Health Organization stated a series of health goals as part of its long-range plans in the "Health for All by the Year 2000" initiative and the challenge was taken up by health officials in the European Union, the United States, and elsewhere. The health goals for the United States were stated in reports from the office of the Surgeon General in 1979, and again in 1991 and 2000. Examples of goals are reduction by specified amounts of perinatal mortality rates, unplanned teen-age pregnancies, smoking prevalence, sexually transmitted diseases. See also *HEALTHY PEOPLE 2000*.

health indicator A directly measurable variable that reflects the health status of the population. Health indicators include infant and perinatal mortality rates, incidence rates of notifiable diseases that are reported with reasonable completeness, disability days measured by medical certification for sickness absence from school or work, cancer incidence as recorded and reported by a cancer registry, records of certain specific prescribed medications, records of causes of death, the pro-

portion of certified deaths for which adequate medical records exist, and others. Some indicators may be measured in terms of their presence or absence, for instance some health related legislation and availability of sickness and medical and hospital care insurance.

health inequalities See HEALTH DISPARITIES.

health information system A set of methods and procedures to compile and disseminate all types of statistics on population health, i.e., HEALTH INDICATORS, sometimes personal health data. See also INFORMATION SYSTEM.

health insurance Often more accurately called medical insurance or sickness insurance, this is a system for financial protection of individuals and families against the costs of medical and hospital care for illness and injury by paying these costs from a collective fund derived from taxation or other revenue, or individual insurance premiums, or some combination of these. Health insurance may work in several ways. Often it is a fringe benefit of employment with the premium paid by the employer or shared between employer and employee. It may be a collective system or group insurance, as in the "lodges" that preceded comprehensive tax-supported national health insurance programs in Britain (the National Health Service), Canada (Canadian Medicare), many European nations, New Zealand, and Australia. In the United States, health insurance is fragmented among many private insurance companies, group health insurance, and, for some people such as the elderly, the indigent, and native Americans, agencies of the US government.

health maintenance organization (HMO) A variety of health care organization that arose in the United States, comprising groups of physicians and other health care professionals who provide therapeutic care and sometimes preventive medical screening services for enrolled persons and family groups but seldom provide insurance coverage for health-promotion and counseling services. HMOs may be nonprofit or profit-making organizations. They usually have clinics affiliated with hospitals that allocate beds to the enrolled members who need inpatient care. The services are provided for fixed fees with contractual limitations on referrals for more specialized services than those the HMO can provide, a situation that can cause frustration and dissatisfaction for patients and their physicians.

health manpower (health workforce, health human resources) development An educational and training initiative of the World Health

Organization and of many nations, aimed at increasing the supply of physicians, nurses, and other professional workers in the health sector in rich and low-income countries, where cultural, economic, political, and other barriers sometimes impede recruitment, training, and retention of physicians, nurses, medical technicians, and the like.

health measurement scales Health is multifaceted, and to measure each facet objectively is a daunting task. Specific measurement scales are available to assess mobility, ability to dress, wash, negotiate stairs, shop for essentials, etc., using, for instance, the ACTIVITIES OF DAILY LIVING (ADL) SCALE; other measurement scales assess neurological and mental status, with questions and tests of memory, mood, emotional status, usually by means of ordinal or nominal scales on a survey instrument. All such scales recognize that "health" is not directly measurable.

health outcomes In evaluating the performance of health services, it is best to make use of objective indicators. Several of these are alliteratively identified as death, disease, disability, discomfort, disruption, and dissatisfaction. Death and disease are measured by mortality and morbidity rates, disability by means of the ADL or equivalent scales, discomfort by the amount of medication required to obtain relief of symptoms, disruption by the extent to which health problems impair capacity to engage in normal work and social activities, and dissatisfaction by such indirect unobtrusive measures as broken appointments, requests to change health care providers, surveys of patient satisfaction, and various others.

health plan A term often used to describe personal and family insurance coverage for the costs of medical and hospital care. It really means medical insurance plan.

health planning A prominent activity of all health departments is short-term, medium-term, and long-range planning. Important considerations are RESOURCE ALLOCATION, priority setting, distribution of staff and physical facilities, planning for emergencies, extremes of demand and unforeseen contingencies, and preparation of budgets for future fiscal periods with a feasible time horizon, often 5 years ahead, sometimes as far ahead as 10 or even 15 years, recognizing that it takes this long to develop new systems and train skilled health professionals, so it is desirable to attempt prediction of future needs for specialized professional staff and their resource needs. See also SCENARIO.

health policy A set of principles formally agreed to by elected and/or appointed health authorities at the national, regional, or local level. Health policy may be initiated by professional workers in the health system, by politicians, or by both. The purpose may be to guide health planning and health systems development to meet specified health needs; to provide specified programs and services; to ensure a consistent basis for the regulation, implementation, administration, and provision of health services, consistent with stated aims and objectives; to enhance efficiency and effectiveness; to control escalating costs; to advance a political agenda; or, often, to achieve some combination of these aims. Health policies require continuous monitoring and evaluation to remain consistent with underlying societal values and resource limitations to facilitate evolution in response to changing needs of the population.

health professional A gender- and status-neutral term for anyone professionally trained in a health science discipline who provides services for patients or clients or the public in a health care system or service. The term applies to all whose competence has been assessed by appropriate methods, e.g., physicians, nurses, sanitarians, dietitians, epidemiologists.

health promotion The policies and processes that enable people to increase control over and improve their health. These address the needs of the population as a whole in the context of their daily lives, rather than focusing on people at risk for specific diseases, and are directed toward action on the determinants or causes of health. Health promotion is action oriented and based on public policies, for instance provision of facilities such as bicycle pathways, recreational parks to encourage healthy behavior, and public meeting places to encourage social interaction; and deterring health-harming behavior by providing smoke-free zones. See OTTAWA CHARTER FOR HEALTH PROMOTION and HEALTH EDUCATION.

health protection A useful term to describe important activities of public health departments, specifically in food hygiene, water purification, environmental sanitation, drug safety, and other activities in which the emphasis is on actions that can be taken to eliminate as far as possible the risk of adverse consequences for health attributable to environmental hazards, unsafe or impure food, water, drugs, etc.

Health Protection Agency The Health Protection Agency (HPA) is an independent body that protects the health and well-being of the British population. The Agency plays a critical role in protecting people from infectious diseases and in preventing harm when hazards involving chemicals, poisons, or radiation occur. Its activities are described at http://www.hpa.org.uk/.

health-related quality of life A HEALTH STATUS INDICATOR that provides a proxy measurement of the UTILITY or value of a particular health state. Like utility, it is usually measured on a scale from zero to one, and assessed in conjunction with self-perceived or observed physical, social, and emotional function of individuals. In practice it is assessed by questionnaire or interview, using a rating scale if possible, rather than open-ended questions.

health research An all-encompassing term that some engaged in it prefer to use (rather than medical or biomedical research) to describe all forms of biological, behavioral, and/or social science research on all aspects of human health and disease.

health resources All resources concerned with the health sector, that is, buildings, equipment, supplies, personnel, and educational and communications material involved in protecting the public from hazards to health, preventing disease, and treating the sick.

Health Resources and Services Administration (HRSA) The US government agency that oversees federally funded and administered health resources and services. The range of its roles and responsibilities is displayed at http://www.hrsa .gov/.

health risk A general term for any form of hazard or risk to health.

health risk appraisal (HRA) Syn: health hazard appraisal. The systematic assessment of a person's chances of falling ill or dying of specified conditions that can be predicted with some reliability on the basis of risk factors (assessed by epidemiological evidence). HRA begins by considering each person's actuarial risks based on age and sex, with adjustments to allow for increased or reduced risk of coronary heart disease, tobacco-related cancers, and other known determinants of reduced or enhanced longevity.

health sciences The scholarly activities that contribute to the professional knowledge, skills, and expertise of members of the health professions. These are the raison d'être of a medical, dental, or nursing school, school of public health, etc. Health sciences include basic sciences, anatomy, physiology, biochemistry, microbiology, immunology, pharmacology, clinical sciences, medicine, surgery, obstetrics and gynecology, psychology, psychiatry, therapeutics, social and behavioral sciences, epidemiology, biostatistics, and, to round out the education, biomedical ethics, history of medicine, and sundry other scholarly activities. Selected technical terms from all these disciplines can be found in this dictionary.

health sector Conceptually and for planning purposes, society is sometimes considered to be made up of sectors: the health, educational, housing, transport, defense, law enforcement, commercial and industrial sectors. It is an imperfect categorization because of overlaps and omissions, but it is nonetheless useful. In terms of budgetary allocation and employment in the wealthy nations, the health sector is among the largest and most expensive.

health services A vague, general, all-embracing term for all health care services collectively.

health services research All aspects of research aimed at evaluating health services. These aspects are concerned primarily with OUTCOMES but also with the process by which health services are provided and with their organizational and administrative structure. The principal disciplines involved include epidemiology; statistics; economics; social, behavioral, and management sciences; clinical sciences; and other fields, such as ethics and law.

health status The degree to which a person (or specified group) can fulfill usually expected roles and functions physically, mentally, emotionally, and socially. Any departure from the usually expected status is an indication that disease is present. Health status can be assessed clinically by asking questions and conducting a physical examination and/or by health status indicators or health measurement scales.

health status indicator Any criterion that can be used to assess the health status of a person or specified group. Commonly used criteria include the presence or absence of symptoms (malaise, cough, breathlessness, pain, and a host of others); presence or absence of physical signs (fever, elevated pulse rate, blood pressure, etc.); or presence or absence of abnormal findings of radiological or laboratory tests. Some particular health status indicators exist, such as QUALITY-OF-LIFE SCALES and SICKNESS IMPACT PROFILES. A popular survey instrument to measure health status is the SF36, a 36-item health questionnaire. At the level of communities, health status is assessed by such measures as incidence or prevalence of indicator diseases (diarrhea, malaria, etc., in low-income tropical countries; untreated hernia, refractive errors in upper-income countries); health care and obstetric coverage, etc. See also HEALTH INDICATOR.

health survey A SURVEY, which may be conducted by face-to-face or telephone interview or by a self-completed questionnaire, and/or physical examination and special tests to investigate aspects of health and disease, risk factors and determinants of health, use of and satisfaction with health care services, etc. There are many varieties and levels of complexity, from very simple brief sets of questions and/or cursory physical examinations, to detailed studies of samples of the general population, as in the US NATIONAL HEALTH AND NUTRITION EXAMINATION SURVEYS (NHANES) and similar national sample surveys in the United Kingdom, European Union, Canada, and other countries.

health system The word "system" is most often used in the context of the economic, fiscal, and political management method that nations use to run the national health care services. It can also refer to a local or regional group of organized health services. "Health system" is defined in the WHO Report for 2000 as all the activities whose primary purpose is to promote, restore, or maintain health.

health team The group of health professionals who provide care for persons and populations. Ideally, every patient in a modern multispecialty hospital or clinic should be cared for by such a cohesive team, but often in reality the "team" is an ad hoc group that is loosely structured, rather than a cohesive team in which members work in harmony with one another, each with a well-defined role and responsibilities. In public health services, teamwork may often be more coherent, as in epidemic investigation, environmental health, caring for problem families, and many other specialized tasks of local, regional, and national public health services. A health team may also be centered on a patient or on a specific disease; for instance, persons with diabetes are the central members of the team that is responsible for maintaining them in metabolic balance.

health visitor A British term for a public health nurse. Health visitors in the past gave much of their professional attention to maternal and child health care, especially home visits to women who had recently given birth. Now they also care for elderly, infirm housebound and chronic sick people. The term is used in some middle- and low-income countries, such as Pakistan, to describe frontline health care workers who are trained to assess health status and provide simple guidance on management of common health problems.

health worker Usually a synonym for HEALTH PROFESSIONAL but can have a more inclusive flavor, when it describes untrained hospital staff, such as porters, cleaners, and food handlers.

healthy active life expectancy The average amount of time an individual can be expected to live in a state of good health and without disability, based on actuarial and epidemiological data.

healthy city, healthy community An initiative of the European Regional Office of the World Health Organization that originated soon after the ALMA-ATA Conference and Declaration in 1978 and spread to cities and communities worldwide. The aim is to enhance the quality of life by making communities conducive to healthy living, providing resources and facilities for recreation; easy access to settings for exercise, sport, and physical activity, such as swimming, bicycling, and walking; and designing dwellings that are amenable to good living rather than just stultifying and depressing places to live. There is much emphasis on SUSTAINABLE DEVELOPMENT. The success of the healthy cities movement in Düsseldorf, Toronto, Dakar, and several other pioneer cities encouraged expansion to cities in more than 50 countries, rural communities, and island states. The initiative faded when many communities perceived that it provided excuses for national governments to download tasks and programs that had previously been financed by national or state budgets.

healthy life year (HeaLY) A composite indicator incorporating mortality and morbidity into a single number similar to the DALY but without adjustment for age differences.

Healthy People 2000 A US PUBLIC HEALTH SERVICE report published in 1990 that set out some specific goals and targets to be achieved by 2000, using health-promotion and disease-prevention strategies and tactics. The document outlined the roles and responsibilities of government agencies, the health sector, industry and other sectors of society, and individuals. It was adapted in modified form by public health leaders in other nations.

Healthy People 2010 A revised version of the US PUBLIC HEALTH SERVICE document of 1990, published in 1000, outlining health goals and targets to be achieved by 2010. This is part of an ongoing activity that focuses on policies and plans to improve the health of the American people, with periodic revisions in the light of changing information about health status and health needs. For details, see http://www.healthypeople.gov/ Goals for 2020 are currently being developed.

healthy worker effect The effect of prior selection, observed in the early stages of studies of workers in industries exposed to occupational hazards. Because unhealthy people are more likely to be rejected and healthy people are more likely to be recruited, the sickness and death rates initially may be lower in the exposed workforce than in the general population.

healthy year equivalents An abstract measure of health-related quality of life that incorporates sets of preferences for individual life expectancy and preferences for states of health, used mainly in CLINICAL DECISION ANALYSIS.

hearing aid An electronic device to amplify sound waves, preferably designed to amplify sound of specific frequencies associated with particular kinds of deafness identified by audiometric tests. Hearing aids offer immense benefits to many people with hearing impairment, but they are not a universal panacea, especially for people whose impairment mainly affects specific sound frequencies. Cochlear implants are an alternative, albeit a costly one, and not always readily accessible.

hearing impaired A description of a partially deaf person that is useful because it emphasizes the fact that deafness is an impairment of the sensory apparatus or of the nervous system that without correction by a hearing aid can lead to a disability of hearing. Deaf people can be handicapped and at risk because they cannot hear warning signals and are often unable to take part in conversations, listen to music, or enjoy others of life's pleasures.

hearing loss An objectively measured assessment of hearing that uses audiometric tests to map the actual frequencies on which acuity of hearing is impaired or hearing is absent altogether.

hearsay rule An informal rule in organizations, as well as courts of law, that statements based on remarks or comments by third parties cannot be accorded complete credibility unless it is possible to verify them independently.

heart attack A lay expression, often meaning an acute, perhaps fatal, episode of myocardial infarction, with severe chest pain and/or erratic heart action (fast, irregular pulse).

heart disease A general term that covers atherosclerosis, coronary heart disease, hypertension, rheumatic heart disease, and congenital heart disease. Heart disease is the leading cause of death worldwide, and it is to a considerable extent preventable. Modern multispecialty clinics and hospitals often have specialized staff to deal with each aspect, and with age-related problems, so there are pediatric cardiologists, specialized vascular surgeons, cardiothoracic surgeons, etc.

hearth The base of a furnace or fireplace. The extent to which combustion is complete and emissions contain suspended particulate matter depends on oxygen flow to the hearth. An inefficient hearth, as well as the type of fuel combusted, may be the source of air pollution.

heat cramps Muscle pain caused by sodium loss in sweat that may be the first sign of the body's inability to cope efficiently with physiological adjustment to a hot, moist environment or to sustained physical activity, as in a lengthy sporting contest, such as a soccer match, on a hot day.

heat exhaustion A severe reaction to working in a hot, humid environment in which sweating has led to dehydration without cooling, as well as loss of sodium and other electrolytes, vasodilation has not helped to cool the body, and cardiac and circulatory efficiency is impaired.

heat island An urban region that retains heat during hot weather, where night-time temperatures remain high, and refreshing evening breezes are imperceptible.

heat stress Physiological distress caused by exertion in excessively hot and humid environmental conditions, manifest by flushing, sweating, exhaustion, etc. A high HUMIDEX reading is more dangerous to the cardiovascular system than high ambient temperature per se, especially if there is also a high level of SMOG.

heat stroke The end stage of malfunction of the body's physiological regulatory mechanisms under extreme heat stress, manifested by a sharp sustained temperature rise, circulatory collapse, central nervous system damage, loss of consciousness, and death, unless effective intervention is immediately available.

heat syncope A state of collapse and usually loss of consciousness associated with exposure to excessive heat. Maintenance of fluid intake is important in preventing this condition.

heat wave An extreme weather event in which there is a prolonged period of above-normal temperatures. "Prolonged" means anything from a few days to a few weeks; "above normal" means above the expected averages for that place at that season. Heat waves may be accompanied by other climatic events, for instance episodes of severe SMOG in large urban regions, and the combination of heat and smog is dangerous to health for infants, the elderly, and persons with chronic cardiovascular or respiratory disease. Severe heat waves can cause heavy mortality even in otherwise favorable living conditions. For instance, a heat wave in western Europe in 2003 killed an estimated 25,000, mostly infirm elderly people or frail infants. The climate models of global warming scenarios suggest that heat waves will increase in frequency and severity in coming decades.

heavy metal A metal with a high atomic weight. The term is not precisely defined, but in the context of public health, it is conventionally understood to include those that have adverse effects on human health, i.e., antimony, arsenic, bismuth, lead, and mercury. Other metals, heavy and otherwise, have adverse effects, too, including chromium, nickel, and, of course, the radioactive metals. Because it is vague, the term is better avoided.

hebdomadal mortality rate Syn: neonatal mortality rate. The mortality rate in the first week of postnatal life. The numerator is the number of infants born alive who die before the end of their first week of life, and the denominator is the number of live births in the same year.

Heimlich maneuver A potentially life-saving first-aid technique to deal with an obstructed airway by applying firm pressure to the hypogastrium (upper abdomen) with a clenched fist clasped in the other wrist. This can usually produce enough air pressure to dislodge a bolus of food in the hypopharynx, but it must be done carefully to avoid fracturing ribs, especially in the case of elderly people with fragile bones. This technique was developed by the American thoracic surgeon Henry Heimlich (b. 1920).

Helicobacter pylori A bacterium that is implicated in the etiology of gastritis, peptic ulcer, and possibly gastric cancer. The organism, which can be detected in the gut of a high proportion of humans, is either an initiator or a cofactor in causing peptic ulcer. Antibiotic treatment to eradicate the pathogen leads to improvement and cure of peptic ulcer. The role of this pathogen in gastritis and peptic ulcer was discovered by the Australian physicians Robin Warren (b. 1937) and Barry Marshall (b. 1951). They received the Nobel Prize for their work on this in 2005.

helminth A generic name for a parasitic worm, which anatomically may be a ROUNDWORM, a flatworm, a segmented TAPEWORM, or a HOOKWORM. The science of helminthology is a large component of PARASITOLOGY, particularly fascinating because of the complex ecology and the complex life cycles of many parasitic worms.

help line A telephone line, generally a free call, open 24 hours 7 days a week, to provide advice, guidance, referrals, etc., for people experiencing various kinds of social and/or emotional problems. Help lines have become commonplace in almost all large communities, often staffed by volunteers, perhaps with backup provided by a trained social worker.

Helsinki, Declaration of A set of guidelines on acceptable conditions for medical research involving human participants (research subjects) that was approved by delegates to a meeting in Helsinki of the World Medical Association (WMA) in 1964; this declaration was the response of the WMA to the findings of the Nuremberg trials of Nazi war criminals, that led to the NUREMBERG CODE. The Declaration of Helsinki has been reviewed and revised at several subsequent meetings of the WMA, and is considered to be the gold standard statement on desirable conditions for all forms of research involving human subjects. The COUNCIL FOR INTERNATIONAL ORGANIZATIONS OF MEDICAL SCIENCES (CIOMS) and many national organizations sponsoring medical research have drafted guidelines and codes of conduct derived from the Helsinki declaration. These apply in all situations involving research with human participants. See http://www.wma.net/e/policy/b3.htm for the current version of the Declaration of Helsinki and discussion of its revisions.

hematology The medical specialty dealing with diseases of the blood and blood-forming organs.

hematopoietic system The body system concerned with production, metabolism, circulation, and eventual destruction of circulating blood cells that have reached their natural life expectancy. The main components of the system are the bone marrow, spleen, and lymphatic glands.

hematuria The presence of blood in the urine.

Hemlock Society A society that originated in the United States and has spread to other nations to promote EUTHANASIA for the incurably ill who seek to end their lives to avoid a painful period of terminal suffering for themselves and their nearest and dearest. In 2003, the Hemlock Society changed its name to End-of-Life Choices, and in 2004, End-of-Life Choices merged with Compassion in Dying. The organization is now known as Compassion and Choices. Information about it and the methods it advocates is at http://www.compassionandchoices.org/.

hemodialysis Removal of toxic metabolic products from circulating blood by passing the blood through a semipermeable membrane outside the body. This is used to treat renal failure and some other conditions, but long-term, chronic dialysis can lead to electrolyte disturbances, anemia, and aluminum toxicity causing dementia.

hemoglobin The oxygen-carrying red pigmented protein compound contained in red blood corpuscles in all mammals, including humans.

hemolysis Destruction of red blood corpuscles by processes that fragment them while usually leaving them in circulation, so the fragments clog up other organs, such as renal glomeruli and tubules, as well as causing hemolytic jaundice. Hemolysis can be caused by chemical toxins, by the action of pathogens such as the malaria parasite, and various other conditions, mostly serious.

hemolytic disease of the newborn A condition caused by incompatibility of fetal red cells and maternal immunoglobulin G antibodies produced in response to fetal antigen. Severe cases (the condition called erythroblastosis fetalis) occur with Rh incompatibility between mother and fetus; prevention of this is a priority of good-quality obstetric care. It can be prevented by the timely administration of immune globulin.

hemolytic-uremic syndrome A dangerous complication of *ESCHERICHIA COLI* O57:H7 infection, with hemolytic anemia, thrombocytopenia, and renal failure that can be fatal, especially in small infants.

hemophilia A hereditary sex-linked condition due to a defective clotting mechanism that results from deficiency of an essential clotting factor, usually FACTOR VIII. It passes only from mothers to their sons, but also can occur as a random mutation. Many hemophiliac patients who rely on Factor VIII to prevent bleeding were infected with HIV/AIDS and with hepatitis C before screening tests for these diseases were developed to detect them and prevent use of contaminated blood.

hemorrhagic disease of the newborn A neonatal disease caused by deficiency of vitamin K, which is usually synthesized in adequate amounts by commensal organisms in the gastrointestinal tract but can occur when these organisms are not present. It can be prevented (and treated) by parenteral injection of vitamin K in neonates.

Henle, Friedrich Gustav Jacob (1809–1885) A German pioneer histologist and pathologist, who made many original observations, notably about the microstructure of kidneys. He was at the interface of the miasma theory and the germ theory of disease causation and in *Von den Miasmen und Kontagien* (*On miasmata and contagion*, 1840), he enunciated three of the four postulates later adopted by ROBERT KOCH and often inappropriately called Koch's postulates.

Henle-Koch postulates Syn: Koch's postulates. First formulated by the German pathologist FRIEDRICH GUSTAV JACOB HENLE (1809–1885) and adapted and modified by the German bacteriologist ROBERT KOCH (1843–1910), these are four criteria that usually suffice to confirm the causal relationship of a pathogenic organism to a specific infectious disease. The postulates are: 1. The agent must be demonstrable in every case of the disease; 2. The agent is not present in other diseases; 3. After isolation in culture, the agent must be able to produce the disease in experimental animals; and (added by Koch) 4. The agent can be recovered from the experimental animal. All four postulates can be demonstrated with many bacterial diseases but have not been confirmed in some in which a causal connection may have to be inferred from other evidence, e.g., HIV/AIDS.

hepatitis Inflammation of the liver. This has many possible causes, including virus infections, bacterial infections, and various chemicals, including alcohol. The word is often used without qualification to mean viral hepatitis. Hepatitis A is transmitted by the fecal-oral route via contaminated water. Hepatitis B is transmitted from mother to infant and in blood and body fluids. The other alphabetically designated varieties, hepatitis C, D, E, F, etc., are each immunologically and epidemiologically distinct, are mainly transmitted by way of contaminated blood or blood products, and were discovered when they declared themselves clinically in epidemics related to transfusions or parenteral injections.

hepatitis vaccines Identified hepatitis viruses include hepatitis A; B; non-A non-B, now called hepatitis C; D, also called delta hepatitis virus; E; F; and G. Hepatitis A and E are transmitted by the fecal-oral route, the others by blood or body fluids. Because of molecular (immunological) differences, vaccines must be prepared individually to protect against each variety. Vaccines are now available against hepatitis A, B, and D (hepatitis B vaccine is partially protective against this). No vaccines were available for protection against other varieties of hepatitis as of 2005. See http://www.cdc.gov/idu/hepatitis/vaccines.pdf for further details.

heptachlor A cyclodiene pesticide in the same family as aldrin, dieldrin, and chlordane that was found in 1983 by the EPA to be too toxic for all uses except underground termite control. Later it was found to be associated with increased incidence of leukemia and genital dysplasia.

herbalist A specialist in the treatment of disease by the use of herbal remedies. This is an ancient traditional practice, often using remedies that have been successfully used for centuries.

herbal remedies A range of folk medicines, many of them empirically discovered hundreds of years ago to be effective, derived from or consisting of portions of plants. Some of the plants are domestically cultivated, such as foxglove, from which digitalis is derived; others, such as the cinchona bark from which quinine is derived, grow wild and are gathered by folk healers. In many cultures, knowledge about the efficacy of herbal remedies is carefully preserved and handed on by oral tradition from one generation to the next. Since about the middle third of the 20th century, modern pharmacologists have systematically studied traditional herbal remedies, seeking to identify and refine their active ingredients, and have added to the pharmacopeia many useful drugs to treat and prevent disease. Controlled trials have revealed that, although some herbal remedies are effective, many are ineffective apart from a placebo effect, and some are harmful. Some traditional herbal remedies, for instance rauwolfia, have been adopted and patented, and have become profitable for pharmaceutical corporations.

herbicide A chemical compound that is toxic to and kills plants, sometimes selectively. A group of broad-leaf herbicides that are polyaromatic hydrocarbon compounds, such as AGENT ORANGE, and commercial preparations of 2,4-D are highly effective but are also harmful to human health. 2,4-D is classified by the International Agency for Research on Cancer as a possible human carcinogen. Its use for cosmetic purposes on lawns is deprecated.

herd immunity The resistance of a community or group to the invasion and transmission of an infectious pathogen. It occurs when a sufficiently high proportion of members of the community are immune because of prior infection or immunization, leading to a very low probability that an invading pathogen will encounter a susceptible host. This is computable, based on the product of the number of susceptible persons in the population and the probability that they will encounter a source of contagion, i.e., an active case or infectious contact. Thus, herd immunity is a statistical probability rather than an actuality. It is the extent of resistance of the population to the invasion and spread of an infectious agent, and it is based on the agent-specific immunity of a high proportion of the population. The proportion that must be immune to achieve herd immunity varies according to the infectious agent, its transmission characteristics, the spatial distribution of immunes and susceptibles in the population, and other ecological and environmental factors. Full understanding of herd immunity requires familiarity with advanced theoretical statistics.

herd immunity threshold An important concept in infectious disease epidemiology, this is the proportion of immune persons in a population, above which the incidence of new cases of a specific infection declines and eventually ceases altogether. This threshold varies according to the characteristics of the infectious pathogen. It is expressed mathematically as

$$H = 1 - 1/R_0 = (R_0 - 1)/R_0 = (\gamma T - 1)/\gamma T$$

where H is the herd immunity threshold, R_0 is the BASIC REPRODUCTIVE RATE, γ is the INFECTION TRANSMISSION PARAMETER, and T is the total population.

heredity The passing on of biological (genetic) characteristics from one generation to the next, which is a consequence of the transmission of specific genes from either of the biological parents, each of whom contributes half the genes to the offspring.

heritability, heritable Terms used rather loosely to describe conditions such as undue susceptibility to infections with a strong familial tendency, without specifying whether they are inherited as genetic traits or the consequence of familial, behavioral, or environmental factors.

herniated intervertebral disk A condition usually caused by heavy lifting in ergonomically inefficient ways, in which a portion of the shock-absorbent nucleus pulposus that separates each vertebra from those adjoining it is extruded into the spinal canal, where it can exert pressure on the spinal cord or nerve roots, causing persistent pain, e.g., sciatica, and sometimes paraesthesia and/or muscle weakness. It is often occupational in origin.

heroin Diamorphine. A highly addictive derivative of OPIUM, one of the principal illicit drugs, and the basis of a lucrative drug-trafficking underground industry controlled by criminal gangs who obtain it from poppy plants grown by peasant farmers in Afghanistan and Myanmar (Burma), and transport it from there to the industrial nations in Europe and North America, where they market it. Heroin addiction is a serious public health problem, aggravated in many nations by the emphasis on punitive, rather than preventive and therapeutic approaches, to its control. Heroin is available in the United Kingdom and most of the European Union for palliative care of patients with severe pain but is not legally available in the United States or Canada.

herpes A group of conditions due to related viruses that cause irritating, usually acutely painful skin lesions. The name is derived from a Greek word meaning "creep" and refers to the tendency of the skin eruption to creep along the skin surface.

herpes genitalis See GENITAL HERPES.

herpes simplex This is caused by the herpes simplex virus type II. It is usually a perioral infection, and tends to recur, often associated with an acute upper respiratory infection, such as a common cold.

herpes viruses A class of viruses that can cause diseases, including genital herpes, herpes simplex, and herpes zoster. The EPSTEIN-BARR VIRUS that causes infectious mononucleosis and Burkitt's lymphoma and the CYTOMEGALOVIRUS also belong in this family of viruses.

herpes zoster Syn: shingles. A skin eruption that is manifest as painful inflammatory or vesicular lesions in a particular dermatome. Herpes zoster often occurs in older people or those with impaired immunity, due to reactivation of varicella virus that has been dormant since childhood infection. The neuralgic pain and related sleeplessness and insomnia can persist for many months, even years. See also GENITAL HERPES.

heterogamy Sexual reproduction in species with female and male zygotes (HETEROZYGOTES).

heterosexual transmission Transmission of infection by means of heterosexual intercourse.

heterozygote An individual (or organism) with two different alleles at the same locus on each chromosome; inheritance of the trait associated with that locus is determined by the dominant allele.

heuristic method A method of reasoning that relies on a mixture of empirical observation and theory, often unproven, to arrive at a solution that may or may not be correct and cannot be proved to be either correct or false.

hierarchy Arrangement of entities in an ordered sequence from low to high, least to greatest, smallest to largest, etc.

hierarchy of evidence The CANADIAN TASK FORCE ON THE PERIODIC HEALTH EXAMINATION (1994) reviewed published work on the efficacy of preventive methods, and devised a method to assess the quality of the evidence, as follows:

I. (Best quality) Evidence from at least one properly designed RANDOMIZED CONTROLLED TRIAL (RCT).
II-1. Evidence from well-designed controlled trials without randomization.
II-2. Evidence from well-designed COHORT or CASE CONTROL STUDIES, preferably from more than one center or research group.
II-3. Evidence from multiple time series with or without the intervention; dramatic results from un-

controlled experiments, e.g., first use of rabies vaccine in 1885, penicillin in the 1940s.
III. Opinions of respected authorities based on clinical experience, descriptive studies, reports of expert committees, consensus conferences, etc.

It is not always possible to achieve complete scientific rigor; partly because sometimes randomized trials may not be feasible or may be unethical.

hierarchy of needs The theory of self-actualization of the American psychologist Abraham Maslow (1908–1970), who conceptualized an ascending hierarchy of needs, beginning with the basic requirements for self-preservation (food, shelter, clothing); safety and security; order, structure, and a degree of certainty or predictability about life; then, important but somewhat less essential needs, the need to belong to a family or other stable unit; the need to be loved and to love; the need for self-esteem; and finally the need for self-actualization, i.e., to become what one wants to become in life.

high altitude disease Syn: altitude sickness and MOUNTAIN SICKNESS. Acute high altitude disease affects people who are physiologically adapted to life at sea level or relatively low altitude when they ascend rapidly to altitudes above 2,500 to 3,000 meters, caused by hypoxia and electrolyte imbalance, with various combinations of cardiovascular, respiratory, neurological, gastrointestinal, and musculoskeletal symptoms, potentially fatal in persons with impaired respiratory or cardiovascular function, but usually subsiding within a few days as the body adapts to reduced atmospheric pressure and oxygen concentration.

high blood pressure See HYPERTENSION.

high density lipoprotein (HDL) High density lipoprotein cholesterol, which transports cholesterol to the liver for excretion in bile and is generally protective against the formation and progression of vascular atherosclerosis. For males, the optimal HDL concentration is 60 mg/dL, and a level lower than 40 mg/dL carries an increased risk of coronary heart disease. Contrast LDL cholesterol, which enhances the risk of atherosclerosis. See LOW DENSITY LIPOPROTEIN (LDL).

high risk group A defined population subgroup that research has shown to be more likely than others to suffer from a condition of interest. For instance, many epidemiological studies have shown that cigarette smokers have higher incidence and death rates from lung cancer than do nonsmokers; smokers therefore are a high risk group for lung cancer. The term should be used with tact and care to avoid stigmatizing or "blaming the victim."

Hill's criteria The British medical statistician Austin Bradford Hill (1897–1991) identified eight criteria that can be used to help distinguish statistically significant associations that indicate causation, i.e., an association in which a cause produces an effect. The criteria are as follows:

1. Strength of the association, i.e., the size of the risk, as measured by appropriate statistical tests.
2. Consistency, i.e., the association is replicated in different settings and using different methods.
3. Specificity, i.e., a single specific putative cause produces a specific effect.
4. Dose-response relationship, i.e., an increasing amount of exposure to an agent, either in amount or duration, increases the risk of disease.
5. Temporal relationship, i.e., exposure to the cause always precedes the effect.
6. Biological plausibility, i.e., the relationship accords with currently accepted understanding of pathophysiological processes.
7. Coherence, i.e., the association is compatible with current understanding of theory and practice.
8. Experiment, i.e., the condition can be prevented or relieved by the regimen of an experiment, e.g., a randomized controlled trial.

Hippocrates of Cos (c. 460–377 BCE) The "father of medicine," who founded a school of medicine near Epidaurus in Greece. He and his followers made many important observations and left a record of clinical and epidemiological observations, including *Epidemics*, which is a set of detailed clinical observations on conditions that are mostly communicable, and *Airs, Waters, Places*, which was the first systematic treatise on environmental health. The wisdom demonstrated in this work justifies describing Hippocrates also as the "father of public health."

Hippocratic oath A code of conduct formulated at the school of medicine under the leadership of HIPPOCRATES OF COS (c. 460–377 BCE). The Hippocratic oath probably evolved from simpler affirmations of allegiance taken by priest-physicians at the end of their period of apprenticeship but has survived in much modified form for almost 2,500 years because it set out basic rules of conduct for the physician-patient relationship, dealing with issues such as permitted and proscribed aspects of this relationship, safeguarding confidentiality, and the duty to teach new recruits to the profession of medicine. Throughout the 20th century the oath was much modified, and also was adopted in suitably modified form by other health professions, such as nursing. Other health disciplines such as epidemiology have developed CODES or GUIDELINES for ethical conduct.

Hiroshima The industrial port city in Japan that on August 6, 1945, was the first human settlement to experience the detonation of an atomic bomb. The bomb caused the immediate death of about 80,000 people, death within a few weeks of burns and acute radiation sickness of 10,000, and death of radiation-related cancer and other after-effects of another 60,000 by the end of 1945. Deaths of leukemia and bone, brain, and other cancers raised the total deaths to more than 200,000 in the following 2 decades. See http://www.csi.ad.jp/abomb/.

Hispanic A word used to describe persons resident in the United States whose ethnic origin includes Spanish-speaking (or Portuguese-speaking) ancestors who entered the United States from Latin America.

histamine A biologically active amine secreted by neural, endocrine, and mast cells, released in the body by metabolism and/or allergic reaction. It causes smooth muscle contraction, including contraction of bronchiolar muscles and mucous secretion, causing headaches, asthma, hay fever, and urticaria, and in extreme cases, bronchospasm associated with anaphylactic shock. See also ANTIHISTAMINES.

histogram A chart (graph) commonly used to show visually the distribution of a variable, such as hemoglobin or blood pressure, in a population. The area under the curve is proportional to the numbers, and the base is proportional to the size of the group.

histoplasmosis A systemic mycotic infection usually acquired from soil containing the spores of the causal organism, *Histoplasma capsulatum* or *H. duboisii*.

historical cohort study A COHORT STUDY that makes use of pre-existing health-related facts about members of a defined population who can be classified into exposed and unexposed groups on the basis of information that may have been collected years or even decades earlier. Often such a study requires use of a RECORD LINKAGE system to ensure that the past and present sets of health data refer to the same person.

historical demography Data on population numbers, age distribution, age at marriage, birth intervals, family and household composition, birth and death rates, and age-specific death rates reveal much about the structure and to some extent the function of societies under environmental and other stress, e.g., from famine, war, migrations in past times. Notable studies in this field have been done in the British Isles, Sweden, and Quebec, among other places.

historical epidemiology The study of past patterns of occurrence rates of infectious and chronic diseases, changing diagnostic and treatment methods, considered in the context of contemporary understanding of the nature and causes of diseases and efficacy or otherwise of prevailing preventive and therapeutic methods. Much can be learned from historical comparative studies.

HIV See HUMAN IMMUNODEFICIENCY VIRUS, the retrovirus that causes AIDS.

HIV/AIDS The acronym for HUMAN IMMUNODEFICIENCY VIRUS infection with sufficient degree of clinical damage to cause AIDS, the ACQUIRED IMMUNODEFICIENCY SYNDROME.

HIV tests The tests used to detect the presence of HIV are based on immunological methods. The initial screening test is the enzyme-linked immunosorbent assay (ELISA), which is highly sensitive and specific but requires Western blot or indirect fluorescent assay for confirmation.

HIV transmission The HUMAN IMMUNODEFICIENCY VIRUS (HIV) is a delicate organism that does not long survive outside the body. Transmission of HIV implies contact between mucosae or abraded skin and infected blood or other body fluids, including semen, breast milk, vaginal secretions, saliva (a small but real risk), and urine. Transmission may occur during unprotected heterosexual or homosexual intercourse, during vaginal delivery or breast feeding, and by way of infected blood or other body fluids, semen, saliva, vaginal secretions, or in infected body tissue, e.g., organs or tissue that is transplanted from an infected to an uninfected person. Contaminated blood is an important transmission vehicle among illicit intravenous drug users. The frequently long incubation period between primary infection with HIV and the onset of clinically diagnosable AIDS means that the virus is often transmitted from an infected, but symptom free, person to others, whether by the sexual route, needle sharing by INTRAVENOUS DRUG USERS, during childbirth, breast feeding, or by some other means. This accounts for much of the explosive growth of the worldwide pandemic of HIV/AIDS since the disease first emerged in 1981. There have been several tragic surges in the epidemic, caused by use of HIV-contaminated blood and blood products in the early 1980s. See http://www.unaids.org for details.

HLA See HUMAN LEUKOCYTE ANTIGEN.

HMO See HEALTH MAINTENANCE ORGANIZATION.

Hodgkin disease A malignant disease of the lymphatic system, i.e., a lymphoma, identified by and named for the British physician Thomas Hodgkin (1798–1866). Definitive diagnosis depends on the presence of characteristic malignant cells. A causal infectious pathogen has been suspected but never demonstrated, despite much epidemiological study.

hold and treat ordinance A common municipal ordinance that applies the POLICE POWER of public health to restrain and treat persons with contagious diseases, by force if necessary.

holism A word coined by the South African statesman J. C. Smuts (1870–1950) to describe the notion that fragments tend to coalesce to form a whole. Smuts applied it to political fragments, but the concept has broadened to encompass all fragments that tend to unite into larger entities. The concept of holism further implies that the properties of the parts are influenced or determined by their relationship to the whole entity. This concept is important in holistic medicine.

holistic health An imprecise concept from alternative medicine purporting to cover the totality of physical and mental well-being in the context of prior life experiences, present way of life including diet, exercise, relationships with others, and future aspirations. Persons in good holistic health are supposedly fit and happy, relate well to others in and outside their family, perform work effectively and efficiently, enjoy recreational pursuits, are in control of their lives, and have planned for and are optimistic about the future. The ideal is admirable, but the concept lacks realistic solutions to the occurrence of diseases that might best be dealt with by early detection. See also WELLNESS.

holistic medicine Usually a synonym for varieties of alternative medicine, sometimes purporting to produce HOLISTIC HEALTH. It often mixes elements of Ayurvedic, herbal, and other medical systems. It became popular in the late 20th century among people who followed unconventional ways of living.

Holmes, Oliver Wendell (1809–1894) American physician, poet, and philosopher who crusaded against PUERPERAL SEPSIS. Like IGNAZ PHILIPP SEMMELWEIS, he discovered that puerperal infection was prevented when the obstetric attendant observed strict personal hygiene, washing and scrubbing hands and wearing clean clothes, to minimize the risk of contaminating the raw uterine tissue. He published his findings in the *New England Quarterly Journal of Medicine and Surgery* in 1842–43, but, like Semmelweis, he was greeted with hostility from his colleagues.

holoendemic A term applied to an infectious disease that is recurrent or becomes chronic, for which a region's high prevalence of infection begins in infancy or early childhood, persists throughout childhood, and thereafter reaches a stage of equilibrium, with adults less often than children showing signs of infection. The term is most often applied to malaria endemicity.

home birth Conduct of labor and childbirth at home, supervised by a MIDWIFE, or in the United Kingdom and the Netherlands until the recent past, a family doctor. Provided dangerous complications such as prolapsed umbilical cord or severe postpartum hemorrhage do not occur, home birth is usually safe, exposes the mother and neonate to less risk of cross-infection than a hospital or birthing center, and is said to be a valuable bonding experience for other family members in attendance. Dangerous obstetric complications can occur, even in apparently low-risk women, so home birthing is safest when well-equipped and staffed obstetric services are readily available and accessible.

home care Syn: domiciliary care. The medical, nursing, or other health-related care of ill, infirm, or disabled persons in their own homes as contrasted with care that is provided in an institutional setting, such as a hospital or nursing home. For conditions that can be as effectively managed in the home, this is less costly than institutional care, as well as emotionally less disruptive for the sick persons and their families.

home care services A wide range of medical care and social services that are available in many communities to meet the needs of infirm, elderly, chronically disabled, and housebound persons, including, for instance, MEALS ON WHEELS, home visits by public health nurses to mothers and newborn infants, domiciliary midwifery in some communities, homemaker services, etc.

home health care programs A generic term for domiciliary medical and nursing care that is provided as part of a formal program, e.g., a feature of some prepaid health care plans. Home nursing services are the most widely used aspects of most such health care programs.

homelessness A perennial problem in an unequal society in which people unable to pay for accommodation, or who lack the mental, emotional, or financial resources to maintain a dwelling to provide them with shelter, are forced to rely on charitable hostels for shelter or live on the street. Homelessness can result from poverty and chronic unemployment or from the inability to maintain a

dwelling because of mental or emotional illness, alcohol or substance misuse, or other chronic disability. Its prevalence in affluent societies such as those in the United States and Europe is partly a consequence of the DEINSTITUTIONALIZATION of psychiatric services and demolition of institutions that formerly provided long-term custodial care, and reveals the indifference of the general public and its elected representatives, who may blame the victims rather than try to help them. See also ASYLUM.

homeopathy A system of medical care founded by the German physician Christian Friedrich Samuel Hahnemann (1755–1843) in Leipzig in 1796, based on the theory of "like curing like," i.e., giving sick people a minute dose of a drug that produces symptoms resembling those of the disease they appear to have. Thus, if the disease causes vomiting and diarrhea, it is treated with a high dilution of a drug that causes vomiting and diarrhea. This might "work" sometimes with acute gastrointestinal infections that respond to emetics and/or purgatives but is less likely to be successful in treating conditions such as congestive heart failure and chronic arthritis. Despite this, the doctrine of homeopathy has found favor with enough people to remain an acceptable treatment regimen, even in these days of evidence-based medicine. Among its devotees are some members of the British royal family, an earlier member of which founded the Royal Homeopathic Hospital in London. One notable feature of modern homeopathic medicine is its reliance on extremely dilute solutions of the active ingredient. This suggests that when the treatment works, it does so either in response to as-yet-undiscovered physiological processes or by the power of suggestion. The desensitizing methods used by allergists resemble aspects of homeopathy in that they involve minuscule and slowly increasing doses of allergens.

homeostasis The physiological processes that by way of autoregulatory feedback loops and other mechanisms maintain the internal environment of the body in balance at near-constant (normal) levels of temperature, blood chemistry, etc., regardless of external environmental conditions, and are generally essential to the maintenance of efficient bodily function.

homicide Deliberate killing of another human, an act of interpersonal violence that is common enough in some socially distinct sections of society to be recognized as a public health problem. INFANTICIDE, practiced since antiquity in some cultures as a form of population limitation, is one form. Homicide is a prominent public health problem among young urban males in deprived communities such as the slum GHETTOES of some cities in the United States and is often conducted by paramilitary death squads in many protracted low-intensity violent armed conflicts in low-income countries in Africa, Latin America, and elsewhere.

homograft A tissue or organ graft that is immunologically identical to that of the host. Most often this is a graft of skin from elsewhere on the body to close a deficiency caused by injury, loss of skin due to burns, etc.

homophobia Pathological antipathy and hostility toward HOMOSEXUALS, manifested by hate, violence, discrimination, and denial of human rights.

homosexual Syn: GAY (male), lesbian (female). A person who is sexually attracted to members of the same sex, rather than to persons of the opposite sex. Homosexuality appears to be inherent, rather than an acquired behavioral characteristic, but its underlying cause is not known. Genetic factors, birth order, family dynamics, and neurophysiological mechanisms have been postulated, but there is no persuasive evidence for any of these. Estimates of its prevalence range from less than 1% to 5% or more of the population. In single-sex institutions such as prisons and armed forces, homosexual relationships arise among persons normally heterosexual, then disappear on resumption of life in a community with two sexes. Acceptance, i.e., tolerance, of homosexuals has varied considerably throughout history, related to the culture, religious beliefs, and the toleration or condemnation of alternative ways of living and behaving. In some Western democratic nations, there is increasing tolerance for homosexuality and other alternative lifestyles, which became more visible than previously in the late 20th century, coinciding with the HIV/AIDS epidemic, which took a heavy toll and drew attention to the high proportion of gay men who were distinguished creative and performing artists, but considerable bigotry, intolerance, persecution, violence, and hate crimes against homosexuals still occur. The doctrines of the Catholic and some other churches, much of Islam, and some other religions may seem to encourage intolerance and contribute to discrimination and violence against homosexuals.

homozygote A cell or individual possessing identical alleles at the same locus or loci on chromosomes, a condition described as homozygous.

hookworm A nematode parasitic roundworm, *Ankylostoma duodenale* or *Necator americanus*, that survives by attaching to the epithelial lining of the intestine, usually in the duodenum or small intestine, and feeding on the host's blood, often causing severe anemia.

horizontal transmission In contrast to vertical or mother-to-child transmission, horizontal transmission occurs when infectious pathogens, e.g., HIV, pass from one person to another in the same generation, generally by heterosexual or homosexual intercourse.

hormesis A beneficial adaptive reaction to repeated low doses of an agent that has harmful effects at higher doses. The reaction was empirically applied as long ago as in Renaissance Italy by the infamous noblewoman Lucrezia Borgia, who took small incremental doses of poisons to acquire some resistance to their effects before using these poisons on political victims. In the 1960s it was studied quantitatively in reactions to low doses of ionizing radiation and then found to apply quantitatively to some poisonous chemical substances. The effects may include enhanced health, accelerated growth, and more efficient reproduction.

hormonally active substances See ENDOCRINE DISRUPTORS.

hormone A chemical compound, usually complex in structure, that is produced by an endocrine gland and secreted into the bloodstream, where it acts on specific organs, tissues, or cells as a regulator, or promoter, of an essential bodily function. Steroid hormones are lipid molecules that enter the target cells. They include the sex hormones. Other hormones are amino acids or chains of amino acids. An example of these is INSULIN, which can be synthesized. Most steroid hormones are extracted from glands that secrete them or from genetically modified cultures.

hormone replacement therapy (HRT) The use of female sex hormones, generally estrogen and progesterone preparations, to relieve menopausal symptoms, such as hot flashes or flushes, vaginal dysplasia, and loss of or decline of libido, and to retard the onset of chronic conditions, such as heart disease. Although many women and their physicians are convinced that HRT is an effective therapeutic method, the evidence from randomized controlled trials is not persuasive. The risks include a small increase in incidence of cancer of the uterus and some cardiovascular diseases. For details, see http://www.nlm.nih.gov/medlineplus/hormonereplacementtherapy.html.

hospice An institution or other setting that provides care for the dying or incurably ill. This usually consists of palliative care comprising physical, psychological, social, emotional, spiritual, and sometimes financial and legal support. Hospice care existed in medieval Europe in convents and monasteries and was revived in modern times, initially in Britain under the leadership of the British nurse, social worker, and physician Cicely Saunders (1918–2005).

hospital An institution with facilities for diagnosis and treatment of medical, surgical, and/or obstetric conditions, with an organized professional staff of physicians, nurses, other health professionals, and support personnel, offering inpatient care and often ambulatory care, too.

hospital-acquired infection See NOSOCOMIAL INFECTION.

hospital catchment area, hospital district The region, which may or may not be clearly defined geographically, from which patients attending a hospital are drawn.

hospital discharge abstract system A system for collecting, compiling, and analyzing summary statistical data from hospital records in order to create quantitative profiles of hospital activities, including length of hospital stay in relation to diagnostic categories, case fatality rates, occurrence of complications, NOSOCOMIAL INFECTIONS, etc. Pioneers in the collection and statistical analysis of hospital records include the British nurse Florence Nightingale (1820–1910) and the Hungarian obstetrician IGNAZ PHILIPP SEMMELWEIS (1818–1865). Widely used national systems include the Hospital Inpatient Enquiry (HIPE) in the United Kingdom and the Commission on Professional and Hospital Activities (CPHA) in the United States. Their compiled statistics have many uses, including preparation of CLINICAL PRACTICE GUIDELINES and evaluation of the effectiveness and efficiency of hospital care.

hospital discharge data Summary statistics about all patients separated from hospital by being discharged alive or dead, consisting of personal identifying information, clinical data (diagnosis, treatment, outcome, etc.), length of hospital stay, complications, etc., all of which can be analyzed as part of the process of evaluating hospital care.

hospital visit An administrative and financial term for a billable encounter between a physician and a patient that takes place in a hospital, rather than in a physician's office. It is not usual practice for a physician to charge for each encounter when a patient is receiving ongoing care, but if a patient is seen by another physician in consultation during a hospital stay, that physician may count this as a hospital visit and bill accordingly.

hospital waste Material that may be infected or contain toxic substances and sharp objects that are discarded after use by personnel in hospitals. It includes used wound dressings, human blood, organs and tissue derived from operative procedures, used hypodermic needles and other sharp or cutting objects (sharps), and bloodstained operating room gowns and drapes. Special disposal facilities must be provided for hospital waste. See also HAZARDOUS WASTE DISPOSAL.

host A person, animal, or population group that harbors a disease agent, such as a pathogenic microorganism. In many diseases, the host is the human who harbors the disease agent, but some disease agents have complex life cycles involving an INTERMEDIATE HOST as well as the definitive host in which the disease is manifest.

hotline A telephone number that is accessible for emergencies or for standard information, e.g., about specific health problems, such as sexually transmitted diseases, suicidal thoughts, unwanted pregnancies. It is often a toll-free number. Examples include 911 (or 999) for police, fire, or ambulance and many SAMARITAN SERVICES and the like. See also HELP LINE.

hot spot A slang or jargon term for a NIDUS of infection, lawless or violent community, section of an industrial plant where a hazardous process is conducted, a place from which hazardous material can escape into the environment, or any other troublesome location.

house dust The accumulated detritus of dust mites, desquamated skin and other dead organic matter, animal fur, abraded fragments of carpets and curtains, much of which is allergenic and capable of provoking asthma and other allergic reactions in susceptible persons.

housefly The most common domestic pest fly, *Musca domestica*, which is almost ubiquitous. It is a source of food-borne infection when it feeds on fecal material or other sources of contamination and then carries pathogens to food that has been left where flies can feed on it. Flies are not true disease vectors but passive carriers of many varieties of pathogens.

household A collective term for all the person(s) who occupy a dwelling, usually collaborate in running it, most frequently, although not necessarily, a family unit.

household survey A survey, usually conducted by face-to-face interviews or sometimes by means of self-completed questionnaires, in which households, generally selected by a process of random allocation, are the unit of investigation.

household waste In affluent societies, each household generates a prodigious quantity of waste, comprising meat, vegetable, and other food waste; packaging material; bottles; plastic containers; other plastic wrapping; metal containers, etc. In rural regions, many farms and homes have their own incinerators. Urban areas rely on GARBAGE DISPOSAL METHODS. Safe and effective disposal of household waste requires separation into biodegradable waste, which can be composted, other recyclable waste, and miscellaneous material that requires further treatment.

housing conditions Loosely, these are the specific physical features of dwelling places. More precisely, a set of requirements such as those specified in MODEL STANDARDS that must be met before dwellings are declared fit for occupancy. These include explicit requirements for living space; cooking, washing, and toilet facilities; ventilation, etc.

housing inspector A health inspector (sanitarian) who is responsible for assessing fitness of dwellings for human occupancy.

housing laws A range of national laws and local ordinances intended mainly to protect the lives and health of the occupants of dwellings, especially communal dwellings such as tenements and lodging houses, that set out specific requirements on fire safety, ventilation, sanitation, kitchen hygiene, bedroom occupancy, etc. The details vary according to the jurisdiction.

human development The process by which communities, populations, nations, and persons achieve their optimum level of health, educational attainment, housing, and economic conditions. Human development includes physical, mental, social, emotional, and cultural components.

Human Development Index A composite index used by the World Bank and the United Nations Development Programme (UNDP) that combines indicators on three dimensions: longevity (life expectancy); knowledge (adult literacy rate and average years of schooling); and income (real gross domestic product per capita in purchasing power). The validity of this index is difficult to assess because it attempts to combine three sets of variables in a unidimensional scale, but it may be useful in providing an annual comparison of the health and economic status of regions and nations that can generate discussions about policies affecting health and the economy. The Index is discussed in the 2003 UNDP annual report at http:// hdr.undp.org/reports/ global/2003/.

human ecology The scientific study of the interrelationships among individuals, families, and communities of people, and other living things that share the same living space or environment that takes into account all the interactive ways that relationships among them and their living and nonliving environment, including physical and social living conditions, can affect their well-being and their health. See also ECOLOGY.

human engineering Deliberate, planned, systematic intervention or manipulation of the way people live and interact, e.g., in a workplace, such as an office, aimed at enhancing efficiency.

human experimentation A research study of humans in which the investigator deliberately modifies conditions or circumstances, e.g., by administering an experimental preventive or therapeutic regimen, in order to find out what happens. There are clearly defined ethical principles and rules that must be observed when human experiments are done. The most important rule, which is inviolable and enshrined in the NUREMBERG CODE, is that the INFORMED CONSENT of the subjects (participants) in the research study is absolutely mandatory. Therefore, research involving human subjects must undergo ethical review, by an INSTITUTIONAL REVIEW BOARD (IRB) in the United States and similar bodies in other countries.

human genome epidemiology (HuGE) The intersection of genetics and epidemiology in studies of the distribution and genomic determinants of important diseases, e.g., diabetes and other disorders of metabolism, cancer, cardiovascular disease, osteoporosis, and schizophrenia. The aim is to identify genetic factors that could be manipulated by interventions to prevent or retard progress of conditions attributable to aberrations of the genome. It is the systematic application of epidemiologic methods and approaches to the human genome to assess the impact of human genetic variation on health and disease. The applications include (1) gene discovery; (2) population risk characterization; (3) evaluation of genetic information for diagnosis and prevention (including genetic tests and family history information, both for clinical use and for population screening) and for genome-based therapies. The Human Genome Epidemiology Network (HuGEnet) is a worldwide collaboration that is assessing how genomic variation affects population health. See http://www.cdc .gov/genomics/hugenet/default.htm.

Human Genome Project An ambitious multinational collaborative research endeavor that set out in 1987 to map the entire human genome, i.e., to map all the chromosomes, sequence all the genes, and identify as far as feasible the genes responsible for resistance and susceptibility to diseases such as cancer (as well as many genetically determined diseases, such as cystic fibrosis, Huntington's disease, etc.). The Human Genome Project has had some spectacular successes, and by 2002, two independently working groups of investigators claimed to have sequenced the entire human genome. Many clinicians express skepticism about claims that sequencing the human genome will be a panacea and will make much else in therapeutics irrelevant.

human growth hormone A polypeptide secreted by the anterior lobe of the pituitary gland that controls cell and tissue growth and development. It can be used to promote growth in adolescents who are late passing developmental milestones and has been misused as an illicit performance-enhancing substance by some athletes.

human immunodeficiency virus (HIV) The retrovirus that causes ACQUIRED IMMUNODEFICIENCY SYNDROME (AIDS). It was discovered in 1983 by the French microbiologist Luc Montagnier (b. 1932) and colleagues, after intensive international studies following the first reports of acquired immunodeficiency syndrome in 1981. It is a small, spherical RNA virus that reproduces by invading cells such as lymphocytes that manufacture antibodies and causing them instead to make copies of the virus. There are two serologically distinct types: HIV 1, discovered in 1981, and HIV-2, discovered in 1986. They are geographically circumscribed, HIV-2 predominating in western Africa, HIV-1 elsewhere in the world. The main route of transmission is by sexual contact, but any contact of blood or body fluids between an infected and a susceptible host can lead to infection. It is thought that the virus originated in Africa, perhaps many decades ago, and may have jumped species from monkeys to humans when monkey blood was used ritually or in traditional medicine in Africa. The HIV epidemic spread explosively around the world. The initial epidemic in the United States and Europe occurred mainly among promiscuous homosexual males but was soon followed by blood-borne epidemics among injection drug users who shared needles, and, in an iatrogenic tragedy, in patients such as hemophiliacs, surgical cases, and lymphoma patients who were infected by contaminated blood transfusions. In Africa, Asia, and Central and South America, the main route of transmission is by sexual intercourse. As of 2005, more than 40 million cases and 12 million deaths had occurred as a result of HIV infection.

human leukocyte antigen (HLA) A genetically determined protein that is unique to each individual, inherited according to Mendel's laws. Many diseases are associated with HLA configuration, e.g., cystic fibrosis, celiac disease, ankylosing spondylitis, juvenile rheumatoid arthritis, and insulin-dependent diabetes, and others display gene-environment interaction, e.g., psoriasis, lupus erythematosus, hyperthyroidism, arthritis associated with salmonella infection, etc. HLA testing is used to determine tissue compatibility, i.e., to distinguish self and nonself, to predict whether transplanted tissues and organs will be accepted or rejected by the host.

human papilloma virus (HPV) There are more than 100 strains of HPV. Many are harmless, some cause simple warts. Some cause genital warts, the most common SEXUALLY TRANSMITTED DISEASE. HPV is implicated in causing cancer of the cervix, as well as causing the common wart. See also PAP TEST. See http://www.niaid.nih.gov/factsheets/stdhpv.htm for current information.

human resources development A set of educational and training policies supported by the World Health Organization and other UN agencies intended to maximize the intellectual potential of developing nations. In the health sector, the emphasis has been on professional and technical education and training for primary health care.

human rights A set of moral principles governing human conduct toward other humans, enunciated in the United Nations UNIVERSAL DECLARATION OF HUMAN RIGHTS, the DECLARATION OF THE RIGHTS OF THE CHILD, and other internationally recognized and ratified statements. These principles have evolved from the cultural values of civilized societies and the ideas of philosophers of earlier civilizations and generations. Basic human rights include freedom; equality; autonomy; access to the necessities of life, i.e., water and food, clothing, and shelter; personal security; protection of the law; absence of discrimination; recognition as a person; and freedom from arbitrary arrest, imprisonment, torture, or cruel or inhuman punishment. Health is recognized as a human right in the ALMA-ATA DECLARATION, and by philosophers of public health, but ways to implement this right remain elusive. It is sometimes overlooked that possession of rights implies a duty to uphold the rights, and it is seldom clear who has this duty. The United Nations declarations on rights, e.g., the Declaration of the Rights of the Child, have been signed and ratified by all the nations of the world except Somalia and the United States. See also UNITED NATIONS HIGH COMMISSIONER FOR HUMAN RIGHTS.

human services Syn: people services. A jargon term for publicly supported social services and assistance ("welfare") that came into vogue in the decades of tax cuts and downsizing in the late 20th century, when publicly administered services in many countries were drastically reduced in the mistaken belief that population health would not be jeopardized. As a result, waiting lists have sometimes grown very long, and urgent medical needs may remain unmet.

human settlements A general term for any established collection of dwellings in which people live. The term applies across the whole range from temporary shelters of nomadic hunters to high-density, high-rise apartments in a modern city, but is used mainly in relation to the latter.

human variability A commonplace observation that hardly needs to be mentioned: each human being is immunologically unique, but many biological characteristics, such as hemoglobin, blood pressure, vital capacity, height, and weight, are normally or log-normally distributed. Other aspects of human diversity linked to emotional and social factors are also important in planning health care and educational and social programs.

humidex A numerical score that adjusts ambient temperature to allow for atmospheric humidity. Thus, a summer heat temperature of 30°C with a humidity level of 80% gives a humidex reading of 36°C, which is uncomfortably hot for most people. A high humidex reading and a high pollution level are among the undesirable qualities of summer living in many cities.

humidifier A device to increase atmospheric humidity in an indoor environment, used mainly in cold climates when atmospheric moisture levels are very low. It works by blowing air through a set of filters moistened with water that is continuously replenished from a reservoir.

humidity The atmospheric concentration of water vapor. Absolute humidity is the water vapor expressed as kilograms per cubic meter of air. Relative humidity is the proportion of atmospheric moisture in relation to what there would be if the air were completely saturated with water vapor.

humus Decomposed organic matter in soil, generally aerobic and devoid of structure reminiscent of its biological origins but nutritionally rich in nitrogen and phosphates, and a valuable regenerator of soil in which crops are to be planted. Humus sometimes contains pathogenic organisms or spores, e.g., those of tetanus, botulism, actinomycosis, etc.

hunger The desire for food that can be a pleasant sensation under normal circumstances but can be very unpleasant, even painful, if not satisfied in a timely manner. Hunger is a dominant feeling, both physiological and emotional, in STARVATION and FAMINE.

hunger strike A form of nonviolent protest against conditions, used for instance by political prisoners who refuse to eat in order to publicize the cause they believe in, using what they may perceive to be the only means available to them. Prolonged hunger strikes can be fatal, so prison authorities sometimes attempt to avert the risk of death by forced feeding of hunger strikers.

hunter-gatherers Human groups, usually nomadic or seminomadic, who subsist by hunting, trapping animals, and gathering fruits, berries, roots, etc., rather than through agriculture and animal husbandry. Until the development of agriculture and fixed human settlements about 10,000 BCE, all humans were hunter-gatherers. Nomadic hunter-gatherers are less vulnerable to infections transmitted via the air or fecal-oral route than are people in fixed settlements. The study of PALEOPATHOLOGY suggests that nutritional deficiency was rare before the introduction of agriculture, after which dental health began to deteriorate, bone growth was sometimes retarded, and tuberculosis and other diseases became evident in the archeological record.

Huntington disease A fatal progressive degenerative neurological and mental disease described by the American physician George Huntington (1850–1916) with onset in early or middle adult life that is inherited as a single-gene autosomal dominant characteristic with complete penetrance. A screening test for the presence of the gene is available and raises troubling ethical questions for members of affected families, and often for their attending physicians, because a positive test is a death sentence, and some people prefer not to know their fate. More information is available at http://www.ninds.nih.gov/disorders/hunt ington/huntington/htm.

hurricane Syn: typhoon, cyclone. A severe weather event in which warm air over an ocean develops a rapid circular movement, with very high wind velocity (to 250 km/hour or more), becomes laden with water vapor, and creates storm surges. The combination of high winds, very heavy precipitation, and storm surges causes flooding that has a destructive effect on human settlements, especially on low-lying land at or close to sea level. For instance, hurricane Katrina in August 2005 flooded the city of New Orleans and caused approximately 1,000 deaths and billions of dollars in damage in the region, including the destruction of public health and other infrastructure.

hybrid The offspring of genetically dissimilar parents.

hydatid disease The condition caused by hydatid cysts that form in the lungs, liver, brain, and elsewhere when larvae of the canine tapeworm *Echinococcus granulosa* lodge in these organs. This tapeworm passes the adult phase of its life cycle in the intestine of canines (dogs, wolves, foxes), which ingest it when they eat the flesh of animals in which the larval and cyst stages are passed. The intermediate hosts are herbivores that ingest the eggs deposited on grass in canine feces. Humans are accidental intermediate hosts who ingest eggs deposited in dogs' feces, so hydatid disease occurs predominantly among shepherds, farmers, etc., who work with dogs that herd their sheep. Hydatid disease was formerly common in countries where sheep-herding is a large part of rural economy, e.g., Iceland, central Asia, Australia, and New Zealand. Educational campaigns aimed at breaking the life cycle by ensuring that dogs do not eat raw offal and improving the personal hygiene of farmers, etc., has led to eradication from Iceland, and near-eradication in Cyprus, Australia, and New Zealand.

hydrocarbons A large group of chemical compounds containing hydrogen and carbon atoms in many possible combinations. When hydrogen and carbon combine alone, they form coal, methane, natural gas, petroleum, or a series of aliphatic or aromatic compounds. When hydrogen and carbon combine with other elements, such as chlorine, nitrogen, phosphorus, etc., the range of compounds increases enormously, and include proteins, long-chain fatty acids, and innumerable industrial chemicals.

hydrochloric acid (HCl) A colorless liquid solution of hydrogen chloride that is powerfully acidic, capable of dissolving many metals, and releasing hydrogen while doing so. It occurs in very dilute solution in gastric digestive juices, where it contributes to digestion of dietary proteins.

hydroelectric power generation A form of renewable energy production, considered "clean" because it does not produce harmful emissions, as do carbon-based fuels. Hydroelectric dams may drown fertile river valleys that were previously the habitat for large populations that have been displaced to environments less capable of sustaining them, although they also provide water storage for irrigation of previously parched land. In tropical and subtropical regions, dams and irrigation schemes may extend the range and habitat for disease vectors, including mosquitoes and snails. The positive and negative side effects of hydroelectric dams are more often considered in long-range planning now than they were in the early 20th century.

hydrogenation The chemical process of hydrogen bonding with other elements or molecules that occurs in, or as a by-product of, many industrial processes. The simple hydrogen compounds of industrial and medical importance include hydrogen peroxide, hydrogen sulfide, hydrogen cyanide, and the halides (chlorides, bromides, iodides, fluorides).

hydrogen peroxide (H_2O_2) A colorless liquid with strong oxidizing power, used as a disinfectant and bleaching agent.

hydrogen sulfide (H_2S) A colorless poisonous gas with a characteristic smell of rotten eggs, produced by anaerobic decomposition of organic matter, that occurs in some natural gas and oil deposits, where it is an ingredient of SOUR GAS that poisons cattle and sometimes people.

hydrologic cycle The processes of movement of water in nature, i.e., evaporation, precipitation, uptake on land, runoff to the sea, important to all living things that require water for their survival.

hydrology The scientific study of water, its chemistry, physics, distribution, etc.

hydrophilic A compound that has an affinity for water.

hydrophobia Aversion to water. See RABIES.

hydroponics Growth of plants in a liquid nutritive medium, rather than in soil. Increasingly used to grow vegetables out of season in climates and environments where they do not naturally grow and for the indoor cultivation of illicit plants, especially marijuana. Hydroponic vegetables look extremely healthy and usually are but may sometimes be deficient in minerals.

hygiene The principles and practices dealing with preservation of good health. Hygiene involves values that determine individual and collective behavior. These values include a commitment to cleanliness, especially cleanliness in food handling, sanitary disposal of excreta and other noxious waste, elimination of vermin, and prevention of pollution. Hygiene, as the ancient Greeks understood, includes a commitment to preserving physical fitness through exercise, a balanced diet, and regular rest and sleep. Hygieia was the goddess of health in Greek myths. Other early civilizations in

China and India flourished in part because they too understood elementary principles of hygiene. See also SANITATION.

hygrometer An instrument for measuring humidity or the moisture level in the air.

hyperactivity An abnormal level of physical activity, muscle movement, restlessness, etc., that is sometimes a feature of emotional disturbance, especially in childhood, and may occur also with use of some drugs, e.g., Benzedrine and derivatives. See also ATTENTION DEFICIT HYPERACTIVITY DISORDER (ADHD).

hyperbaric Pressure significantly elevated above the normal prevailing level. The term is applied particularly to high atmospheric oxygen pressure, as used to treat conditions in which oxygen uptake by the lungs is impeded, e.g., CARBON MONOXIDE poisoning; and to high air pressure, used to prevent and treat DECOMPRESSION SYNDROME.

hyperbaric chamber An enclosed boiler-shaped pressurized container large enough to enclose an adult, who can be viewed through a window and whose physiological functions are recorded as the air pressure and oxygen concentration in the chamber are raised. It is used to treat decompression injury and CARBON MONOXIDE poisoning.

hyperbaric injury Exposure to environments greatly exceeding normal atmospheric pressure, e.g., in deep sea diving or a hyperbaric chamber, can cause a variety of vascular injuries, including intraocular damage impairing eyesight and intracranial damage, such as cerebral hemorrhage, if the pressure is increased too rapidly. Middle ear and paranasal sinus damage also occurs. NITROGEN NARCOSIS due to greatly increased dissolved nitrogen concentration in serum is a dangerous condition among deep sea scuba divers. BAROTRAUMA is a risk if the pressure is subsequently reduced to normal too rapidly.

hyperendemic A description of a disease that is constantly present in a population at a high level of incidence and prevalence, usually affecting all age groups.

hyperlipidemia Abnormally high concentration of serum lipids, a condition that occurs with high-fat diets, and may also be genetically determined or the result of using some drugs.

hypersensitivity pneumonitis An allergic-inflammatory pneumonitis, e.g., FARMER'S LUNG.

hypertension Syn: high blood pressure. This very common condition is often associated with stress of occupational or emotional origin, but in the common form called essential hypertension, its causal mechanism is incompletely understood. However, empirical associations with electrolyte (salt) intake, low birth weight, obesity, emotional stress, physical inactivity, and age-related hardening of the arteries have been clarified by much research throughout the past century. Normal adult blood pressure is 90 to 135 mm Hg systolic and 50 to 90 mm Hg diastolic. Blood pressure greater than 140/90 mm Hg is considered hypertensive and below this but above 120/80 mm Hg is prehypertensive. Untreated hypertension tends to get worse and carries a high risk of complications, including stroke, heart attack, and retinal and renal damage. If detected early, hypertension generally responds well, often to nonpharmacological regimens, such as yoga and exercise, as well as to antihypertensive medication.

hyperthermia Abnormally high body temperature prolonged to an extent that endangers life.

hyperthyroidism Syn: Grave's disease, after the Irish physician Robert Graves (1797–1853). A condition in which excess thyroxine is produced, manifested by elevated metabolic rate, often accompanied by exophthalmos.

hypochondria Persons with this disorder believe that they are afflicted with serious illness. They interpret normal body signals as ominous symptoms of serious disease and have an obsessive concern about bodily functions, such as bowel movements. Persons with hypochondria make others around them suffer too, and consume disproportionate amounts of health care resources.

hypothermia Abnormally low body temperature, a dangerous, life-threatening condition caused by exposure to prolonged cold and/or evaporative cooling while wearing wet clothes in a cold wind. It is a common cause of death in immersion in cold water, e.g., victims of torpedo attacks on ships in the North Atlantic during World War II.

hypothesis A conjecture that can be tested and (potentially) refuted. See also NULL HYPOTHESIS.

hypothyroidism A condition in which inadequate thyroxine secretion occurs, usually associated with IODINE DEFICIENCY DISORDERS, a condition with marked geographic distribution in alpine regions, where there is a deficiency of iodine in food and water. This causes MYXEDEMA in adults and cretinism in infants and children, associated with sluggish intellect that becomes irreversible if left untreated. This condition is dramatically responsive to enhanced iodine intake, usually as iodized salt, recognized as one of the most successful public health measures available.

hysteria An uncommon condition recognized by the ancient Greeks that was given this name by HIPPOCRATES OF COS, who attributed it to a "wandering uterus" and recommended sexual intercourse to cure it. SIGMUND FREUD thought it was associated with repressed sexuality and noted that it more often affected women than men. Its manifestations may include bizarre neurological symptoms that are expressed dramatically and sometimes respond to treatment by hypnosis. It can occur as a sequel of childhood sexual abuse or as one form of post-traumatic stress disorder.

hysterical epidemic See BEHAVIORAL EPIDEMIC.

I

IARC See INTERNATIONAL AGENCY FOR RESEARCH ON CANCER.

iatrogenic disease Disease resulting from the actions of a physician or other health professional. This usually means conditions specifically caused by following medical advice, using prescribed medications, or surgical interventions, and does not necessarily include NOSOCOMIAL INFECTIONS or other medical mishaps and misadventures. Iatrogenic disease is often preventable by adhering to procedures of proven efficacy and safety established by evidence-based medical practice.

Ibn Ridwan (998–c. 1061) An Egyptian physician and scholar who rose from humble origins to become chief physician of Egypt and the guardian of public health, emphasizing the importance of hygiene and a clean domestic and urban environment. He was among the Arab scholars who helped to preserve and transmit to Renaissance Europe the writings of HIPPOCRATES OF COS and Galen.

ICD See INTERNATIONAL CLASSIFICATION OF DISEASES.

ICD number The code number that identifies a specific diagnostic entity in the INTERNATIONAL CLASSIFICATION OF DISEASES. The level of precision in identification increases with the number of digits coded to identify a condition.

ice Street name for an addictive preparation of METHAMPHETAMINE that is smoked undiluted or mixed with tobacco. It produces rather prolonged intense euphoria, often followed by depression and paranoid feelings when the effect subsides.

iceberg phenomenon A common situation in clinical practice, where only a small proportion of cases of important diseases, the tip of the iceberg, are seen at an early stage in the natural history when intervention can achieve prevention, cure, or relief of symptoms. The metaphor of the tip and the submerged part of an iceberg is apt even in tropical countries; few people are unfamiliar with the concept. The proportion of missed cases varies. For some malignant neoplasms, such as cancer of the cervix, prostate, and breast, the size of the submerged portion has decreased with improved screening methods; for adult-onset diabetes, the submerged portion is about 50%; for psychiatric disorders, it may be as much as 75% to 80%; and for hypertension, it may be as high as 90%.

ICU See INTENSIVE CARE UNIT.

ID The widely used abbreviation for identifying document(s). Photo ID includes a photograph.

IDDM See INSULIN-DEPENDENT DIABETES MELLITUS.

identifying data The set of information that identifies an individual as precisely as possible. The uniqueness of each individual is established by fingerprints, DNA profile, and/or iris scan. Many RECORD LINKAGE systems, as well as hospital and other health care record systems, including billing systems, prescription records, etc., use unique identifiers to avoid the possibility of confusing one person with others who have the same name. Identifying data usually include personal and family names, or a code representing these names, a sequence of eight digits for birth date (year, month, day), and another code for sex (male or female). Additional information may include birthplace, mother's maiden name, and father's first and last names.

identity 1. An individual's sense of self, i.e., the characteristics that are unique to each person. 2. The data and information used to identify an individual, e.g., recent photographs, fingerprints, detailed description, DNA profile, and/or documents such as passport or driver's license with identifying personal information such as full name and Social Security number.

identity theft The illicit acquisition of the personal identifying data of another individual, usually for criminal purposes. All custodians of personal data files, including those in public health and its numerous specialties, must be on their guard against this crime.

idiopathic Descriptive of conditions with no known cause or obscure pathogenesis.

idiosyncrasy A distinctive personal characteristic, especially one that is peculiar or abnormal, e.g., one that induces an atypical drug reaction or an inappropriate emotional response. Some idiosyncratic drug reactions are genetically determined.

IDU See INJECTION (OR INTRAVENOUS) DRUG USE.

illegal immigrant Syn: Undocumented alien. A person residing and often working in a country without official permission. Economic imperatives, political persecution, wars, evasion of law enforcement agencies, and other factors impel an estimated several million in the United States and comparable numbers in the European Union and other rich countries to cross international borders from their homelands to seek work, usually in the underground economy. There is also illegal immigration into low-income countries. In all countries, illegal immigrants include girls and women pressed into the sex trade and hourly rate wage earners in SWEATSHOPS and in unskilled occupations, e.g., in the hospitality industry. They are at high risk of many health problems and may carry and transmit communicable diseases to those they contact in their work or lodgings.

illegitimacy The status of a child born out of wedlock, formerly a stigmatizing condition but in most modern societies a status that is tolerated and socially accepted.

illicit drug A drug that is used despite legal sanctions against its use. In the past, the term has applied to narcotics, such as heroin, opium, etc., but now it also applies to performance-enhancing steroid preparations used by athletes and aspiring athletes.

illiteracy Inability to read and write, usually because of lack of education in how to do so. The prevalence of FUNCTIONAL ILLITERACY, i.e., inability to read well enough to follow simple written directions, varies from about 5% to 20% in apparently literate societies with allegedly universal education at least through grade school. Functionally illiterate persons can recognize numbers and street signs but are unable to read newspapers, books, or labels on supermarket purchases, med-

ications, etc. This is a potentially serious disability. Illiteracy is a social problem with serious implications for public health in some countries and cultural or ethnic groups in which girls and women are deprived of education, especially when pregnancy or sickness requires the ability to follow written instructions about actions needed to preserve health. In these cultures, it is a marker for social barriers that impede public health initiatives, such as family planning programs.

illness The subjective sensation of experiencing a diseased state.

illness behavior Syn: sickness behavior. Illness, especially when it is chronic, obliges people to seek help, placing them in a dependent position with family and health care workers. In doing so, people adopt a SICK ROLE. This is a normal consequence of ill health and may facilitate the work of those involved in care of the sick, but it can erode autonomy, infantilize adults, and put them in a position of dependency and obedience to the sometimes arbitrary orders of everyone in the health care hierarchy, from eminent specialists to teenage receptionists and hospital porters. It can be prolonged, even perpetuated, and in these cases it becomes a harmful complication of disease and disability that retards recovery. Health care workers need to be aware of this phenomenon and avoid its undesirable effects on the outcome of health care. See also HEALTH BEHAVIOR.

illness theories Usually called theories of illness, these are the concepts people use to explain what they perceive to be wrong with their health. Ancient theories include the influence of evil spirits, witchcraft, the wrath of a vengeful god. Ancient Greeks and medieval Europeans held a humoral theory, that character was determined by the balance among four "humors"—phlegm (phlegmatic), choler, or yellow bile (choleric), blood (sanguine), melancholy, or black bile (melancholic)—and that many diseases arose because of imbalances among these humors. The theory and concept of CONTAGION is ancient: it was epitomized in stigmatizing of lepers and others with disfiguring skin diseases. A superstitious belief in the contagiousness of cancer and mental disorders hindered advances in their investigation and care until the 1800s. The miasma theory, that some diseases were caused by an ill-defined emanation from rotting organic matter, persisted into the mid-19th century. The miasma theory was supported by the observed association of malaria with swamps. The germ theory has ancient origins but did not become dominant until the discovery of microscopic organisms. It is abundantly confirmed when the HENLE-KOCH POSTULATES are fulfilled. Scientific advances since the late 19th century have identified many biochemical, metabolic, and hormonal causes of disease. The theories of SIGMUND FREUD and others seek to explain mental, emotional, and personality disorders and some physiological manifestations of disease on the basis of tensions between subconscious and conscious thought. Some important diseases, such as multiple sclerosis, remain unexplained.

illumination Syn: illuminance. Energy in the form of visible radiation that falls on a surface or an object, measured in lumens per square meter. In schools, workplaces, public buildings, city roads, and pathways, specified illumination standards are often required for safety.

image 1. The representation of an object that is produced when electromagnetic radiation passes through it or is reflected from it. Visible images are formed when light impinges on the retina, and various forms of images are produced by photography, microscopes, electron microscopes, x-rays, etc., and can be viewed, e.g., on fluoroscopic screens or suitable radiosensitive film. 2. The perception of personal characteristics by the self and by others, which may be similar or different. See also BODY IMAGE.

imaging Syn: diagnostic imaging. A visual image produced by ultrasound or by radiological scanning using x-rays, tomography, computerized axial tomography (CAT or CT scan), or nuclear magnetic resonance imaging (MRI or NMR). MRI exposes the body to larger doses of ionizing radiation than does a CAT scan, especially when radioactive isotopes are used, but neither form of scanning is considered a serious source of ionized radiation, and the clinical benefits of diagnostic precision considerably outweigh the possible harms.

imago 1. The final ("perfect image") developmental stage of an insect after it has undergone all its metamorphoses. 2. In psychoanalysis, the subjective image that individuals form of persons who have significantly influenced their emotional development.

immersion syndrome Syn: immersion foot, trench foot. Peripheral vascular lesions, especially of the feet, caused by lengthy periods of working with feet in cold water or soggy wet socks and boots. This is an occupational disease of outdoor and farm workers in cold damp conditions and was a common disability of soldiers engaged in trench warfare in World War I. More extensive prolonged immersion or working in wet clothing in cold conditions can cause more generalized vascular damage, but hypothermia is a frequent outcome.

immigrant A person who migrates to and settles in a country other than that of birthplace and upbringing. Immigrants often differ culturally and sometimes in health-related behavior from persons born and raised in the country. Categories include legal immigrants who may acquire citizenship rights (including access to health care, education for their children, and other social benefits); ILLEGAL IMMIGRANTS, who do not have citizenship rights and often work in SWEATSHOPS or similar unhealthy conditions; and migratory, itinerant, and guest workers, who have temporary visitor status rather than permanent settler status. These latter groups may not only have health problems of their own, but sometimes may be a health danger to others, harboring contagious diseases such as tuberculosis that SCREENING medical examination identifies in legal immigrants. Migration may be voluntary or involuntary, the latter group being REFUGEES or INTERNALLY DISPLACED PERSONS. Immigrants often have health problems different from those of the people among whom they settle.

immigration The movement of people into a country as IMMIGRANTS, an important determinant of population structure. This shapes the social fabric in nations when influx of many immigrants over a relatively brief period can transform the demographic and social profile, as in the United States in the late 19th to early 20th centuries, the United Kingdom, Australia, Canada, and western Europe in the middle and late 20th century. Migrations have occurred in most human societies. As the world's population quadrupled in the 20th century, residents of some countries perceived social, housing, employment, and health-related problems associated with immigration, and legal and physical barriers have been created. After the middle of the 20th century, the US Immigration and Naturalization Service responded to economic and political pressure and began limiting unimpeded entry of immigrants. Similar actions have been taken in the United Kingdom, the European Union, Australia, and Canada. SCREENING for contagious diseases such as tuberculosis and HIV infection has also become more rigorous. These measures have not stopped ILLEGAL IMMIGRANTS, who sometimes include persons with serious contagious disease, who also may be victims of unscrupulous employers, forced to do difficult and dangerous work for long hours and very low pay, with further adverse health consequences.

immission A German word for all forms of environmentally harmful emanations from industrial sites, covering with one word atmospheric pollutants, noise, vibration, ionized and nonionized radiation on any wavelength, unpleasant or noxious odors, etc. There is no equivalent word in English that describes collectively or individually all the diverse forms of harmful environmental influences on health.

immune response The reaction of the host's immune system to antigen in an invading (infecting) pathogenic organism, or to foreign protein, as in transplanted organs or tissues. The response is humoral and local; antibody is produced by dermal lymphatic tissue (T cells) and by B cells, which are a type of lymphocyte. Antibody combines with antigen in an antigen-antibody complex to inactivate or neutralize antigen. This defensive mechanism often effectively controls infection.

immune system The organs and dermal tissues that produce and maintain immune responses (reactions) to foreign antigens. These are strategically dispersed in portions of the hemopoietic blood-forming tissues in bone marrow, where leukocytes and T-helper cells are produced. Other immune tissues include dermal cells that produce immunoglobulin, lymph nodes, spleen, and thymus. Immune tissues are sensitive to ionizing radiation and to immunosuppressing drugs that are used to prevent reactions to transplanted organs and tissues.

immunity Resistance to infection, usually because of the presence of ANTIBODY that protects the individual from harm by the pathogenic organism responsible for the infection. Species-specific NATURAL IMMUNITY exists when an organism is inherently resistant to a pathogenic organism; e.g., humans have natural immunity to the virus of canine distemper, which is lethal for dogs. Immunity may be acquired through previous exposure of the host to a pathogen, leading to production of ANTIBODIES in response to the alien protein. Depending on variations in host-agent interaction, active immunity may be lifelong or transient. PASSIVE IMMUNITY is conferred by an antibody that has been produced in another host and acquired naturally by transfer from mother to infant, or artificially by injection of ANTISERUM or IMMUNOGLOBULIN.

immunity from prosecution An indemnity, for instance of government agencies, from legal action that might otherwise be taken by individuals or groups to right what they perceive to be a wrong or harm they have suffered. This can protect public health departments and their officials from legal action, e.g., when adverse reactions to immunization occur. Under some circumstances, corporations also may be deemed immune from prosecution for harms due to their actions.

immunization Syn: vaccination. The artificial induction of active immunity by introducing into a vulnerable host the specific antigen of a pathogenic organism, usually by parenteral injection, sometimes orally, as with oral POLIOMYELITIS vaccine, or intranasally, as with live attenuated influenza vaccine. The antibody may be contained in a culture of live attenuated or otherwise modified organisms that have retained their antigenicity but lost their capacity to cause disease. Passive immunization refers to transfer of maternal antibodies via the placenta or breast milk, or artificially using immune or hyperimmune globulin. Passive immunization is not long-lasting because the antibodies undergo metabolic breakdown. Vaccines are prepared from live attenuated pathogens maintained in culture media or otherwise modified organisms, or from killed organisms that retain antigenicity. Immunization against some pathogens is possible by using purified protein extract or genetically modified variations. Smallpox VACCINATION, the first effective form of immunization, came into general use in the early 19th century after the English physician Edward Jenner (1749–1823) published *An Inquiry into the Causes and Effects of the Variolae Vaccinae* in 1798. Jenner's work was among the most important contributions to public health of all time. Smallpox vaccination uses VACCINIA virus, which has the same antigenic properties as virulent SMALLPOX (variola) virus.

immunofluorescence A procedure for identifying protein molecules and tracking their metabolic pathway by means of antibody containing a fluorescent compound.

immunoglobulins Large protein molecules that contain antigen-binding regions where foreign antigen is inactivated. Humans have five types of immunoglobulin (Ig), designated IgG, IgA, IgM, IgD, and IgE, identifiable by electrophoresis and by the structural and functional differences that enable them to bind with and therefore inactivate different varieties of foreign protein or antigen. IgA occurs on cell membranes and in mucus secretions. It comprises 10% to 15% of the body's total immunoglobulin and is reduced in the presence of conditions that impair immune responses, e.g., HIV infection. Immunoglobulin G (IgG) comprises about 80% of the body's immunoglobulin. It occurs in serum and forms part of secondary immune responses.

immunology The scientific study of immunity, its determinants, mechanisms, etc., and their role in defending the body against infection and invading foreign protein, including transplanted organs and tissues.

immunosuppression Inhibition or drastic reduction of immune response that is produced by radiation-induced damage to hematopoietic tissue, by certain drugs and toxic chemicals, and by the action of certain microorganisms, notably HIV, and some overwhelming bacterial infections, e.g., acute streptococcal and meningococcal septicemia.

immunotherapy A treatment regimen used by allergists to desensitize people so they can better tolerate allergens.

immunotoxicity The property of a drug or toxic chemical that poisons the immune system.

impact assessment Formal study of a public health intervention that usually focuses on the intermediate objectives in the continuum of process, impact, and outcome. Impact measures are usually short term and process oriented, such as immunization coverage rates linked to an intervention like a vaccination program, and that logically precede long-term outcomes, such as reduced incidence rates of vaccine-preventable disease. The term is also applied to assessment of effects that can be expected, or that have occurred, as a result of significant changes in an environment or habitat but usually is applied to midcourse and short-term evaluations and may focus on whether objectives have been or are being achieved. Impact assessment is preferably outcome oriented, rather than process oriented, but meaningful outcome measures are not always feasible or available.

impact factor In medical and scientific journals, the impact factor is a measure of the timeliness and frequency with which original articles in a specific journal are cited by authors of articles in other journals that are indexed in the SCIENCE CITATION INDEX, a publication of the Institute for Scientific Information. It is regarded by many editors and editorial management committees as a measure of the "importance" of particular journals, and to some extent this is true: journals such as *Nature*, *Science*, *Lancet*, *British Medical Journal*, *JAMA*, and *New England Journal of Medicine* have a high impact factor; but there is debate among science and medical journal editors about the significance of this.

impact fraction A generalized measure of POPULATION ATTRIBUTABLE RISK that takes into account both risk factors and protective factors, as well as multiple levels of exposure, differing responses to exposure, etc. This measure is used to formulate and evaluate public health policy.

impaired driving A widely used legal and medical term to describe drivers of vehicles who are incapable of driving with safety to themselves and

others, usually because their skill and judgment have been impaired by alcohol intoxication, other substances, or disease. Impaired driving is a cause of 10% to 30% or more of deaths and serious injuries in road traffic crashes, so it is a serious public health problem.

impaired professional A physician, nurse, or other health professional person whose intellectual capacity, judgment, or technical proficiency has been damaged by drugs or disease.

impairment A physical or mental defect of function or structure in a body system or organ that usually, but not necessarily always, leads to a DISABILITY and sometimes to a HANDICAP. Impairments may affect sensory, motor, intellectual, mental, and emotional functions in many possible combinations and may be acute short-term and temporary or chronic, including permanent. The INTERNATIONAL CLASSIFICATION OF FUNCTIONING, DISABILITY AND HEALTH lists the possible varieties.

impartiality Even-handedness, objectivity in all dealings, a behavior pattern embodied in the ethical principle of EQUITY or distributive justice, an important ethical principle in public health.

Imperial Cancer Research Fund This large UK independent charitable foundation has merged with the Cancer Research Campaign to form Cancer Research UK. It is a foundation that supports fundamental research, clinical trials, etc. It derives its funds from bequests, revenue from shops run by volunteers, and government grants for sponsored research. See http://www.cancerresearchuk.org/ for details.

imperial units The traditional system of weights and measures in much of the English-speaking world and some other nations, consisting of tons, pounds, ounces, etc.; miles, yards, feet, inches; gallons and pints, with other units, such as furlongs and gills, that became obsolete longer ago. The imperial system was superseded by the simpler and more efficient metric system in most nations several generations ago, and in scientific notation has been superseded by SYSTÈME INTERNATIONAL (SI) units of measurement. (See Appendix for conversion tables.)

implant The use of surgical techniques to replace a defective body organ or tissue, such as an opaque lens or a malfunctioning cochlea. Tissue matching is not an essential prerequisite for these procedures because immunosuppressive drugs make this unnecessary, but rigorous testing for HIV and other infections is required. Before this became routine, there were occasional tragedies when recipients were infected. Another medical disaster occurred when CREUTZFELDT-JAKOB DISEASE was transmitted to recipients of cadaveric dura mater.

implied consent The situation in which a patient or client submits to procedures, etc., but has not provided formal informed consent. A person who responds to questions in a telephone survey is granting implied consent to participate in a study. A patient who offers an arm and a vein for a physician to withdraw a sample of blood is implying consent to the procedure. Implied consent is ethically, morally, and legally insufficient when the consequences of the procedure could be harmful. For instance, if the blood is to be tested for HIV infection, the possible consequences of a positive test, e.g., loss of employment and insurance benefits, are so serious that it is essential to obtain informed consent formally and in writing.

impotence Inability to achieve or to sustain an erection for long enough to perform successful sexual intercourse with insertion of the penis into the vagina and ejaculation of semen. The causes include impaired blood supply to erectile tissue, due to arteriosclerosis; some neurological diseases; psychological and psychosexual problems; and various medications, drug, and/or alcohol use. Heavy smoking, which can cause erectile dysfunction, is another possibility. Although it bends the truth slightly, antismoking campaigns and posters that mention the risk of impotence as a consequence of smoking may be a deterrent to youths who might otherwise become tobacco addicts. Impotence, also known as ERECTILE DYSFUNCTION DISORDER, has become a popular diagnostic category since the development and aggressive marketing of Viagra and other drugs to enhance potency.

imprinting A form of learning in early life, especially of animals and birds, but also a determinant of some aspects of human behavior, such as the expression of affection, which develops under the influence of interaction between mother and infant.

impulse 1. The signal transmitted along a nerve fiber, induced by the movement of ions. 2. In physics, the product of a force and the duration of its action. 3. In psychology, a spontaneous emotion or action in response to an emotional stimulus.

imputation The process of replacing missing values in a large-scale epidemiological or social research study, when all other relevant parameters and values are known for an individual subject, by inserting an "average" or other plausible value. The process is of course arbitrary and subject to various biases and errors and must be disclosed in reporting the results.

inborn errors of metabolism A group of genetically determined disorders in which an ENZYME required for normal metabolism is defective, causing it to malfunction; is inactive; or is missing altogether. They can often be treated by dietary regimens that take into account their inability to carry out a specific metabolic function because of the missing or defective enzyme involved in that particular metabolic pathway. Examples include phenylketonuria and cystinuria. Most inborn errors of metabolism are inherited as recessive characteristics.

inbreeding Syn: consanguinity. Mating and production of offspring by people who are closely related genetically. In domesticated animals and in plants, inbreeding is deliberately practiced to enhance desired qualities, such as strength, beauty, and speed. In humans, the closest varieties of inbreeding, parent-offspring mating and sibling mating, are categorized as INCEST, which has been recognized since ancient times and in almost all cultures as harmful because it is associated with high frequency of abnormal offspring. More remote inbreeding, e.g., marriages of first cousins, is widespread in some south Asian populations and among Trobriand Islanders and European aristocracy. The evidence on possible harm to offspring is equivocal and is being actively studied.

incapacity A word used mainly in legal medicine, referring to the absence of testamentary capacity, i.e., not "being of sound mind" or possessing the ability to testify in court or write a legally sustainable will. The word is also used to describe inability to control a motor vehicle because of impaired mental, neurological, or physical capacity.

incest Sexual intimacy between close blood relations, i.e., siblings, parent and child, uncle-niece, aunt-nephew. Incest has long been TABOO in most societies and is the subject of myths, legends, and literature, e.g., Sophocles' *Oedipus* trilogy. In some communities it has been empirically associated with a high frequency of abnormal offspring. It was customary and approved in the families of the pharaohs in the Egyptian dynastic period. If an underage person is one of the partners, it is criminal sexual abuse. If incest leads to pregnancy and childbirth, the risk of genetic defects in the offspring is greater than in mating among unrelated couples, especially if both partners carry a recessive gene for a deleterious inherited characteristic. The prevalence of incest varies according to cultural values. In Western societies it is often identified in criminal proceedings in cases of sexual abuse, but its true prevalence is unknown. In the Middle East and the Indian subcontinent, as many as 50% of marriages are of first cousins and uncle-niece pairs, and there appear to have been no major adverse genetic effects on health as a result. See also INBREEDING.

incidence In epidemiology, the occurrence of new events or cases. This is expressed as an absolute number, or as a RATE when the POPULATION AT RISK is known or can be reliably estimated and related to a specified period of time, so incidence rate=number of new cases in a specified period÷person-time at risk in this period. More loosely, as in many vital statistical measures, the average or mean population at risk during the period is commonly used as the denominator. A multiplier, 10^n, is used to produce a rate that is a whole number rather than a decimal fraction.

incineration Controlled burning of domestic or industrial waste, widely used as a method to dispose of waste. This is preferably done in a furnace or stove to maximize efficient combustion and minimize the volume of toxic fumes and smoke.

incinerator A domestic or industrial receptacle for combustion of waste material. The emissions from incinerators, especially industrial incinerators, may contain toxic ingredients such as dioxins. Thus, industrial incinerators often must comply with environmental standards to ensure that the combustion of toxic products is conducted under conditions such as very high temperatures that ensure complete combustion and destruction of the toxic ingredients.

inclusion bodies Particles that occur in many somatic body cells, believed to be viruses undergoing morphological changes in the course of absorption into the body.

income The extent to which individuals or groups have command over access to necessary and desired goods and services, usually estimated from the amount of financial or material resources accruing to an individual, a group, or a nation over a specified period.

income distribution The way national income is allocated or divided among all who receive income from labor, goods, services, capital investments, government or other pensions, etc.

income elasticity The capacity of personal income to adjust to financial demands, distinguishing between necessities (shelter, food, clothing, etc.) and luxuries or discretionary spending.

income levels, World Bank classification The WORLD BANK classifies nations into four groups (low-, lower-middle-, upper-middle-, and high-income countries) based on estimated gross national income (GNI) per capita, using equivalents of US dollars and ignoring fluctuating exchange rates. At 2002 US dollar values, LOW- AND MIDDLE-INCOME COUNTRIES had an annual per capita GNI of less than US\$735; that of lower-middle-income countries was in the range of US\$736 to 2,935; upper-middle-income countries, US\$2936 to 9,075; and high-income countries, US\$9,076 or more.

incompetence Inability to perform expected tasks. Professional incompetence is a designation of physicians, nurses, etc., who are unable to perform essential tasks expected of them. Personal incompetence may be due to physical impairment or handicap, or to a mental, emotional, or personality disorder. Professional and personal incompetence may lead to public health problems. The purpose of professional qualifying examinations and periodic reassessment now widely used is to ensure that the public is protected from incompetent workers.

incremental costs The difference between marginal costs of alternative courses of action. In a more precise sense, the difference between the lowest possible estimated cost and the cost of the program or service that was implemented.

incubation The process of maintaining fertilized eggs, bacteria, etc., in an environment that enables them to grow, develop, mature, hatch, or, in the case of bacteria, reproduce.

incubation period The period that elapses between invasion of a pathogenic organism and the first appearance of clinical manifestations of infection. In VECTOR-BORNE DISEASES, the incubation period in the vector is the time between entry of the pathogen and the point at which the vector becomes infective, i.e., the pathogen has completed developmental stages in the vector, which then carries viable pathogens that can infect new hosts in the next stage of the pathogen's life cycle.

incubator A device that provides a microenvironment favorable to the growth and development of organisms such as bacteria or fertilized eggs.

independent variable In a research study, the characteristic, quality, or entity that is hypothesized to influence DEPENDENT VARIABLES that are being measured.

index 1. An alphabetical listing of key words and phrases in a book, listing the pages on which related information can be found. 2. A rating scale or scoring system. Many such rating scales are used in public health, the social sciences, and epidemiology to assess physical function, mental capacity, quality of life, severity of pain, and general health. See for example ACTIVITIES OF DAILY LIVING (ADL) SCALE and QUALITY-OF-LIFE SCALES.

index case The initial case in a communicable disease outbreak that spreads person to person. In genetics, the PROPOSITUS, i.e., the individual whose condition first draws attention to a genetic trait.

indexes of social health Several methods have been developed to assess the social well-being and extent of social pathology in a community. Some rely on available facts in existing records of public agencies, such as people receiving social assistance, food aid, and income subsidies, and other economic indicators. Some use data on social pathology, such as calls to the police to settle domestic disputes, reports of vandalism, child neglect. These may be combined with demographic data, such as density of occupancy and proportion of old people living alone, from census reports, to identify "high-risk" neighborhoods where public health nurses can intervene to help minimize untoward outcomes. See also JARMAN INDEX and TOWNSEND SCORE.

indexing 1. Automatic adjustment of salaries, wages, and pensions to adjust for changes in the cost of living. 2. The process of entering information about individuals on a rating scale. 3. The process of entering items such as bibliographic details in an index.

Index Medicus The bibliographic search and retrieval system maintained by the NATIONAL LIBRARY OF MEDICINE that has recorded titles and authors of original articles and names of a very large number of serial journals of biomedical sciences, in English and other languages, since 1879, when it was established as the National Library of Medicine's "Index Catalogue" by the physician, public health pioneer, and librarian JOHN SHAW BILLINGS (1838–1913). For many years, the *Index Medicus* was published in monthly, quarterly, and annual volumes. Now it can be searched online at http://www.nlm.nih.gov (the Web site of the National Library of Medicine).

Indian Health Service An agency of the US Department of Health and Human Services that provides preventive and therapeutic health care for members of indigenous population groups. The service includes hospitals, clinics, outreach services, etc. Details are available at http://www.ihs.gov.

Indian Medical Service (IMS) The network of preventive and therapeutic services established in India during the period of British colonial occupation, primarily for the benefit of the occupiers.

Medical scientists and physicians of the IMS made important contributions to identification and control of tropical vector-borne and other diseases. It was the origin of the contemporary All-India Institutes and other outstanding health research institutions in India, as well as the medical and public health services of modern India. Similar services were established by other European powers, such as the Dutch in their Indonesian colonies and the Germans in Africa, and some advances in tropical diseases came from these sources.

indicator An attribute that can be used to measure and/or record an event, process, or phenomenon.

indicators of health Syn: health indicators. A term covering all forms of data on population health, notably life expectancy, infant and child mortality rates, cause-specific mortality and morbidity, sickness absences from work and school, health care resources, facilities, utilization rates, case fatality and complication rates, immunization rates, teenage pregnancy rates, and data on health-related behavior, such as cigarette smoking rates, use of automobile seat belts, etc.

indigence The condition of financial destitution and lack of resources of food, clothing, and shelter that are necessary to sustain life. Indigence predisposes to many medical problems. It may be due to disabling disease, or in countries with inadequate medical insurance such as the United States and many poor nations, it may be caused by pauperization from the costs of disabling disease.

indigenous population The people who were present in a country before it became colonized by people from another, generally more aggressive, culture in possession of weapons that enabled them to take over the territory previously occupied by the indigenous population. The indigenous population has usually been present since that region or territory was first occupied by humans, i.e., it is an aboriginal population, often nomadic hunter-gatherers. Colonization almost always has caused major disruption of the habitat and way of life of indigenous populations and has given rise to many serious and intractable health problems among most of them.

indirect costs 1. Syn: overhead costs. The cost of administration, buildings and maintenance, rental of premises, heat, light, water, etc. 2. In disease costing, the losses in production, well-being, etc., imposed by the occurrence of disease or injury, as distinct from direct treatment costs.

indirect transmission This term describes several ways in which infection can pass from cases to susceptibles, including airborne transmission, as by droplet spread; transmission by a common vehicle, such as contaminated water, food, cooking utensils; and vector-borne transmission, as with mosquito-borne or tick-borne diseases. Transmission of infection may occur from an active case, a carrier, or a healthy contact.

individualism A philosophical belief and political ideology that gives primacy to the interests of the individual, rather than the interests of the community, perhaps even the family. A prevalent belief system in many democratic nations that can have undesirable consequences if circumstances such as serious epidemics or natural disasters require collective social action.

individual rights See HUMAN RIGHTS.

individual risk, susceptibility See RISK.

indolent disease A term used to describe a condition that continues for a prolonged period, usually years rather than months, without significant progression, remission, or recovery; often a synonym for chronic disease. Some infections are indolent. Examples include certain mycotic or fungus diseases, some cases of chronic tuberculosis, and some varieties of mental disorder.

indoor air pollution An environmental health problem of dwellings and other buildings in several kinds of human settlement, resulting from the presence of air pollutants, such as emission products of combustion, toxic fumes, etc., and inadequate or inefficient ventilation. Indoor air can become contaminated with emissions from BIOMASS FUELS, TOBACCO smoke, vapors from volatile solvents, carpet adhesives, insulating material, etc. Many large office buildings and multistory high-rise apartment towers are tightly sealed against the elements and rely on heating and air conditioning to control the indoor climate. Indoor air pollution occurs if ventilation is inadequate or inefficient and air stagnates, leading to elevated concentration of carbon dioxide, toxic fumes, etc., to cause the SICK BUILDING SYNDROME. Buildup of carbon monoxide from carbon fuel space heaters is far more dangerous and occasionally causes death of an entire family.

indoor relief A form of social assistance in the United States, a term that is mainly of historical interest, describing assistance to inmates of almshouses and poorhouses that required recipients to reside in designated institutions in order to retain eligibility for benefits.

induced abortion An abortion brought about by deliberate intervention, rather than a natural occurrence. This may be done, especially in some developing countries, by the pregnant woman herself under unhygienic conditions that lead to infection and death of more than half a million women annually. In countries where induced abortion is legal, it has a mortality rate close to zero.

induction The form of logical analysis that proceeds from observation of particular events or circumstances to creation of a "rule" or "rules" about underlying processes that could explain the observed phenomena. Another name for this is "generalization from the particular." There is no infallible method of logical reasoning that will actually do this, but conceptually bright ideas, scientific breakthroughs, and statistical inference are examples of inductive reasoning. Contrast deduction, which is "particularizing from the general."

induction of labor A procedure to initiate or accelerate labor and childbirth when prolonging a pregnancy would expose the fetus or mother or both to undue risk. Medical or surgical methods or a combination may be used for this purpose. Useful answers to questions about induction of labor for expectant mothers are at http://www.childbirth.org/articles/labor/induction.html.

induction period See LATENCY, LATENT PERIOD.

inductive learning An educational method based on logical reasoning from observations to the underlying natural laws that explain the observations. It has been used in some health-promotion programs, but it is a rather time-consuming and costly method.

industrial hygiene The art and science devoted to recognition, evaluation, and control of the environmental factors and stresses that occur in or are related to the workplace and working conditions that may cause sickness, impaired health and well-being, discomfort, and inefficiency among workers or others in the communities located near a workplace. The industrial hygienist anticipates, treats, and controls unhealthy working conditions and seeks to protect and enhance the health of workers. The term dates to the early days of the industrial revolution, when working conditions in many factories were appallingly bad. It is almost synonymous with OCCUPATIONAL HEALTH but may differ in putting greater emphasis on protecting and improving workers' health.

industrialization The process of change from an agrarian to an industrial economy that uses - machines to generate energy, manufacture and transport goods, and move people speedily between their dwellings, workplaces, and recreational settings. These processes usually cause environmental destruction and pollution of air, water, and land with the waste products of industrial development.

industrial pollution Pollution of air, water, soil, or food that is of industrial origin.

Industrial Revolution The transition from an agrarian economy to an economy based on the use of coal-fired machinery to manufacture an increasingly wide range of goods. The process began in Britain in the 18th century after the invention of the steam engine. It progressed rapidly throughout the 19th century and extended to the rest of western Europe, the United States, and Japan, then to the former Soviet Union. A wave of modernizing industrialization occurred in India, Brazil, Mexico, Indonesia, Thailand, China, and some oil-rich nations in the late 20th century period of GLOBALIZATION.

industrial waste This term is usually applied to waste products and by-products of industrial processes. Some industrial waste, as in the petrochemical industry, is extremely toxic. Industrial waste is usually collected and disposed of in ways separate from those used for domestic waste, but many industrial waste sites are poorly controlled and a source of serious environmental pollution.

industrial worker Syn: manual worker, blue-collar worker. A person who works in a factory, mine, forestry, fishing, or other occupation requiring considerable physical and often not much intellectual effort. Industrial work is often repetitive, as on assembly lines in factories, requires strenuous physical effort, and may be dangerous, e.g., deep sea fishing, underground mining. Modern machinery has reduced the heavy physical work required in the past by many kinds of industrial workers. The work does not usually require many years of education or academic excellence, so it is a common "choice" for people who did not do well in school. The occupational hazards, including the risk of injury and premature death, can be considerable. Contrast clerical or WHITE-COLLAR WORKER.

inequalities in health Syn: health disparities, gap. The differences in levels of HEALTH INDICATORS associated with and often correlated with inequalities of socioeconomic levels. These inequalities are related to the effects of educational, housing, environmental and occupational factors, gender, and ethnicity, and to behavioral factors, such as differences in exposure to cigarette smoking and other risk factors. Differences in values, such as belief in the virtues of physical exercise and

access to and ability to pay for sporting facilities, also play a part. Psychoneuroimmunological factors related to self-esteem may influence the risk of conditions that relate to hierarchical position in clerical and professional occupations, favoring those at the highest occupational levels over those below them in health risks as well as in income, but housing conditions, crowding, and exposure to infectious pathogens, educational opportunities, ease or difficulty of access to health care services, and the like, are usually more important. See also SOCIAL CLASS and SOCIOECONOMIC STATUS (SES).

inert gas Syn: noble gas. Helium, neon, argon, krypton, xenon, and radon, all of which occur in trace amounts in the atmosphere, and all of which share the quality of being difficult to combine chemically with other elements or chemical compounds, thus the name "inert," although this name is discouraged in favor of "noble" because most do form compounds and also have important industrial uses or are biologically important, e.g., radon as a marker for radioactivity.

infamous professional conduct The phrase used to describe several kinds of bad behavior by a physician or other health professional in the United Kingdom and nations with similar medicolegal systems. It includes sex with a patient, prescribing or providing narcotics without appropriate medical indication, falsifying financial records, etc. In law it may apply to any gross violation of fiduciary duties. The penalty is usually permanent or temporary revocation of the license to practice.

infancy In lay usage, an imprecisely defined period from birth to the age when a child is toilet trained and/or can feed, dress, and wash without the help of a parent or older sibling. Statistically the term is more narrowly defined (see INFANT).

infant Strictly speaking, a child between birth and 1 year of age. In common usage, the age range is more loosely defined, describing a child between birth and an age when independent activity, such as walking, feeding, and washing, can be performed.

infant botulism See INTESTINAL BOTULISM.

infant formula Artificially manufactured substitutes for human breast milk, usually made from powdered or dehydrated cow's milk with additives, etc., to create a mixture (formula) that mimics human breast milk as closely as possible. Most are marketed in dry form and reconstituted by adding water and warming. Provided kitchen hygiene is scrupulously observed, the risk of contamination with dangerous pathogens is small, but it is often difficult or impossible to ensure freedom from pathogens in low-income countries. See also FORMULA FEEDING.

infant health A fairly sensitive indicator of the quality of a nation's health and social support systems is the state of infant health, measured by infant and perinatal mortality rates, mortality rates from infectious diseases in the second 6 months of life, and data on early development, especially growth rates and the ages at which infants reach developmental milestones.

infanticide Deliberate killing of an infant, usually newborn. In some ancient and even in some contemporary societies, this has been an acceptable practice, the nearest alternative to effective contraception. In most nations it is a crime, perpetrated usually by a desperate young woman with an unwanted pregnancy, but selective survival of male infants continues to be encouraged in some countries, with or without selective female infanticide. Disparities in the male:female sex ratio revealed by censuses in China and much of south Asia could be explained by the prevalence of female infanticide, abortion of female fetuses detected by ultrasound, and selective loss of female infants from neglected illnesses and poor nutrition.

infantile paralysis See POLIOMYELITIS.

infant mortality rate (IMR) Strictly speaking, the proportion of liveborn infants dying before reaching their first birthday. In practice and in vital statistical tables, IMR is defined as the ratio of the number of deaths in a year of infants—i.e., children aged less than 1 year—to the number of all liveborn infants in that year. Conceptually, UNICEF defines it as the probability of dying between birth and age 1 year, expressed as a rate per 1,000 live births. Although the IMR is neither a true rate nor a proportion, in common and professional usage, it is always called a rate.

infant nutrition The ideal nutritional substance for infants is human breast milk (unless the mother has HIV). If human breast milk is not available, INFANT FORMULA is the next best thing, provided it is prepared under suitably hygienic conditions. Some infant formula manufacturers have been more concerned about the commercial success of their product than about its suitability and freedom from contamination with pathogenic organisms. Resolutions passed by the World Health Assembly, the United Nations Children's Fund, and nongovernmental organizations concerned for infant and child well-being since the middle 1980s have put some moral pressure on infant formula manufacturers to act responsibly, and there have been

some improvements in this state of affairs, but it is not yet ideal.

infection The invasion of a susceptible host by a disease agent (a pathogenic organism) that can develop and proliferate and usually, but not necessarily, causes overt disease. Pathogenic organisms include viruses, bacteria, mycoses (fungi), protozoa such as the malaria parasite, and metazoa such as fleas, lice, and many intestinal parasites. Infection may be unapparent, i.e., subclinical, or manifest as anything from mild illness to fulminating, overwhelming, and rapidly fatal disease. See GRADIENT OF INFECTION.

infection control The measures taken by public health physicians, epidemiologists, hospital infection control officers, and others to contain the spread of infections. These include promotion of hygiene (hand-washing), barrier techniques, DISINFECTION, STERILIZATION, ISOLATION, QUARANTINE, the use of prophylactic antibiotics, IMMUNIZATION, etc. Infection control is an ESSENTIAL PUBLIC HEALTH SERVICE.

infection transmission parameter The proportion of all possible contacts between infectious cases and susceptibles that lead to new infections, an important concept in EPIDEMIC THEORY. See also MASS ACTION PRINCIPLE.

infectious disease See COMMUNICABLE DISEASE.

infectious mononucleosis Syn: glandular fever, the kissing disease. A viral disease, most often seen among adolescents and young adults, caused by the Epstein-Barr virus (EBV), transmitted in saliva or by direct contact; usually a mild illness, but it sometimes persists for months. It may be a cause of some cases of chronic fatigue syndrome. The relationship to lymphoma is uncertain and inconsistent. See http://www.cdc.gov/ncidod/diseases/ebv.htm.

infectivity 1. The capability of a disease agent to invade, survive, and multiply in a host. 2. The proportion of exposures to an infectious agent that result in an infection.

inference The process of logical reasoning that combines observed phenomena with accepted truths or axioms in order to formulate generalizable statements. Statistical inference applies the process to data sets with calculated degrees of uncertainty. CAUSAL INFERENCE, often applied to results of epidemiological research, is the process of logical reasoning that must often rely on accumulated circumstantial evidence to reach conclusions about cause-effect relationships.

infertility Inability to become pregnant, e.g., because of a malfunction in the fertilization process due to defective sperm or ova or anatomical abnormality, such as occluded fallopian tubes.

inflammation The defensive reaction of the body to an infection, an irritant, chemical or physical injury, or degenerative process, such as development of atheromatous plaques in atherosclerosis. The characteristic features of inflammation are heat, swelling, pain, and flushing due to increased blood flow through inflamed tissue, but in low-grade and indolent inflammatory processes, not all these features are apparent. Inflamed cells release histamine, which causes the blood vessels to dilate and produce fluid exudate. Kinins and prostaglandins are also released. Leukocytes (phagocytes) congregate in the inflamed tissues, and an IMMUNE RESPONSE occurs.

inflation A persisting increase in prices of essential goods, such as food, accompanied by demand for increased wages and salary to cover the rising prices. In free market economies, it is accepted as a fact of life that annual inflation rates of as much as 2% are "normal" and can and should be absorbed without harm to the national economy. Inflation increases at a significantly greater rate when any or several among the range of possible pressures on the economy is present, such as war, sharp reduction or scarcity of essential resources of food or energy, or increase of money supply. The consequences can include an accelerating inflationary spiral, which can have a serious impact on public health services with fixed budgets and staff on fixed salaries and wages.

inflation index Syn: cost of living index. A numerical indicator of the extent of inflation, usually calculated from data on the prices for specific goods and services, comparing current prices with those at fixed times in the past.

influenza Syn: flu, grippe. An acute infectious disease primarily of the respiratory tract caused by the influenza virus. Epidemic influenza is a serious infectious disease that often has a high case fatality rate. It usually occurs at intervals of several decades in pandemic form and more frequently in epidemics confined to a country or region. It is due to a virulent and highly infectious form of the influenza A virus, resulting from a mutation of the virus associated with antigenic shift. Persons possessing antibodies from exposure to previously circulated antigens may have limited resistance to a mutant strain. In intervals between epidemics and pandemics, cases occur sporadically, usually due to infection with viruses of influenza B or C, which do not cause epidemic spread. See also AVIAN INFLUENZA. For details on international regulations, current outbreaks, and vaccinations, see http://www.who.int/csr/disease/influenza/en/.

informal economy The system of barter, i.e., trading based on exchange of one set of goods for another without money changing hands, and a wide variety of cash transactions not officially identified to goods and services taxation agencies, e.g., transactions stemming from advertisements in the classified columns of newspapers, notices on bulletin boards, etc. See also GRAY MARKET.

informatics The study of information, information systems, and the use of processing, storage, retrieval, and analytic methods used to deal with information, including the use of computers, machine intelligence, and all other aspects of information management. Informatics is used in public health services to process data from vaccination programs and send reminder notices when booster doses are due, and in similar applications with other target populations.

information Facts (data) that have been arranged and/or transformed in order to provide the basis for analysis and interpretation and (ideally) transformation into knowledge. Information on public health is summarized in many ways for transmission to and use by public health officials, to ensure that policies, programs, and day-to-day decisions are rationally based.

information system In general, the combination of data sources and the methods and procedures used to process, analyze, store, retrieve, transmit, and display these data. In the health sector, the vital and health statistics derived from all sources that inform administrators, managers, health service professional staff, and the public about health needs, health resources, use of services, costs, and outcomes of sickness episodes and interventions to prevent and treat sickness and injury.

information technology (IT) A field of science and technology that has made spectacular advances in the past half century and continues to do so. The advances in computers, including miniaturization, advanced circuitry, fiberoptics, and communications satellites, have transformed society, facilitating collection, processing, transmission, and storage of information on a scale and with a scope that were unimaginable half a century ago.

information theory A theory in mathematics and logic that deals with the nature, methodology, effectiveness, and accuracy of information gathering, processing, analysis, transmission, and use.

informed consent In research involving human subjects, their voluntary consent, or the consent of a responsible proxy, such as a parent or legal guardian, is absolutely essential. This has been universally accepted since the NUREMBERG CODE (1948) spelled out the details of the procedure. Consent must be voluntary, freely given, after the subject or patient has been fully informed and offered a choice; there must be no coercion, duress, undue influence, or penalties for withholding consent; and there must be a right to withdraw at any time. A fundamental feature is ensuring that patients and research subjects understand all the implications of consenting. This important process should be mandatory as a preliminary to all preventive and therapeutic interventions in the health service field. It is a legal necessity as well as an ethical requirement. The CIOMS Guidelines for Research Involving Human Subjects (revised 2002) and the draft guidelines for ethical review of epidemiological studies (2005) specify many items of information that must be conveyed to and understood by research subjects as part of the process of granting consent to participate in research. See http://www.cioms.ch for details.

infrared radiation Electromagnetic radiation with a wavelength that is too long to be visible to human eyes, i.e., 0.8 microns to 1 mm. Although it is invisible, it emanates RADIANT HEAT, and it can penetrate fog or haze that scatters visible light waves. Infrared radiation is used in night vision goggles and the equipment that enables large passenger aircraft to land safely in thick fog.

infrasound Vibrations in the air that occur at a frequency too low to cause audible sound but that may be perceived by tactile vibrations. If prolonged or occurring with high energy, infrasound can be destructive, e.g., to the masonry and fabric of buildings.

infrastructure This term generally means the fixed physical resources of an organization, such as its buildings, equipment, facilities for transport, and communications. Sometimes the term also includes the numbers and grades of human resources, that is, the staffing structure and the budgeted funds to pay salaries, wages, fringe benefits, and pensions.

infusion A solution or suspension, usually of an organic substance, such as an alkaloid, prepared by immersing it in hot water. Tea is an example. Many herbal remedies are infusions of herbs.

ingenuity gap The disparity between the technical knowledge and expertise needed to solve environmental, social, and behavioral problems, especially those created by modern industrial civilization, and the knowledge and expertise that currently exist. A variation on the theme is the gap between the knowledge and expertise that are readily available in rich industrial nations and those that are accessible and available to people in low-income countries, where they are needed and would materially enhance life quality and survival chances. The term was coined by the Canadian political scientist Thomas Homer-Dixon (b. 1956). See also CAPACITY BUILDING.

ingroup A sociological term for people who perceive themselves as participants in social, cultural, political, or other shared activities, because they either are involved in decision-making or have the capacity to influence decisions in some way, such as being able to vote in assemblies of representatives of the group.

inhalable particles Airborne particles 25 microns or smaller can be inhaled. Those larger than 10 microns are normally deposited in the upper respiratory tract. Particles smaller than 10 microns can penetrate to the bronchi; particles smaller than 2.5 microns can penetrate to and lodge in the alveoli. These are responsible for most of the pathogenic effects, e.g., of PNEUMOCONIOSIS.

inhalant Fumes or an aerosol suspension of a medicinal agent, taken in an inhalation. Inhalants are widely used to treat symptoms of asthma. These are often self-administered and may be overused, especially by children and teenagers, who sometimes experience dangerous cardiovascular adverse reactions attributable to excessive doses of bronchodilators.

inheritance Qualities passed on from parent(s) to child(ren); a rather vague term that can mean genetic characteristics inherited according to MENDEL'S LAWS, characteristics acquired by social imprinting from parent(s) or others in early childhood, or behaviorally, by mimicking parents or others. The word also means a bequest received from a deceased relative.

inhibition 1. In biology, suppression or cessation of a function, e.g., a neurological, endocrinological, or enzyme-mediated activity. 2. Reduced or prevented muscle activity by conscious or sometimes by subconscious action. 3. In psychology and psychoanalysis, restraint of an instinct, e.g., sexual attraction, by moral, ethical, or legal constraints.

initiator In the language of behavioral scientists in the educational field, an initiator is a creator of an innovation, i.e., a new idea or practice that is progressively adopted by others. See also INNOVATORS.

injection drug A drug that is taken into the body by injecting it into a muscle or a vein. In common usage, the term often applies to illicit drug use.

injection (or intravenous) drug use A term almost always used in the context of illicit drug use, often self-administration, perhaps with shared needles and enhanced risk of blood-borne HIV and other infections.

injunction A court-ordered legal process that restrains an individual or group from taking action that otherwise they would, or might, take.

injury Damage caused by external force applied to the body. The "force" may be physical, e.g., direct penetrating or blunt trauma, heat, a chemical substance, or, more loosely speaking, it may be an emotive force, such as libelous or slanderous language directed against a person or group. In the context of taxonomy and classification, the word "injury" is preferred to "accident" in the ICD and in official documents, such as those of the WHO. Premature death and permanent disability as a result of injury are very large public health problems everywhere, including low-income countries as well as affluent nations. Injury is a particularly common public health problem among children, and among adolescents and young adults, predominantly males.

injury prevention An important aspect of public health. The term applies to injury prevention in traffic, industry, school, home, and recreational settings. Injury prevention is conducted through education, behavior change, elimination or minimizing of environmental and occupational hazards, and use of warning signs and labels, protective clothing, and safety equipment.

inmate A rather pejorative word for someone who resides in an institution, especially a custodial institution, such as a prison or secure mental hospital.

inner city An ill-defined term describing the central business and commercial zone of a city, sometimes used when this zone has decayed as businesses and commercial activity have relocated to suburban malls with more abundant car parking facilities. The inner city then may become a wasteland of slum housing whose occupants often have multiple social and health problems. However, large general hospitals were usually located in inner cities in earlier times, and many remain there. A further stage of GENTRIFICATION has occurred and has revitalized and renewed the prosperity of many formerly decayed inner city zones.

innovation-diffusion theory A theory to explain the way innovative ideas and concepts spread through society or portions of society, such as members of the medical profession. The theory describes the conceptual framework and the role of community and professional leaders, word of mouth, and communication methods such as the Internet, television, and other media.

innovator(s) The person(s) in the population who first use(s) a new idea, behavior, or practice. The concept is regarded as an important aspect of dissemination of new ideas and beliefs in health promotion and health education. In the theory of health promotion and health education, innovators are those who first adopt the creative ideas of INITIATOR(s), which are spread by disseminators to early (and late) adopters.

innumeracy Lack of comprehension of numbers, what they signify, and how to add, subtract, multiply, and divide.

inoculation See VACCINATION.

inpatient A sick, injured, or convalescent person who occupies a bed in a hospital.

insanity A term in lay and legal language to describe a mental disorder severe enough to impair the capacity to make essential decisions or to be responsible for criminal conduct. Psychiatrists have discarded the word in favor of PSYCHOSIS, which is a more precise designation for sufficiently impaired capacity to make decisions. The law recognizes temporary insanity, but the psychiatric identification of this condition is sometimes hotly debated in law courts.

insect A member of the phylum *Arthropoda*, class *Insecta*, a large class of segmented arthropods, animals with head, thorax, and abdomen and an exoskeleton, usually with three pairs of legs and two pairs of wings on the thorax. Typically they have antennae and segmented eyes that are anatomically and physiologically different from mammalian eyes. Many insects live in symbiosis with other species, including humans, and some play an essential role in human economy, e.g., by pollinating fruit and flowers, but others are agricultural pests, competing against humans for cultivated crops, or domestic pests that foul stored food. Some insects are disease carriers, either passive carriers, such as flies and coc roaches, or active disease VECTORS, in which pathogenic microorganisms undergo essential developmental stages before they can be transmitted to the human host for the next stage of their life cycle, where they cause human disease. Some insects cause disease directly, for example by infesting the skin or through poisonous bites or chemical sensitivity. In numbers of species and in biomass, insects are the dominant class of animal life forms on earth.

insecticide A substance that kills insect pests. There are several well-defined categories, including systemic poisons and nerve poisons, such as the acetylcholine inhibitors, which are sometimes harmful to human health. See also PESTICIDE.

INSERM Institut National de la Santé et de la Recherche Médicale. The French national institute for health and medical research, roughly equivalent to the NATIONAL INSTITUTES OF HEALTH (NIH) in the United States or the MEDICAL RESEARCH COUNCIL (MRC) in the United Kingdom. See http://www.inserm.fr for details.

in-service training An educational method, especially in nursing (including public health nursing), in which those who are learning are at the same time assisting in providing health care.

insolation A measure of the amount of exposure to solar (actinic) radiation, which varies with latitude, being greatest at the equator and lowest at the poles.

insomnia A common SLEEP DISORDER, consisting of sleeplessness or insufficient sleep to satisfy metabolic needs. It may take any of several forms: inability to fall asleep, wakefulness after a brief and insufficient period of sleep, or repeated wakeful periods during hours normally spent asleep. The causes include environmental factors such as noise, uncomfortable conditions for sleeping, anxiety, depression, and physical conditions, such as urinary frequency.

instar The intermediate stage of insect molting, usually between two larval stages or between the larva and imago stages.

instinct An inherent, perhaps genetically determined behavior, in contrast to a learned behavior. Instincts explain much of the stereotypical behavior of insects, animals, and birds. Human instincts are a topic of debate. There is an instinct for self-preservation that behavioral scientists believe may be made manifest in aggressive behavior, and there is a reproductive or sex instinct. In urban civilized society, learned behaviors are used to suppress or control instincts that might otherwise be disruptive to social harmony, but this is often difficult with adolescent youth and helps to account for many teenage pregnancies and cases of sexually transmitted diseases in young people.

Institute of Medicine (IOM) A nonprofit membership organization, established by the US National Academy of Sciences in 1970, that identifies, studies, and reports on medically relevant issues and problems, including many in the field of public health. The 1988 report *The Future of Public Health* is among many important documents produced under IOM auspices. For details and current activities, see http://www.iom.edu/.

institution 1. An edifice accessible to the public that provides services of some kind, e.g., health services. 2. In the social sciences, an established component of social structure composed of socially or culturally assigned meanings, roles, norms, customs, etc., as in the institution of the family, organized religion, or legal and political systems.

institutionalization The process of becoming dependent upon an institution for care and social support or of placing someone in such a facility. Also, the process of an attitude or behavior being perpetuated in an organization, as in INSTITUTIONAL RACISM.

institutional neurosis A psychiatric disorder in which a person confined for a long period in a hospital, mental hospital, or prison assumes a dependent role, passively accepts the paternalist approach of those in charge, and often develops symptoms and signs associated with restricted horizons, such as increasing passivity and lack of motivation to cooperate in rehabilitation. See also ILLNESS BEHAVIOR and SICK ROLE.

institutional racism Syn: systemic racism. A situation in which staff members in an institution, such as a hospital, government department, educational establishment, or police force, share a collective prejudicial attitude toward members of a racial or ethnic group different from their own. This attitude tends to be communicated to new staff members and thus to be perpetuated. It may be localized to a particular site, but sometimes it pervades an entire organization, such as all or most of the components of a health care or law enforcement system.

institutional review board (IRB) The term used in the United States for the standing committee of a hospital, medical school, or other health service facility that is responsible for reviewing proposals to conduct research that involves human subjects and plays a role in other ways, for instance overseeing fiscal affairs..

instrumental error A systematic measurement error caused by faulty or inaccurate measuring instruments, defective reagents, etc.

insulation Protective layer against fluctuations in external conditions or circumstances, or a protective shield for the outside world against harm from what is beneath or behind the insulation. Insulating material may itself be harmful to health; e.g., asbestos that was used for many years to insulate against heat or cold is a carcinogen, as are PCBs used as electrical insulators.

insulation workers This term usually applies to workers who install or remove asbestos insulation and are at risk of asbestosis, asbestos-induced lung cancer, and mesothelioma. It also describes workers in the electric cable industry, where occupational risks include exposure to synthetic rubber compounds associated with bladder cancer or vinyl chloride associated with hemangiosarcoma.

insulin An essential hormone produced by the β islet cells of the pancreas. It is a polypeptide that plays an essential role in carbohydrate and fat metabolism; encourages the uptake, utilization, and storage of lipids as triglycerides; and prevents the breakdown of protein. Insulin is required to treat type 1 or insulin-dependent diabetes.

insulin-dependent diabetes mellitus (IDDM) Syn: juvenile diabetes, type 1 diabetes. It is important to detect and treat this disease as early in its natural history as possible because if it is untreated or inadequately treated and other risk factors, such as hypertension, exist, renal, retinal, and other complications are more common and often more serious.

insurance An economic and financial system to provide protection from costs incurred by loss of earning capacity, premature death, or various other mishaps, by making individual payments into a collective pool from which funds are drawn as needed by individuals to pay in whole or in part for required services or goods. This system is widely used in all Organization for Economic Co-operation and Development (OECD) nations and some others, to provide insurance against the costs of medical and hospital care and pharmaceutical remedies. In most nations where they exist, medical and hospital insurance systems are publicly administered, universal, and at least partly tax supported, but in these respects, as in many others, the United States is an exception, providing only partial publicly financed tax-supported insurance for the elderly, the disabled, and persons on welfare.

integrated pest management (IPM) A system for dealing with pests intended to reduce and ultimately eliminate the use of ecologically harmful pesticides, i.e., herbicides and insecticides, and to replace them with crop and livestock management methods that do not require toxic or harmful pesticides. The philosophy is to use chemicals only when absolutely necessary, rather than to use them as a first resort, as is now often the case.

integrated pollution prevention and control A system established in the European Union that operates at the planning stage of a proposed development and begins by considering how the proposed development could affect ecosystems and human health, taking into account the necessary measures to eliminate as far as possible any adverse effects that the development might have. High priority is given to measures intended to prevent pollution or contamination of the air, water, soil, and food. This system came into operation in the European Union following a legislative directive in 1996. See http://europa.eu.int/comm/environment/ippc/.

integrated prevention and control of disease A strategy advocated in primary care that combines active prophylaxis of conditions, such as respiratory infections, sexually transmitted diseases, and other communicable diseases, with interventions to treat and cure these diseases. An equivalent strategy has been developed for major noncommunicable disorders in the COUNTRYWIDE INTEGRATED NONCOMMUNICABLE DISEASE INTERVENTION (CINDI) project, modeled after the Finnish North Karelia project, now active in more than 20 countries under WHO auspices.

integrated vector management (IVM) A set of evidence-based, decision-making procedures for the planning, delivery, and evaluation of sustainable combinations of vector control measures with a measurable impact on transmission risks. This began in the Eastern Mediterranean Region of the WHO and has been adopted everywhere that vector-borne diseases are a problem. The combination of interventions has a sequential hierarchy, starting with locally suitable environmental management and personal protection, to which may be added biological control and, as a final resort, chemical interventions toward the desired level of transmission risk reduction. IVM includes both vector control interventions and the assessment and regulation of other sectors (e.g., irrigation, transport, urban planning, and development); it considers all options for intersectoral action and applies the principle of decision making at a level as close as possible to the community. IVM is compatible with health sector reform, in particular decentralization, and emphasizes economic aspects of the various options, including synergies resulting from their combination. For details and current status, see http://www.emro.who.int/rbm/PDF/GlobalStratFrameIVM.pdf.

integrated waste management A system of waste disposal in which all parties participate in the decision-making process to arrive at workable solutions to the problems of waste disposal.

integration Blending and linking together of individuals and groups in ways that are intended to minimize or eliminate differences and their potentially adverse effects on members of some groups.

As applied to people in heterogeneous populations, the process is fraught with social and emotional tensions, and its ultimate success or failure may depend on a combination of political leadership and the presence or absence of other causes of social tension. One important outcome of successful integration is usually improved health levels among previously disadvantaged groups. In the health care system, horizontal integration links a group of hospitals, clinics, or health departments that all offer more or less comparable services in order to reduce administrative overhead costs, and vertical integration links a hierarchy from generalized to superspecialized health care services.

integrity 1. In biology, the state of being whole, intact, with all bodily systems functioning and, by implication, capable of withstanding threats, e.g., from invading pathogens. 2. In ethics, this is one of the virtues. It means morally honest and resistant to temptation or dishonorable conduct.

intellectual property A creative work, such as poetry, literature, or musical composition, or a device or invention that can be patented or copyrighted. Legally, the term applies to patents, trademarks, designs, copyright, and other tangible and original products of the human intellect. The intellectual property system offers incentives by recognizing and rewarding inventors and creators for their endeavors, encouraging research and development. The system contributes to a balance between inventors' rights and the public interest. The World Intellectual Property Organization (WIPO), an agency based in Geneva, Switzerland, oversees protection of intellectual property in 182 member states. WIPO has implemented agreements of great importance to essential drug availability and affordability. The combination of inventors' rights and the rules of the World Trade Organization can lead to decisions with adverse implications for public health, as in the case of generic drugs to prevent or treat endemic and epidemic diseases in low-income countries. The rules require that intellectual property rights be protected, typically for 20 years, and this can impede transfer of technology to low-income countries in great need of it.

intelligence A multifaceted set of functions of the cerebral cortex that includes the ability to understand and interpret sensory input, synthesize ideas and concepts, and implement appropriate action based on all relevant input and stored memory ("experience"). It can be measured or assessed in several ways by standard tests and clinical procedures.

intelligence quotient (IQ) An indicator of individual intelligence developed by the French psychologist Alfred Binet (1857–1911) that uses specialized tests of verbal and numerical capacity and ability to grasp abstract concepts, comprehend relationships, and cope with unusual intellectual challenges. The validated test instruments, e.g., the WECHSLER SCALES for adults and for children measure several dimensions of intelligence. It is essential to ensure that individual(s) being tested are culturally familiar with the examples and concepts used in test items, but even so the validity of IQ tests is sometimes questioned.

intensive care The provision of life support facilities and monitoring equipment by medical and nursing staff, with a high ratio of staff to patients, to persons who are critically ill or injured.

intensive care unit (ICU) The acronym is widely used. Patients in ICU are more vulnerable to nosocomial infections than are less severely ill or injured patients, especially if their immune systems are compromised. Thus, the ICU is a setting for preventive, as well as therapeutic, care.

intention to treat analysis A strategy used in RANDOMIZED CONTROLLED TRIALS that aims to prevent bias due to loss of participants by including all participants in data analysis, whether or not they completed the intervention given to the group of which they were a member. Bias caused by failure to adhere to the protocol may otherwise cause one group to show differences from the baseline data that are unrelated to the effects of the intervention.

interdisciplinary teamwork A frequently used approach to problem solving in public health, in which professional staff from several disciplines work collaboratively on complex cases, such as those involving public or personal health problems associated with poverty, unemployment, or ethnic tension, preferably with case conferences and periodic assessments of progress. Examples include a team comprising a nurse, social worker, psychologist, representative of a religious faith, and physician.

interest group See PRESSURE GROUP.

interferon The name given to the first identified effective antiviral agent. Interferons are actually a class of naturally occurring substances in the body that help to regulate immunity and have an inhibitory action on reproduction of some viruses.

intergovernmental organization (IGO) A standing or ad hoc institution, committee, or agency, usually established at the initiative of the United

Nations, with representatives drawn from all or most UN member states. UN agencies are intergovernmental organizations.

Intergovernmental Panel on Climate Change (IPCC) A group of natural, physical, and biological scientists, with economists, political scientists, etc., that has worked under the auspices of the United Nations since the late 1980s on studies of factors affecting worldwide and regional trends of climate patterns, seeking to identify the determinants of climate change, predict future climatic trends, and reach conclusions that can be used by policy-makers to inform decisions about appropriate courses of action to adapt to and mitigate climate change. See http://www.ipcc .ch for current status reports and regional and global projections.

intermediate host The animal, insect, or occasionally human in which an infectious pathogen passes a developmental stage preceding the adult stage. Insects such as mosquitoes, ticks, and blackflies; freshwater snails; animals; and fish are usually the intermediate hosts of pathogens that cause human disease. One exception is HYDATID DISEASE, in which sheep, and sometimes humans, are the intermediate host of a helminth that passes its adult stage in canines.

intern Specifically, a recent medical or health science graduate who is gaining experience under supervision in a hospital or other health care setting. In more general terms, an apprentice in any professional setting, e.g., an intern in a legislative assembly.

internally displaced persons The term used by the UNITED NATIONS HIGH COMMISSIONER FOR REFUGEES (UNHCR), the INSTITUTE OF MEDICINE (IOM), and other agencies to describe persons who have been forcibly uprooted from their homes and habitat by violent armed conflict or by disasters, such as floods, earthquakes, or prolonged droughts, and remain within the borders of their own country. If they cross the border, they are designated as REFUGEES.

internal validity See VALIDITY.

international agencies and organizations A general term for any and all agencies in the international field, including multilateral, bilateral, and intergovernmental agencies.

International Agency for Research on Cancer (IARC) A large, semiautonomous division of the World Health Organization based in Lyon, France, that initiates, conducts, and sponsors a range of research studies of cancer, including fundamental research on the molecular biology, immunology, genetics, etc., of cancer, epidemiological studies, assessment of carcinogens, and efficacy of therapeutic regimens. See http://www .iarc.fr for details.

International Bank for Reconstruction and Development See WORLD BANK.

International Classification of Diseases (ICD) A systematic arrangement of all specific names, diagnostic labels, etc., for health-related conditions, i.e., diseases, injuries, and routine procedures, into groups according to their mode of causation, or body system affected, with numbers assigned to each. The terminology and details of grouping are determined by internationally representative experts who report to their governments and to the World Health Organization, which publishes periodic revisions at intervals of approximately 10 to 15 years. The 10th revision, called the *International Statistical Classification of Diseases and Related Health Problems* (ICD-10), was approved by the World Health Assembly in 1989, published in 1990 and had come into general use in most nations by 2003. This has 22 chapters and more than 1,000 specific categories with room for expansion. See http://www3.who.int/icd/vol1htm2003/fr-icd.htm.

International Classification of Functioning, Disability and Health (ICF) Sometimes known as ICIDH-2, this is the revised and updated version of the INTERNATIONAL CLASSIFICATION OF IMPAIRMENT, DISABILITY, AND HANDICAP, originally published in 1980. The ICF, published in 2001, corrected some discrepancies in the original classification system and underwent a title change, at least partly because of emotional and political arguments against use of the words "impairment" and "handicap." Impairments are now called "limitations of body function or structure," disability has become "activity limitation," and the new term for handicap is "restriction of participation." Full details and discussion are available at http://www.who.int/classifications/icf/en/.

International Classification of Health Interventions Originally called the International Classification of Procedures, this is a listing of approved names and descriptions of diagnostic and therapeutic interventions that is suitable for use in summary statistics compiled by national and regional agencies in the health field. See http://www .who.int/classifications/ichi/en/.

International Classification of Health Problems in Primary Care (ICHPPC) This taxonomic system allows for use of PROBLEM ORIENTED MEDICAL RECORDS, instead of or as well as ICD diagnostic categories and is oriented to the kinds of problems encountered in physicians' offices in rich industrial nations such as the United States and Australia. The use of problems, rather than precise diagnostic categories, is both a strength in recognizing inability to identify many underlying disease processes encountered in primary care and a weakness in introducing many sources of inaccuracy and bias in analysis of the activity of physicians in primary care. Many of its rubrics are only marginally useful or irrelevant in primary care in developing countries.

International Classification of Impairment, Disability, and Handicap (ICIDH) Now superseded by the INTERNATIONAL CLASSIFICATION OF FUNCTIONING, DISABILITY AND HEALTH (ICF), this is a taxonomy and numerical coding system for all forms of impairment, disability, and handicap. It has had considerable favorable impact on the perception of disability and handicap by professional staff in the health services.

International Classification of Primary Care (ICPC) The official classification system of the World Organization of National Colleges, Academies and Academic Associations of General Practitioners/Family Physicians (WONCA), prepared in collaboration with working groups from WHO and WONCA. This comprises reasons for encounter, diagnostic categories, and interventions (treatments, referrals, etc.). Its complexity is a deterrent to widespread adoption, but where it has been used, it has provided much valuable data for detailed analysis of aspects of the process and outcome of primary medical care. A summary of the classification is available at http://www.adfammed.org/online_resources/ICPC_Wonca_brochure290304.pdf.

International Classification of Procedures (ICP) The official classification of diagnostic and therapeutic procedures, now called INTERNATIONAL CLASSIFICATION OF HEALTH INTERVENTIONS.

International Committee of Red Cross and Red Crescent Societies The worldwide consortium of humanitarian societies based in Geneva. It arose from the initiative of the Swiss banker Jean Henri Dunant (1828–1910), who established the International Red Cross Society after witnessing the horrific plight of victims of the battle of Solferino in 1859. The purpose of the Red Cross was originally to provide aid and comfort to war wounded and prisoners of war. It has broadened to include provision of aid in natural disasters, such as earthquakes and famines. For details and current activities see http://www.icrc.org/eng.

International Council for Control of Iodine Deficiency Disorders (ICCIDD) A nongovernmental organization founded in 1986 to reduce and ultimately eliminate iodine deficiency disorders, by assisting governments and international agencies to establish and sustain programs of salt iodization (by adding potassium iodate to salt in the regions of the world where deficiency is endemic, leading to cretinism and myxedema). Iodine deficiency is the most common preventable cause of brain damage in the world, with more than 2 billion people in 130 countries at risk. The ICCIDD provides expertise to assist in monitoring, using urinary iodine levels for this purpose, and to ensure that the programs are sustainable. The organization's program was later broadened to include addition of dietary micronutrients to prevent malnutrition. The activities and status are summarized at http://www.iccidd.org and in the newsletter at http://www.iccidd.org/newsletter/newsletterindex.html.

international health The branch of public health practice concerned with health problems that transcend national frontiers to affect regions or the entire world, and that is primarily devoted to health care problems of developing (low-income) nations. It incorporates elements from clinical specialties, notably pediatrics, obstetrics, and emergency medicine; includes ideas from cultural anthropology, economics, politics, social demography, management sciences, etc.; and aims to elevate levels of health indicators in developing countries and regions to approximately the level of rich industrial nations, using strategies and tactics, including social and gender development, as well as traditional public health approaches, such as health education, nutritional enhancement, vaccination programs, primary care services, etc.

International Health Regulations The formal set of regulations adopted by the World Health Assembly in 1969, aimed at ensuring greater effectiveness in the control of serious communicable diseases that often occur in epidemic form and cross international borders. The revised regulations, approved by the World Health Assembly in 2005, cover essential epidemic surveillance and control procedures, requirements for immediate notification of dangerous outbreaks, isolation, vaccination, and effective treatment, where applicable. Details and information about current epidemics are at http://www.who.int/csr/ihr/en/.

International Labour Organization (ILO) The agency established by the League of Nations after the conclusion of the Peace Conference that attempted to resolve the world's problems after the World War I. The ILO was one of the few positive achievements of the Peace Conference. It has greatly helped to improve working conditions in industry and agriculture, applying pressure to limit dangerous working conditions and child labor, improve working conditions for women, provide social security for workers, and much else. See http://www.ilo.ch for details.

International Monetary Fund (IMF) A United Nations agency founded in 1946 to maintain international financial cooperation and stability, promote trade, and assist poor nations with short-term loans at times of financial crisis. The IMF advises on ways to achieve financial stability, but some of its approaches, i.e., those requiring STRUCTURAL ADJUSTMENT (a collaborative program with the WORLD BANK), can impose conditions that disrupt local economies and cause hardship for people in low-income countries.

International Nomenclature of Disease A systematic comprehensive taxonomy aimed at listing all the accepted names of all diseases, procedures, etc., compiled under the auspices of the Council for International Organizations of the Medical Sciences and the World Health Organization. The criteria for official names include specificity, absence of ambiguity, simplicity, and that the name be self-descriptive. The aim is to produce a master list of officially recommended names that all agree would comprise an official taxonomy. Unfortunately, budget cuts led to suspension of this WHO project.

International Organization for Migration (IOM) The main intergovernmental organization concerned with migration, established in 1951 to assist in resettling many millions of people displaced from their homes and habitats by wars in many parts of the world in the preceding decades. It is based in Geneva. In 2005, it had 109 member states and 24 states with observer status. IOM is dedicated to promoting humane and orderly migration. It provides services and advice to governments and migrants, promoting international cooperation on migration issues and the search for practical solutions to migration problems. It provides humanitarian assistance to migrants and INTERNALLY DISPLACED PERSONS in need, and works closely with governmental, intergovernmental, and nongovernmental partners. See http://www.iom.int/ for details.

International Organization for Standardization (ISO) The worldwide private federation that is often incorrectly called the International Standards Organization because of its acronym. Its aim is to reach agreement on many kinds of standards, ranging from scientific and technical standards to those related to commercial goods and services, such as credit cards. Members of the federation are representatives of national groups fulfilling this function. The member organization for the United States and Canada is the American National Standards Institute (ANSI).

International Programme on Chemical Safety (IPCS) A joint initiative of the United Nations Environmental Programme, the International Labour Organization, and the World Health Organization aimed mainly at reducing risks of exposure to toxic substances in the workplace, by establishing safe exposure levels and occupational hygiene standards.

International Standards Organization (ISO) See INTERNATIONAL ORGANIZATION FOR STANDARDIZATION (ISO).

Internet The communication network of computers that transmits data, text, and pictures all over the world by electronic signals from one computer to others, using telephone lines and modems or wireless systems and satellite receivers. The most widely used features are e-mail, which from modest beginnings in the early 1980s has expanded at a prodigious rate, so by early in the 21st century, an estimated 800 to 900 million people used it regularly for work or recreational purposes; and the WORLD WIDE WEB, an enormous, amorphous repository of information that is stored on WEB SITES in various classified ways that facilitate retrieval more or less systematically. The Internet has become an integral part of public health practice, replacing the telephone as the means of communication, for instance for contagious disease outbreak notification and for many other purposes.

internment Confinement of people in a camp or prison-like custodial institution, usually aliens in times of war and prisoners of war. Conditions in internment camps can be unhealthy. International agreements, not always respected, give the Red Cross and other neutral agencies rights of access and sometimes of intervention to ensure humane treatment of internees.

interobserver variation Sometimes called observer error, but "error" is an inappropriate word for this phenomenon. A pervasive problem in all observational studies is that when two or more people examine a patient, an x-ray, an electrocardiogram, a microscopic slide of tissue, blood cells, or other natural phenomena, they do not always agree on what they see and on its significance. The prevalence and magnitude of observer variation can be considerable. When experienced and competent specialists such as radiologists or hematologists examine a series of chest x-rays or blood slides, they may report different findings in 5 to 15 cases per 100. The differences of opinion are not always clinically important but have serious consequences if a life-threatening lesion is overlooked.

Observer variation can be devastating for candidates if their answers to examination questions are assessed by a careless, opinionated, or incompetent examiner. Discovery of very high rates of variation in grading of examinations prompted the use of objective tests.

interpersonal skills Syn: people skills. Ability to communicate with, identify with, and relate easily to others, regardless of their social and cultural background. This is regarded as an important asset of public health workers and other kinds of health professionals, often mentioned in job descriptions and the like, but objective assessment is often difficult to assess.

interpersonal violence Syn: intentional violence. A general term sometimes used in statistical tables for assault, rape, murder, and other forms of intentional violence directed against others.

intersectoral action A term espoused by health-related and other international agencies meaning action that involves several sectors of society, for instance action by the health, education, housing, and local government sectors to enhance community health.

interval cancer A cancer that develops after a cancer screening test, such as a PAP SMEAR or a mammography examination, and before the next scheduled screening or physical examination.

intervention A general term covering any and all actions taken by health professionals aimed at preventing, curing, or relieving a health problem.

intervention strategy A formally designed plan of action to deal with a health problem, usually at a community or population level.

intervention study A formally designed scientific study, often using epidemiological methods, aimed at assessing or evaluating the effects of an intervention strategy.

interviewer's manual The set of instructions that interviewers are required to follow when conducting interviews in a survey. A hallmark of quality in research based on personal interviews is the development and use of an interviewer's manual that is often very detailed and is used to train interviewers before they begin their work.

interview schedule A survey instrument used to deliver a formal, carefully designed sequence of questions to the subjects of an investigation, such as a household survey of health status, use of medical services, or health-related behavior. Under ideal circumstances, interview schedules are designed by experts in this activity, pretested on a small sample, and pilot-tested in the field to assess acceptability and validated by requestioning a sample of those already interviewed. In the highest-quality interview-based research studies, all interviewers are carefully trained to ask questions in a standardized manner and required to follow the procedures laid out in an interviewer's manual.

interview survey A SURVEY in which respondents are asked questions in face-to-face interviews, i.e., orally, rather than replying to written questions. This has the advantage that respondents do not know what questions are to come when responding to a particular question, so their answers are unlikely to be influenced by their perception of what the interviewer would "like" them to say or really wants to know. Thus, interviews are a good method of assessing attitudes, beliefs, values, and opinions. On the other hand, they are labor intensive and therefore more costly compared with self-completed questionnaires.

intestinal botulism Syn: infant botulism. A dangerous condition resulting from ingestion of spores of *Clostridium botulinum*, which grow and produce the toxin. This can cause fatal toxicity, or the floppy infant syndrome with poor muscle tone, respiratory insufficiency, etc. One mode of infection is ingestion of the *C. botulinum* spores in unpasteurized honey, which is sometimes given to infants or used to sweeten the soother (pacifier) intended to quiet the infant.

intestinal flora The microorganisms that normally inhabit the gastrointestinal tract, mainly the small and large intestines. Most are commensal or, in some instances, symbiotic, e.g., synthesizing vitamin K, which is essential to prevent capillary hemorrhages. Pathogenic organisms can also inhabit the gut, where they may cause disease or provide a nidus of infection for others to whom the pathogens are transmitted, commonly during food-handling.

intimacy A close emotional relationship. In legal parlance, "intimacy" is a euphemism for sexual intercourse. An intimate partner is a spouse or person who shares a long term sexual relationship.

intoxication A condition in which the function of the brain and/or other vital organs is impaired by the action of a toxic substance. The term covers impairment caused by prescribed or illicit drugs, workplace exposures, etc., as well as alcohol used to excess.

intraobserver variation Syn: intraobserver error. Differing readings of the same phenomenon by the same observer on second or other subsequent review. With chest x-rays, the same observer reports different findings on re-examination of the same set of x-rays about once in 20 films; i.e., the intraobserver variation rate is about 5%.

intraocular pressure The pressure of the aqueous fluid in the anterior chamber of the eyes. The pressure is elevated in GLAUCOMA.

intrauterine device (IUD) A contraceptive method that relies on the presence inside the uterus of an object made of plastic or metal that prevents implantation of the fertilized ovum. An IUD is believed to work by thickening the mucus around the cervix, thereby acting as a barrier to the passage of sperm. An IUD may cause a state of chronic low-grade inflammation and sometimes causes an offensive vaginal discharge. The method is frowned upon by those who believe human life begins at conception. However, it has the advantage of being permanently in place, so it provides protection against pregnancy through unplanned or casual acts of sexual intercourse.

intrauterine growth retardation A condition in which fetal development proceeds more slowly than normal, developmental milestones are reached later than expected, and prospects of delivery of a healthy full-term infant are diminished. It is defined as weight less than the 10th percentile for a given gestational age. It is caused by malnutrition, maternal disease, and placental abnormality. It may be associated with increased risk of cardiovascular disease and hypertension in later life. See also BARKER HYPOTHESIS.

intravenous drug user Usually abbreviated to IVDU or IDU. A term mainly applied to persons who use illicit street drugs, often under unhygienic conditions. Sharing needles with other users is a common feature of the subculture of IVDUs. Consequently, there is a high risk of transmitting blood-borne infections, including HIV and hepatitis B and C. Because many such persons finance their addiction by crime or prostitution, they may constitute a public health risk to others as well as endangering their own health.

intrinsic incubation period The period required for the development of a parasite or pathogen in a definitive host before the parasite or pathogen can be transmitted to or infect the intermediate host. For instance, the intrinsic incubation period for malaria in the human host is 7 to 30 days, varying with the type of malaria parasite. There is a PREPATENT PERIOD of about 6 to 16 days from the bite of an infected mosquito to appearance of the parasites in peripheral blood, then usually an additional period during which premonitory symptoms

occur. There is a wide range of intrinsic incubation periods for parasitic infections with hemoflagellates, helminths, etc.

intubation Insertion of a tube into a bodily orifice. The term is usually applied specifically to the insertion of a laryngeal tube to ensure adequate ventilation of the lungs in unconscious patients or as part of anesthetic procedures.

intuition Capacity or ability to understand a principle or abstract concept, sometimes one that has eluded others, without the exercise of conscious reasoning or thought. Intuition is sometimes regarded with suspicion as a dubious way to arrive at decisions, but creative scientists, such as the British biologist and Nobel laureate Peter Medawar (1915–1987) have emphasized the importance of intuition in the initiating stages of original scientific discoveries. See also SCIENTIFIC METHOD.

invasive procedure A diagnostic or therapeutic procedure involving penetration of the body's integrity, as by insertion of a needle, an incision through the skin, or use of an endoscopic device. Invasive procedures always carry some risks, for example, of introducing infectious pathogens.

inverse care law The availability of good medical care tends to vary inversely with the needs of the population served. This inverse care law operates more completely where medical care is most exposed to market forces, and less so where such exposure is reduced. This "law" is based on observations published by the British general practitioner Julian Tudor Hart (b. 1927) in 1971. It is described at http://www.sochealth.co.uk/history/inversecare.htm.

inverse square law The mathematical law formulated by Isaac Newton (1642–1727) stating that the gravitational attractive force diminishes inversely as the square of the distance between the bodies. The same law applies to natural phenomena, such as ionizing radiation and illumination of a surface by a source of light, and these applications of the inverse square law are important in setting standards for exposure to ionizing radiation and illumination of workplaces.

inversion layer An atmospheric phenomenon in which the temperature increases with increasing altitude, rather than the reverse, which is the usual disposition whereby layers of warm air occur below layers of colder air. Inversion layers can trap humid, perhaps smoggy, air and thus cause an environmental condition that is hazardous for people with chronic respiratory disease.

in vitro Descriptive of a procedure or test of biological material that is conducted in a laboratory setting using tissue cultures or reagents but not an actual living organism.

in vitro fertilization (IVF) Fertilization of an ovum under laboratory conditions, using the mother's ovum obtained by laparoscopic extraction, and sperm (usually obtained by masturbation or by aspiration from the vas deferens); after observation of the first few cell divisions, the fertilized ovum is implanted in the mother's uterus. Multiple pregnancy is a common outcome.

in vivo Descriptive of a procedure or test that makes use of living organs, or living animals, in which the biological processes involved can be directly observed.

involuntary smoking A more suitable term than "passive smoking" to describe inhalation of air contaminated by tobacco smoke.

iodine (I) A halogen element, a brownish crystalline solid that is an essential element for human metabolism. Iodine is required for the production of thyroxine. In regions where iodine is deficient, or where iodine uptake is inhibited by enzymes in vegetables such as kale where this is large part of the diet, IODINE DEFICIENCY DISORDERS, cretinism and myxedema are a common public health problem.

iodine deficiency disorders (IDD) This term refers to all the effects of iodine deficiency on growth and development in human and animal populations, which can be prevented by correction of the iodine deficiency. These effects include miscarriages, stillbirths, congenital abnormalities, varying degrees of fetal brain damage, including cretinism, goiter, dwarfism, and impaired mental function at all ages. Usually iodine deficiency is due to the absence of environmental compounds containing iodine salts. This is most common in alpine regions. Another possible cause is a diet rich in green leafy vegetables, such as kale, which contain an enzyme that blocks iodine uptake by the thyroid gland. The end result is the same in both situations: "congenital" thyroid deficiency or cretinism, associated with mental retardation, stunted growth, goiter, characteristic facial appearance, and slow metabolism. In adults the main manifestation is myxedema and goiter, often with extreme thyroid enlargement. Both conditions respond to supplementary iodine, and in infants and children this can prevent permanent intellectual damage.

ionizing radiation Electromagnetic radiation with wavelength shorter than 10^{-7} meters. These wavelengths comprise x-rays, gamma rays, and cosmic rays. All have some properties of waves, e.g., travel at the speed of light, and some characteristics of high-energy penetrating particles, which may be the basis for their biological activity, which can be mutagenic, teratogenic, and carcinogenic.

IPCS See INTERNATIONAL PROGRAMME ON CHEMICAL SAFETY.

iron (Fe) Metallic element that possesses the capacity to be magnetized, is an essential element in the production of hemoglobin, and is very widely used in many industrial applications, especially in the manufacture of steel.

iron deficiency anemia A condition caused by inadequate intake of dietary ingredients containing iron compounds and/or chronic continuing iron loss in slow bleeding, as from peptic ulcer, severe menorrhagia, hookworm disease, or other chronic blood loss. The features include pallor, lassitude, weakness, and debility. The treatment is replacement iron, but treating the underlying cause to prevent further blood loss is of equal or greater importance.

iron lung The lay term for the type of respirator invented by the American industrial hygienist Philip Drinker (1893–1972). This works by encasing the body in an airtight cylinder (the iron lung), within which the air pressure is alternatively raised and lowered, producing suction that causes lungs to inflate and pressure that deflates the lungs, thus mimicking the process of inhalation and exhalation when respiratory muscles are paralyzed, e.g., by POLIOMYELITIS. In the severe polio epidemics from the 1930s to the early 1950s, the use of iron lungs saved many lives.

irrigation 1. The use of canals, trenches, sprinklers, etc., to provide water to arid regions. The water may be drawn from a river (e.g., the Nile), a reservoir, artesian well, etc. Prolonged use can adversely affect soil chemistry and ultimately can render a fertile region unproductive. 2. In many surgical and other therapeutic procedures, sterile saline is often used to cleanse or wash an infected wound or other lesion.

irritant A substance that causes irritation and often inflammation, especially of mucous membranes and surfaces. It may be solid, liquid, or gaseous, and is commonly acidic or alkaline.

ischemic heart disease A condition in which restricted blood flow or oxygen supply to the heart muscle (myocardium) impairs its efficiency. Often this causes cramp-like ischemic pain, angina pectoris, or myocardial infarction, which is often fatal.

It is usually caused by CORONARY HEART DISEASE but can have other causes, including severe anoxia. It can be detected by medical history taking, physical examination, electrocardiography, or screening procedures embodying all these. It is sometimes treated by coronary artery bypass graft surgery. The risk of occurrence can often be reduced by low-cholesterol diet, exercise, and avoidance of smoking.

island population A genetically isolated population, sometimes literally on an island although the term applies to any discrete population group that breeds (intermarries) only with others who belong to the group. Some ethnic groups that seek to preserve their ethnic identity behave as island populations even when living in an urban area among many other people Characteristically, island populations have a limited gene pool, within which harmful recessive characteristics may exist and be expressed increasingly, often in the phenotype after several generations.

ISO See INTERNATIONAL ORGANIZATION FOR STANDARDIZATION (ISO).

isocyanide A compound of nitrogen and carbon with an organic or inorganic radical that is the basis for important industrial chemicals, including pesticides, some of which are highly toxic. For example, methyl isocyanate was responsible for the industrial disaster in BHOPAL, India, in 1984.

isolate n. 1. A pure culture of an organism. 2. In genetics, a population group with a relatively limited gene pool, in which mating takes place only within the group.

isolation 1. In microbiology, the separation of one microorganism from others, usually by using serial cultures that favor the growth of one over others in the mixture. 2. In communicable disease control, separation or segregation of infected persons or animals from others for the period of communicability of the infectious agent that they harbor, in order to prevent the spread of the agent to other persons who may be susceptible to it or may spread the agent to others. Several forms of isolation are recognized and used according to the nature of the disease and the infectious agent that causes it. UNIVERSAL PRECAUTIONS are applied when an infectious pathogen could be transmitted in contaminated blood or body fluids. Strict isolation requires segregation of an infected patient in a private room; use by all attending medical and nursing personnel of gown, gloves, face mask, and goggles; and use of disinfectants before leaving the room. Contact isolation is not quite as strict, permitting more than one infected patient to share a room; mask, gown, and gloves are desirable. Respiratory isolation and tuberculosis isolation require similar precautions, but use of gloves is not essential. Enteric precautions, drainage/secretion precautions, and blood/body fluid precautions are required for patients with enteric infections or possibly infected discharging wounds, etc., and necessitate strict hygienic disposal of infected fluids or feces. See also QUARANTINE.

isoniazid A powerful antibiotic discovered and widely used in the 1950s, especially useful in the treatment of tuberculosis, until resistant organisms became prevalent.

isotopes Two or more forms of the same element that have the same atomic number but differ in mass number because they possess different numbers of neutrons in their nuclei. They have identical chemical and biological properties. In nature, many elements occur as mixtures of two or more isotopes. Radioisotopes, i.e., radioactive compounds, can be used to trace the passage of compounds containing the element through the biological transformations of metabolism, etc.

Itai-Itai disease A disease first identified in Japan, with renal osteodystrophy due to cadmium toxicity, which causes severe bone pains. Itai-Itai means "ouch-ouch."

IVDU See INTRAVENOUS DRUG USER.

ixodid ticks The common name for the family of ticks (*Ixodidae*) that carry the rickettsia causing ROCKY MOUNTAIN SPOTTED FEVER, SCRUB TYPHUS, several other rickettsial diseases, and some varieties of hemorrhagic fever. The ticks live on grass before seeking a blood meal from wild ungulates, domesticated goats and sheep, or humans.

J

jab The colloquial term used by physicians, nurses, the general public, and the media in Britain to describe an immunizing injection or other parenteral medication, derived from the warning remark of the physician or nurse, "Just a little jab," as the needle is about to penetrate.

Japanese encephalitis A common form of AR-BOVIRUS encephalitis in south and east Asia, an acute inflammatory viral infection, caused by a fla-vivirus, transmitted by Culex mosquitoes. It is prevented by vector control and elimination or exclusion of mosquitoes from contact with human hosts. Epidemics were formerly common during wet seasons of high mosquito prevalence. A vaccine developed in Japan is used to protect children and is recommended for those planning extended visits to endemic rural regions.

jargon A mixture of technical terms and slang used by members of a profession or trade that is intelligible to those in the field but partly or wholly incomprehensible to others. Anthony Murphy, quoted in the Preface to the *Dictionary of Epidemiology*, described it as "obscure and/or pretentious language, circumlocutions, invented meanings, and pomposity delighted in for its own sake." The jargon of psychiatry and related fields is called "psychobabble." Some jargon words and phrases ultimately enter standard dictionaries, but in the interests of clarity and comprehension, it is preferable when possible to avoid using jargon.

Jarman index A scoring system developed by the British general practitioner Brian Jarman (b. 1933) for the level of social deprivation in a community, using census data on percentages of old people living alone, single-parent families, children younger than 5 years of age, unskilled and unemployed persons, ethnic minorities, over-crowded dwellings, changes of address in previous year, etc. Although a valid indicator, it is not generally accepted outside the United Kingdom, and there it is less widely used than other scales, such as the TOWNSEND SCORE.

Jehovah's Witnesses A Christian sect whose members' beliefs may adversely affect their health and sometimes that of others. Their best-known belief entails refusal to accept blood transfusions. Devout Jehovah's Witnesses prefer to die rather than receive a blood transfusion, and, unless compelled by court order, they also deny transfusion for dependent children. The refusal of Witnesses to accept blood helped to motivate research on blood transfusion substitutes before the recognition that HIV and hepatitis B and C can be transmitted by blood and blood products.

Jellinek formula A formula proposed by the British physician E. M. Jellinek (1890–1963) to estimate the prevalence of chronic alcohol abuse based on the proportion of necropsies in which cirrhosis of the liver is revealed. The formula is flawed by SELECTION BIAS and has no scientific validity.

Jenner, Edward (1749–1823) The British country doctor who is credited with observing that inoculating or scarifying the skin with calf lymph infected with cowpox could prevent SMALLPOX, the procedure for which he coined the word VACCINA-TION. Jenner's work derived from the testimony of a local farmer, Benjamin Jesty, that milkmaids who had experienced cowpox did not get small-pox and from the introduction into England by Lady Mary Wortley Montagu (1689–1762) of "variolation" with dried secretions from healing small-pox blebs, which she had learned when living in Constantinople. Jenner's account, described in *An Inquiry Into the Causes and Effects of the Variolae Vaccinae* (1798), was influential in spreading the practice of VACCINATION throughout the world. See also ERADICATION OF DISEASE.

jet lag A sleep disorder familiar to all who travel across multiple (usually three or more) time zones in jet aircraft, caused by the discordance of circadian rhythm and local time at destination. It takes about 1 day for each hour of time zone difference between origin and destination of the journey to readjust to local time. A trans-Atlantic flight from the east coast of the United States to Paris or Geneva (6 hour time zone difference) ideally requires a recovery period of 5 to 6 days before sleep rhythm, mood, and intellectual functions return to normal.

jigger A variety of flea, *Tunga penetrans*, that burrows into the skin, usually on the feet, causing painful swelling.

Jim Crow laws State laws introduced mainly in the southern United States after emancipation of slaves, intended to establish permanent de facto segregation with all its adverse consequences, including those affecting health. They were declared unconstitutional by the US Supreme Court in 1954. The term derives from a line in a Kentucky min-strel song, not from the name of a person.

jimson weed an evil-smelling seasonal herb that is particularly common in the southern states of the United States. It contains several alkaloids, including atropine and hyoscine, and is used both medicinally (e.g., to treat rheumatism and asthma) and as a hallucinogen. It is harmful to fetal development and has been classified by the FDA as a toxic substance.

job analysis A set of procedures in OCCUPATIONAL HEALTH/MEDICINE and ENVIRONMENTAL HEALTH in which the activities that a worker undertakes are studied to identify and correct potential sources of occupational risk. It may consist only of a documentary study of tasks or include ergonomic studies, direct observation of working conditions, interviews, or combinations of these.

job description A formal statement of the tasks expected of persons in particular positions in a workforce comprising many varieties of specialties, technologies, etc. By extension, a statement of the roles, tasks, and responsibilities expected of any worker in any organization.

Johannesburg Summit See WORLD SUMMIT ON SUSTAINABLE DEVELOPMENT.

Joint Commission on Accreditation of Healthcare Organizations (JCAHO) A nonprofit organization sponsored by the American Medical Association, the American Hospital Association, and specialist associations of physicians and others that sets and maintains standards of care in American health care institutions, periodically inspecting each to ensure that standards are upheld. The organization began in 1951 as an oversight body to monitor quality of care in American hospitals and has extended its range to cover ambulatory care, health maintenance organizations, and the like, although as yet not significantly to public health agencies. See http://www.jcaho.org/ for details.

Joint United Nations Programme on HIV/AIDS Formerly the United Nations Special Programme on AIDS, this program is a direct responsibility of the UN Secretary General, in recognition of the global reach, number of cases and deaths, and unprecedented spread of the HIV/AIDS pandemic. It has direct functional connections with other UN bodies, including the International Labour Organization, United Nations Children's Fund, United Nations Development Programme, United Nations Population Fund, United Nations High Commissioner for Refugees, United Nations Office on Drugs and Crime, the World Food Programme, the United Nations Educational, Scientific and Cultural Organization, the World Bank, and the World Health Organization, collectively known as the ten cosponsors. UNAIDS is responsible for collecting, analyzing, and disseminating statistical data on AIDS and HIV infection, guiding and facilitating AIDS prevention and control programs in many countries, and advocating for greater emphasis on this huge public health problem. As of January 2006, HIV/AIDS has affected more than 42 million people and caused more than 12 million deaths. For more information and details, see http://www.unaids.org.

Jones criteria A set of criteria defined by the American cardiologist T. D. Jones (1899–1954) to confirm the diagnosis of RHEUMATIC FEVER, a formerly common systemic disease that was a sequel of acute pharyngitis caused by hemolytic streptococcal A infection and was almost always followed by chronic valvular heart disease. The criteria were revised and updated in 2000. They include streptococcal pharyngitis, fever, inflammatory arthritis of one or more large joints, elevated sedimentation rate, chorea, carditis, or mitral or other valvular incompetence (preferably confirmed by echocardiography); the criteria are useful now mainly in low-income countries and among deprived social groups in whom cases of rheumatic fever occasionally occur. The revised criteria approved by the American Heart Association in 2004 are at http://circ.ahajournals.org/cgi/content/full/106/19/2521?ck–ck. See also STREPTOCOCCAL INFECTION.

Jones, Mary Harris (1830–1930) An activist and advocate of human rights known as "Mother Jones," she played a major role in helping to reduce and eventually eliminate child labor and inhumane and unhealthy working conditions in factories, mines, and SWEATSHOPS in the United States.

joule The energy required to exert a force of one newton for a distance of one meter. At the earth's surface it is the amount of energy required to lift one kilogram 10 centimeters. It is named for the British physicist James Prescott Joule (1818–1889).

journal club A group of professionals—physicians, health scientists, and the like—who meet to discuss and critically review articles they have recently read in specialized journals in their fields of expertise. The frequency of meetings, their formality, and the extent to which members merely inform one another or critically review and discuss what they have read vary considerably. At its best, a journal club is a powerful learning tool, perhaps especially in acquainting members with cutting-edge developments in fields other than their own.

j-shaped curve A distribution curve relating risk on the Y axis to exposure level on the X axis, in which the lowest risk is associated with a moderate, rather than minimal, level of exposure. An example is the relationship of daily alcohol consumption to all-cause mortality rates, in which modest alcohol consumption is associated with lower mortality rates than total abstinence from alcohol, whereas heavy alcohol consumption leads to higher death rates. In the words of the Victorian ballad, "A little of what you fancy does you good." Interpretation of j-shaped curves may be confounded by competing risks, selection bias, and other factors.

jumping genes Mobile segments of DNA that occur in some chromosomes, associated with altered genetic activity, insertion or deletion sequences, and other features of instability.

junk DNA Segments of DNA that have been detected in the genome but have no known function. The term indicates a degree of arrogance on the part of scientists, who seem to be saying, "It has no use because we haven't discovered a use for it."

junk foods Typically, mass marketed manufactured food that has a high carbohydrate (sugar) and fat content but few essential nutrients. Marketed in attractive packages emphasizing style over substance, convenience over cost, flavor over nutritional content and food value, these appeal to people in a hurry who snack rather than dine. They are disproportionately costly but are consumed in huge quantities at entertainment venues such as sports arenas and cinemas, by preteen and teenage children at and after school, and by people watching television, where many junk foods are advertised. Examples include candy, hot dogs, potato chips, pretzels, donuts, and carbonated sweetened beverages. Because of high carbohydrate and TRANS FAT content and the fact that many who consume junk foods get insufficient exercise, frequent consumption of such foods contributes to JUVENILE OBESITY and obesity in adults, and thus is a public health problem. See also FAST FOOD.

junkie A slang expression for an addict to an illicit drug who relies on prostitution or petty theft to finance the addiction. More generally, a junkie is someone who is uncritically infatuated with a popular cause or a pastime, such as a particular style of popular music.

junk science A derogatory term for aspects of scientific inquiry and inference for which critics say the evidence is flawed or the interpretation of the evidence and conclusions based on it are unjustified. The term has been used mainly by hostile critics of particular varieties of scientific investigation, including critics of epidemiological evidence linking various exposures to outcomes such as cancer,

and critics of climate scientists who have concluded from available evidence that the earth's climate is changing as a consequence of human activities. When the accusation of "junk science" is leveled against articles in peer-reviewed journals, it is important to ascertain whether the accuser has a vested interest in discrediting the work.

just cause Credible grounds for legal action, e.g., to remedy irresponsible toxic waste disposal.

justice In BIOETHICS, justice is one of the basic principles, meaning fairness, impartiality, equity. It includes the concept of DISTRIBUTIVE JUSTICE, and application of AFFIRMATIVE ACTION when this is desirable or necessary. In all aspects of law, including law relating to public health problems, justice means seeking the truth and basing judgements on evidence rather than on the eloquence of arguments for differing points of view. See also EQUITY.

juvenile A person below the age at which he or she is legally permitted to act independently of parental or other authority. This is variously defined as 16, 17, 18, 19, or 21 years, most often 18 or 21 years, but it varies according to jurisdiction and sometimes other circumstances. Clear definition is essential because of legal constraints in the health sector, as well as in the education system and other sectors of society, on what juveniles may do, and what others may do to or for them without the consent of parents or guardians. See also AGE OF CONSENT.

juvenile delinquency Antisocial behavior by youths that is defined as falling within the range of concern to law enforcement authorities, such as vandalism, destruction of property, shoplifting, petty theft, taking and driving a car belonging to someone else, and assault (especially when carried out by a gang attacking one person). Law enforcement authorities mete out punishments of varying severity. Ideally, youths who get into trouble with the law in these ways should be screened by a child psychiatrist because a significant proportion of them are emotionally disturbed and require psychiatric care rather than punishment and retribution.

juvenile obesity A growing public health problem in affluent nations, where children spend less time playing energetic games and more time passively watching television, often snacking on JUNK FOODS while doing so. In the United States in the early 21st century, the prevalence reached 20%, and it is higher in some ethnic groups. It is also common in the European Union and among adolescent children of affluent parents in China, India, and other industrializing nations.

K

kala-azar Syn: visceral leishmaniasis. Kala-azar comes from two Hindi words meaning "black fever." It remains a common tropical disease in India, Bangladesh, Pakistan, and the Middle East and occurs also in North Africa and elsewhere around the Mediterranean. It is caused by a protozoan parasite, *Leishmania donovani*, transmitted by sandflies that also infect dogs, rodents and other mammals. Prevention requires environmental control of the habitat of canines, rodents, etc., and protection of infants, children, and domestic pets from sandfly bites. Fine-mesh bed nets impregnated with insecticide can protect infants and children from sandflies as well as mosquitoes. Treatment with pentavalent antimony compounds is a specific and usually reliable cure. See also LEISHMANIASIS.

kaolin Hydrated aluminum silicate used to make fine china and in medicines for diarrhea.

KAP Acronym for knowledge, attitudes, practice, three attributes assessed in family planning surveys that are frequently used by demographers to provide baseline information before the program begins and to evaluate the success of established programs. Sometimes the acronym is KABP, for knowledge, attitudes, beliefs, and practice. These attributes may be used for surveys other than family planning, for instance, AIDS surveys.

Kaplan-Meier estimate A nonparametric method of compiling survival tables named for two American statisticians, E. L. Kaplan (b. 1920) and P. Meier (b. 1924). It is based on calculation of survival probabilities, allows for missing observations, and yields a reliable estimate of survival rates that can be used to compare outcomes of two or more treatment methods.

Kaposi's sarcoma An indolent cutaneous malignant condition described by the Hungarian dermatologist Moritz Kaposi (1837–1902). This was formerly rare outside the Mediterranean region but has become common where the HIV/AIDS pandemic has spread. Its occurrence is a marker of severe immunosuppression.

karyosome The resting phase of nuclear chromatin in the nucleus of a cell.

karyotype The chromosomal constitution seen in a somatic cell nucleus.

Kawasaki syndrome A condition of unknown etiology first identified by the Japanese pediatrician Tomisaku Kawasaki (b. 1920) in the late 1960s. It occurs worldwide, causing fever, measles-like symptoms and signs, and coronary artery dysplasia, usually resolving without lasting damage. It is believed to be a retrovirus disease, an idiosyncratic reaction to staphylococcal or streptococcal infection, or an allergic reaction to dust mites or cat fleas.

keloid Exuberant overgrowth of scar tissue accompanying and following wound healing. It occurs most frequently in persons with pigmented skin and can be severely disfiguring.

kelvin The SI unit of temperature, in which 0K is absolute zero, i.e., $-273.15°C$. Named for the British physicist Baron Kelvin, William Thomson (1824–1907).

Kepone See CHLORDECONE.

keratin A protein that occurs in and forms the outermost layer of skin, and is the main ingredient of hair, nails, and horns, including those of the reindeer and rhinoceros. The protein does not enhance male sexual potency, despite the widely held belief that leads to slaughter of rhinoceroses for their horns. Repeated friction or pressure on skin leads to profuse keratin formation in corns and calluses.

keratitis-conjunctivitis A severe inflammatory ocular condition that is often occupationally related, e.g., to the use of arc welding equipment without adequate shielding of the eyes from ultraviolet radiation or to vitamin A deficiency or trachoma. All forms of the condition endanger eyesight, and all are preventable.

keratomalacia Softening and loss of translucency of the cornea, caused by severe vitamin A deficiency, which eventually leads to blindness unless vigorously treated with vitamin A.

keratosis Increased production of keratin caused by exposure to ultraviolet radiation (solar keratosis); sometimes called *hyperkeratosis* and a precursor of squamous cell skin cancer. Other forms of keratosis include seborrheic keratosis and, before penicillin, keratosis associated with arsenical treatment of syphilis.

kerosene A petroleum distillate of relatively low volatility that is used mainly for cooking and space heating. In confined spaces, combustion can be a cause of carbon monoxide poisoning.

ketones A family of organic chemicals in the carbonyl group, produced by oxidation of alcohols. They include ACETONE, produced by incomplete metabolism of fats in severe diabetes and other metabolic upsets that give rise to the characteristic fruity odor of KETOSIS.

ketosis Biochemical intoxication caused by accumulation of acetone in the blood, causing a characteristic odor on the breath, usually as a result of unstable or uncontrolled DIABETES.

keyhole surgery See LAPAROSCOPIC SURGERY.

Keynesian economics An approach to adjustment of national economic planning to offset the harmful social consequences of recession or depression, proposed by the British economist John Maynard Keynes (1883–1946). Keynes advocated dealing with economic recession by deficit budgeting and injection of money into social programs aimed at boosting employment.

killed vaccine A vaccine prepared from killed pathogenic organisms, i.e., viruses or bacteria, that although dead retain their inactivated toxins and antigenic properties.

killer cells Large granular lymphocytes that are part of the body's immune defense mechanism. They take part in recognition and destruction of malignant cells as well as alien pathogens.

kiln An oven for heat treatment of many kinds: cooking, curing pottery, manufacturing alloys and many other compounds, extraction of sulfur from petroleum, destruction of toxic substances such as PCBs, etc. Depending on the construction, the fuel used, completeness of combustion, and temperature achieved, kilns may or may not be the source of severe atmospheric pollution.

kilobase The unit of length of a strand of DNA or RNA, comprising 1,000 base pairs.

kinesiology The scientific analysis of motor and sensory functions in the limbs, which is applied in ergonomics, prosthetics design, rehabilitation medicine, sports medicine, and physiology.

King's Evil Syn: scrofula, lymphadenopathic tuberculosis. A very rare condition today but one that was common in medieval Europe; it caused disfiguring red swelling over the affected glands and was popularly believed to be cured or relieved by the touch of the monarch. In medieval Europe, many kinds of skin lesions, including psoriasis and other noncontagious conditions, probably were lumped together and imprecisely described as King's Evil.

Kinsey Reports Two reports on human sexual behavior produced under the supervision of the American psychologist Alfred C. Kinsey (1894–1956) that had a considerable influence on shaping attitudes toward human sexuality. The reports, *Sexual Behavior in the Human Male* (1948) and *Sexual Behavior in the Human Female* (1953), were based on in-depth interviews with relatively small, selected samples, and the results have dubious generalizability, but they had a sensational impact, among other things because of their estimates of the prevalence of homosexuality, which were later found to be exaggerated. They were the first documents on human sexuality to achieve wide circulation and open discussion, thereby leading to loosening of previously existing reticence and inhibition about discussing sexuality, even between spouses or physicians and their patients.

kinship A group of people who are genetically closely related by ties of blood and marriage or its equivalent, i.e., parents and children, siblings, cousins, aunts, and uncles.

kissing bug The reduviid bug, a large beetle, often living in walls of adobe houses, that transmits Chagas disease, the South American TRYPANOSOMIASIS. Its nocturnal bite feels like something brushing against the skin, thus the name "kissing." Infection occurs when bug feces contaminate mucosal surfaces or abrasions due to scratching the site of the bite.

Kitasato, Shibasaburo (1852–1931) Japanese bacteriologist who is credited by some authors with the discovery of the PLAGUE bacillus *Yersinia pestis* and who helped to clarify the mechanism of antitoxic immunity in work on the tetanus toxin.

Klebs, Theodor Albrecht Edwin (1834–1915) German bacteriologist, discoverer of the bacillus responsible for diphtheria, whose name is remembered in the genus *Klebsiella*.

Koch, Robert (1843–1910) German bacteriologist, a founding figure of medical bacteriology, who was responsible alone or with collaborators for the discovery of many important pathogenic bacteria, using high-quality microscopes and newly developed methods of bacterial staining and culture (some of which he invented). His discoveries included the pathogens responsible for anthrax, cholera, and tuberculosis, and in travels to India and Africa, he did seminal work on many other diseases, including plague, malaria, African trypanosomiasis, and rinderpest. He was awarded the Nobel Prize for Physiology or Medicine in 1905.

Koch's postulates Named for the German bacteriologist ROBERT KOCH (1843–1910), these criteria confirming that an agent such as a bacterium causes a disease should be attributed in part to Koch's contemporary FRIEDRICH GUSTAV JACOB HENLE (1809–1885). Purists call them the HENLE-KOCH POSTULATES. The postulates are: The organism must be present in every case and must be isolated, cultured, and identified; it must produce the disease when a pure culture is given to a susceptible animal; and the organism must be recoverable from the animal.

Koplik spots Little red spots that appear on the buccal mucosa in the premonitory stage of many cases of MEASLES, first described by the American physician Henry Koplik (1858–1927). Today they are not considered an important diagnostic sign, although they can be useful in infants and small children with heavily pigmented skin on whom the measles rash is less clearly defined.

Korean hemorrhagic fever Syn: hantavirus disease. A bunyavirus infection with wild rodents as the usual host, transmitted to humans in aerosolized rodent droppings, causing fever, hemolysis, and renal failure in severe cases. It has long been endemic and occasionally epidemic in the Far East, and came to the notice of Westerners in the 1950s during the Korean War.

Korsakoff psychosis A toxic encephalopathy usually caused by chronic ALCOHOLISM that leads to amnesia and a tendency to fabricate implausible anecdotes to fill the memory gaps. Named for the Russian neuropsychiatrist Sergei Korsakoff (1853–1900).

kosher A word describing food prepared according to rules that devout Jews observe. Animals must be slaughtered, prepared for cooking, and eaten according to rules set out in the books of Leviticus and Deuteronomy. These rules forbid eating pork, bacon, and other meats derived from pigs, proscribe meals that mix meat and milk or milk products, and have several other mandatory features. Some of these rules may originally have been based on empirical observations about the relationship of certain foods to disease, e.g., of pork to trichinosis. Muslim halal rules are similar.

Krebs cycle A biochemical sequence identified by the German, British-naturalized biochemist Hans Krebs (1900–1981) that is the essential feature of carbohydrate metabolism. It is the basis for aerobic metabolism in plants, humans and other mammals, and many microorganisms. It is mediated by mitochondrial enzymes and is the process whereby carbohydrates are transformed in the process of glycolysis to produce energy.

Kübler-Ross stages of dying The process of psychological adjustment to impending death described in 1969 by the Swiss-American psychiatrist Elizabeth Kübler-Ross (1926–2004). The five stages are denial, anger, bargaining, depression, and acceptance.

kurtosis The extent to which a bell-shaped curve is peaked.

kuru The fatal neurological disease caused by PRIONS, i.e., a SPONGIFORM ENCEPHALOPATHY, that occurred among members of the Fore tribe in the New Guinea highlands and was transmitted by ritualistic eating of the brains of tribe members who had died of the disease. It is probably extinct now that the cause has been identified and culturally determined ritual cannibalism has ceased. Daniel Carleton Gajdusek (b. 1923) correctly connected the relationship of kuru to the ingestion of brain tissue contaminated by prions and earned a Nobel Prize for that work in 1976.

kwashiorkor Syn: protein-energy malnutrition. A severe nutritional disease of infants and small children caused by protein deficiency. In a dialect spoken in Ghana, the word means "deposed child," recognizing that the disease occurs when a child is weaned and a new baby begins breast feeding, because the weanling's diet is deficient in protein. The features include failure to thrive, wasting, marasmus, and susceptibility to infection. The prevalence varies and rises at times of scarcity. The condition was described in 1935 by the British pediatrician Cicely Williams (1893–1992).

Kyoto Protocol Syn: UN Framework Convention on Climate Control. An internationally agreed upon set of staged reductions in atmospheric emissions of combustion products of carbon-based fuels, formulated at a meeting of heads of state in Kyoto, Japan, in 1997. Climate scientists and public health experts believe this is an essential measure to help allay the most dangerous adverse environmental and human health effects of climate change. Nations that ratified the protocol agreed to reduce carbon emissions to 1990 levels by 2010. This is only a token reduction, insufficient to have meaningful environmental or health benefits, but it has great symbolic value. Nevertheless, it has been resisted by interest groups representing the energy and transport sectors. The Kyoto Protocol had been ratified by enough industrial nations to come into force in 2005. Japan, the United States, and Australia have not ratified it, and some nations that have ratified have not yet enforced it. See RIO DECLARATION and WORLD SUMMIT ON SUSTAINABLE DEVELOPMENT. Information regarding the UN Framework Convention on Climate Change is available at http://unfccc.int/essential_background/convention/items/2627.php.

L

label 1. A notice, such as a pharmacist's instructions on a bottle of pills. In some jurisdictions this must state the generic or pharmacological name of the medication. In some countries, the label or a package insert must warn about adverse effects and emergency management of overdose. 2. In NOSOLOGY and DISEASE TAXONOMY, the diagnostic or "disease label" assigned to a condition. 3. In medical jargon, a "label" is the name of a disease or a diagnostic category that is, figuratively speaking, attached to a patient—a depersonalizing process that designates a person by a disease label: stroke, diabetic, bronchitic, epileptic, arthritic, and many more. All imply imperfection to some degree and many carry a stigma.

labeling 1. Pharmaceutical preparations, much edible merchandise, and foodstuffs are required by law in most nations to display a label describing the ingredients, including additives and preservatives. 2. In the health, education, and law enforcement sectors, "labeling" means using words or phrases to describe types of persons encountered in that sector. To be labeled "diabetic" or "hypertensive" diminishes the humanity of the person so labeled; and labels such as "AIDS victim," "alcoholic," "cripple," and "neurotic" are stigmatizing or demeaning.

labile Variable, changeable, responsive to outside influences, a term applicable to moods, the reactions of chemicals and biological preparations to heat and of crowds to provocation by persuasive speeches, and other phenomena.

laboratory A place (room, building) equipped for scientific experiments and/or routine physical chemical and biological tests and/or for production of vaccines, drugs, etc. Laboratories may be dangerous: the hazards include exposure to toxic chemicals, pathogenic organisms, and ionizing radiation. Safe staff practices, storage of reagents, and shielding of radioactive materials are important.

laboratory worker Syn: laboratory technician. An occupational group comprising professionally and/or technically trained staff in hospital laboratories, diagnostic clinics, public health services, environmental surveillance, etc. Significant occupational risks arise in some laboratory work, notably exposure to BIOHAZARDS, IONIZING RADIATION, and toxic chemicals.

labor force The proportion of the population in each age group who are economically active as employers, self-employed, employees, and unemployed. This is an indicator of the proportion of the population who are eligible and available for work. Factors affecting this include school leaving age, numbers proceeding to higher education, retirement age, facilities for infant and child care, and motivation of mothers with dependent children to join or return to the workforce.

labor force participation rate An index of employment levels in nations that maintain statistics on numbers actively employed as a proportion of all people in the specified age groups eligible for employment, usually ages 15 to 64 years, 18 to 64 years, or whatever the age range is between leaving school and retiring, with adjustment for numbers or proportions receiving disability pensions.

labor-management relationship This can be a tense relationship because of differing objectives. Management aims to prosper by minimizing costs and enhancing efficiency; workers aim to ensure that their work is adequately rewarded, that working conditions do not endanger health, and that they are provided long-term security. These dissonant aims are at the root of many industrial disputes. Issues affecting the health of workers frequently arise in these relationships.

labor market The workforce and the industrial, commercial, domestic, and foreign industries that employ them. Globalization has complicated their interactions and introduced additional fluctuating economic, social, political, and environmental factors into this "market." Health conditions, such as the presence or absence of endemic and epidemic disease, and perceptions of the health hazards associated with some occupations may further complicate the picture.

labor movement An organized collective activity of workers who aim to improve their working conditions, secure stable incomes, and ensure retirement and other benefits, including insurance against the cost of work-related disabilities and their treatment. The labor movement gathered momentum throughout the first 100 years of the industrial era and remained vigorous in most industrial nations through the latter part of the 20th century, except when inhibited by totalitarian regimes or antilabor legislation. One of the principal concerns of the movement is to improve the safety and reduce the health risks associated with many occupations.

labor room Syn: labor ward. The section of a hospital where women are supervised during labor and delivery of their infants. In the past, labor rooms were dangerous places because of the risks of PUERPERAL SEPSIS. In the late 20th century, labor rooms began to be superseded by BIRTHING CENTERS.

lactation The hormonally mediated and controlled secretion of milk by the mammary glands.

lactose A carbohydrate, the disaccharide sugar that occurs in milk.

lactose intolerance Syn: lactase deficiency. An inherited inability to digest lactose, and therefore milk and many dairy products, usually caused by inability to synthesize the enzyme lactase. It is a common metabolic condition among many non-Caucasian peoples, that is, people of African, Asian, Native American, and Mediterranean origin.

Laënnec's cirrhosis The form of cirrhosis of the liver associated with nutritional deficiency that can occur in chronic alcoholism, first described and linked to chronic alcoholism by the French physician René Laënnec (1781–1826), who also invented the stethoscope.

lakh A Hindi and Urdu word for 100,000. It is included in this dictionary because it appears as the denominator for many rates in public health documents from India, Pakistan, and Bangladesh. A crore, 10 million, is 100 lakhs.

La Leche League An international organization founded in 1956 by mothers who wish to breast feed their infants, and to promote breast feeding among others. This organization is active in North America and Europe and offers educational material on aspects of infant care and development. Details of its policies and programs are at http://www.lalecheleague.org/.

Lamarckism The French naturalist Jean Baptiste Lamarck (1744–1829) proposed a theory that acquired characteristics such as athletic prowess could be inherited. The concept has resurfaced from time to time, for instance, in the "master race" doctrines of the Nazis and the Stalinist-inspired beliefs and fabricated genetic evidence of the Soviet biologist Trofim Lysenko (1898–1976).

Lamaze technique The approach to labor and childbirth of the French obstetrician Fernand Lamaze (1891–1957) that relies on breathing, relaxation, and exercises, rather than drugs, to minimize pain associated with the process of labor.

landfill A widely used method of garbage disposal that consists of dumping garbage on waste land, such as a quarry, open-cast mine, or swamp. Ideally, this is evenly spread, compacted, and covered with a layer of soil After decomposition and settling, which takes several years, the site can be beautified with playing fields or, if local zoning laws permit, converted for commercial or even residential use. Decomposing organic matter in landfill sites generates methane, and monitoring for methane concentration should be obligatory, but seldom is. Sometimes methane is harvested and used as fuel. Noxious odors and toxic fumes are a hazard of many landfill sites. Other hazards include toxic material in garbage that can leach into aquifers; proliferation of pests such as rats; and ecosystem disruption if the landfill was formerly a stage on the flight path of migratory birds or habitat for endangered species. Landfill sites in many jurisdictions are subject to increasingly strict regulation, with innovations such as separation of garbage into recyclable and other categories and safeguards to protect sensitive ecosystems and minimize harm to the environment. In many low-income countries, human scavengers risk their health to collect whatever they can salvage for reuse or sale. See also HAZARDOUS WASTE DISPOSAL.

landmine Indiscriminate war weapon of which the victims are often not combatants in an armed conflict but innocent bystanders, including children who are killed or maimed while playing and farmers attempting to cultivate land that has been mined. Many millions of landmines were scattered in combat zones in southeast Asia, Angola, Mozambique, Yugoslavia, and Afghanistan, and in the demilitarized zone separating the two halves of the Korean Peninsula. Their terrible toll led to organized efforts to prohibit their use, spearheaded by the International Campaign to Ban Landmines (ICBL), which was awarded the 1997 Nobel Peace Prize. The ICBL initiative culminated in an international UN convention and treaty to ban landmines, the Ottawa Treaty, approved by the UN General Assembly in 1999. This has been ratified by more than 80 nations but not the United States. The activities of the ICBL are described at http://www.icbl.org.

Landsat A series of orbiting satellites that map the earth's resources and incidentally reveal seasonal variations in vegetation, plankton growth on lakes, etc., associated with the prevalence levels of vectors, such as mosquitoes, blackflies, and ticks.

language barrier In the health sector, a common problem is inability of health workers and those they serve to communicate because they speak different languages. This occurs, for instance, with immigrant and refugee communities. It is often compounded by a CULTURAL BARRIER, partly due to differing values associated with the cultural origins of each language and partly due to other inherent cultural differences.

laparoscopic surgery Syn: keyhole surgery. A surgical innovation, also called minimally invasive surgery, introduced for abdominal and joint surgery in which a small incision is made through which a fiberoptic instrument (laparoscope, arthroscope) is introduced into the peritoneal, pleural, or joint cavity, enabling the removal of diseased organs, damaged ligaments, etc., without operative trauma and prolonged postoperative recovery with all the risks of nosocomial infection and other misadventures associated with admission to a hospital.

laparoscopy Use of a fiberoptic instrument to view the peritoneal cavity, widely practiced in gynecology, e.g., for tubal ligation, and by surgeons for many abdominal surgical procedures.

larva One of the developmental stages between egg and adult of arthropods.

larva migrans Human infection by the larval phase of animal and avian nematode parasites, such as canine hookworm or lumbrical worms. The larval worms usually penetrate the skin, causing itching and a rash, but cannot complete their life cycle because humans are a dead-end host. Visceral larva migrans can occur with toxocariasis, and this is very serious if it affects the eyes.

larvicide A pesticide that kills larvae, commonly used to kill the aquatic larvae of mosquitoes. This may be a poison added to water or a liquid, such as kerosene, that reduces surface tension so mosquito larvae cannot adhere to the surface to breathe, so they drown.

laser Acronym for light amplification by stimulated emission of radiation. Lasers emit a powerful, precisely directed, single-color, coherent beam of light. This has high energy that can be used medically, e.g., to treat retinal hemorrhage. Lasers have many industrial uses and are used also to direct ordnance and to impair the vision of adversaries in armed conflicts. Lasers can cause blindness due to retinal damage and severe burns if mishandled.

Lassa fever A lethal hemorrhagic fever caused by a FILOVIRUS. It occurs mainly in equatorial West Africa, first reported from Lassa, northern Nigeria, in the 1950s. It affects an estimated 100,000 to 300,000 people annually and causes 5,000 deaths, but in severe epidemics the case fatality rate can exceed 50%. The virus was isolated in 1969. It is a zoonosis with wild rodents as the primary host, but the natural history of the virus and possible vectors have not yet been adequately investigated. It is a potential weapon in biological warfare. Control requires isolation and universal precautions. See http://www.cdc.gov/ncidod/dvrd/spb/mnpages/dispages/lassaf.htm.

latchkey children School-age children whose parents work until after the school day has ended and who therefore must go home to an empty house and fend alone for varying periods until their parents return. Latchkey children may be victims of parental neglect and are at risk of many kinds of misadventure during repeated periods alone.

latency, latent period The period between exposure to a disease agent and the appearance of clinical symptoms and signs of the disease. The term is used mainly in relation to the effects of exposure to environmental and occupational agents, such as ionizing radiation and asbestos. It is analogous to but not a synonym for INCUBATION PERIOD, which implies a biological process of agent-host interaction in which the agent multiplies. A biological process may be involved in latency, but the agent does not multiply or reproduce like a pathogenic organism.

latent heat The quantity of energy stored as heat by an object, such as a container of warm water, that can be released or is emitted into the environment by conduction, convection, or radiation.

latex The sap from various plants, including the rubber tree, that forms a rubbery substance when dry. By extension, the same word describes synthetic rubber substitutes, especially those that are refined and used to manufacture surgical gloves, condoms, etc. Some users develop latex allergy, which can be intractable enough to enforce a change of occupation or brand of condoms.

Latin square A statistical research design of columns and rows in which each experimental unit is assigned a position in a column and row, and each can occur only once in each column and row. It is used mainly in agricultural research. It is useful in reducing confounding effects, for instance, of seasonal variation in intervention studies of respiratory disease.

latrine A toilet or private place to void the bowels, usually a communal toilet in an army camp. It may be a pit privy, a chemical toilet, or one that uses water-carried sewage disposal. In many past military campaigns, inadequate latrine sanitation and hygiene led to more deaths and disability from fecal-oral infectious disease than did armed combat.

laughing gas Nitrous oxide, N_2O, an anesthetic agent first used by the British scientist Humphry Davy (1778–1829) and his friends as an intoxicant that made people laugh uncontrollably. It was adopted by the American dentist Crawford Long (1815–1878) and others for dental and obstetric anesthesia. In the 1970s, it once again had a vogue as a mood-modifying substance among fringe groups, including members of the gay community in some American cities, but fell from favor when some users had severe cardiovascular episodes after its use.

lavage Washing, rinsing, or irrigation of a wound, ulcer, or body cavity.

Laveran, Charles Louis Alphonse (1845–1922) French parasitologist and tropical disease specialist, who in 1880 discovered the presence of malaria parasites in the blood and recognized that these were the cause of malaria. He was awarded a Nobel Prize for his work in 1907.

law A rule or general principle. There are several varieties. 1. Laws of nature (such as the law of gravity), which are regarded as axioms or proved by observation or experiment. 2. Manmade laws include common law, established by custom and tradition, often on the basis of morality; statute law, based on legislation enacted by the elected representatives of the nation; and case law, based on precedents established by decisions in courts of law. Public health laws are based on statutes that have been enacted in many nations to protect the health of the public, and case law based on decisions rendered by courts in numerous cases in which lawyers have successfully (or otherwise) argued, e.g., for damages incurred by working with asbestos, drinking water contaminated by toxic pollutants, etc. In modern industrial nations, especially the United States, environmental health protection has depended heavily on law courts that have argued TOXIC TORTS and other matters affecting health.

law of large numbers The statistical law described by the Swiss mathematician Jakob Bernoulli (1654–1705) stating that the accuracy of a sample mean is increased, and the standard error is reduced, as the sample size, i.e., the number studied, is increased. Thus, a large sample size is more likely to be representative of the universe population studied than a small sample size. In reality, the sampling method is more important to validity than is the sample size.

lay reporting A health information system used mainly in countries where professionally trained health workers are in short supply. Using standard case definitions for surveillance, the emphasis is on identifying gross manifestations of threats to health by asking lay reporters (community leaders, school teachers, etc.) to record and transmit information about such conditions as high fever with shivers and sweats, bloody diarrhea, fever

with skin rash, watery diarrhea, and malnutrition. Usually only death reports are submitted, but epidemics are also reported, especially those of an unusual nature. See also VERBAL AUTOPSY.

LC50 LC means lethal concentration. The atmospheric concentration of a toxic gaseous substance that is sufficient to kill 50% of exposed experimental animals in a toxicity test.

LD50 LD means lethal dose. In TOXICOLOGY, the dose of a substance that is sufficient to kill 50% of experimental animals, i.e., the lethal dose for 50% of the experimental animals.

LDL See LOW DENSITY LIPOPROTEIN.

leachate The liquid in which soil substances are dissolved during the process of LEACHING.

leaching The process of washing soluble material out of a solid substance; the liquid containing these dissolved solids is called LEACHATE.

lead (Pb) A dense, malleable metal that has many industrial uses both in its metallic form and in organic compounds, and almost all of which are poisonous. Lead was used from 6000 BCE until the middle or late 20th century in domestic utensils, water pipes, molding, roofing, etc. Lead forms poisonous salts with "soft" acidic water, and its use in water supply systems is now prohibited. Calcium compounds can be added to drinking water to reduce acidity and the risk of lead leaching in localities with old housing served by lead pipes. Lead is also used in accumulator batteries. Inorganic and organic lead compounds are widely used in paints and pigments, as additives to gasoline, and for many other purposes. See also LEAD POISONING.

lead colic The combination of constipation and paroxysmal colicky abdominal pain that occurs often in cases of LEAD POISONING, for example, from ingesting lead-based paint, or ingesting lead salts as an abortifacient.

lead poisoning Lead disrupts calcium metabolism, hemoglobin synthesis, and neural function. The symptoms include anemia, abdominal colic, and, most important, impaired neurological function, which in infants and children can cause long-term, probably permanent, damage, including mental retardation at high exposure levels, and cognitive deficits detectable by neuropsychological tests among children with relatively low background lead exposure levels. This effect has been confirmed in cohort studies in several parts of the world. The toxic effects of lead were known to the Roman scholar Pliny the Elder (23–79 CE) and described by the British physician George Baker

(1722–1809), but it took persuasive scientific evidence of neurological damage to children and persistent public outrage to induce legislators to enact moderate safeguards by the late 20th century, and even these were resisted by the lead industry.

lead time The period of time gained when a disease such as cancer is detected early in its natural history as a result of presymptomatic SCREENING, in contrast to not diagnosing it until it declares its presence by causing symptoms or signs.

lead time bias A systematic error introduced when followup does not begin at comparable stages in the natural history of the disease. Lead time bias can occur in comparisons of survival rates for conditions such as cancer when allowance is not made for the stage of the disease when diagnosis was made and treatment begun. Thus, early diagnosis of cases in a SCREENING program and early treatment may or may not influence the survival rate. It may merely mean that the presence of the disease is known for a larger proportion of the person's lifetime.

learning The process of acquiring knowledge and understanding of a subject, concept, technique, or procedure. This process can proceed in any or all of several ways, including rote learning and memorizing, working through problems, performing learning tasks, etc.

learning disability A general term for problems with cognition, intellectual capacity, or emotional states that impair the ability of children to achieve expected educational attainments at the normal age. The varieties include dyslexia, attention deficit hyperactivity disorder, mental impairment, and many other conditions, including very high intelligence that may lead to boredom in regular classes. Defective sensory input (short-sightedness, visual impairments, profound deafness) interfere with ability to learn in a classroom setting but should not be called a learning disability, although the effects may be similar. School health services can detect and identify the causes of many learning disabilities if they have suitable screening measures, and many of them respond to intervention.

least developed country (LDC) An obsolete term for a country at the low end of the scale of gross national product per capita with undeveloped or very rudimentary infrastructure. The preferred term now is low-income country. See also INCOME LEVELS, WORLD BANK CLASSIFICATION.

leech A species of segmented annelid worm, with a cranial sucker adapted for sucking blood, that was used by medieval physicians to treat congested tissues or draw blood from patients. Leeches are used occasionally in modern therapeutics to reduce swelling of congested tissues, especially if caused by blood clots, because the leech's salivary juices dissolve blood clots.

Leeuwenhoek, Antoni van (1632–1723) A Dutch microscopist who ground his own lenses and perfected techniques for magnification up to 200 times, allowing him to visualize very small objects not previously seen. Among the structures he described were red blood corpuscles, spermatozoa, protozoa, intestinal parasites, and possibly some of the larger bacteria.

legal liability A form of ACCOUNTABILITY that has the force of law. Statutory or case law can be used to enforce it. In public health services, authorities or individual professional staff members identified by name and/or duties may or may not be legally liable when mishaps occur. In some jurisdictions and for some purposes, such as immunization services provided by public health departments, no-fault provisions have been written into applicable regulations to protect them from legal liability, and legal mechanisms for compensation may also be specified. Public health officials should be familiar with the procedures and legal provisions in their workplace.

Legionnaires disease Syn: legionellosis. A form of bronchopneumonia caused by an elusive Gram-negative microorganism, *Legionella pneumophila*, that is transmitted person to person and by water vapor in humid environments. The name derives from epidemiological investigations of an epidemic among members of the American Legion who attended a convention in Philadelphia in 1976 and were infected by moist air from a hotel air conditioning plant that was a COMMON VEHICLE for transmission of the pathogenic organism. A nonpneumonic form of the disease, called PONTIAC FEVER, was identified before 1976.

leishmaniasis A protozoan infection of dogs, rodents, and humans, transmitted by sandflies, identified by the British bacteriologist William Leishman (1865–1926). The causative organism, *Leishmania donovani*, causes three varieties of the disease: cutaneous, mucocutaneous, and visceral leishmaniasis. The latter is KALA-AZAR.

Leishman's stain A staining technique invented by the British bacteriologist William Leishman (1865–1926) to render visible the structure of parasites and bacteria, and also red blood cells.

lepromin test A skin test analogous to the TUBERCULIN TEST for *Mycobacterium leprae*, the leprosy bacillus. Now used only in research, not as a diagnostic tool.

leprosy Syn: Hansen's disease, named for the Norwegian physician G. H. A. Hansen (1841–1912). An indolent chronic infectious disease caused by *Mycobacterium leprae* that mainly attacks the peripheral sensory nerves and connective tissue, causing extensive destruction. Formerly common in Europe and Asia, leprosy is now confined mainly to a few regions in tropical countries. The WHO initiated a Leprosy Elimination Programme in 1991. The aim of this program was to reduce the maximum annual incidence in endemic regions to fewer than 1 per 10,000. By 2004, this had been achieved in 110 of 122 countries where leprosy was previously endemic. In 2005, WHO's global Leprosy Elimination Programme moved its operations base from Geneva to the Regional Office for South-East Asia in New Delhi. See http://www.who.int/lep/ for program details.

leptophos One of the organophosphate pesticides first manufactured in 1971, soon discovered to cause a severe demyelinating degenerative neurological disease in exposed workers and therefore banned. Manufacture ceased in 1976, but stocks remained in use in some low-income countries.

leptospira Motile spirilla that are difficult to detect, culture, and stain. Some strains of leptospira cause hemorrhagic fevers and liver and renal failure.

leptospirosis A group of bacterial zoonoses caused by LEPTOSPIRA. These include WEIL'S DISEASE (rat-bite fever), traditionally an occupational disease of sewer workers that is transmitted by rats, an ongoing occupational disease of cane field workers, and a cause of chronic renal failure in endemic areas, where frogs and toads maintain the organism in the environment. Another disease in this family is canicola fever, usually a milder condition, transmitted by dogs.

lesion A portion of an organ or tissue that is diseased or injured, by a wound, ulcer, abscess, tumor, etc.

leukemia A malignant disease of bone marrow that causes excessive production of white blood corpuscles. There are several varieties, acute or chronic, affecting leukocytes or lymphocytes. Acute leukemia rapidly affects red cell and platelet production in bone marrow so patients become anemic and develop extensive hemorrhages and bruising. Resistance to infection is disrupted, and this is a common cause of death. Sometimes in children the onset is so acute that death caused by overwhelming infection may occur before the peripheral blood picture becomes diagnostic. This and other acute forms of childhood leukemia were universally fatal until modern treatment methods with bone marrow transplants, anticancer drugs, etc., made complete cure possible. The underlying cause and pathogenesis are unknown in many cases, but some appear to have a genetic basis and some identified etiological agents include ionizing radiation (in atomic bomb and nuclear accident survivors); benzene; and retroviruses, e.g., human T-cell leukemia virus type I (HTLV-I).

leukoplakia Patchy white lesions on the tongue and upper oropharynx, a premalignant change associated with tobacco, betel chewing, and chronic diseases, such as syphilis.

leukorrhea A white discharge from the vagina; if this is not profuse and there is no offensive odor, it is a normal phenomenon. A profuse, offensive-smelling vaginal discharge occurs with several varieties of infection and/or ulceration, such as the most common, TRICHOMONIASIS.

levonorgestrel A long-acting injectable steroid contraceptive that is usually implanted subcutaneously, where it is slowly released over a period of months, during which it inhibits ovulation. It has a low failure rate and is especially useful in populations in which women wish to limit the risk of pregnancy but may not be able or willing to take the oral contraceptive pill for extended lengths of time. Its trade name is Norplant.

liability An obligation or responsibility that imposes a duty. It may be enforced by law, a LEGAL LIABILITY, and may impose financial obligations. Product liability can impose a legal duty on manufacturers and sometimes those who sell products to comply with set standards and criteria. Professional liability applies to the obligation to maintain standards, e.g., of a licensing body, and to perform expected actions according to these standards, and not to perform actions outside these standards. See also NEGLIGENCE.

lice Plural of louse, parasitic insects that occur in three varieties: head lice, pubic lice, and body lice. Body lice (*Pediculus corporis*) are associated with two louse-borne diseases of great public health importance, louse-borne epidemic TYPHUS and RELAPSING FEVER, both of which were common for centuries, associated with overcrowding, wearing dirty clothes, and lack of access to bathing, washing, and opportunities to put on clean clothes, typically conditions associated with warfare, displacement, poverty, and refugee movement. Head lice (*Pediculus capitis*) commonly infect school children, laying eggs, known as nits, that attach to hair and require combing with a fine-tooth comb to detach them. Children infect one another when the lice move from one child's head to another. Head lice often occur in epidemic form in schools. Pubic lice (*Pthirus pubis*, "crabs") are anatomically different, infest pubic hair almost exclusively, and spread from person to person during sexual intercourse. Head lice and pubic lice, although transmitted person to person by direct contact, do not carry or transmit disease.

license A legal procedure that confers specified rights, duties, and benefits, usually recorded on a certificate or other document granted by a formally constituted licensing board. Many varieties of public health professional require a license to carry on their profession.

licensed practical nurse (LPN) A nurse who has had simple practical in-service training, usually in a hospital or clinic, but has not had the extensive formal education required for licensure as a REGISTERED NURSE.

licensure The statutory or legal process of obtaining a license that confers on a professional person the legal right to practice a profession or trade in the jurisdiction where the license is recognized.

lichen A tenacious form of moss and, by analogy, a skin eruption with this appearance that is sometimes a fungus infection, sometimes an indolent form of skin cancer.

life chances A term favored by some behavioral scientists to describe the interplay of individual or group behavior and environmental factors that may be either protective of or conducive to the occurrence of chronic or infectious diseases.

life course The natural history of human life. A term for conditions that evolve over a large part or all of the life span from infancy, or even from conception, through adolescence, adult life, and senescence, sometimes peaking in early adult life, sometimes in middle age, but generally progressing throughout life as a person grows older. The term is recognition of the fact that the natural history of many chronic diseases and the natural life span of humans are intertwined. See, for example, BARKER HYPOTHESIS.

life cycle The developmental changes undergone by individual members of a species, including fertilization, reproduction, death, and replacement by a new generation. The life cycle is linear for individuals, cyclical for populations. In many species, a succession of cycles is linked by sexual or asexual reproduction. In many parasitic species, the life cycle requires dependence on a definitive host, in which the adult parasite lives and reproduces, and an intermediate host, or sometimes two intermediate hosts, in which the parasite develops during part of its life cycle. In vertebrates, the life cycle is

from fusing of the gametes to the death of the resulting individuals.

life expectancy Syn: expectation of life. The average number of years a person of specified age and sex is expected to live if current trends in mortality rates prevail in the future. It is based on current age-specific mortality rates, and is adjusted by an ACTUARY or other designated official of an insurance company to allow for increased or reduced probability of early death associated with known RISK FACTORS. It is a theoretical concept with wide confidence limits. Each of the parameters has a name and a symbol, e_x for life expectancy at age x, l_x for the number in the hypothetical birth cohort who survive to age x, q_x for the probability of dying at age x, etc. Other adjustments include DISABILITY-FREE LIFE EXPECTANCY and the calculations made by clinicians for HEALTH RISK APPRAISAL (HRA). Life expectancy at birth is a particular aspect that serves as an indicator of population health status. Life expectancy at birth, e_0, is the average number of years that a newborn can be expected to live if current mortality trends continue. This is sensitive to the effect of infant and early child mortality, so it is lower in countries with high infant and early childhood mortality than in upper-income countries where most infants survive. See also COHORT. For US life expectancy tables, see http:// www.cdc.gov/nchs/ fastats/lifexpec.htm.

life signs See VITAL SIGNS.

life skills A set of abilities regarded as essential to effective and efficient functioning in modern urban society, including ability to hold a job, manage money, find and keep accommodation, stay within the law, and form normal social relationships.

life span See LIFE EXPECTANCY.

lifestyle The behavior pattern, customs, and habits of persons or groups, generally considered in the context of consequences for health, and including nature and amount of exercise, dietary habits, and use of tobacco, alcohol, coffee, tea, stimulant and sedative substances (licit or illicit), and recreational time.

life support systems 1. The environment and ecosystems that sustain human populations, including quality of the air, water, soil, disposition of human settlements and food-growing regions, climatic and other fluctuating variables, etc., that influence ecosystem sustainability. 2. The techniques and apparatus used in hospital intensive care services to maintain cardiac and respiratory function, fluid and electrolyte balance, etc., in critically ill and injured persons.

life table An actuarial statistical table of a theoretical birth cohort of 1,000 or 100,000 for each year of age from birth to 100 years, displaying the number who will die before reaching their next birthday, the number surviving, and the probability of individuals surviving and dying. For current US life tables, see http://www.cdc.gov/nchs/products/pubs/pubd/lftbls/lftbls.htm. See also LIFE EXPECTANCY.

lifetime risk The probability, often expressed as a percentage, that at some stage in life a person will develop a designated condition, specifically cancer. There is a lifetime risk of about 25% of getting cancer, and a lifetime risk of about 20% of dying of cancer in upper-income countries. Data are rarely available to compute comparable lifetime risks for populations in developing countries.

light Electromagnetic radiation in the visible wavelength, 400 to 760 nanometers. Adjoining this wavelength are ultraviolet light, which is the range from 400 nanometers down to about 1 nanometer, and infrared, which is 750 nanometers to about 1 mm. Light is required for chlorophyll metabolism and for healthy growth and development of humans and many other organisms.

Likert scale A method devised by the American behavioral scientist Rensis Likert (1903–1981) to categorize and score responses to questions in a survey by arranging them in a hierarchy on an ordinal scale, such as "strongly agree," "agree," "no opinion," "disagree," and "strongly disagree."

limb reduction birth defects Birth defects ranging from minor digit abnormalities to partial or complete absence of upper and/or lower limbs (PHOCOMELIA or amelia), such as among offspring of mothers who used the antinausea drug thalidomide during early intrauterine development.

Lind, James (1716–1794) Scottish physician and naval surgeon who conducted the first recorded CLINICAL TRIAL, to test his hypothesis that addition of fresh fruit, i.e., limes or lemons, to the diet would prevent SCURVY on long sea voyages. Lind is credited with inventing the clinical trial and with initiating a paradigm shift in thinking about dietary deficiency as a cause of disease.

lindane Hexachlorocyclohexane, also called benzene hexachloride (BHC), a powerful insecticide, endocrine disruptor, and neurotoxin, and a suspected carcinogen. It is used, among other things, to treat head lice. Its toxicity and possible carcinogenicity are uncertain. For details, see http://www.nlm.nih.gov/medlineplus/druginfo/medmaster/a682651.html.

linear accelerator An apparatus to accelerate charged particles, e.g., for radiological examination or for some forms of radiotherapy. Unless properly shielded, operators of linear accelerators risk harm from exposure to ionizing radiation, e.g., malignant disease, birth defects.

linear regression The simplest form of regression model, in which a random variable y is related to variable x according to the formula $y = \alpha + \beta x + \varepsilon$, where α is the intercept, β is the slope of a regression line, and ε denotes random error. In practice, this model works by fitting a series of data points to the regression line. It is frequently used in public health applications.

linear relationship A relationship between two variables such that when one changes by a specific amount, the other changes by a directly proportional amount, either in the same or in the reverse direction.

linkage The process of connecting things to each other. Two important varieties in the health field are genetic linkage and record linkage. GENETIC LINKAGE is the tendency of two genes that occur close together on the same chromosome to be inherited together. RECORD LINKAGE is a method of relating information in one set of personal records to information in other sets.

Linnaean classification The classification system used originally for all species in the plant kingdom, subsequently for all biological organisms. It is a binomial system, in which the first part is the generic name of the organism and the second is the specific, or species, name. All organisms are arranged into the general type of organism, the genus (plural: genera), and each unique member of the genus, the species. At a higher level, genera belong to a class within a phylum (plural: phyla), then come families and ultimately kingdoms. The classification was invented by the Swedish botanist Carl von Linné (1707–1778). See also TAXONOMY.

lipids A naturally occurring family of fatty or oily organic chemicals, not soluble in water, but they are soluble in organic solvents. They consist of long-chain hydrocarbons, fatty acids, phospholipids, steroids, and various others. They are important dietary ingredients in foods containing fat, and are essential in many aspects of human metabolism, e.g., providing energy stored as fat, the ingredients for synthesis of steroid hormones, and lipoproteins.

lipoprotein Chemical (biochemical) compound of lipid and protein. Lipoproteins form the cell membrane in most body cells. Some lipoproteins are enzymes, and some play an important role in transporting fats and in cholesterol metabolism. All human cells need fats and cholesterol to build cell membranes and to organize their structure and protein enzymatic systems. Lipoproteins in the blood carry fats around the body. Chylomicrons carry fat from the intestines to the liver and to fatty tissue. Very low density lipoproteins carry synthesized glycerol from the liver to fatty tissue. Low density lipoproteins ("bad cholesterol") carry cholesterol from the liver to body cells. High density lipoproteins ("good cholesterol") collect cholesterol from body tissues and return it to the liver.

liquefied petroleum gas (LPG) Usually a mixture of light, volatile hydrocarbons that liquify under pressure but vaporize and ignite when the pressure is reduced. They include propane and butane, which are extensively used as fuels for heating as well as for internal combustion engines.

liquid scintillation counter See SCINTILLATION COUNTER

Lister, Joseph (1827–1912) The British surgeon who applied the discoveries of bacteriologists, notably LOUIS PASTEUR, using a carbolic acid spray as an ANTISEPTIC to control bacterial infection in labor wards and operating rooms. While this was an inherently clumsy, less elegant approach to infection control than asepsis (i.e., hand-washing and sterilizing instruments advocated by OLIVER WENDELL HOLMES and IGNAZ PHILIPP SEMMELWEIS), Lister's methods, unlike those of Holmes and Semmelweis, were widely adopted and led rapidly to a dramatic decline in the incidence of PUERPERAL SEPSIS and fatal or serious postoperative wound infection.

listeriosis The variety of food poisoning caused by *Listeria* species, rod-shaped, motile aerobic bacteria commonly transmitted in milk and milk products, especially cheese and yogurt. Infection causes a low fever, gastroenteritis, and, in about 25% of cases, meningoencephalitis. In late pregnancy and in neonates, it can be dangerous. It responds to ampicillin and gentamicin. Prevention requires rigorous food and kitchen hygiene, pasteurizing milk and milk products, and thorough cleaning and cooking of all suspect food.

literacy The quality of being literate, able to read and write. There are wide variations. Some people can only read labels on price tags, train or bus timetables, instructions on packaged food or bottles of medicine, and newspapers consisting mainly of pictures and large headlines (functional literacy). A higher level of literacy is required to read serious prose, poetry, or scientific journals, although this does not necessarily mean that advanced literacy always confers ability to follow simple written directions, such as labels on bottles of medicine or dietary instructions.

literacy rate The rate, usually expressed as a percentage, of people who are functionally literate, i.e., able to read simple instructions and local newspapers. As no time dimension is usually specified, it is a prevalence, strictly speaking, rather than a true rate. The status of girls and women is reflected in a country's literacy rate, which correlates inversely with infant and child mortality rates. Nations and communities with low female literacy rates have high infant and child mortality rates.

lithium (Li) A silvery, low-density metal, lithium is the basis for important chemical compounds including ceramics, plastics, lubricants, and mood-modifying drugs for manic-depressive illness. Lithium compounds are used in long-term treatment of mania, BIPOLAR DISORDER, and prophylaxis of recurrent depression.

lithosphere The earth's crust, comprising rock, shale, gravel, etc., some of which bears minerals or contains pockets of oil or natural gas. Quarries and mines invade only the outermost fringes of the lithosphere, and those who work in them encounter many occupational hazards.

lithotripsy The use of focused ultrasound waves transmitted through the body to cause renal calculi and gallstones to disintegrate, obviating the need for invasive surgery to remove them.

live birth Complete expulsion or extraction from the mother of a living offspring, one that breathes independently, has voluntary muscle movements, etc. WHO defines a live birth as complete expulsion or extraction from the mother of a product of conception, irrespective of the duration of pregnancy, which after such separation breathes or shows any other evidence of life, such as beating of the heart, pulsation of the umbilical cord, or definite movement of voluntary muscles, whether or not the umbilical cord has been cut or the placenta is attached.

liver fluke Several flukes, trematode parasitic flatworms, cause human disease, fascioliasis. They include *Fasciola hepatica* and *Opisthorchis* species. The adult worms live in the biliary tract and have a complex life cycle involving freshwater snails, a free-living stage, and freshwater fish. Humans and fish-eating mammals are infected when they eat raw fish or plants that are contaminated by infective metacercaria, such as watercress or water chestnut.

live vaccine A vaccine prepared from living pathogenic organisms, usually in attenuated form. Examples include measles, mumps, the Sabin poliovirus vaccine, and rubella vaccine.

living will A notarized document specifying actions that a person wants to be taken in his or her interests if illness impairs the ability to communicate wishes about care in the event of a prolonged period of terminal illness. The living will commonly asserts a person's wish not to undergo heroic interventions, such as cardiopulmonary resuscitation. See also ADVANCE DIRECTIVE.

LOAEL See LOWEST OBSERVED ADVERSE EFFECT LEVEL.

loa loa A variety of FILARIASIS that occurs in forest regions of West Africa. It is caused by a nematode filarial worm transmitted by horseflies and produces spongy soft-tissue swellings.

lobbyist A representative of an advocacy or special interest group seeking to influence the opinions and legislative decisions of elected representatives. Interactions between legislators and lobbyists may be benign, but lobbying often is perceived to confer benefits, promises of support from blocks of voters, financial support for re-election campaigns, free holidays and similar benefits, or outright bribes. Yet without lobbying, legislators may lack information to make informed judgments about proposed legislation. Lobbying in the United States has sometimes been more detrimental than beneficial to health and environmental issues.

local air pollution control The system used in the United Kingdom for regulation of localized atmospheric emissions by local government authorities rather than by the national government. This is used mainly as a form of local and, to a lesser extent, regional nuisance abatement. The system works well except when a pollution source downwind from a residential community evades regulation. In the United States and Canada, AIR SHED management is a comparable system.

local government The elected body that is directly responsible for and answerable to the members of a local community. Local governments usually oversee and may politically influence the work and priorities of local public health services.

local (public) health department The organized public health services that relate directly to the people and their public health problems in a local community, such as a municipality or city, in contrast to regional or national public health services and ministries that serve many localities. In many countries, there is no clear definition of "local" or distinction of municipal, district, and regional public health departments. The designation is determined by population and topography.

local public health system/services The system that provides public health services to a specified community, distinguished by inclusion of personal health services such as maternal and child care, treatment for sexually transmitted diseases, home visits to identified vulnerable and high-risk groups, such as isolated infirm elderly people, by public health nurses, dietitians, etc., as necessary for health maintenance to enable people to remain in their own homes rather than move into an institutional setting. In the United States, the response to the Institute of Medicine's report *The Future of Public Health* (1988) has included redefinition of local public health services to include explicit statements about their capacity to provide 10 ESSENTIAL PUBLIC HEALTH SERVICES. For details and discussion, see http://www.phppo.cdc.gov/nphpsp/documents/localmodelstandarsonly.pdf.

lochia The normal healthy vaginal discharge that occurs for about 7 to 14 days in the mother after vaginal delivery of an infant.

lockjaw The colloquial name for TETANUS, specifically the rarely seen, severe, life-threatening disease with facial rictus and muscular spasms that prevent the mouth from opening normally.

locus of control A term used by behavioral scientists to describe the perception that person(s) have regarding who is responsible or accountable for making important decisions. The term is used mainly about a study subject or patient, usually with the implication that the autonomy of the subject or patient is being encroached upon or voluntarily relinquished.

lod score A term used in genetics to describe the logarithm of the odds, i.e., probability, that a gene is linked to or related to the occurrence of a syndrome or disease. A lod score of 3 or more indicates a significant probability of association between a DNA marker and a condition.

log 1. Abbreviation of logbook, a written record of activities, such as a ship's log or a logbook of experiments. Research workers are required by the conditions of many research grants to maintain a complete log of all activities pursuant to their research protocol. 2. Abbreviation of logarithm.

logarithmic transformation The process of converting ordinal values to logarithms.

logging industry This industry harvests trees for timber used in building, furniture manufacture, softwood lumber used to make newsprint, and diverse other products. It is a heavy industry, and is hazardous, with an occupational mortality and serious injury rate among the highest of all occupational groups. It is increasingly perceived as ecologically harmful and often unsustainable because trees are felled and forested regions cleared at rates often greater than the rate at which new growth occurs in replanted regions. Destruction of habitat and species extinction are other negative features of the logging industry, and in tropical regions another consequence is emergence or re-emergence of exotic and dangerous pathogens.

logic The branch of philosophy and scientific reasoning concerned with canons of thought, precise definition, and unique names for tangible objects and abstract concepts, criteria of validity in reasoning, the use of inductive and deductive methods of reasoning, rational classification, and the application of the fundamental principles of underlying sciences (mathematics, physics, biology, etc.). Accepted axioms and assumptions are used as little as possible, the aim being to reason systematically from first principles. Application of logic is a sine qua non of good science.

logistics Coordination of complex operations involving several or sometimes many agents and varieties of operation, primarily in military situations, but the word describes activities conducted to deal with any complex task, such as program development or disaster management.

log normal distribution A distribution in which one variable, x, is the logarithm of another, y.

London smog A notorious episode of SMOG afflicted greater London in late November and early December of 1952, causing an estimated 7,000 excess deaths from cardiorespiratory disease directly attributable to smog generated by widespread domestic use of soft brown coal as heating fuel in the presence of a stagnant air mass. The principal ingredient incriminated in this episode was sulfur dioxide. The concentration of suspended particulate matter was also very high. This episode led directly to improvement of air pollution control in London and elsewhere throughout the United Kingdom. See also LOS ANGELES SMOG.

loneliness The perception of isolation from others that may be real or imagined and causes feelings of sadness, depression, or anxiety. It is a relatively common problem in elderly people whose close kin have died or moved away, and a potentially serious health problem, especially when combined with sensory and/or mobility impairment or depression.

longitudinal study Sometimes a synonym for CO-HORT STUDY, but often loosely used to describe any long-term study in which groups of people are reassessed after an interval or periodically.

long-range planning An essential activity of any complex organization, this is planning with a time horizon extending beyond the immediate budgetary period, usually for 5 years or more or, in more far-sighted organization, for 10, 15, 20, or 25 years into the future. Long-range planning in public health takes account of variables such as demographic projections, in both the population served and the staff serving them, economic forecasts, and predictable trends in social and economic development. It may be unrealistic and infeasible to plan further ahead than 25 years, but longer periods may be justifiable when considering issues of sustainable environments.

long-term care Medical, nursing, and social care of dependent persons over a prolonged period that may be provided by a multidisciplinary team or an individual caregiver, either in the dependent person's home or, more often, in an institution. It can include bedside nursing care, physiotherapy, provision of hot meals, rehabilitation, palliative care, or any combination of these. Long-term care is required for increasing numbers of dependent elderly and infirm people in modern urban societies where many people have no close kin to care for them. Special problems arise in the long-term care of persons with ALZHEIMER'S DISEASE, who may require custodial care to prevent wandering away. NOSOCOMIAL INFECTIONS are a common problem. The provision and economics of long-term care are challenging problems in many nations with aging populations.

long wave radiation Electromagnetic radiation with a wavelength greater than 0.3 microns and in the spectrum of lightwaves a wavelength greater than 0.7 microns. This includes the infrared wavelength, so it is an important consideration in atmospheric heat exchange. See also GREENHOUSE EFFECT.

Lorenz curve A graphical representation of income inequality in which cumulative percentage shares of national income are plotted against cumulative percentages of persons (or households) receiving each percentage of income. Incomes are inequitably distributed in all nations, notably in the United States, where the topmost 1% receive an estimated 25% of national income. The model was developed by the American economist Max O. Lorenz (1880–1962).

Los Angeles smog The haze or smog that afflicts Los Angeles and causes upper respiratory irritation (red, watery eyes, dry cough, etc.). This is a photochemical phenomenon, caused by the effect of solar ultraviolet radiation on oxides of nitrogen in automobile exhaust fumes, producing a combination of toxic and irritant oxides of nitrogen and other compounds and aggravated by high concentration of ground level ozone.

lost to followup The general term for all original participants in a COHORT or other long-term study who cannot or do not take part in further phase(s) for any reason, e.g., death, refusal, being untraceable, or having moved away from the study region.

Louis, Pierre Charles Alexandre (1787–1872) French physician and mathematician, one of the founding fathers of medical statistics and its applications in epidemiology. He wrote *Recherches Anatomico-Pathologiques sur la Phthisie*, a monograph of statistical research based on his analyses of 1,960 clinical cases and 358 pathological specimens from cases of tuberculosis, and taught his statistical methods to several 19th century physicians and epidemiologists from Britain, the United States, and other European countries, including WILLIAM FARR, William Budd, and OLIVER WENDELL HOLMES.

louping-ill A paralytic tick-borne neurological virus disease primarily of sheep that can infect humans, such as farmers. "Louping," an obsolete version of "leaping," refers to convulsive twitching and jumping of affected sheep. The disease can have considerable economic impact when it occurs in epidemic form and is therefore an important veterinary public health problem. It is controlled by eliminating ticks.

louse See also LICE. Wingless parasitic insect, usually species-specific, often selective in body sites that it inhabits. Human body lice can carry two dangerous epidemic diseases: louse-borne TYPHUS FEVER and RELAPSING FEVER. Head lice can occur in epidemic form in schools and institutions, and pubic lice are transmitted most easily during sexual intercourse.

Love Canal A disused canal at Niagara Falls, New York, that became a toxic waste dump for the Hooker Chemical Company. Among the toxic chemicals dumped there were large quantities of PCBs and dioxins, which permeated aquifers and contaminated Lake Ontario, causing an epidemic of reproductive failure in fish-eating seabird colonies as the toxins bioconcentrated in marine food chains. Public outrage arose in the 1970s and early 1980s when residents of nearby homes fell ill and a small localized cluster of birth defects and childhood cancers occurred, although this was never unequivocally demonstrated to be attributable to environmental pollution by PCBs or dioxins. Concern about the toxins released from Love Canal led to legislation that created the SUPERFUND.

low- and middle-income countries See INCOME LEVELS, WORLD BANK CLASSIFICATION.

low back pain A frequent symptom of a problem that can sometimes prove intractable, with any of several causes, including occupationally related musculoskeletal injury. Other causes include gynecological and renal disorders. The cause is hard to diagnose, and often there are legal claims for compensation when the pain is attributed to injury, especially in the workplace. This ranks among the most common causes of compensation claims on occupational insurance policies.

low birth weight A birth weight at or below 2,500 grams. Very low birth weight is defined as birth weight below 1,500 grams, and ultralow birth weight is below 1,000 grams. Birth defects are increasingly common at low birth weights, and many low birth weight infants require prolonged intensive care, which of course is increasingly costly.

low density lipoprotein (LDL) Plasma lipoprotein, comprising phospholipid, cholesterol esters, and triglycerides that transport cholesterol from the intestine to the liver. Excessive amounts of LDL and perhaps associated metabolic defects lead to accumulation of cholesterol and deposition as atheromatous plaques in arterial walls, especially in large vessels, including coronary arteries. The optimum level of LDL is less than 100 mg/dL (2.6 mmol/L); a level above 190 mg/dL (4.9 mmol/L) carries a high risk of atherosclerotic heart disease.

lowest observed adverse effect level (LOAEL) A term used in toxicology. Its self-evident meaning is the lowest concentration of a substance at which adverse effects are observed. Its utility is limited by the small numbers of test animals used in most toxicology studies, generally 20 to 50 per dose group, and resulting uncertainty about the shape of the dose-response relationship at low doses.

low-income group This is usually defined as the lowest decile, or lowest quintile, of household income. The health experience of this group is almost always at the low end of a gradient running from the highest- to lowest-income groups in the same and similar communities.

low-risk behavior Actuaries, epidemiologists, and others who compare health indicators always approve of persons whose behavior as revealed in answers to questions and/or by observation demonstrates low risk, e.g. nonsmoking, exercising regularly, eating and drinking in moderation, always using seat belts when driving, etc.

lumen 1. The SI unit of the amount of light emitted by a source of one candela. 2. The space enclosed by a tubular organ or blood vessel.

lung cancer During the second half of the 20th century, this was the most common killing cancer among men in many Western industrial nations (United States, United Kingdom, Europe), and in the last 2 decades of the 20th century it achieved this unwelcome status also among women, during a period in which the lung cancer death rate had begun to decline among men. These rates and trends reflect the influence of the principal risk factor: cigarette smoking.

lupus Lupus erythematosus, a chronic, recurrent systemic autoimmune disease with hepatic, renal, cerebral, cutaneous, and psychiatric manifestations. Susceptibility to systemic infections makes those with lupus vulnerable to opportunistic pathogens such as tuberculosis. The disease affects women more frequently than men. The course is usually slow, but relentless, deterioration.

luteinizing hormone The pituitary hormone involved in stimulating the formation of corpus luteum, i.e., one of the essential phases in the menstrual cycle.

lux The SI unit of illumination, i.e., one lumen per square meter.

Lyme disease A tick-borne disease caused by a spirochete, *Borrelia burgdorferi*, first identified in the village of Lyme, Connecticut, although it had been recognized and known by other names in Europe for 100 years. Since the identification of the causative organism, cases have been reported from many parts of the world. The principal signs are skin rash, arthritis, and meningoencephalitis. The condition can be treated successfully with doxycycline in the early stages but is often indolent, can become chronic or recurrent, and may cause prolonged disability. Control requires elimination or exclusion of ticks, but because these are carried by wild deer and other feral animals, this is difficult. See http://www.cdc.gov/ncidod/dvbid/lyme/ for details.

lymphadenopathy A pathological process affecting lymph glands that causes them to swell and become easily palpable. Usually this is inflammatory; sometimes it is of neoplastic origin.

lymphocyte The leukocyte (white blood corpuscle) responsible for producing specific immune responses; lymphocytes normally constitute about a third of all leukocytes. Their production is impaired or disrupted in disease states, e.g., HIV/AIDS, by radiation, and by immunotoxic drugs.

lymphogranuloma venereum A syndrome caused by a sexually transmitted infection with *Chlamydia trachomatis* (which also causes ocular trachoma); in recent years, this has been among the most common of the sexually transmitted diseases.

lymphoma Strictly speaking, swelling of lymphatic tissue, but the word is almost always applied to malignant conditions originating in lymph glands. Two main varieties are HODGKIN DISEASE, named for the British physician Thomas Hodgkin (1798–1866), which is probably caused by a virus, and non-Hodgkin lymphoma, which is often associated with exposure to polyhalogenated hydrocarbons, such as herbicides.

lysergic acid diethylamide (LSD) Street-named "acid," an easily manufactured synthetic hallucinogen derived from alkaloids of ergot. Its effects include elevation of mood, followed by sensory hallucinations, delirium, panic attacks, and other aberrant behavior. Its popularity arises from its alleged capacity to induce euphoria, but this is a minor and inconsistent effect.

lysis Disintegration of cells, with rupture of cell walls and destruction of nucleus and other anatomical features. This occurs with cell death; attack on the cell by chemicals, bacterial toxins, etc.; and in autolysis, i.e., dissolution of cells as a natural phenomenon.

M

macrobiotics An alternative lifestyle and dietary regimen distantly based on the oriental concepts of yin and yang (female and male) forces, astrological signs, the "vibrations" that people emanate, and similar concepts that are outside the mainstream of conventional medical and scientific beliefs. The macrobiotic diet has a high vegetable protein intake; avoids animal fats, canned foods, coffee, tea, and refined sugar;

and includes some unconventional ideas, such as avoiding tropical fruits and certain other - vegetables. It has dubious claims to improving health.

macroclimate The climate that prevails over a large geographical region, as contrasted with the MICROCLIMATE of a small circumscribed area or locality.

macroeconomics The study of the behavior of an economic system (e.g., in a market-driven economy or a socialist state) considered as an entity.

macular degeneration An age-related deterioration in the macula, the central section of the retina responsible for receiving and transmitting images of faces, printed matter, and similar fine details. Macular degeneration causes progressive loss of vision affecting the ability to recognize faces and read written material, road signs, and the like, although it is not necessarily accompanied by comparable loss of peripheral vision. It may be caused by vascular lesions, or it is an age-related condition accelerated by toxins including nicotine. Tobacco smoking tends to accelerate macular degeneration.

mad cow disease See BOVINE SPONGIFORM ENCEPHALOPATHY.

madness Syn: insanity, psychosis. Irrational or otherwise deviant conduct associated with a person's loss of contact with reality or other clinical evidence of psychosis. In a more general sense, a mental, emotional, or social behavioral aberration. A nonspecific subjective (and pejorative) diagnostic label preferably replaced by a less emotive diagnostic labelfor a condition that must be explored by careful psychological and psychiatric assessment.

maggot The larval stage of a housefly, blowfly, or green fly that grows in rotting meat or other organic matter. Their presence signifies putrefaction or filth and is an indication to condemn public premises, such as restaurants and rooming-houses. Maggots were formerly and are still occasionally used as a therapeutic method to cleanse suppurating or gangrenous tissue.

magic bullet The term originally applied to SALVARSAN, the arsenical treatment for syphilis derived from chemical compounds related to aniline dyes, by the German microbiologist Paul Ehrlich (1854–1915) in 1909. The term has been generalized and applied to any specifically targeted chemotherapeutic agent that is used to treat a particular disease.

magnesium (Mg) Light, metallic element that burns with an incandescent flame, indicating its affinity for forming chemical bonds. Magnesium is essential in chlorophyll formation, metabolism, and neural and muscular function, so it is one of the elements essential to all living things.

magnetic fields Syn: electromagnetic fields. The zones around power lines, equipment, or systems subject to electric currents. This includes the earth's own magnetic field, the MAGNETOSPHERE.

The magnetic fields around high-voltage electric power transmission lines, domestic appliances, and cellular telephones appear to have biological properties that are not yet fully understood but might include the capacity to alter cellular susceptibility to neoplastic change.

magnetic resonance imaging (MRI) Syn: nuclear magnetic resonance imaging, diagnostic imaging, body scanning. When the human body is exposed to radio frequency waves in a strong magnetic field, an image with the visual illusion of being three-dimensional is produced and can be projected onto a fluorescent screen or preserved on a photographic plate. This is a powerful diagnostic tool for revealing soft tissue configuration in the body. It is widely used as a diagnostic and prognostic aid to detect the presence and assess the progress of neoplastic lesions.

magnetosphere The magnetic field generated by rotation of the earth's molten iron-containing core. This magnetic field surrounds the earth and shields the biosphere from excessive exposure to harmful cosmic ionized radiation, thus protecting all living things. It is a component of the earth's LIFE SUPPORT SYSTEM, essential for population health. Interaction of cosmic radiation and ionized particles with the magnetosphere creates the dramatic and beautiful displays called the aurora in high northern and southern latitudes.

mainstream smoke The portion of tobacco smoke directly inhaled by a smoker, as contrasted with SIDESTREAM SMOKE, that is not inhaled and therefore is a greater environmental pollutant. The toxic and carcinogenic ingredients of mainstream smoke enter and harm the smoker's lungs.

mainstreaming A term to describe provision of health care, educational, and/or social services to specific groups of people with special needs within the existing health and social sectors, rather than in specially designated programs and services. The advantages include economy of resources and staff and avoidance of segregating people with special needs, but the disadvantages may include lack of highly specialized staff required to serve some people's specific special needs. The term is also used to describe application of a policy across an entire system, as in gender mainstreaming, which means application of gender equity throughout the system.

major medical insurance In nations such as the United States that lack comprehensive publicly funded insurance against the costs of expensive medical care for serious or "catastrophic" illness or injury, private insurance carriers offer policies to cover part of the cost of these services. Major medical insurance does not usually cover the cost of health maintenance, screening, or preventive services.

malabsorption syndrome A condition characterized by fatty diarrhea, anemia, weight loss, peripheral neuropathy, and various other symptoms and signs; it is caused by tropical sprue, fistula, or other anatomical abnormality that hastens the flow of intestinal contents, thus not allowing enough time for absorption and digestion of nutriment.

malaria A severe mosquito-borne protozoan infection of the blood and blood-forming organs causing recurrent bouts of high fever due to the destruction of red blood corpuscles by PLASMODIA, malaria parasites. It is one of the world's greatest public health problems, affecting more than 200 million people and killing about 2 million every year, including more than 1 million children. Its long-term effects include hemolytic anemia, and it has devastating effects on other organs and tissues. It is now mainly a tropical and subtropical disease, but historically it has been endemic in cool temperate zones, wherever the anopheline mosquito vectors can exist. Current facts and figures and details of programs such as ROLL BACK MALARIA are at http://www.who.int/topics/malaria /en/.

malaria life cycle The protozoan parasites of the genus PLASMODIUM that cause malaria in humans have a life cycle with a sexual phase in female anopheline mosquitoes and an asexual phase in human hosts. The sexual phase begins in the bloodstream of the human host with formation of microgametocytes and macrogametocytes, which develop into microgametes and macrogametes in the mosquito, where fertilization is followed by development of OOCYSTS, from which SPOROZOITES are released, enter the mosquito's salivary gland, and invade the bloodstream when the mosquito has its next blood meal. In the vertebrate host, the sporozoites invade the liver, undergo SCHIZOGONY and release MEROZOITES that invade red blood corpuscles. Inside red blood cells, merozoites, which appear as their "ring" stage, feed on hemoglobin and grow during their trophozoite phase, and undergo nuclear division (schizogony) to form schizonts. As the mature schizonts release merozoites, the red cells burst, and the fresh merozoites invade more red blood cells, causing the periodic bouts of fever characteristic of malaria that accompany this phase of the life cycle. Destruction of red blood cells causes hemolytic anemia and increasing debility. Some trophozoites develop into gametocytes, ready to invade anopheline mosquitoes when they next take a blood meal. Four different species of *Plasmodium* cause different clinical and epidemiological features of malaria. Various species of *Plasmodium* infect other vertebrates, mostly with a high degree of species specificity.

malaria terminology The common types of malaria are named on the basis of their periodicity, severity, and the specific plasmodium parasite responsible. Thus, benign and malignant tertian, quartan, falciparum, and cerebral malaria are identified. The prevention and control of malaria have generated enough terms to fill a substantial glossary. For example, drug-resistant malaria is classified as RI, RII, or RIII in terms of the extent of parasitemia after specified time intervals from beginning treatment. Periodicity is classified as quartan if the fever recurs every 3rd day, that is on day 1, day 4, and day 7; and as tertian if fever recurs on alternate days, day 1, day 3, day 5, etc. Stable malaria occurs year-round and varies little with changing seasons. Unstable malaria fluctuates widely. Usually, but not necessarily always, the incidence of new cases is greatest in the wet seasons. Several levels of endemicity have been recognized and categorized on the basis of the prevalence of enlarged spleens in children 2 to 9 years of age. Although this classification is no longer routinely used, it is offered here because it appears in much of the older published work on malaria. Hypoendemic means an enlarged spleen rate, of less than 10%, in children aged 2 to 9 years of age; mesoendemic means an enlarged spleen rate of 11% to 50%; hyperendemic means an enlarged spleen rate over 50% in children, usually over 25% in adults; and holoendemic means an enlarged spleen rate over 75% in children and a low adult rate. However, confounding variables abound, so modern malaria specialists regard enlarged spleen rates as a crude and unreliable measure of the impact of malaria on populations. Evidence from thick blood films and polymerase chain reaction tests provide better indicators of prevalence and endemicity. See the WHO Glossary at http://www.who.int/topics/malaria/en/ for details on these and other terms used in malariology.

malariology The scientific study of malaria, including the molecular biology of malaria parasites, the immunologic study of host-parasite interactions, the entomology of anopheline mosquitoes, the epidemiology of malaria, including mathematical models of epidemic and endemic malaria, use and evaluation of preventive and treatment regimens, and the quest for vaccines, as well as for effective treatment regimens. Few diseases have generated such sustained intense study, which is fitting since this is one of the world's largest unsolved public health problems.

malathion One of the organophosphate insecticides, used in mosquito control programs after DDT resistance developed. It has relatively low toxicity compared with other organophosphates, but it is a cholinesterase inhibitor, and acute poisoning can cause neurotoxic symptoms (paresis, paralysis of cranial and peripheral nerves). Its use has been restricted in some countries and in others, including the United States and Canada, it is an insecticide of choice for mosquito control programs. See http://www.epa.gov/pesticides/op/malathion.htm for details on uses, toxicity, etc.

male climacteric Syn: male menopause. Diminution of male libido, sometimes accompanied by psychogenic symptoms, such as mood swings resembling the menopause. ERECTILE DYSFUNCTION DISORDER often accompanies and may be the first symptom of the condition, and this often has a specific cause, such as arteriosclerosis or diabetes.

malformation A general term for any gross anatomical deformity, such as neural tube defect, phocomelia, conjoined twins, cardiac septal defects, imperforate anus, and many more conditions. Malformations are congenital, sometimes with known causes, such as early prenatal exposure to viruses such as rubella, environmental toxins such as dioxin, pharmaceutical drugs such as thalidomide, or chromosomal or genomic abnormalities. Often the cause is unknown.

malignancy, malignant condition Malignant means evil, bad, and as an adjective, this is the usual meaning in medicine and public health, applicable to many conditions. In a specific sense, "malignancy" means malignant neoplasm, pathological aberration of cell growth that leads cells to develop and proliferate abnormally and invade and destroy normal tissues and organs. See also CANCER, CARCINOMA, and NEOPLASM.

malingering Fabrication or simulation of symptoms with intent to deceive, for instance in lawsuits for damages resulting from occupational injury, or to avoid military service. Malingering is not a mental disorder, but malingerers may sometimes be mentally disturbed. The condition costs insurers and society considerable sums of money. The label "malingerer" should not be lightly applied because the appearance may cloak a serious and treatable psychological disorder.

malnutrition Literally bad nutrition because of inadequate intake of nutriment or lack of some essential dietary ingredient, such as protein, mineral or vitamins. Common varieties include protein-calorie malnutrition (KWASHIORKOR), vitamin A deficiency, vitamin C deficiency, and more extreme forms that occur in FAMINE, MARASMUS, and STARVATION. Specific varieties due to vitamin deficiencies are prevented and treated by dietary supplements; famine and mass starvation require urgent intervention and usually international aid.

malocclusion A dental condition in which teeth do not come into effective contact for proper mastication of food. There are many varieties and causes, some associated with deformities of the jaw or facial bones, some with abnormal eruption of primary or secondary dentition, some with imbalance between the size of teeth and the space for them to fit in the jaw bones. Malocclusion can impair mastication and digestion and predisposes to gum disease, but the undesirable effects of malocclusion are often cosmetic, rather than harmful to physical health.

malpractice A form of behavior of a health professional, usually a physician, that deviates far enough from what is regarded acceptable to constitute misconduct because it is dishonest, unethical, unprofessional, or incompetent. Malpractice includes sexual exploitation of patients, misuse of drugs, and medical negligence and is often punishable by revoking of medical license.

Malta fever, Mediterranean fever See BRUCELLOSIS.

Malthusian Adherence to the beliefs of the English clergyman and amateur economist Thomas Robert Malthus (1766–1834), who expounded his ideas in *An Essay on the Principle of Population* (1798). Malthus applied a simple demographic analysis to show that populations tend to grow exponentially, whereas essential resources, especially food supplies, increase arithmetically, leading to increasing imbalance of population and food supplies, making it desirable, if not essential, to limit human reproduction, to aim for ZERO POPULATION GROWTH, as contrasted with unrestrained family size and population growth. Malthus' dire predictions did not materialize because Europeans expanded into the Americas and Australasia where populations were able to escape starvation and more food could be grown. However, Malthus' predictions may prove reliable if countries experience a DEMOGRAPHIC TRAP.

mammogram An image of the anatomical structure of the breast produced on a photographic plate by low intensity x-ray, used to screen for breast cancer.

mammography Use of a mammogram to examine a woman's breasts for evidence of cancer. The commonly used method involves x-ray mammography, low-penetration soft tissue radiological examination, which exposes a woman to only a minimal dose of ionizing radiation. An alternative, THERMOGRAPHY, which relies on measurements of radiant heat emanating from the breast, is less reliable and is seldom used. Mammography is recommended for women in the second half of their reproductive life, roughly age 30 to 50 years, at 2-year intervals and less frequently for the following 20 years. Evaluations have shown the value of mammography in early diagnosis to reduce breast cancer mortality. Indications and other information are at http://www.nlm.nih.gov/medlineplus/mammography.html. See also SCREENING.

managed care A form of fiscal management of medical services used by HEALTH MAINTENANCE ORGANIZATIONS and other health care organizations to allocate referral and treatment services. The effects on personal care should be imperceptible to patients, but sometimes excessive bureaucracy and rigid rules based on diagnosis-related groups about referrals can impede freedom of physicians and patients to select the optimum choice for individuals. The rapidly rising costs of managed care in the United States have caused concern to insurers and governments. Many comparative studies have shown that managed care in the United States is more costly than comprehensive tax-supported medical care services because of high administrative overhead, and that outcomes are usually inferior.

management The art, science, and technique of getting things done by deployment of material and human resources in a systematic manner, and monitoring how, and how well, they are done. Management is often equated with ADMINISTRATION, managers with administrators. The distinction is that administration is concerned with objectives and aims, strategy and tactics, and management deals with how to implement these, how to get things done.

management by objectives Syn: results-based management. The approach to management that functions by setting specified objectives, targets, or aims, and proceeds by assessing the extent to which these are achieved, making suitable adjustments in the event of partial or total failure to achieve them. Measurement or quantifying of work output is implicit in the procedures.

manager The designated official responsible for management in an organization. This official generally works with and supervises the persons responsible for carrying out assigned tasks and reports to a higher authority, such as a director of operations.

mandate In the health sector, a commission, or explicit statement of empowerment for a professionally qualified person to perform a designated service or fulfill a requirement.

mandatory procedure A procedure that is required, whether to save life or for statutory or legal reasons.

manganese (Mn) A metallic element, an essential metabolic requirement, required as a cofactor in many enzyme systems by all plants and animals.

Manson, Patrick (1844–1922) British physician and tropical disease investigator. He discovered the filarial worm responsible for filariasis and its mode of transmission by mosquitoes. He made many other important original observations about tropical diseases. He was mentor to RONALD ROSS, who, with the Italian physician B. G. Grassi (1855–1925), clarified the life cycle of the malaria parasite, and he established the London School of Hygiene and Tropical Medicine.

Mantel-Haenszel test A CHI SQUARE TEST developed and refined by the American statisticians Nathan Mantel (1919–2002) and William Haenszel (1910–1998) for use with stratified sample data to control for the effects of CONFOUNDING variables. Mantel and Haenszel developed several other useful statistical methods, e.g., to adjust the ODDS RATIO to estimate relative risk.

Mantoux test Syn: tuberculin test. A skin test for evidence of infection with the tubercle bacillus that produces a region of redness, swelling, and induration in the skin surrounding an intradermal injection of tuberculin, the purified protein derivative (PPD) of the tubercle bacillus about a week after injection. It was developed by the French physician Charles Mantoux (1877–1947).

manure The excreta of domestic animals, cows, horses, pigs, etc., mixed with straw and used as fertilizer. Manure often contains pathogens, viruses, bacteria such as tetanus and clostridial spores, protozoa, or helminth eggs that may pose a risk for farmers and gardeners.

MAO inhibitors See MONOAMINE OXIDASE (MAO) INHIBITORS.

map, mapping 1. A pictorial representation of a country or region, intended to display features of importance, such as topography, location of cities, towns, etc., often presented in several colors or shades to display demographic, epidemiological, or other features that vary from one locality to another (a CHOROPLETH MAP). The process of preparing such a map is mapping or cartography. The term can also describe the representation of relative positions of genes on chromosomes. In epidemiology, SPOT MAPS have played an important role in clarifying routes of transmission ever since they were first used by JOHN SNOW and others in the mid-19th century. 2. The study of behavioral risk factors is sometimes called behavioral risk mapping. This approach is used in focused interventions for such conditions as HIV/AIDS among injection drug users.

marasmus Severe malnutrition that occurs after a period of prolonged hunger and starvation, usually with both protein and calorie shortage and deficiency of vitamins and essential minerals. It occurs in famine, in the advanced stage of certain diseases associated with malabsorption, and in some cases of child neglect.

Marburg disease Syn: African hemorrhagic fever. A dangerous hemorrhagic fever caused by a filovirus possibly carried by African monkeys that was first identified as a specific disease in Marburg, Germany, in 1967. In Central Africa, it has a case fatality rate ranging from 25% to 80%. Like Ebola virus disease, it can occur in epidemic form with very high case fatality rate, as in Angola in 2005. There is no effective antiviral therapy and no approved vaccine, although an experimental vaccine has been shown to be effective in infected monkeys. Information including current surveillance data is at http://www.who.int/csr/disease/marburg/en/.

March of Dimes A charitable foundation founded in 1938 by President Franklin Delano Roosevelt as the National Foundation for Infantile Paralysis to aid victims of POLIOMYELITIS. It relied on small donations collected door-to-door rather than on bequests or large donations. It supported research, including the work of Jonas Salk, that led to the first effective polio vaccine. With the control of epidemic polio myelitis the March of Dimes shifted its focus to support for and research on causes of birth defects. See http://www.marchofdimes.com/ for details.

margin of safety A phrase that may be expressed in general or quantitative terms that indicate safe levels of exposure to, or environmental concentration of, toxic or harmful substances. The slope of the dose-response curve is an indicator of the margin of safety. The more gradual the slope, the greater is the margin of safety.

marijuana Syn: cannabis, THC, pot, weed, grass. The active ingredient is produced from an easily cultivated hemp plant, *Cannabis sativa*, that is soporific, hallucinogenic, and a mood elevator. It is mildly (if at all) addictive, but habitual smoking carries a risk similar to that of tobacco smoking for chronic obstructive lung disease and respiratory cancer, although the risk is less than with tobacco smoking because marijuana smokers seldom smoke as heavily as cigarette smokers. Marijuana, the alkaloid cannabis, which is ingested in cakes or biscuits, and the purified alkaloid tetra-hydro-cannabinol (THC) are illegal in most countries but legal in the Netherlands and available on medical prescription for chronic pain in a few other countries, including Canada.

marker Indicative of the presence of a factor, influence, phenomenon, etc. See also BIOMARKER.

market A physical or conceptual setting where goods and/or services are negotiated and traded. Markets can have advantages for consumers who can seek the best available price but can have disadvantages such as protectionist policies, trade secrets, and monopolies. Many economists say that a free market is the most democratic way to conduct human affairs, but exceptions are recognized, and many philosophers and practitioners of health care and public health believe that a free market is not the best way to conduct health services. For example, it is more important to ensure a secure supply of essential vaccines and drugs by protecting the market than to allow a competitive market system to drive costs down but run the risk of impaired security of supply.

market-basket survey A periodic review of the content, costs, and nutritional composition of the food purchases of "average homemakers" that is used as an indicator of cost of living variations and also provides insights into nutritional intake and public understanding of nutrition. Market-basket surveys are also used to assess the content in foodstuffs of toxic substances, such as arsenic, dioxins. See http://www.cfsan.fda.gov/~lrd/dioxdata.html.

market testing A semiformal or formal test of a product, such as a pharmaceutical preparation, to assess the acceptability of presentation and cost of the product. Not to be confused with a PHASE IV CLINICAL TRIAL.

Markov process A stochastic process in which the conditional probability distribution at any future time is independent of the current state of the process. This mathematical system is named for its inventor, the Russian mathematician A. A. Markov (1856–1922). It is used in economic modeling. In epidemiology, it helps predict the course of pathogen transmission.

marriage counselor A professionally trained person who can intervene when marital partners have problems that threaten to disrupt the marriage and seek help to preserve their union. Some problems have medical or psychiatric dimensions, so there may be a professional interface with physicians in psychiatry, clinical preventive medicine, or other relevant fields.

marsh gas The gas produced by anaerobic decomposition of organic matter in swamps, etc. It may contain any of several odoriferous gases, but its principal component is usually METHANE, which is odorless and flammable.

masked depression A manifestation of clinical depression in which patients compensate for their depressed mood by adopting behaviors that occupy their time as fully as possible throughout waking hours, e.g., they may engage in constant demanding intellectual or physical work. Some creative artists and some scientists mask depression in this way.

masking Concealing identity, as with the proverbial burglar's mask. In clinical trials, the process of withholding the identities of study subjects in treatment and control groups, usually described as "blinding." The word "masking" is preferred to "blinding" by some clinical trial specialists on the grounds that "blinding" may be an emotive word.

Maslow's hierarchy of needs A conceptual model of human motivation developed by the American behavioral scientist Abraham Maslow in 1954. The model is based on the premise that much human behavior is goal directed. At the most basic level are needs related to the survival instinct (need for food, shelter, clothing, etc.); then come the need for safety and security, social needs such as family and other SOCIAL SUPPORT SYSTEMS, then what Maslow and others describe as self-actualization needs, i.e., achieving full potential as a person and thus satisfying self-esteem.

mass action principle A basic principle in infectious disease epidemiology that expresses in a mathematical formula some important predictive variables influencing the course of epidemics. These variables relate the anticipated course of an infectious disease epidemic to the number of susceptible persons in the population, the number of current infectious cases, the incubation period or SERIAL INTERVAL, which is the period between analogous phases of two successive waves of the epidemic, and the INFECTION TRANSMISSION PARAMETER, a constant for each specific infectious disease. The relationship is expressed in a formula:

$$C_{t+1} = C_t \times S_t \times r$$

where C_{t+1} is the number of new cases one serial interval in the future, C_t is the number of current cases, S_t is the number of susceptibles, and r is the infection transmission parameter.

massage Any among a variety of methods of kneading, pounding, stroking, pulling, or pushing parts of the body, primarily the limbs, as a form of therapy. Physiotherapists and massage therapists carry out a sequence of such maneuvers to treat aches, pains, strains, sprains, other soft tissue injuries, generally not reinforcing their ministrations with drugs. Critical evaluation shows that massage therapy is effective for many such conditions and for others, including pain management in advanced cancer, and it is rarely harmful.

mass casualties A term to describe the large numbers of dead and injured victims of a natural or manmade disaster. Situations involving mass casualties call for special methods and procedures, including provision of shelter, methods to dispose of the dead, emergency professional staff and infrastructure support, such as transport and communication facilities, TRIAGE to sort victims into those who can be helped by FIRST AID, evacuation to a tertiary hospital, compassionate handling of next of kin, and anticipation and amelioration of post-traumatic stress disorder.

mass media The printed press, newspapers and magazines, radio, television, and Internet sites that purvey news, information, misinformation, and all shades of opinion. Mass media provide a platform for dissemination of essential health information, so public health officials, health educators, and others need to know how to work with and use them and to be aware that they tend to sensationalize health issues and concerns, emphasize "newsworthy" items, and generate spurious controversies, which may be a disservice to health concerns and the general public.

mass medication Delivery or administration of a preventive or therapeutic regimen to the entire population or to selected portions of it. Examples include the addition of iodine to table salt in regions where there is known to be iodine deficiency; the addition of sodium fluoride to reservoir water, which is often deficient in fluoride; and mass vaccination campaigns against contagious diseases. Although it may be reminiscent of a paternalist past era of public health practice and is sometimes resisted on ideological or ethical grounds, the benefits of mass medication outweigh these possible disadvantages.

mass observation A method of assessing crowd behavior by actually observing, for instance, spectators at a sporting event; used in market research to assess popularity of products and to assess health-related behavior, such as hygienic practices, prevalence of smoking, seat belt use.

mass spectroscopy A method of assessing the molecular structure of substances by ionizing and passing them through an electronic beam in the case of liquids or a spark in the case of dry material.

master-file The file containing the original records relating to an event or process.

mastitis Inflammation of breast tissue, a common condition among breast-feeding women.

mastoiditis Inflammation of the mastoid sinus, an acutely painful and potentially dangerous complication of middle ear infection that can occasionally give rise to osteomyelitis or meningitis.

masturbation Sexual self-stimulation, a common human behavior associated with much adolescent guilt and angst. It is usually harmless but can have adverse psychological consequences. In 1997, the US Surgeon General remarked that masturbation is free from risk of sexually transmitted diseases and pregnancy and should not be condemned as an adolescent activity. Although scientifically valid, the remark implied approval, which was morally unacceptable to some, and the Surgeon General was forced to resign.

matched pairs A research design in which pairs of subjects are matched on as many criteria as feasible, other than the variable(s) under study, in order to minimize the effect of confounding variables. For instance, in a clinical trial, pairs could be matched for sex, age group, and occupation. A matched pairs design includes a matched pairs analysis, which can further contribute to the control of extraneous and confounding variables.

matching The process of establishing criteria for comparing individuals and groups that includes a careful search for similarities among individuals, as well as differences, that might contribute to or reduce the risk of confounding variables that vitiate the results of analysis. Matching may be done with individuals or with groups or grouped data. At its simplest, matching employs basic criteria (age, sex, occupation) and may include ethnicity, place of residence, income, dietary practices, or many other selected variables according to research design requirements.

maternal and child health (MCH) The branch of health services that focuses on mothers and their children. This is an extremely important component of public health sciences and practice, comprising many facets of health promotion and protection, disease prevention before and during pregnancy, safe care throughout labor and delivery and during the postpartum period and subsequently, especially through the early childhood years. It also involves curative personal services, which may be provided by family physicians, pediatricians, and nurses. Providers of MCH may be members of a LOCAL (PUBLIC) HEALTH DEPARTMENT, a HEALTH MAINTENANCE ORGANIZATION (HMO), independent fee-for-service health care providers, or alternative health care practitioners. The emphasis is on promoting and protecting health: monitoring growth and development, advising on infant feeding, nutrition counseling throughout childhood, ensuring that infants and small children receive vaccinations, etc.

maternal care A vague term that generally means care of women during late pregnancy, labor, and the immediate postpartum period. The emphasis is, or should be, on protecting the health of both mother and infant.

maternal deprivation A SYNDROME of physiological and behavioral aberrations observed in infants and children, attributable to insufficient or inadequate motherly nurturing. The features include delay in reaching developmental milestones, lack of ability to relate easily to others, and antisocial conduct, some features of which are observed in primates, as well as humans. It was described and identified as a syndrome by the British psychiatrist John Bowlby (1907–1990). The reality of the syndrome has been validated by recent observations of orphans in Romania and abducted children forced into armed conflicts in Africa.

maternal mortality Syn: maternal death. Death of a woman while she is pregnant or within 42 days of the termination of a pregnancy, regardless of the duration of the pregnancy and its mode of termination. For classification purposes, maternal death is further divided into: 1. Late maternal death, i.e., death of a woman from direct or indirect obstetric causes more than 42 days but less than 1 year after the termination of the pregnancy. 2. A pregnancy-related death is death of a woman while she is pregnant or within 42 days of the termination of pregnancy irrespective of the cause of death. 3. A direct obstetric death is death due to obstetric complications of pregnancy. 4. An indirect obstetric death is death resulting from a cause that existed before the pregnancy and is not aggravated by the physiological effects of the pregnancy. More than half a million women a year worldwide die of pregnancy-related causes, predominantly in developing countries. Many are caused by uncontrolled bleeding and/or infection, often a complication of botched abortions. Anemia is a common predisposing cause in low-income countries. Three widely used measures of maternal mortality are maternal mortality ratio, maternal mortality rate, and lifetime risk of maternal death. Maternal mortality ratio, i.e., the number of maternal deaths in a specified time period per 100,000 live births during the period, is most often used. The maternal mortality rate is the number of maternal deaths in a specified period per 100,000 women of reproductive age during the period. Lifetime risk of maternal death takes into account both the probability of pregnancy and the probability of dying as a result of that pregnancy and is cumulative over a woman's reproductive years. An approximation is the maternal mortality rate multiplied by the average length of a woman's reproductive life, which is 35 years.

maternal mortality ratio (MMR) The risk of dying of puerperal causes, i.e., associated with pregnancy, labor, childbirth, or the postpartum period, expressed as a ratio per 100,000 births, or less often as a "rate" per 100,000 women of reproductive age. Puerperal causes are mostly clearly defined, although the postpartum period is not. For statistical purposes, the WHO defines "postpartum" as any time up to and including 42 days after the termination of pregnancy, regardless of the duration of the pregnancy. The denominator is the number of live births in the same period in the same administrative or statistical jurisdiction. This is a complex statistic. The numerators and denominators do not correspond, notably when death is associated with abortion, which is the most common cause of maternal mortality in low-income countries. Discussion is at http://www.who.int/reproductive-health/publications/maternal_mortaity_2000/challenge.html.

mathematical model A representation of a biological process, system, or relationship by means of a mathematical equation or set of equations, often involving several random variables. The model usually consists of a mixture of variables and one or more associated constants or parameters. A model that does not involve random variables is deterministic. Models can be used to explain complex processes and to predict possible future trends, for instance in the incidence of diseases. In public health, mathematical models of communicable disease epidemiology were developed by WILLIAM FARR, RONALD ROSS, and others, and improved by later workers to plan and evaluate control measures for epidemics of malaria, influenza, HIV/AIDS, and other diseases. Models have been developed for cancer control, cardiovascular disease control, and other health programs.

matron The British term, now obsolete, for the head nurse or senior nursing officer in a hospital.

matrix 1. The substance of an organ or tissue. 2. The array of columns and rows in a table.

Max Planck Institutes The German institutes named for the physicist Max Planck (1858–1947) that support fundamental and applied research in a wide range of natural, biological, and medical sciences. The funds come partly from the public purse and partly from grants and contracts provided by the private sector, foundations, and donations.

maximum allowable concentration (MAC) One of several ways to display the criteria of safe levels of exposure to a hazardous or toxic process, chemical, etc., that can be used to establish the acceptability of working conditions. Expert committees of the World Health Organization, and

in the United States, the Occupational Safety and Health Administration (OSHA) have used a combination of laboratory and field tests and empirical observations to determine MACs, and in many countries these are written into official regulations with penalties for violation. MACs are often interpreted as a license to contaminate to the allowable level, rather than as an incentive to clean up the workplace environment.

maximum tolerated dose (MTD) The maximum dose of a substance that can be tolerated without adverse effects. This may be either a single dose or a daily intake level, depending upon the rate at which the substance is metabolized and/or excreted.

MCAT Medical College Admission Test, an intellectual screening procedure that is the first requirement of most medical schools in the United States, usually accompanied by other selection procedures, such as interviews with applicants who perform satisfactorily on the MCAT.

McKusick classification A classification of congenital conditions such as deformities and inborn errors of metabolism established by the American geneticist Victor McKusick (b. 1921) that is described and discussed in a landmark monograph *Mendelian Inheritance in Man* (1966). Every inherited disease identified in McKusick's classification is assigned a MIM NUMBER, and this number has been universally adopted by human geneticists. Frequent revisions have ensured that the McKusick classification remains abreast of advances in clinical and molecular genetics.

MD Officially the abbreviation for the academic degree of doctor of medicine; in practice, the abbreviation for "medical doctor," regardless of the exact nature of professional qualifications.

Meals on Wheels A widely used service in many countries, providing a meal, usually a hot meal, once a day, for elderly and housebound infirm persons, under the auspices of local public health or social services or a voluntary agency.

mean See MEASURES OF CENTRAL TENDENCY.

means test Assessment of financial resources and ability to pay for medical, social, and certain other services, e.g., subsidized housing, that are provided free or with subsidy for indigent persons. In the United States, means tests are used to assess eligibility for MEDICAID, FOOD STAMPS, and certain other services paid from public funds. Similar systems exist in many other nations.

measles A highly infectious virus disease that has been and still is responsible for very high case fatality rates among infants and young children who are vulnerable to bronchopneumonia as a complication if they are malnourished and not vaccinated. Adults exposed for the first time in their life to measles are also vulnerable. Measles was one of the most effective biological weapons that Europeans unwittingly deployed in the conquest and colonization of the Americas. It has been almost entirely eliminated from upper income nations since the introduction of measles vaccine, now usually given in combined doses with mumps and rubella vaccine (MMR VACCINE). See http://www.nlm.nih.gov/medlineplus/measles.html for information on current status, recommended vaccine requirements, and other details.

measles vaccine A live attenuated measles virus vaccine is preferable to the earlier killed virus vaccine developed by the American virologist and Nobel Prize laureate John Enders (1897–1985). It is heat labile so must be refrigerated until immediately before it is used. Preserving the COLD CHAIN is essential when this vaccine is given in the field in developing countries.

measurement properties and terminology The properties to be considered in relation to any measurement are ACCURACY, PRECISION, RELIABILITY, REPEATABILITY, REPRODUCIBILITY, and VALIDITY. Accuracy and precision are often confused but are distinct and different. Accuracy means the degree to which a measurement or estimate represents the true value of the attribute being measured, whereas precision is the degree of detail in the measurement. Reliability means dependability; and repeatability or reproducibility refers to the closeness with which a sequence of measurements of the same entity agree with each other.

measurement scale Any of the available ways to categorize data is called a measurement scale. Available ways include the dichotomous scale, either of two alternatives, positive or negative; the nominal scale, which arranges data into unordered categories, such as race, religion, country of birth; the ordinal scale, in which data are arranged in ordered qualitative categories, such as income levels or socioeconomic status; the interval scale, which arranges data on a quantitative basis at specified systematic intervals, such as Celsius or Fahrenheit temperature scales, ages, or dates of birth; and the ratio scale, in which values run from one fixed point to another, e.g., zero to infinity, that is used to measure and compare heights, weights, blood pressure, and some other variables.

measures of central tendency A general term for several parameters related to the distribution of variables around some "central" value. These parameters are the MEAN, MEDIAN, and MODE. The

median is the value at the point where exactly half the values in a set are higher and half are lower when all the values in a set are arranged in sequence. The mode is the most commonly occurring value in the set. The mean can be one of three kinds: the arithmetical mean is the sum of all the values in a set divided by the number of values in the set; the geometric mean is calculated by adding the logarithms of all the values in the set, dividing by the number of values, and taking the antilogarithm of this number; and the harmonic mean is the sum of the reciprocals of the values in a set, divided into the number of values in the set.

measures of disease occurrence These include measures of INDICATORS of disease, symptom clusters, risk-related behaviors, and OUTCOMES, death, disease, disability, etc. The measures conventionally used are INCIDENCE rates and PREVALENCE. In many situations there is a possibility of confusion between incidence rates and prevalence and also between RATES and RATIOS. It is important always to specify precisely and to be aware of problems such as the distinction between rates and ratios.

measures of dispersion The extent to which a series of measurements vary around a central value is signified by the STANDARD DEVIATION when the data are normally distributed. The difference or distance between the highest and lowest value is called the range.

mechanical transmission The transmission of pathogenic organisms by an animate or inanimate vehicle, carrier, or vector in which the pathogen does not undergo any form of development. For instance, houseflies carry fecal-oral pathogens on their feet, and house pets carry ticks and fleas, which may not necessarily multiply on the animal carrier before transmission to a human host.

Médecins du Monde A voluntary organization of health professionals predominantly but not exclusively in low-income, French-speaking nations, that aims to develop long-term capacity to meet the health needs of the people, rather than focusing solely on immediate crises.

Médecins sans Frontières (MSF) This private, nonprofit voluntary organization, also known as Doctors Without Borders, was founded in 1971 by a small group of French physicians. It has become the world's largest independent medical relief organization with sections in 18 countries. MSF is at the forefront of emergency health care and care for populations with endemic diseases and neglect. In catastrophes, such as armed conflicts, natural disasters, epidemics and famines, MSF provides primary health care, performs surgery, rehabilitates hospitals and clinics, and runs public health programs. Through long-term programs, MSF treats chronic diseases such as tuberculosis, malaria, sleeping sickness, and AIDS. Each year, MSF deploys more than 2,500 medical and support volunteers who join 15,000 locally hired staff to provide medical aid in more than 80 countries. MSF unites direct medical care with a commitment to bearing witness and speaking out against the underlying causes of suffering. MSF's resources originate mainly from private donations, with additional funding from donor governments, the European Union, and such UN entities as the UN High Commissioner for Refugees. MSF is politically neutral and differs from other organizations, such as the INTERNATIONAL COMMITTEE OF RED CROSS-RED CRESCENT SOCIETIES (ICRC), in focusing on the provision of continuing curative and public health services for noncombatants. See http://www.msf.org/ for details.

media See MASS MEDIA.

median See MEASURES OF CENTRAL TENDENCY.

mediation A discussion process aimed at narrowing differences between adversarial parties in industrial disputes that sometimes invokes health concerns in the course of resolving conflict. As a method of conflict management, mediation is used in complex political confrontations and to help to resolve marital and familial conflicts.

Medicaid A US social assistance program established in 1965 and publicly funded jointly from federal and state sources and administered by the states to pay for hospital and medical care of the medically indigent and people whose income level falls below a prescribed ceiling. Details are available at http://www.cms.hhs.gov/medicaid.

medical aide, assistant, auxiliary These terms are used more or less interchangeably to describe a person who provides generally unskilled or minimally trained help to a physician or the professionally qualified staff of a clinic or hospital. By implication, this is help that involves contact with patients or clients, rather than merely clerical assistance, and may include such tasks as preparing injections, applying bandages and dressings, and administering clinical tests (urinalysis, refraction, blood pressure, etc.).

medical anthropology The study of ways in which culture, tradition, and customs determine the occurrence and outcome of illness; the work of traditional healers, healing methods, rituals; how people perceive and react to illness; and many other general and specific ways in which culture and behavior influence health and illness. This is an essential body of knowledge and ideas with which all public health specialists should be acquainted.

medical audit A systematic evaluation of the processes of medical care based on statistical analyses of length of stay, procedures, outcomes, complication rates, etc., in relation to diagnoses, service providers, etc., all aimed at finding ways to enhance efficiency and effectiveness of care.

medical care Care of sickness or injury under the direction of a physician or, more loosely, care provided by any qualified professional person in a health-related institution, clinic, or comparable setting. In this sense, the term has administrative, fiduciary, ethical, and legal, as well as clinical, implications.

medical device An instrument, machine, or apparatus used for diagnosis, treatment, or prevention of disease or injury, e.g., crutches, prosthetic equipment, hearing aid, cardiac pacemaker.

medical entomology The study of insects of importance in medicine and public health. This is a major aspect of many vector-borne tropical disease control programs, in which it is essential to know the details of the vector's life cycle, preferred habitats, and seasonal patterns. Understanding medical entomology is an essential prerequisite to control of vector-borne diseases.

medical ethics The application of ethical principles to situations encountered in medical practice and medical research. See BIOETHICS.

medical examiner An official, usually a physician, who investigates deaths that appear not to be due to natural causes, i.e., violent, unexpected, occurring in industrial settings or in traffic, or possibly due to foul play or self-inflicted. See CORONER

medical geography In the scholarly pursuit of GEOGRAPHY, this is a specialized field that considers the distribution of specific diseases and human characteristics in relation to the geographical and topographical features of regions in a country or in the world.

medical history Syn: history of medicine. The meeting place of the scholarly pursuits of Clio, the muse of history, and Hygieia, goddess of health, this is the study of history as it has been influenced by disease, epidemics, famines, and the scientific, social, political, and cultural history of medicine, nursing, other health professions, and the history of public health. It also includes information about the discoverers of new knowledge in the medical sciences, such as when and where they lived and worked and how they made their discoveries.

medical indigence The status of persons who are sick or injured and lack the resources or insurance to pay for the cost of their treatment. This status is encountered in nations that lack comprehensive publicly funded (tax-supported) medical and hospital insurance programs. Among the nations of the Organization for Economic Cooperation and Development (OECD), the United States has the largest proportion of medically indigent persons.

medicalization A process whereby a normal activity, such as pregnancy and childbirth, evolves into a situation that requires, and even becomes dominated by, specialized medical care. Maternity nurses and midwives aim to prevent this. Other aspects of medicalization include invention of terminology to describe what had previously been considered everyday aspects of life, allied to creation of specialists and therapeutic regimens to "treat" the invented disease entities. Thus, misbehaving adolescents suffer from "oppositional conduct disorder" requiring treatment by psychiatrists and support staff; and age-related declining sexual potency becomes erectile dysfunction disorder, treated by drugs that generate large profits for their manufacturers. Medicalization accounts for an increasing burden of the rising costs of health care.

medically underserved area Syn: medically underserved community. A region or community identified by health agencies, medical associations, or politicians, as lacking an adequate supply of physicians, nurses, hospital beds, or health care infrastructure, to meet health care needs. In some jurisdictions, this designation qualifies such a region or community to receive capital funding for buildings, equipment, and financial incentives to encourage an influx of physicians, nurses, etc.

medical model A term used by sociologists to describe situations in which the conventional actions of physicians (diagnosis, treatment, prognosis) can be applied. See also MEDICALIZATION.

medical officer of health (MOH) Syn: LOCAL (PUBLIC) HEALTH OFFICER, COMMISSIONER OF HEALTH. A physician trained in public health sciences and practice who is responsible for supervising the protection of the people's health in a locality such as a city or a municipality. An MOH requires special skills in epidemiology, environmental, behavioral, and other health-related sciences; public health law; administrative competence; and political savvy. This last quality is a sine qua non: many public health problems have complex political dimensions that engage advocacy groups, political pressure groups, and ambitious politicians in search of election-winning causes.

medical professionalism The form of PROFESSIONALISM that is, or ought to be, a distinguishing characteristic of the medical profession. Its qualities include knowledge of basic and applied medical sciences, technical skill, the virtues of integrity, compassion, altruism, and the quality that the great Canadian physician William Osler (1849–1919) described as equanimity. The same qualities are required to a considerable extent by all public health professionals.

medical record A file of information about a patient that usually consists of several categories of facts: 1. Personal identifying and basic sociodemographic information (name, age, sex, place of residence, occupation, next of kin); 2. Clinical information (symptoms, signs, test results, diagnoses, treatment regimens, progress notes, outcomes); 3. Economic and fiscal details (method of payment, insurance coverage); 4. Administrative data (site, institution, specialty of service); and 5. Behavioral data (evidence on adherence to treatment regimen, keeping or breaking appointments).

Medical Research Council (MRC) The name of the agency in several English-speaking nations that administers medical research funds derived mainly or exclusively from government revenue or outright government grants. The MRC is publicly funded, administered, and accountable. The best known and largest is the UK Medical Research Council. Information about the UK MRC is accessible at http://www.mrc.ac.uk/. The Canadian Medical Research Council was replaced by the Canadian Institute for Health Research (CIHR) in 1997. See http://www.cihr-irsc.gc.ca/. The Australian equivalent is the National Health and Medical Research Council (NHMRC), accessible at http://www.nhmrc.gov.au. In France, L'Institut National de la Santé et de la Recherche Médicale (INSERM), accessible at http://www.inserm.fr, largely fulfills this role.

medical subject headings (MeSH) The generalized and precise terms used as keywords by the librarians of the NATIONAL LIBRARY OF MEDICINE and increasingly in other medical libraries to index the topics contained in articles listed in the *Index Medicus*. All are now included in the NLM's computerized data base, facilitating rapid searches for precise information. For details, see http://www.nlm.nih.gov/mesh/meshhome.html.

medical waste Used dressings, bandages, surplus blood and tissues from laboratory tests, used hypodermic needles, vials that contained injectable medications, etc. Much of this is hazardous waste and must be safely and securely disposed. It is often incinerated, but this requires special high-temperature methods if correctly done because regular low-temperature incineration may release toxic dioxins, furans, and other dangerous emission products.

Medicare A US federal government program to provide public funds to help pay for the medical and hospital care of persons 65 years of age and older, and others such as invalid pensioners entitled to Social Security benefits. Established in 1965, Medicare is federally administered. It has many detailed stipulations. For details see http://www.medicare.gov.

medication A general name for any preparation, medicine, pill, ointment, etc., that is applied, ingested, or injected in order to cure an illness or relieve its symptoms.

medicine 1. The profession and calling concerned with care of the sick, including care by skilled professional staff, lay healers, and family members. "Medicine" is a wide-ranging field of human activity, not confined to the profession that requires a university education. 2. A medication that is taken to treat a sickness. 3. The scientific study of disease and its determinants. In some traditions, the highest role of medicine is to preserve health and prevent disease, but in modern affluent nations, the profession of medicine is overwhelmingly dedicated to treating the sick, and this absorbs more than 95% of all health-related expenditure.

Medicines and Healthcare Products Regulatory Agency The British government agency that is responsible for assessing and regulating proprietary and over-the-counter pharmaceutical products, medications, medical devices, and other health care products. Details of its activities and conclusions are at http://www.mhra.gov.uk.

meditation A mental and emotional state sometimes described as concentrated relaxation, in which the meditating person empties the mind of troubling thoughts and feels at peace with others and with social and physical conditions in the environment. Meditation is advocated as a way to treat anxiety states, some forms of depression, stress-related conditions such as hypertension, and sometimes other physical conditions. Practitioners of YOGA are able to enter a trance-like state when meditating, and in this state, very slow heart rates and respiration have been observed, indicating that under some circumstances, meditation can slow metabolism significantly. See also BIOFEEDBACK.

medium 1. A nutrient broth or jelly that is used to grow cultures of microorganisms. 2. An intermediate or intervening entity. 3. (adj.) Pertaining to quantities and qualities midway between extremes.

MEDLARS Acronym for medical literature analysis and retrieval system, a service provided by the US NATIONAL LIBRARY OF MEDICINE in the 1960s, since superseded by MEDLINE and other more advanced computer-based search and retrieval systems.

MEDLINE The computerized online data base of the NATIONAL LIBRARY OF MEDICINE that contains data on authors, titles of articles, volume and pages numbers of journals in which articles appear, and covering all items listed and recorded in the *Index Medicus* since 1966. MEDLINE and its searchable data base PUBMED, derived from MEDLARS, are comprehensive, searchable data bases of medical and scientific publications. Others include Embase, *Science Citation Index*, the COCHRANE COLLABORATION, and SocioFILE. See http://www.ncbi.nlm.nih.gov/entrez/query.fcgi for details and access also to related sites.

mefloquine An antimalarial quinine derivative that is often effective when malaria is resistant to chloroquine. It can be used to treat falciparum malaria. However, it has serious adverse effects for some people, must not be taken during pregnancy, and is associated with major mood and personality disorders and even episodes of psychotic violence, so it must be used with caution and preferably under close medical supervision.

megacity Syn: megalopolis. A very large urban agglomeration. It may be a single city that has simply continued to grow and expand in all possible directions, usually upwards with multiple high-rise dwellings, as well as laterally, sprawling over formerly open countryside as in many American cities; or it may be the fusion of two or more existing cities, as in Tokyo-Yokohama, or the region sometimes called BosWash, in the northeastern United States encompassing Boston, New York, Washington, and various intervening cities, large ones such as Philadelphia and smaller ones such as Hartford and New Haven. Megacities often have outgrown essential infrastructure, including sewers and public transport, and have citizens with multiple social and public health problems.

meiosis Cell division unique to gonads in which pairs of chromosomes in germ cell precursors are segregated into the two daughter (i.e., haploid) cells, a complex two-stage process of division that leads to formation of male and female gametes that will transmit hereditary characteristics to the next generation after fertilization. In humans, only oocytes in the ovaries and spermatocytes in the testes undergo meiosis.

melancholia An archaic term for DEPRESSION. The word is derived from two Greek words meaning "black bile," implying that the liver is the seat of the problem, and it evokes the humoral theory of disease causation.

melanin The dark brown pigment produced in response to solar radiation by melanocytes in the skin, the retina, and hair. It provides protection from exposure to ultraviolet radiation.

melanoma A neoplasm of the melanocyte cells, almost always malignant and often extremely so, with a propensity to invade and metastasize widely. People with little natural melanin pigment, such as those of northern European origin, who live in subtropical regions exposed to intense solar radiation are particularly vulnerable to malignant melanoma.

melatonin The hormone involved in the sleep-wake cycle, derived from serotonin and produced in the pineal gland and retina. Melatonin secretion is greatest at night and lowest by day. It is part of the control mechanism of the reproductive cycle in many animals. It reputedly helps overcome JET LAG and relieve the associated sleeplessness.

melena Black stools, the appearance of stools containing partly decomposed blood, caused by hemorrhage higher up in the gastrointestinal tract than the rectum or descending colon.

melioidosis An uncommon bacterial infection caused by *Burkholderia pseudomallei* that may occur in agricultural workers in many parts of the world with indolent symptoms of pulmonary congestion and consolidation, or may be relatively symptomless. It is acquired from infected soil or contact with infected animals. It responds to broad-spectrum antibiotics.

meltdown The consequence of catastrophic overheating in the core of a nuclear reactor. This has partially happened in nuclear power plant accidents at THREE MILE ISLAND and CHERNOBYL, and it is believed that in theory a severe catastrophic meltdown could cause widespread and penetrating melting and vaporizing of the environs of a nuclear power plant.

meme A word coined by the British geneticist and biological scientist Richard Dawkins (b. 1941) to describe the cultural "inheritance" of behaviors transmitted from generation to generation by a combination of oral tradition and stored information in libraries, etc. The combination of genes and memes determine the characteristics of members of a nation or community.

memory 1. A complex neurological and psychological phenomenon located in the cerebral cortex, comprising short-term and long-term memory, sensory and psychological associations, as with sights, sounds, smells. Many aspects are poorly understood, despite decades of research. With advancing age, memory often becomes partly defective, with progressive loss of ability to recall names or recognize faces. Memory loss is a consistent feature of dementia. Some memories are retained, others lost or suppressed, and retrieval is fraught with uncertainty, even controversy in the case of FALSE MEMORY SYNDROME. 2. In computer science, "memory" is the programs and data (information) stored on magnetized disks or tape.

memory loss A generic phrase for several neurological and psychological conditions. A benign form is the common problem of many people past middle age who have progressively increasing difficulty recalling names and associating them with familiar faces. Encephalopathy due to drugs, alcohol, toxic chemicals, brain damage of vascular origin, amnesia, Alzheimer's disease and other organic brain diseases are more serious causes, and psychiatric disorders are an additional group.

menarche The developmental milestone in female life marked by the onset of menstruation. Other pubertal changes—enlargement of breasts, broadening of hips, etc.—proceed over a period of several years around this event. Menarche has occurred at progressively younger ages since the late 19th century for reasons not fully understood, probably including improved nutrition.

Mendel, Gregor (1822–1884) The Austro-Hungarian monk and botanist who worked out the mathematical laws of genetics, essentially applications of probability theory. Mendel observed and recorded results of breeding garden peas of different configuration, demonstrating that the characteristics of the second generation derived equally from both parent plants. He published his findings in 1866 in an obscure journal, where they remained unnoticed until 1900. His work is commemorated in the term "Mendelian genetics" for the inheritance patterns he described.

Mendelian randomization A development in genetic epidemiology based on Mendel's second law that inheritance of one trait is independent of inheritance of other traits. It uses common genetic polymorphisms that are known to influence exposure patterns (such as propensity to drink alcohol) or have effects equivalent to those produced by modifiable exposures (such as raised blood cholesterol concentration). Associations between genetic variants and outcome are not generally confounded by behavioral or environmental exposures. This means that observational studies of genetic variants have properties similar to INTENTION TO TREAT ANALYSES in randomized controlled trials.

Mendel's laws The laws of Mendelian genetics, established by Gregor Mendel, govern the inheritance of many single-gene characteristics and influence inheritance of complex multigene characteristics. The law of segregation states that an inherited characteristic is controlled by a pair of alleles that separate and are incorporated in different gametes. The law of independent assortment states that separated factors are independent of each other when gametes form. Single-gene disorders are uncommon but may be sex-linked, recessive, or dominant characteristics.

meningitis Inflammation of the meninges, the endothelial lining of the brain and spinal cord. This is almost always an acute life-threatening disease caused by bacteria or viruses. Some forms, e.g., acute meningococcal meningitis, can occur in epidemics, characteristically in army camps, and can be prevented by type-specific vaccines. Meningococcal meningitis is a major problem in parts of Sub-Saharan Africa. Other important varieties are caused by *Haemophilus influenzae*, tuberculosis (uncommon), and several viruses. Meningitis can occur as a complication of many other infectious diseases.

meningococcal diseases Infections caused by the bacterium *Neisseria meningitidis*, formerly called meningococcus. This organism is often resident in the nose or pharynx, and can become highly infectious and cause epidemics in confined communities such as military barracks and residential schools. It can cause meningitis, pneumonia, and, less commonly, septicemia and septic arthritis. All usually respond well to antibiotics; a vaccine was developed in 2005.

menopause The milestone in a woman's life marked by the cessation of MENSTRUATION and often by an array of associated symptoms, including mood swings and vasomotor changes (hot flushes or flashes) that may persist for months or years. The symptoms may be partly determined by cultural factors but are also due to hormonal withdrawal and vasomotor malfunction. Menopausal symptoms may be at least in part culturally determined. Women in some cultures do not appear to get significant unpleasant symptoms. In affluent nations, HORMONE REPLACEMENT THERAPY (HRT) is popular and is claimed to relieve many of the symptoms, as well as to reduce the impact of postmenopausal osteoporosis.

menorrhagia Pathologically excessive loss of menstrual fluid, which includes a considerable amount of blood, often sufficient to cause iron-deficiency anemia.

menstrual cycle The monthly rhythmic maturation and discharge from the ovary of an ovum ready for fertilization, accompanied by hormonally mediated fluctuation of the uterine lining in preparation for implantation of a fertilized ovum.

If fertilization does not occur, the ovum and the uterine lining are discharged, along with some blood, in MENSTRUATION.

menstrual period The shedding of the mucosal lining of the uterus that occurs in the absence of fertilization, which normally occurs with a regular periodicity of 28 days.

menstruation The normally regular hormone-controlled 28-day cycle during a woman's reproductive years, in which ovulation occurs, and, if fertilization does not take place, the lining of the endometrium is shed, along with menstrual blood. The monthly loss of blood and uterine epithelial tissue is called menses. For some women, menstruation is preceded by mood swings; for a few it is painful or distressing, associated with cramping pain and heavy blood loss that rarely is severe enough to cause anemia.

mental handicap Syn: mental impairment, incompetence, retardation. This term covers a large group of disorders with many possible causes in which intellectual function is inadequate to some degree. A person who is mentally handicapped may be so little affected as to pass unnoticed in everyday life; may require help to negotiate simple transactions, such as shopping or traveling on public transport; or may be unable to function independently, sometimes with associated physiological malfunctions, such as lack of control of bladder and bowel, and loss of social inhibitions, and may therefore require partial or continuing care in a custodial setting.

mental health Syn: mental hygiene. The branch of health care and public health concerned with prevention and control of diseases of the mind. It is classified as conditions in which brain function is affected from birth or as a consequence of environmental or other factors that operate after birth. It includes various levels of mental retardation; conditions in which the affected person retains intellectual contact with the real world, loosely classified as neuroses; conditions in which the affected person lives in a world that has lost contact with reality, loosely classified as psychoses (see PSYCHOSIS); and conditions in which the affected person's previously intact intellectual and emotional functions are lost, progressively or suddenly, loosely classified as DEMENTIA.

mental health services The multidisciplinary, multisectoral array of personnel and facilities to promote, protect, and restore good mental health. They include institutional and community-based public and private services involving the active participation of psychiatrists, psychologists, and social workers. There are custodial and noncustodial mental hospitals, psychiatric services based in general hospitals, and mental health services such as distress centers and hotlines run by local health departments and private voluntary agencies. Privately practicing physicians and psychiatrists and many community-based agencies that care for persons with particular diseases and their families are generally not regarded as components of mental health services, despite involvement in aspects of mental health care. See also DEINSTITUTIONALIZATION, HALFWAY HOUSE, and entries for specific mental disorders.

mental hospital An institution that provides care and shelter for people with mental, emotional, and personality disorders, sometimes severe enough to require custodial care. Mental hospitals have a long tradition, dating back at least to Pergamon in Asia Minor (350 BCE). Until the middle of the 19th century, there was almost no effective treatment for most of the inmates of such hospitals. Among their problems and challenges, an important one was the maintenance of good hygiene and sanitation. Influenced by the philosophy of DEINSTITUTIONALIZATION, large custodial mental hospitals have been closed in many countries since the 1970s, and their patients removed to smaller residences or discharged to community care, despite the fact that such care often is inadequate. Cross infection remains a problem in institutions for the mentally retarded.

mental impairment Syn: mental retardation. The condition in which reduced mental, emotional, and/or intellectual capacity renders individuals unable to function fully or normally in society. Depending on the severity of their condition, they require varying degrees of familial and/or social support, and, in the most extreme cases, institutional care. This miscellaneous group of conditions has many possible causes, including congenital conditions such as DOWN SYNDROME, FETAL ALCOHOL SYNDROME, HYPOTHYROIDISM (IODINE DEFICIENCY DISORDERS [IDD]). Prevention is possible for IDD, and fetal alcohol syndrome is preventable if alcohol intake can be controlled.

mentor In Greek mythology and Homer's *Odyssey*, Mentor was the guide and counselor for Odysseus's son Telemachus. Educators and others have adopted the word to describe a formal or informal attachment between a teacher and a student or small group of students that goes beyond mere teaching or tutoring to include advice and guidance about many other issues and problems encountered by students. The process is described as mentoring and is widely used in graduate level education in public health among other fields of higher professional education.

men who have sex with men A nonjudgmental term favored by members of the gay community and HIV/AIDS advocates to describe homosexual and bisexual men who are often at high risk of sexually transmitted diseases, including in particular HIV/AIDS.

mercury (Hg) Silver-colored metallic element, liquid at room temperatures, with many uses, in scientific instruments, amalgams with other metals for dental fillings, and in compounds in drugs, pigments, explosives, and pesticides. Elemental mercury and its inorganic and organic compounds are almost all extremely toxic to nerve tissue and have been responsible for several episodes of mass poisoning, including MINAMATA DISEASE, caused by eating fish or shellfish contaminated by methyl mercury in industrial effluent in Minamata Bay, Japan.

mercury poisoning Syn: erethism. A disease affecting the central nervous system, mucosal surfaces of the mouth, and the skin caused by environmental or occupational exposure to mercury or many of its compounds. These may be ingested, inhaled, or absorbed through the skin. Many mercury compounds bioaccumulate, for example, in Minamata Bay, Japan, where industrial effluent containing methyl mercury salts bioaccumulated in zooplankton and crustaceans and caused the condition called MINAMATA DISEASE. In the 18th and 19th centuries, mercury salts were used to treat fur for hats; the workers often developed neurological and psychiatric symptoms, hence the saying "mad as a hatter."

merozoite The stage in the human phase of the malaria parasite in which parasites are released to invade red blood corpuscles, either after sporozoites entering from the mosquito's salivary gland have completed their development in parenchymal cells of the liver, or after mature trophozoites have produced and released them in the blood.

mescaline A hallucinogen derived from a cactus that grows in the southwestern United States and Mexico. It was used in religious rituals by pre-Columbian civilizations and is used by some modern substance abusers, often in a mixture with marijuana to induce a hallucinatory "high." It is addictive, and repeated or prolonged use can induce psychosis.

MeSH Acronym for medical subject headings used by the National Library of Medicine to compile entries in the *INDEX MEDICUS*. The MeSH headings are derived from the keywords used in the abstracts or summaries of articles published in indexed journals. Some journals include MeSH headings, rather than keywords, with STRUCTURED ABSTRACTS of published articles. The MeSH headings can be seen at http://www.nlm.nih.gov/mesh/meshhome.html.

mesothelioma A highly malignant neoplasm of pleural or peritoneal membrane, most often caused by exposure to asbestos, that occurs after a very long latency period, usually several decades. It sometimes occurs several decades after exposure to relatively low concentrations of asbestos dust.

messenger RNA (mRNA) The template message required for protein synthesis of DNA.

meta-analysis The critical review and analysis of multiple studies of a causal relationship or a therapeutic or preventive regimen that yields a quantitative aggregate summary of all the results. It is a systematic, organized, and structured evaluation of a problem and of methods used in earlier studies of the problem. It is preferable to include only studies in which there are similar study and control group populations, similar design, methods, and procedures. The aim is to identify and evaluate the overall trend in the pooled results of all studies included in the meta-analysis. It is most often applied to sets of RANDOMIZED CONTROLLED TRIALS (RCTs), but is also used to pool the results of CASE CONTROL and COHORT STUDIES. There is a qualitative element when the studies are critically assessed and their rigor or lack of it is taken into account. See also POOLING and SYSTEMATIC REVIEW.

metabolic diseases A general term for diseases in which normal metabolic processes are upset or disrupted in some way. The causes include inborn (genetic) errors of metabolism leading to absence or malfunction of an essential metabolic process, hormonal dysfunction, and mineral or vitamin deficiency states. Examples include phenylketonuria, diabetes, and thyroid dysfunction.

metabolism The biochemical processes responsible for transformation of nutritional intake into energy to maintain bodily activity, storage as fat for transformation and use as energy at a later time, and excretion of waste products produced during the biochemical transformation of food into energy, otherwise known as metabolic transformation.

metal fume fever An occupational disease with fever, cough, and shortness of breath caused by exposure to the fumes of molten copper or suspended atmospheric copper dust. It occurs also with exposure to the fumes or dust of other metals, such as nickel or chromium, although these produce other and more severe symptoms.

metals Elements and mixtures of elements (alloys) characterized by strength, hardness, ability of many to conduct an electric current, usually a high melting point (mercury is an exception, liquid at room temperature). Some, such as calcium, iron, copper, magnesium, and manganese, are essential trace elements in human, animal, and/or plant metabolism; and others, such as lead, mercury, and arsenic, are extremely toxic. Essential metallic trace elements also may be toxic if large quantities are ingested.

metaphase The second phase of cell reproduction, during which the chromosomes are aligned along the equator of the cell, preparatory to division of the nucleus.

metastasis The pathological process by which malignant cells multiply in organs or tissues that are separate from the original site of the malignant condition, as distinct from spread by invasion of organs and tissues adjacent to the original site. It is not clear whether metastatic cells arise in the primary site and migrate via the bloodstream or lymphatic vessels, or the malignant process initiates neoplasia at the site of metastases. Perhaps both processes occur.

meteorology The study of weather, factors that influence it, and ways to predict its future course. Weather has been recognized as a determinant of health since Hippocrates (4th century BCE). In a time of drastic climate change, such as the early 21st century, the connection of weather to health has become stronger and more relevant to public health than ever before. Increasing concern about weather forecasting in the current period of climatic instability has been accompanied by increasing precision and reliability of meteorological instruments, notably satellite observations that enable accurate tracking of the path of extreme events, such as HURRICANES. Current conditions and forecasts are available at http://www.arl.noaa.gov/ready/cmet.html and from the World Meteorological Association at http://www.wmo.ch.

methadone A synthetic analgesic, with properties resembling those of heroin but less addictive, that is used to treat heroin addiction.

methadone maintenance A method of treatment aimed at weaning heroin addicts from their addiction. It does so, but may be at the cost of creating methadone addiction. To be effective, maintenance methadone must be combined with psychotherapy and social support.

methamphetamine A methylated derivative of amphetamine, a powerful central nervous system stimulant that induces wakefulness and hyperactivity and is therefore a recreational drug, widely used illicitly with street names such as speed, uppers, and CRYSTAL METH. It is often combined with other illicit DESIGNER DRUGS in powerful and dangerous mixtures. Prolonged or repeated use can induce psychotic states resembling paranoia. It is easily synthesized, so "laboratories" to make it have proliferated, and illicit use has become a serious public health problem.

methane (CH$_4$) Syn: marsh gas, fire damp. The simplest hydrocarbon in the paraffin series, an odorless, flammable gas, explosive when mixed with air. Methane is formed by decomposing vegetation. It is released by heating coal and sometimes occurs in large pockets in underground coal mines, where its release can trigger disasters caused by explosion of the gas. In permafrost regions, large quantities are stored in frozen form that could be released as permafrost thaws during the process of GLOBAL CLIMATE CHANGE.

methemoglobin Transformation of oxyhemoglobin to form ferric oxide, rather than ferrous oxide, under the influence of chemicals such as acetanilide or potassium chlorate. This prevents the action of hemoglobin in oxygen–carbon dioxide transfer at the cellular level. In the bloodstream, its blue color causes a characteristic bluish color of the lips, ear lobes, etc., called methemoglobinemia.

Methicillin-resistant *Staphylococcus aureus* (MRSA) An antibiotic-resistant strain of *Staphylococcus aureus*, also called multiple-resistant *S. aureus*, that has proliferated widely, especially in hospitals, where it is responsible for increasing numbers and proportions of antibiotic-resistant NOSOCOMIAL INFECTIONS.

methionine An essential amino acid that is present in many proteins.

methodology The scientific study of methods. This word has evolved from a pretentious alternative to "method" or "methods" to become accepted standard usage when describing in detail how a research study has been conducted.

methods and procedures An essential prerequisite of all research projects and of descriptions of these projects that are prepared for scientific peer review, and ethical review if required, is a detailed, comprehensive account of what will be or was done (the methods) and how (the procedures). It is these aspects of the work that are often collectively described as "methodology."

methoxychlor An insecticide used as a substitute for DDT, less toxic, with a shorter half-life and therefore a useful alternative.

methyl alcohol Syn: methanol, wood alcohol, rubbing alcohol. The simplest of the alcohols, CH$_3$OH, a colorless liquid, poisonous when ingested even in small quantities, used as an industrial solvent. The effects of ingestion include irreversible damage to the optic nerve, causing blindness.

methyl bromide A colorless, odorless volatile gas used as a soil fumigant and insecticide. Human exposure causes irritation of mucosal surfaces, nausea, vomiting; prolonged exposure leads to neurological damage, including paresis, confusion, and visual and other sensory disturbances.

methyl chloride A colorless sweet-smelling gas at room temperature, an intermediate product in some chemical processes, used as a propellant in production of foam plastics and formerly as a refrigerant. It is a central nervous system depressant and causes mental confusion, convulsions, and ataxia; prolonged exposure to low concentrations can cause these effects to become permanent.

methyl isocyanate An extremely toxic precursor used in insecticide production that was responsible for one of the worst industrial accidents ever reported, when it escaped from a Union Carbide plant in Bhopal, India, in 1984.

methyl mercury A highly toxic ingredient of waste products of mercury compounds used in industry. Mercury discharged in industrial effluent contaminates aquifers, water courses, etc. and is biotransformed by bacteria in marine and some freshwater food chains to methyl mercury. This has a long half-life. It was the agent responsible for MINAMATA DISEASE.

methyl tert-butyl ether (MTBE) A colorless volatile liquid used as a gasoline additive to improve efficiency of combustion and reduce emission products.

Metropolitan Life tables Beginning in the 1930s, actuaries and statisticians of the Metropolitan Life Insurance Company prepared and published LIFE TABLES and much other useful statistical information based on analysis of data about their policy holders. This included information about relationships among variables, such as age, sex, weight, height, blood pressure, visual acuity, occupation, place of residence, and tobacco and alcohol use. Policy holders were not, of course, a random sample of the general population, but despite this limitation the Metropolitan Life tables were widely used for many years because they were often the only source of approximately normative data on ranges in body weight and blood pressure. They have been superseded by more representative data from the NATIONAL HEALTH AND NUTRITION EXAMINATION SURVEYS (NHANES) of the US National Center for Health Statistics.

metropolitan statistical area Also called standard metropolitan statistical area (SMSA). The term used by the US Census Bureau to describe the administrative and statistical region embracing a city and its immediate environs that is designated in statistical tables of population, etc., at times of the periodic census.

miasma theory A theory that had considerable currency during the 18th and 19th centuries as a way to explain the origin and propagation of some epidemic diseases, particularly cholera. The theory was that the cause was miasma, an ill-defined emanation from rotting organic matter. The theory derived empirical support from the observed distribution of malaria and yellow fever in marshy regions, until it was discovered that these are mosquito-borne diseases.

microbe A general term for any living thing that is below the limits of visibility with the naked eye, usually including all bacteria, sometimes referring only to pathogenic microorganisms. Because of its lack of precision, the word is best avoided in scientific discourse.

microbiology The scientific study of microorganisms, embracing BACTERIOLOGY, the study of bacteria; MYCOLOGY, the study of funguses and molds; and virology, the study of viruses.

microclimate The climatic conditions in a small circumscribed setting, often implying more benign conditions than those that are usual in the region because of favorable local influences, e.g., the climatic conditions in a valley exposed to sunlight and sheltered from cold winds.

microeconomics The study of individual economic units and their interactions, including the theory of producer, consumer, and market. This aspect of economics deals with how consumers choose to allocate and use their financial resources, and with decisions of manufacturers of goods and purveyors of services regarding the goods and services in a society or nation.

microfiche A method that was widely used to store miniaturized documentary records by photographic reproduction. On a microfiche, a typescript page occupies only a few square millimeters of film. A special microscope projection screen is required to read the stored information, and reading can be a tedious process if many pages have to be scanned, but microfiche was universally adopted as a space-saving measure in libraries all over the world, although now often superseded by computerized records that are more easily and efficiently stored.

microflora A word sometimes used to describe the miscellaneous commensal microorganisms that inhabit the gastrointestinal tract, or more loosely, any colony of micro-organisms.

micronutrient A general term for vitamins and minerals that are essential nutrients required in only tiny amounts as part of daily dietary intake.

microorganism An organism that is visible only under a microscope. Microorganisms occur in prodigious numbers and varieties. They include viruses, bacteria, mycoses (fungi), and unicellular and multicellular microscopic organisms such as many varieties of phytoplankton and zooplankton that are the simplest forms of plant and animal life. Some microorganisms are essential to life, and others are pathogenic.

microwave Electromagnetic radiation in the wavelength ranging from about 30 cm to 1 mm, from radio waves almost to the infrared end of the visible spectrum. The main biological effect is to generate heat in tissues (thus its use in microwave ovens). Microwave length radar has been accused of causing sterility and mental disorders, although the charges are unproven.

midbrain The portion of the brain between the forebrain, containing the cerebral cortex, and the hindbrain. The midbrain is rich in neural transmitting tissue, i.e., nerve fibers and the roots of important cranial nerves, as well as the part of the brain that processes sensory input in many vertebrates. The midbrain is less developed in humans than in other vertebrates.

middle class An imprecise and much abused term. In medieval times, middle class meant people who made their living from trade, in contrast with landowners and the hereditary aristocracy, who were above them; and serfs, landless peasants, wanderers, gypsies, and vagrants, who were below them in social standing. The looser usage began in the industrial era. Social classifications such as the British REGISTRAR GENERAL'S OCCUPATIONAL CLASSIFICATION into five SOCIAL CLASSES imply that the middle classes are skilled clerical and technical workers, but the term seldom has this degree of precision in everyday usage.

middle ear The air-filled cavity between the external auditory meatus and the organs of hearing, the cochlea and its adnexum in the bony cavities in the skull. Air pressure is equalized with atmospheric pressure by the eustachian tubes so the ear drum vibrates when sound waves reach it.

midlife crisis A psychological ailment of contemporary society, characterized by self-absorption, anxiety, and the realization by professional people that they may have achieved their peak in occupational attainment and life satisfaction, that the future may contain more frustration than achievement. This may predispose to or precipitate some stress-related and emotional disorders, so intervention may be justifiable when the condition is identified.

midwife Traditionally, a woman who attends and assists other women during labor and delivery of a neonate, customarily a woman who has had children herself and/or observed and assisted at previous deliveries, and is therefore aware of what normally happens during childbirth. Traditional village midwives, especially in rural regions, have attended women in labor for many centuries, and this calling has accumulated useful empirical knowledge about the conduct of difficult labor, but prevention of puerperal infection was seldom part of this. Provision of basic education in hygiene and aseptic practice, an initiative of some nongovernmental organizations and of WHO, reduced the magnitude of the problem. A safer long-term solution is formal training programs for nurse-midwives and traditional birth attendants.

midwifery The ancient craft practiced since prehistoric times by a MIDWIFE, i.e., a female who assists a woman during labor and delivery. Most modern midwives are formally trained, often in nursing care. Some equivalent to professional training to supplement tradition, custom, and common sense can improve the conduct and safety of childbirth among traditional midwives.

mifepristone An antiprogesterone agent that sensitizes the myometrium to prostaglandin-induced contractions and softens and dilates the cervix. It can be used as an abortifacient in early pregnancy and in medically induced abortion to about 20 weeks' gestation.

migrant workers Workers, usually in the agricultural sector, who move from place to place as the demand for work fluctuates, often seasonally. Many thousands move across North America and Europe in this way every year. They often have health problems related to their way of life and occupational risks to which they are exposed, for instance from exposure to agricultural PESTICIDES. Often they are inadequately protected by occupational and environmental health legislation and regulations, and their children may suffer from lack of medical care and lack of access to adequate education. Many migrant workers live away from home and family for long periods, so sexually transmitted diseases including HIV are another hazard, especially in Sub-Saharan Africa.

migration Movement of people from their country of origin to another country in which they settle, usually permanently. This is a significant demographic factor influencing population structure in many nations. People migrate mostly in search of a more favorable environment or because economic, environmental, ecological, political, or other factors have made their place of origin no longer comfortably habitable, so called "pull-push" factors. Since the latter part of the 19th century, migration has greatly increased in magnitude and range, leading to unprecedented mixing of previously separate gene pools, and contributing to many social, economic, and cultural challenges for migrants and host communities and nations, especially in low-income countries such as in Sub-Saharan Africa.

milk The nutrient fluid secreted by mammary glands that gave the name to the vertebrate class *Mammalia*. Each mammalian species secretes milk with a composition that is biochemically and immunologically suitable for the infants of that particular species, which is why human breast milk is more nutritious for human infants than is cow's milk. Milk is an excellent culture medium for many pathogenic organisms, so precautions such as PASTEURIZATION or boiling must be implemented to protect infants, children, and all others who drink milk for nutrition or refreshment.

Millennium Development Goals A set of eight goals adopted at the UN Millennium Summit in September 2000 to alleviate conditions for more than a billion people in the world who were living in extreme poverty. Several of these goals have implications for public health, and four have explicit health targets: 1. Eradicate extreme poverty and hunger; 4. Reduce child mortality and achieve a two-thirds reduction in mortality in those younger than 5 years, by 2015; 5. Improve maternal health and reduce by three-quarters the maternal mortality ratio, by 2015; 6. Combat HIV/AIDS, malaria, and other lethal diseases, including halting and reversing incidence and death rates from HIV/AIDS, malaria, and other lethal diseases, including tuberculosis. See http://www.developmentgoals.org for a full account and discussion of the millennium development goals.

Millennium Ecosystem Assessment A United Nations initiative to assess the state of the earth's sustainability, conducted by working groups of experts in relevant disciplines, which aims to produce an inventory of global life support systems and their status at the beginning of the new millennium. Reports of the assessment have been released in stages beginning in early 2005. See http://www.millenniumassessment.org for details.

MIM number The American medical geneticist Victor McKusick (b. 1921) conceived the McKusick classification and assigned a five-digit number to each condition he described in his landmark monograph *Mendelian Inheritance in Man* (MIM); these numbers, in fields with blank spaces to allow for new discoveries in Mendelian genetics, have been adopted by clinical geneticists worldwide as the numerical taxonomic system for inherited disorders.

Minamata disease A disease identified in the fishing community of Minamata, Japan, in 1953, with gross physical deformities, mental retardation, and neurological deficit among infants born to mothers whose diet had contained a high proportion of shellfish and seafood. It was caused by poisoning with methyl mercury salts formed by biotransformation from mercury discharged into Minamata Bay by a chemical plant, consumed by plankton, and bioconcentrated in the marine food chain to produce a fetotoxic food item when consumed by pregnant women.

mind Essentially an abstract concept, the word used to describe the sentient parts of the brain responsible for intellectual function; emotions; ability to conceptualize, formulate creative thoughts, and translate these into tangible form, for instance as physical structures, works of art, musical compositions, or literary works.

mind-body medicine See PSYCHONEUROIM-MUNOLOGY.

mine A place where minerals are extracted from the earth. Two main varieties are underground mines and open-pit mines. The former are often dangerous, and the latter often disrupt and disfigure the natural environment. See also LANDMINE, MINER, MINE SAFETY, and MINING INDUSTRY.

miner A worker in the MINING INDUSTRY. In many varieties of underground mine (especially coal mines), this is among the most dangerous occupations that exist. There is ever-present risk of death or serious injury in collapsing mine shafts; explosions due to buildup of flammable gases, principally methane; floods and drowning when the mine shaft penetrates an underground aquifer; and chronic disabling lung diseases, notably pneumoconiosis, that shorten life. In addition, some minerals are toxic, for example lead and uranium.

mine safety Miners have among the highest occupational mortality and morbidity of any group, so there has long been concern about identifying and reducing the hazards. Pliny described lead poisoning and the hazards of asbestos exposure in the first century of our era. The risks of exposure to toxic minerals such as mercury were described by the 16th century German mineralogist Georgius Agricola (1494–1555). The British chemist Humphry Davy (1778–1829) invented the safety lamp, which reduced the risk of fires and explosions in coal mines. In the early 20th century, dust reduction by water sprays reduced the risk of

miner's PNEUMOCONIOSIS. Caged birds, typically canaries, were used as sentinels until chemical and electronic sensors to detect toxic gases and reduced oxygen supply were developed. Modern mine safety includes specialized engineering equipment and studies, ventilation controls, chemical sensors, ergonomics, and psychosocial factors.

mineral fibers Fibers that originate from nonliving matter. The best known is ASBESTOS. Artificial mineral fibers are made from glass, plastics, etc. Mineral fibers, unlike some natural ones, are not allergenic, but some, especially asbestos, have other harmful biological effects.

mineral supplement A dietary supplement added to formula feeds, other manufactured foods, or regular diets. Additional "mineral" content is often combined with vitamins. The most widely used minerals include iron, magnesium, and calcium. Iron supplements sometimes help persons with iron-deficiency anemia, but iron is more often taken in pills. Calcium is added to milk, orange juice, etc. Magnesium is seldom required as a supplement unless foods containing chlorophyll are unavailable. Iodine (not a mineral) is added to table salt. Various other supplements are also used. See http://www.nlm.nih.gov /medlineplus/vitaminsandminerals.html for indications and details.

minimum data set The basic information required to assemble simple vital statistics, together with the accepted terms and definitions used when compiling these statistics. The minimum data set includes the essential information for birth and death certification, and for statistics on primary, secondary, and tertiary medical care. Several countries have established criteria for a minimum data set. In the United States http://www.cms .hhs.gov/quality/mds30/ provides general guidelines on data required for MEDICARE and MEDICAID; comparable sets have been developed in the United Kingdom, Australia, and for many specialized aspects of health care services.

minimum lethal dose The minimum dose of test substance required to kill experimental animals, usually mice.

mining industry A large, heterogeneous, diversified industry concerned with extracting and refining all forms of minerals. Extraction and refining involve many health hazards, some arising in the extraction of minerals (see MINER), others in refining ores and control of toxic emissions from smelter stacks, and others in disposing of the residue that may be toxic and is almost always harmful to the environment.

Minnesota Multiphasic Personality Inventory (MMPI) A validated screening test used in psychological assessment. It contains detailed questions on preferences and aversions, concepts such as introversion-extraversion, motivation and personal goals, and questions that probe for evidence of abnormalities, such as schizophrenia, paranoia, depression, and anxiety.

minor A word used mainly in the United States to describe a young person who is legally barred because of age from some of the privileges and services available to adults, such as driving a car, purchasing and consuming alcoholic beverages, and obtaining contraceptive advice without parental consent. The legal definition of a minor is usually a person younger than 16 or 18 years. Public health officials must know the legally defined ages of minors in their jurisdiction. Minors are not prohibited by law from consensual sexual acts, and the age at which these begin seems to be getting lower.

minority A word with several meanings. In public health, it usually means a specified societal group that may be small in numbers and therefore considered to have limited political influence, such as homosexuals or members of certain ethnic or religious groups. A VISIBLE MINORITY is one that is readily recognizable because of skin color or other distinguishing external characteristics, such as mode of dress or culturally determined behavior. In some communities, so-called visible minority groups constitute a substantial majority.

miscarriage A pregnancy that aborts early in gestation, generally a spontaneous or naturally occurring event attributable to disease, fetal malformation, etc., rather than artificial intervention. It is estimated that as many as 30% of all pregnancies end in natural spontaneous miscarriage.

mission statement A summary of the purpose for which an organization or agency exists. It is usually a carefully composed statement and is preferably brief and unambiguous.

mitochondrion (Plural: mitochondria) Organelle inclusions in the cytoplasm that play a role in cellular respiration and energy production.

mitosis Somatic cell division in which the nucleus divides into two daughter nuclei, each of which contains the same number of chromosomes and genes as the parent nucleus and cell.

MMPI See MINNESOTA MULTIPHASIC PERSONALITY INVENTORY.

MMR 1. Mass miniature radiography, a widely used screening procedure for tuberculosis for many years but uncommon today. 2. Measles,

mumps, rubella vaccine. This is recommended by the US Centers for Disease Control and Prevention and by many other authorities for routine immunization of infants and children against these three diseases. For details on dosage and timing, see VACCINE-PREVENTABLE DISEASE. 3. Maternal mortality ratio. These alternative interpretations of a set of initials illustrate the pitfalls of written or oral communications that use initials or acronyms rather than spelling out in full what is meant.

MMR vaccine A combined vaccine of live attenuated measles, mumps, and rubella vaccine given in two doses by intramuscular injection at 12 months and 3–4 years of age. Evaluations show that the combination protects against all three infectious diseases. A British report of an association between MMR vaccine and autism has been shown to have no foundation in fact. A rare side effect is allergy to the egg protein vehicle in which it is contained.

MMWR See *MORBIDITY AND MORTALITY WEEKLY REPORT*.

mobile program A public health program, such as community-wide vaccination or screening procedure, that moves about in the catchment area, commonly in a truck or van.

mobility 1. Movement of persons from one place to another, described as geographical mobility, or from one social, economic, or occupational group to another, described as social mobility. Often there is a combination. Geographical mobility implies movement within, rather than between, countries, so it differs from MIGRATION. 2. In clinical medicine and physiotherapy, mobility means ability to move joints. 3. The word is also used to describe ability to move around in the home and in public, such as to go out to shop or visit friends and neighbors.

mode See MEASURES OF CENTRAL TENDENCY.

model 1. A small-scale replica or reproduction of a physical structure. 2. A theoretical (usually mathematical, often computerized) equation or simulation, abstract representation, or the formal expression of a theory. 3. A replication in an animal population of a human disease, such as an environmentally related respiratory disease. 4. The alternative scenarios set out in GAME THEORY. The several meanings indicate that models have many applications in many aspects of human existence, including applications in public health science and practice. MATHEMATICAL MODELS of epidemics are a valuable way to predict their probable course, plan control methods, and formulate policy, including its economic aspects.

model standards A set of guidelines or criteria for a specific activity or service. There are several examples in public health. For instance, a detailed set of specified health objectives for the United States is one of the initiatives of *HEALTHY PEOPLE 2000* and *2010*. In collaboration with the American Public Health Association, the US Office of Disease Prevention and Health Promotion established expert groups to draw up specific health objectives, many with specified quantitative targets, to be achieved by specified dates. These objectives and targets generated discussions and plans about actions required to achieve the desired outcomes.

mold Growth of fungus or mycotic organisms on organic matter such as food or on the upholstery, carpets, etc., of households. Some molds metabolize to produce antibiotics such as PENICILLIN and some contain allergens.

molecular biology The study of biology at the level of the molecular structure of biological units, cells, and the genes and chromosomes they contain. This branch of science has burgeoned since the discovery of the molecular structure of the DNA molecule and the HUMAN GENOME PROJECT.

molecular epidemiology The application of the techniques and methods of molecular biology in epidemiological practice and research. For instance, DNA typing is used to track the movement of specific strains of pathogenic agents through a population. Molecular epidemiology has proved a useful method for studying the pathogenesis of neoplasia and mutagenesis. It is best thought of as a method and level of analysis rather than a specific discipline. See also BIOMARKER.

molecular genetics The application of molecular methods to the study of genetics. This branch of science has advanced rapidly since the HUMAN GENOME PROJECT successfully located many genes and began to identify their functions. Applications of genetic engineering have been successful in plant and animals, have led to development of innovative vector control methods using genetically modified mosquitoes, and have begun to make theoretically possible some interventions and actions in human genetic disorders that previously were not feasible. As of 2005, the possible benefits of intervention in human disease are potential rather than actual. For current status, see http://www.ncbi.nlm.nih.gov/About/primer/genetics_molecular.html.

molluscum contagiosum A cutaneous virus disease transmitted sexually or by other direct contact; it heals spontaneously, except in the presence of HIV/AIDS, when it may disseminate.

Monday morning syndrome A term applied to several work-related conditions in which return to the workplace after a short interval away is associated with recurrence of symptoms. Examples include the recrudescence of respiratory symptoms of BYSSINOSIS on re-exposure to cotton dust and of severe headache on renewed occupational exposure to NITROGLYCERINE. The term is also used to describe an alcohol-induced hangover following a weekend of heavy drinking.

MONICA An acronym for Multinational MONItoring of trends and determinants in CArdiovascular diseases, a multicenter, multinational epidemiological study of coronary heart disease, hypertension, and other cardiovascular diseases, sponsored by the World Health Organization, with support from national research funding agencies in the United States, United Kingdom, European Union, and elsewhere, established in 1979. The MONICA project has tracked trends and identified and measured risk factors for coronary heart disease, stroke, etc. See http://www.ktl.fi/monica/ for a summary of the project and links to details.

monitoring Routine, often episodic measurement, performance analysis, or supervision of a process, activity, or function with the aim of detecting and correcting change or deviation from desirable levels. Data are usually collected, analyzed, and recorded. The monitor or monitoring agent may or may not have the role and responsibility to fine-tune the process, activity, or function aimed at correcting departures from desired levels. The distinction between monitoring and SURVEILLANCE is that the former is often episodic or intermittent, whereas the latter is ongoing and continuous, and implies a greater commitment to interpret and disseminate the information obtained.

monoamine oxidase (MAO) inhibitors A group of drugs sometimes used to treat depression that are slow acting and cumulative in their effect. They can interact with certain proteins and amino acids, e.g., tyramine, to cause a sudden and potentially catastrophic rise in blood pressure.

monoclonal antibody Antibody made from cloned organisms, i.e., all with identical DNA. The main uses of monoclonal antibodies are in specific anticancer therapy and immunosuppression.

monoculture 1. A term used in agriculture, horticulture, and forestry to describe cultivation in which all plants come from the same or closely similar genetic strain, usually one that has been especially bred to produce a desired end, such as larger fruit, more marketable lumber, etc. There can be a problem if the uniform genetic composition renders the entire crop vulnerable to a pest, such as fungus infestation. Monocultured crops and plantations of trees also have the effect of reducing biodiversity in the region where they are being cultivated. 2. In sociology, the term is occasionally used to describe a society that is secluded from outside influences and shielded from factors that tend to promote human diversity.

monogamy Marriage or an equivalent relationship of two partners, generally of opposite sexes, with the implied understanding that it is a lifelong arrangement. In modern Western countries, a common variation is serial monogamy, in which partnerships remain stable for a relatively limited time, then break up and are superseded by new partnerships.

mononucleosis A blood disorder, generally viral in origin, in which abnormal mononuclear leukocytes proliferate. Infectious mononucleosis (the "kissing disease") is a common variety, caused by the EPSTEIN-BARR VIRUS, which is also associated with BURKITT'S LYMPHOMA.

monosodium glutamate (MSG) A sodium salt of glutamic acid manufactured from soya bean extract widely used as a preservative and flavor-enhancing agent in foodstuffs. Some people are hypersensitive to it and experience severe vasomotor episodes of flushing and hypotension.

monosodium methane arsenate A pesticide used to control infestations of bark beetle in softwood lumber. It is environmentally persistent and may have serious adverse effects. It is a suspected carcinogen, possibly implicated in childhood cancer.

Monte Carlo fallacy Syn: gambler's fallacy. The false belief that the likelihood of a specific event occurring is inversely related to the elapsed time or number of trials of enabling conditions since the previous occurrence of the event. This belief is false because it ignores the facts of probability theory. The name derives from the conduct of gamblers at Monte Carlo.

Montreal Protocol An international agreement to phase out the production and use of ozone-destroying substances, negotiated in Montreal, Canada, in 1986 under the auspices of the United Nations Environmental Programme, revised several times since to extend the scope to other ozone-destroying substances in addition to CHLOROFLUORO-CARBONS (CFCs). The 2000 revision of the protocol is at http://hq.unep.org/ozone/Montreal-Protocol/Montreal-Protocol2000.shtml.

mood Syn: affect (n). The subjective feelings or emotional state of an individual, e.g., happy or sad. An individual's mood can profoundly influence sensory perception, intellectual function, reaction time in a crisis, and a variety of other physiological functions.

mood disorder Syn: affective disorder. A term for any aberration of mood that leads to abnormal emotional states. The most common mood disorder is DEPRESSION, which is now among the most common causes of disability, and another common and important form is BIPOLAR DISORDER.

mood-modifying substances A general term for illicit street drugs that act by elevating or otherwise altering emotional states (mood) or are hallucinogenic. Most have harmful effects, e.g., on cardiovascular, respiratory, and/or neuropsychiatric function. Examples include LSD, cannabis, Benzedrine, and derivatives.

morals Syn: morality. The accepted norms and standards of conduct of a society, community, or nation. Some are virtually universal features of human societies, such as prohibition of murder, rape, and incest. Many relate to bonding relationships based on the FAMILY and/or on the beliefs and teachings of a religion. Although these tend to remain stable over prolonged periods, they are not immutable. For instance, from at least the 19th century until after about the middle of the 20th century, it was considered immoral for an unmarried couple to live together, but by the late 20th century, it had become commonplace for couples to live together, sometimes for some years before marrying. By the late 20th century, it had become morally acceptable to many Europeans and Americans for homosexual couples to live openly in society. Morals are important determinants of personal and population health, e.g., in rules about sex education and influencing attitudes and practice of public health measures, such as provision of clean needles and condoms for prison inmates, in recognition of the existence in that population of illicit drug use and homosexual relationships that if ignored contribute to the uncontrolled spread of HIV infection.

moral values Values based on deeply held beliefs such as those derived from or associated with religious convictions. Moral values typically are expressed as judgments of whether specific behaviors or situations are right or wrong. Moral values may have beneficial or harmful health consequences, for example related to sexual behavior, where they may inhibit promiscuity and reduce the risk of sexually transmitted diseases, or may lead to public policies, such as prohibition of effective contraception, that are inimical to the reproductive health of girls and women. See also VALUES.

morbidity Sickness, the state or condition of being unwell.

Morbidity and Mortality Weekly Report (MMWR) The weekly publication of the US Centers for Disease Control and Prevention, containing cumulative summaries of numbers of cases of reportable (notifiable) diseases, i.e., communicable diseases of public health importance, as well as short reports of current interest about conditions of public health importance. The data are almost entirely about domestic US conditions, but occasionally there are reports and discussion about conditions occurring elsewhere in the world. See http://www.cdc.gov/mmwr/ for current issue. Many other countries produce equivalent timely reports as a feature of their public health systems. WHO's bilingual *Weekly Epidemiological Record (WER)/Relevé Épidémiologique Hebdomadaire (REH)* provides surveillance information for the entire world.

morbidity survey A community-based inquiry into the prevalence of symptoms, existence of chronic disability, use of medications, etc., usually conducted by asking questions in interviews or by means of self-completed questionnaires. This may be a modest local inquiry or a large-scale, long-term national investigation, such as the household interview surveys of the US National Center for Health Statistics.

mores Social customs that have become established through long practice that has made them akin to traditions. See also CUSTOM and FOLKWAYS.

Mormons Members of a religious sect (the Church of Jesus Christ of Latter-Day Saints) with world headquarters in Salt Lake City, Utah, with several interesting health-related characteristics. Many Mormons are vegetarian, all men are required to perform missionary duties that may include service in low-income countries, where they provide educational and health care facilities while also seeking converts. Their beliefs include opposition to family planning, as well as interest in tracing the ancestry of converts, which led to the establishment of a comprehensive data base on genealogy with information on family lineages from many parts of the world where the church has recruited new members.

morning-after pill Syn: emergency contraception. A medication that can be taken soon after an act of unprotected sexual intercourse in order to prevent pregnancy from occurring. A traditional, but often ineffectual, method was the use of a uterine stimulant that, if taken or inserted in the form of vaginal pessaries, could induce termination of a very early pregnancy. Medically acceptable methods rely on high-dose hormone preparations, either an estrogen-progestin combination or progestin alone. See also MIFEPRISTONE.

morphine Syn: morphia. A purified extract of opium that is a powerful pain reliever and mild soporific. It is addictive, and occasionally it is used as an illicit drug of abuse.

mortality The condition of cessation of life. The medical statistician WILLIAM FARR (1807–1883) said of mortality statistics, "Death is a fact; all else is inference," by which he meant that accurate ascertainment of the fact of death, and information about the age at which it occurred, were the most powerful of all vital statistical data.

mortality rate Syn: death rate. A general term for rates compiled from data on the number of deaths in relation to a specified population at risk. Several common variations are crude mortality rate, age-, sex-, and cause specific mortality rates, and adjusted mortality rates. See also RATE, RISK, and ADJUSTMENT.

mortality risk The risk, or odds, that death will occur. See RISK.

mosaic In genetics, the occurrence in an individual of two (or more) distinct cell lines, derived from the general meaning of the word, i.e., a picture made by joining small pieces of different colors together in a pattern. The word has several other scientific uses, e.g., to describe the pattern of rods and cones in the retina, and certain virus diseases of plants.

mosquito A ubiquitous winged insect species that lays eggs on or in water where larvae develop and metamorphose into flying adults, almost all of which are a nuisance and many of which are dangerous to humans because they are vectors of many MOSQUITO-BORNE DISEASES. Many mosquito species can OVERWINTER, i.e., hibernate either as adults or larvae, and resume life and breeding when the weather warms again. Two principal families of mosquitoes are ANOPHELINES, which are vectors for plasmodia, the malaria parasites, and CULICINES, which can carry many disease agents, including larval filarial worms, the viruses of dengue, yellow fever, several varieties of viral encephalitis, and hemorrhagic fevers. Only the female mosquito requires blood feeds, so only the female mosquito spreads mosquito-borne diseases. Control of many diseases requires control of mosquitoes, e.g., by use of larvicides, insecticides, environmental control by draining swamps, eliminating places where stagnant water can accumulate, use of mosquito-proof screens, bed-nets, etc.

mosquito-borne diseases A large heterogeneous collection of diseases have in common the fact that mosquitoes are the vectors. They include viral, bacterial, rickettsial, protozoan, and metazoan diseases, the most important of which include dengue, Japanese encephalitis, malaria, and filariasis. Mosquito control and preferably eradication are therefore high priorities of public health services. For more information, see http://www.cdc.gov/ncidod/diseases/list_mosquitoborne.htm.

motion sickness The nausea and vomiting that have made sea voyages miserable for countless travelers from time immemorial, long car trips a penance for many children and their parents, and air travel unpleasant for some passengers and those seated near them. It is caused by sensory impulses that bombard the vestibular nerve with signals conflicting with the evidence of other senses about the body's position in space. It is a significant occupational health problem in many settings, e.g., maritime services and the aeronautics and aerospace industries.

motor neuron disease A progressive degenerative disease of the motor neurons of unknown etiology, affecting first the peripheral nerves and progressing upward to attack respiratory and swallowing muscles, at which stage it becomes life threatening and ultimately fatal. Because of its relentless progression and the inevitably unpleasant protracted mode of death, motor neuron disease has led to debates about assisted suicide and euthanasia, with advocates of the disabled and of the right to life being opposed by victims and members of their families.

motor vehicle accident (MVA) One of the most prominent modern public health problems, the cause of a high proportion of premature deaths, especially among young adults, and a great deal of prolonged, sometimes permanent disability. Motor vehicle accidents have been the subject of a great deal of research, covering epidemiological features, i.e., risk factors, evaluation of design and engineering details to make cars safer, design and use of seat belts and air bags, road design, behavioral and social science studies of driver behavior, and emergency surgical care of critically injured traffic victims. Considerable progress has been made in recent decades in improved automobile and road safety design features, reducing unsafe driving practices, e.g., with teen driver education programs, medical screening of older drivers, severe penalties for IMPAIRED DRIVING, and improved separation of high-speed traffic from other public highway users. New problems have arisen with increasing use of off-road vehicles. Many of the public health problems of motor vehicle accidents that are being effectively tackled in rich industrial nations are resurfacing in developing countries as these become motorized. The word "accident" implies an event over which people have no control, and as many such events are predictable and preventable, TRAFFIC CRASH is a preferred term, but it has never gained wide currency.

mottling Dental mottling, a disfiguring discoloration of dental enamel that is caused by excessive dietary intake of fluoride salts, usually because of unusually high concentration of fluoride salts in the environment, usually in the soil.

mountain sickness Syn: altitude sickness. The cardiovascular, respiratory, and neural symptom complex that occurs when a person physiologically adjusted to life at or near sea level ascends rapidly to high altitude (2,500 meters or more). The symptoms include headache, nausea, vomiting, breathlessness, and feelings of ill-defined distress. The cause is oxygen lack. If ascent to high altitude is gradual, cardiovascular adjustment and manufacture of red blood corpuscles to compensate for reduced oxygen transport lead to alleviation of symptoms after a few days.

mouse 1. A small rodent, a household pest and occasional source of human disease, e.g., rickettsial pox, transmitted to humans by mites that infest mice. Mice are a favorite laboratory animal, used in genetics, and to test toxicity or the virulence of pathogens. 2. The tracking and pointing device used to activate computer programs, e.g., in searching the WORLD WIDE WEB.

moxibustion A Chinese traditional medical method in which heat is applied to designated points on the body by burning an herb held near or attached to an acupuncture needle inserted in the skin.

MRC See MEDICAL RESEARCH COUNCIL.

MRFIT See MULTIPLE RISK FACTOR INTERVENTION TRIAL.

mRNA See MESSENGER RNA.

MRSA Initial letters for methicillin- or MULTIPLE-RESISTANT *STAPHYLOCOCCUS AUREUS*. Sometimes "M" refers specifically to methicillin.

multinational corporation Syn: transnational corporation. A conglomerate commercial and industrial organization with offices and branch plants in many parts of the world, usually with its nominal headquarters in a rich industrial nation such as the United States, Switzerland, or nations of the European Union. Some organizations of this nature have evaded laws and regulations on occupational safety and health by relocating factories from nations with rigorous standards to developing nations lacking such high standards, and some corporations have enough political influence to shape laws to suit their ends. Several have annual gross income and capital resources greater than those of most low-income nations, and these and others can influence national policies, including many with implications for the public health.

multiphasic screening The use of several or a whole battery of SCREENING tests to search for early evidence of a wide variety of preventable diseases and precursors of disease. The process is often automated. It may begin with a self-completed questionnaire entered into a computer and using a touch-screen or keyboard for responses, followed by a set of routine body measurements (height, weight, etc.); a wide range of blood tests, respiratory function tests, chest x-ray, electro cardiogram, and other tests. Economies of scale may make this approach worthwhile, but false-positive results may lead many people to be subjected to further costly tests and needless anxiety.

multiple chemical sensitivities The perhaps nonexistent "disease of modern civilization," said to be caused by reaction to many environmental contaminants, such as carpet adhesives, industrial solvents, miscellaneous air pollutants, and other substances that stimulate allergic responses and other symptoms, such as headaches, insomnia, skin rashes, and digestive upsets. The condition was identified and named by CLINICAL ECOLOGY specialists, and many physicians dispute its existence.

multiple regression A set of statistical techniques used, e.g., in sociological and epidemiological analyses, when many variables are involved. The tests commonly used include linear regression analysis and logistic regression analysis.

multiple-resistant *Staphylococcus aureus* **(MRSA)** A widely used term (and abbreviation); also termed methicillin-resistant *S. aureus* for infection with strains of the *S. aureus* that do not respond to any commonly used antibiotics. The resistant strains have proliferated widely because the organism is ubiquitous, and commonly used antibiotics have been environmentally disseminated following their use in animal husbandry, as well as to treat human disease. For further information, see http://www.cdc.gov/ncidod/dhqp/ar_mrsa.html.

multiple risk factor intervention trial (MRFIT) Known by its acronym, this large randomized trial of preventive interventions initially was thought to demonstrate the inadequacy of preventive interventions, such as cholesterol-lowering

regimens, because death rates were not significantly different between the groups with and without intervention. However, more detailed analysis revealed that apparent similarity of intervention and control groups was due, in part at least, to contamination of the control group by publicized intervention methods that many adopted, although it was not meant to be part of their regimen; and that intervention did significantly reduce death rates from coronary heart disease, but the death rates due to violent causes, such as traffic crashes and suicide, were significantly elevated in the intervention group, raising the possibility that lower cholesterol levels were associated with adverse modification of mood. A brief description and formalities for access to data sets from the MRFIT studies are at http://www.nhlbi.nih.gov/resources/deca/descriptions/mrfit.htm.

multiple sclerosis A chronic, progressive, and ultimately fatal neurological disease of unknown etiology (despite decades of intensive research). Its main pathological feature is progressive demyelination of peripheral nerves and the central nervous system. Epidemiological features include geographic distribution mainly in high latitudes, female preponderance, and an association with a bewildering array of probably irrelevant infectious diseases of the patient, family members, pets, etc. It has some features suggestive of an autoimmune reaction, but as of 2005, no single disease agent or process has been implicated.

multiproblem family A term used by social workers and others to describe a family or household containing two or more members with a variety of social, psychological, and/or other problems, e.g., with law enforcement agencies. Health problems are frequently part of the picture, and sometimes dominate it.

multistage model A model used mainly in studies of cancer that postulates several stages in the origin and development of disease.

multistage sampling The use of random sampling methods in several stages, e.g., first to select regions previously defined administratively or geographically, then to select households, and finally to select individual household members.

multivariate analysis A set of analytic techniques used when a series of variables are studied simultaneously and it is necessary to know how the variations in value of one set of variables relate to and interact with others among a large number of variables. There are several popular methods with well-developed statistical procedures that can be used with each. These include correlation and regression analysis, discriminant function analysis, logistic regression, and others. Software packages are available for many of these analytic methods.

mumps A contagious viral disease that has been recognized since antiquity (it was described by Hippocrates in the 4th century BCE). It causes fever and characteristic swelling of the parotid glands and sometimes other glands, including the pancreas and the testes, both of which can be permanently damaged, leading to diabetes and male sterility, respectively. Live attenuated mumps virus vaccine, usually combined with measles and rubella vaccine, is used to prevent infection. Detailed information is available at http://www.nlm.nih.gov/medlineplus/mumps.html.

Munchausen syndrome Syn: factitious disorder. A bizarre symptom complex first described by the British physician Richard Asher (1912–1969) in which patients repeatedly present with convincing stories they have fabricated to persuade physicians to operate on them or otherwise invasively intervene. The public health significance arises from patients with this attention-seeking disorder consuming prodigious amounts of scarce medical resources, depriving others more in need of such resources.

murine typhus A flea-borne rickettsial disease native to rodents (rats, mice, etc.) transmitted to humans by fleas that defecate rickettsia while sucking blood.

Murray Valley encephalitis An arbovirus encephalitis prevalent along the River Murray in Australia, transmitted to humans from pelicans and other aquatic birds by mosquitoes in wet seasons when lagoons form along the river banks so human and avian habitats are closer together than in dry seasons.

muscular dystrophy A group of mostly inherited disorders of neuromuscular function in which there is progressive loss of muscle power, usually associated with defects of muscle protein.

musculoskeletal disorders A miscellaneous group of inflammatory and degenerative disorders of joints and bones that include osteoarthritis, rheumatoid arthritis, gout, osteoporosis, and several other conditions that collectively have been found in most community health surveys to be responsible for the largest single contribution to chronic disability.

mushrooms A large family of fungi that includes some, e.g., truffles, regarded as rare and precious delicacies, others that are a dietary staple and culinary and gastronomic delicacy for good foods, and others again that are poisonous, some extremely so. One variety, *Amanita phalloides*, is a particularly nasty poison that slowly and inexorably causes necrosis of the liver, and others, sometimes called magic mushrooms, are hallucinogenic, producing substances with effects that resemble those of LYSERGIC ACID DIETHYLAMIDE (LSD) or MESCALINE.

mustard gas Dichlorodiethyl sulfide, an oily, volatile liquid that was used in World War I and several times in warfare since then as a WEAPON OF MASS DESTRUCTION, albeit on a small and localized scale. Mustard gas has also been used therapeutically to treat some varieties of aggressive malignant disease, such as acute leukemia.

mutagen An agent that causes MUTATION, i.e., permanent alteration of the sequencing in base pairs of chromosomes, leading to a change in inheritable characteristics that is often abnormal or incompatible with survival, thus causing fetal death or miscarriage. Other mutations produce live offspring with anatomical or other abnormalities of varying degree of severity. Mutagenic agents include ionizing radiation, some pharmaceutical preparations, e.g., THALIDOMIDE, and some substances of considerable commercial importance, including certain broad-leaf herbicides, such as AGENT ORANGE.

mutation An abrupt change in the RNA-DNA structure that leads to the production of offspring qualitatively different from parents. There are many varieties. Some are lethal, but others may either enhance or diminish the capacity of offspring to adapt to their environment. Those that enhance capacity confer an evolutionary advantage upon the offspring, i.e., they are more likely to survive and reproduce, leading to an increase in their number in the next generation.

MVA See MOTOR VEHICLE ACCIDENT.

mycobacteria A family of rod-shaped bacteria that retain their stain when washed in acid, and thus are called acid-fast bacilli. They include *Mycobacterium tuberculosis*, which is the causal organism of tuberculosis, and *M. leprae*, the causal organism of LEPROSY.

Mycobacterium tuberculosis The microorganism that causes most cases of TUBERCULOSIS. It is a slow-growing aerobic gram-positive, acid-fast, rod-shaped bacterium. It can survive for long periods in dry, dusty, dark, and damp environments but can grow and reproduce only in living organisms such as humans. The ZIEHL-NEELSEN STAIN is used to identify it. Formerly very common worldwide, it remains widespread in populations afflicted by poverty, poor nutrition, and overcrowding. In the late 1950s, streptomycin and isoniazid were effectively used antibiotics in tuberculosis control programs in industrial nations, but resistance developed; later-generation antibiotics are now used but multiply resistant organisms are common.

mycology The study of molds and funguses.

mycoplasma A family of amorphous infectious agents with some characteristics of viruses that are responsible for sundry respiratory infections, including some coryza-like diseases and some that have symptoms and signs resembling pneumonia.

mycosis Fungus infection. This may be systemic, e.g., mycosis of the lungs, or topical, the most common varieties of which are athlete's foot and paronychia.

mycotoxins A miscellaneous group of poisonous substances, mostly alkaloids, produced by fungi. They may act by ingestion, inhalation, or absorption through the skin, and include some of the most poisonous substances known, e.g., the toxin of the toadstool *Amanita phalloides*.

myelinopathy A pathological aberration affecting the myelin sheathes of nerve fibers. Several forms of this occur, e.g., toxic damage caused by industrial solvents etc., and degenerative neurological diseases.

myocardial infarction Necrosis of a portion of heart muscle due to oxygen lack, usually caused by occlusion of a coronary artery by atherosclerosis or thrombosis, or both. This is a common life-threatening condition that occurs in the advanced stages of coronary heart disease and is among the most common causes of death in many Western industrial nations. It is increasingly common in many industrializing nations, such as India, and indeed worldwide, except in Sub-Saharan Africa.

myoglobin The heme protein constituent of muscle cells that takes up oxygen from the hemoglobin molecules in the blood.

myxedema The clinical condition produced by HYPOTHYROIDISM, characteristically causing an immobile, expressionless face, coarse skin, slow pulse, and sluggish intellect. It can be due to iodine deficiency or to deficient production of thyroxine, and usually responds well to treatment with thyroxine; but in regions where iodine deficiency is common, correcting the deficiency is the best treatment.

myxomatosis A lethal viral disease of rabbits, deliberately introduced to control the plague of rabbits in Australia. Observations of the progress of the epidemic provided opportunities for epidemiologists to study host-agent-environment interactions, from which valuable lessons were learned for subsequent application in human epidemics. Evolution of generations of rabbits that were resistant to myxomatosis was observed after several years.

N

nanotechnology Construction and use of devices comprising only a few molecules that can be used to manipulate structures at the atomic level. Nanotechnology has potential applications in repair of damaged tissues and organs.

naphtha A general name for any liquid hydrocarbon derived by fractional distillation of petroleum, usually higher alkene fractions with 9 or 10 carbon atoms.

naphthalene A liquid compound of two benzene rings with a pungent odor; used as an insecticide. It is toxic in high doses and can cause hemolysis, hepatocellular necrosis, and other severe effects.

narcotics Substances that are central nervous system depressants, inducing drowsiness, sleep, unconsciousness, or coma, depending upon the dose, if ingested or injected. Some, including barbiturates and phenothiazines, are legal, prescribed drugs; others, notably opium and heroin, are commonly purveyed as illicit drugs.

narratology A word used by family physicians to describe systematic critical study of patients' medical histories and how these are told to attending physicians. Analysis of how patients tell their stories can be related to their medical disorders in predictable ways. This may be a useful way to identify and classify chronic disabling disorders, but cultural factors can cause confusion.

nasopharyngeal cancer Malignant neoplasm affecting the mucosa of the nose, sinuses, pharynx;

associated with exposure to carcinogens such as tobacco, emission products of biomass fuels, formaldehyde fumes inhaled by those in occupations such as woodworking and mortuary work. Another important cause is infection with the EPSTEIN-BARR VIRUS (EBV). EBV is a mosquito-borne virus and therefore nasopharyngeal cancer (affecting lymphatic tissue) due to EBV has a pronounced geographical distribution that correlates with the distribution of the mosquito vectors, notably in Central Africa, where the association was first identified. See BURKITT'S LYMPHOMA.

National Academy of Sciences (NAS) A nonprofit organization of distinguished scientists in the United States (with some foreign members by invitation). It was chartered by an act of Congress in 1863 with the mission of advising the US administration on scientific matters. It publishes many papers and scholarly reports in its *Proceedings* and has subdivided into several academies and other bodies. The NATIONAL RESEARCH COUNCIL was established under charter to the NAS in 1916, and the INSTITUTE OF MEDICINE, an organization for medical scientists invited into the NAS, was established in 1970. The NAS mission is to advance the cause of science and technology in the public interest. See http://www4.nationalacademies.org/nas/nashome.nsf for details. Many other nations have similar bodies, for instance the ROYAL SOCIETY in the United Kingdom.

National Ambient Air Quality Standards (NAAQS) A set of standards issued by the US Environmental Protection Agency (EPA) specifying maximum permissible levels of sulfur and nitrogen oxides, carbon monoxide, suspended particulate matter, ozone, and lead. They are designated as primary standards, i.e., maximum levels compatible with protecting population health. The standards were last modified in 1990. See http://www.epa.gov/air/criteria.html for US criteria. The Clean Air Act, as amended in 1990, requires the EPA to set national ambient air quality standards for pollutants considered harmful to health, and secondary standards to protect public welfare: protection against decreased visibility and damage to animals, crops, vegetation, and buildings.

National Cancer Institute One of the largest agencies of the US NATIONAL INSTITUTES OF HEALTH; it sponsors and funds research on cancer causes and prevention. This was the first condition-specific NIH institute, established in 1937. Its program grants support a nationwide network of cancer centers where the emphasis is on both treatment and research, and it supports many specific project grants. Its activities include oversight of a program of surveillance and end results of treatment. All are described at http://www.nci.nih

.gov/. Similar agencies exist in several other countries, for instance the National Cancer Institute of Canada, information about which may be seen at http://www.ncic.cancer.ca.

National Center for Complementary and Alternative Medicine (NCCAM) An agency of the US NATIONAL INSTITUTES OF HEALTH, established in 1991 (as the Office of Alternative Medicine), with a mandate to assess and conduct research on all aspects of complementary and alternative medicine, safety and efficacy, identification of active ingredients in traditional herbal remedies, underlying physiological mechanisms of yoga, and meditation therapy. See http://nccam.nih.gov/.

National Center for Health Statistics The division of the US CENTERS FOR DISEASE CONTROL AND PREVENTION that is concerned with the collection and analysis of health statistics, i.e., national and some state data on mortality, morbidity, hospital discharge statistics, national health surveys, and the NATIONAL HEALTH AND NUTRITION EXAMINATION SURVEYS (NHANES). It publishes many documents on these and other important sets of health statistics. Links to all these activities are available at http://www.cdc.gov/nchs/default.htm. There are equivalent organizations in many other countries. The Canadian equivalent is the CANADIAN INSTITUTE FOR HEALTH INFORMATION, at http://www.cihi.ca. The British equivalent is the OFFICE FOR NATIONAL STATISTICS, at http://www.statistics.gov.uk formerly the Office of Population, Census and Surveys.

National Death Index A computerized register of US death certificate data that began in 1979. It follows the earlier model of the CANADIAN MORTALITY DATA BASE (1950). It preserves death certificates on microfiche and uses RECORD LINKAGE for epidemiological and other analyses.

National Health and Nutrition Examination Survey (NHANES) A series of population sample surveys of the health and nutrition status of the American people that evolved from the National Health Interview Surveys that began in 1957. These surveys have continued in several series since the first NHANES in the late 1970s and early 1980s. They have provided the most comprehensive sets of normative data available anywhere in the world, much of it available on CD-ROM and on the Web site http://www.cdc.gov/nchs/nhanes.htm.

national health insurance A system for public funding of the costs citizens incur when they require personal medical and hospital care. Many nations provide at least partial support from the public purse for some of their citizens, and in many OECD (Organization for Economic Cooperation and Development) nations personal medical care and hospital costs are wholly or partly publicly funded. This has been an evolving process since it was introduced by the German Chancellor Otto von Bismarck (1815–1898) in 1883–1884. The British NATIONAL HEALTH SERVICE (NHS) introduced in 1948 provides comprehensive tax-supported personal and hospital care, but financial constraints and rising costs have eroded some aspects, and fees are now charged for some aspects of care. By the late 1980s, all European Union nations and all OECD nations except the United States had comprehensive publicly funded personal health care services, usually with the proviso that people pay additional personal expenses.

national health planning A general term for planning by governmental agencies and other stakeholders (patient advocate groups, health insurance carriers, professional organizations of physicians, nurses, other health workers, etc.) for short- and long-term health planning at the national level. In many respects this activity never ceases. New problems and issues constantly arise and contingencies to deal with them must be considered. National leaders often convene ad hoc planning groups because specific or general issues requiring action have surfaced.

National Health Service (NHS) The health care system of the United Kingdom, established in 1948. It is a comprehensive tax-supported system of personal primary care by family doctors (general practitioners), specialist care by hospital-based consultants, and a public health service organized in municipalities and regions. The original organization and financing arrangements were worked out between the postwar Labour government and representatives of the British Medical Association, hospital-based specialists, and independent general practitioners. There have been many reorganizations and reforms, including formation of independent private "trusts" for regional organizations of general practitioners and consultants and administrative flexibility. See http://www.nhs.uk/ for comparisons with health care systems in other nations, including the United States and European nations. The overall per capita costs of the British NHS are consistently well below those of the United States, and its outcomes in terms of mortality rates, hospital major procedure adverse complications, etc., are generally superior, a fact repeatedly demonstrated in many studies. Its long waiting times for many procedures and excessive bureaucracy are often criticized.

National Highway Traffic Safety Administration The US government agency in the US Department of Transportation that receives and implements recommendations about measures aimed at reducing death, injury, and financial costs attributable to traffic crashes, i.e., enhancing highway safety. Examples of its initiatives include action against driving under the influence of alcohol or drugs, drafting legislation on automobile seat belt and motorcycle crash helmet use, mandatory recall of automobiles when defective design features are discovered, and education on road traffic safety. See http://www.nhtsa.dot.gov/ for details.

National Institute for Health and Clinical Excellence The agency of the UK National Health Service that monitors performance and outcomes of medical, surgical, and preventive health care, publishes reports, and issues guidelines on best practices. See http://www.nice.org.uk/ for details.

National Institute for Occupational Safety and Health (NIOSH) The division of the CENTERS FOR DISEASE CONTROL AND PREVENTION that is responsible for conducting research and making recommendations about the epidemiology, prevention, and control of diseases and injuries that are associated with occupations and the workplace environment. Its mission and activities are described at http://www.cdc.gov/niosh/homepage.html.

National Institute of Allergy and Infectious Disease (NIAID) The agency of the US NATIONAL INSTITUTES OF HEALTH that conducts and sponsors research on diseases caused by infectious pathogens, disorders of the immune system, allergies, and related problems. There are special groups that focus on major important specific diseases, including tuberculosis, malaria, and HIV/AIDS. See http://www.niaid.nih.gov/default.htm for details of programs and activities.

National Institute of Environmental Health Sciences (NIEHS) This is a major agency of the US NATIONAL INSTITUTES OF HEALTH; based in Research Triangle, North Carolina. Its mission is to study and control the causes of premature death, disease, and injury due to all environmental causes. It conducts and sponsors a wide range of multidisciplinary biomedical research programs and projects. For details see http://www.niehs.nih.gov.

National Institutes of Health (NIH) The largest, wealthiest, most effective research-oriented agency of the US government, administratively an agency of the DEPARTMENT OF HEALTH AND HUMAN SERVICES (DHHS). It comprises several Institutes that focus on specific categories of disease: cancer, cardiovascular and respiratory diseases, infectious diseases including HIV/AIDS, allergic conditions, arthritis and rheumatism, conditions associated with aging, eye diseases, etc. Some of the Institutes have mandates that go beyond sponsorship of research. For example, the John E. Fogarty International Center for International Health sometimes has a quasi-diplomatic role, and the National Institute of Environmental Health Sciences, based in Research Triangle, North Carolina, conducts standard-setting studies. Most of the Institutes have their headquarters in Bethesda, Maryland. For more information, see http://www.nih.gov, where current organization, major activities, new initiatives, official reports, and more, are accessible.

National Library of Medicine Administratively part of the NATIONAL INSTITUTES OF HEALTH, this is the most comprehensive collection of medical journals and books in the world, established by JOHN SHAW BILLINGS (1838–1913) during the 30-year period (1864–1895) that he supervised the collection in the office of the Surgeon General. Much of the collection is accessible online. It includes the organizational framework for MEDLINE and for the NATIONAL NETWORK OF LIBRARIES OF MEDICINE. See http://www.nlm.nih.gov/ for details. The Canadian equivalent is the CANADIAN INSTITUTE FOR SCIENTIFIC AND TECHNICAL INFORMATION, at http://cisti-icist.nrc-cnrc.gc.ca/cisti_e.html, which maintains a comprehensive collection of Canadian and other scientific serial publications and occasional reports.

National Network of Libraries of Medicine (NN/LM) An electronic data base linking medical libraries throughout the United States and Canada that includes almost 5,000 libraries and retrievable reference collections, making this a very rich resource for references. For North American users, some interlibrary loan facilities may be available, and photocopy services are available for a fee to anyone. The network is accessible via http://nnlm.gov.

National Research Council (NRC) The advisory body of the US NATIONAL ACADEMY OF SCIENCES, established in 1916 with responsibility for coordinating research findings and government policies to implement these findings. The INSTITUTE OF MEDICINE is a major component of the NRC, with the mission of providing leadership and direction for medical and health-related research and implementing relevant policies. See http://www.nationalacademies.org/nrc/. Other countries have similar organizations, for instance Centre National de la Recherche Scientifique (CNRS) in France.

National Rifle Association A politically influential organization dedicated to promoting gun ownership and safe use in the United States. Its mandate is based on the second amendment to the US Constitution (1791) asserting the right of all citizens to bear arms. In the modern, urban United States, access to and unrestrained use of powerful modern FIREARMS has made death and serious injury caused by guns a prominent public health problem, especially among young men. See http://www.nra.org/.

National Science Foundation An agency of the US government that functions autonomously at arm's length, as a foundation to support research and the dissemination of research findings over a wide range of physical and biological sciences, for example with financial support for educational television programs. See http://www.nsf.gov/.

National Screening Committee The British agency responsible for assessing screening methods and advising the government about which screening methods and programs to adopt, the target groups for which they are most appropriate, and similar details. For information about this committee and its program, see http://libraries.nelh.nhs.uk/screening.

National Toxicology Program The program that sets the exposure limits and safety standards applicable to environmental exposures to chemicals used in industry and agriculture and for domestic purposes in the United States, as mandated by the Occupational Safety and Health Act. It sponsors and conducts studies of putative toxic substances, carcinogens, etc., and produces many reports and recommendations. See http://ntp-server.niehs.nih.gov/ for details.

Native American The term used in the United States to describe person(s) of indigenous origin. Other terms are used elsewhere in the Americas; for instance, in Canada indigenous persons are members of First Nations communities, and there, as elsewhere, tribal or other ethnically identifying names such as Navajo, Inuit, and Cree are also used. Generally, Native American health indicators such as life expectancy compare unfavorably with those of white Americans. Some conditions, notably diabetes and arthritis, have high prevalence among Native Americans.

natural childbirth An approach to the management of labor first proposed and implemented in 1933 by the British obstetrician Grantley Dick Read (1890–1959), described in *Childbirth Without Fear* (1933) and modified by many others. It is based on the notion of preventing pain by eliminating fear of labor pains, thus encouraging relaxation to facilitate easier delivery, which was also claimed to reduce perinatal complications and birth injury. The LAMAZE TECHNIQUE is a modification by the French obstetrician Fernand Lamaze (1891–1957) that uses a combination of instruction in exercises and orientation to the events that occur during labor. No randomized controlled trials have ever been done to determine whether natural childbirth does reduce the risk of some complications of labor and the postpartum period.

natural disaster As distinct from a manmade disaster, this is a natural phenomenon, such as an earthquake, tsunami, avalanche, landslide, flood, hurricane, tornado, forest fire, over which humans usually have little, if any, control. Some so-called natural disasters have roots in human actions. For instance, mudslides occur on steep mountainsides that have been cleared of trees, leaving nothing to hold the soil after heavy rain or snow-melt. Many natural disasters have implications for population health, such as disruption of water purification and sewage systems, and some, notably earthquakes and tsunamis, can cause great loss of life.

natural experiment A term applied to John Snow's study of the cholera epidemic in south London in 1854, in which he made use of information about the differing sources of private water supplies to many households, in some of which cholera had occurred and in others of which it had not. The concept of a "natural experiment," in which a real-life situation is observed and studied systematically, has been applied to many other conditions. Examples include observations of child growth and development before, during, and after a period of wartime food rationing, which showed that the balanced diet of British food rations was nutritionally superior to prewar diets; reduced lung cancer mortality rates among former smokers who quit; reduced traffic crash mortality when speed limits were lowered and enforced during a fuel crisis in the 1970s; and increased head injury mortality when some states relaxed requirements for motorcyclists to wear safety helmets.

natural gas Underground deposits of flammable gaseous hydrocarbons, varying in composition but usually mainly methane, used as fuel. Natural gas occurs in strata with oil, but deposits may consist almost entirely of gases. Some varieties of natural gas, such as SOUR GAS, which is gas containing large proportions of hydrogen sulfide, are extremely toxic.

natural history The descriptive study of living organisms, i.e., plants and animals, in their normal habitat. See also ECOLOGY.

natural history of disease Applied to the description of a disease, this term means the way the disease evolves and progresses, particularly in the absence of intervention. Abundant information about the natural history of many chronic, long-term, progressive and recurrent diseases reveals

that they have several stages: stage of pathological onset; presymptomatic stage; and clinical stage when the disease is manifest. The use of SCREENING TESTS in the presymptomatic stage enables early detection of some conditions including certain cancers and cardiovascular diseases, and this may provide opportunities for effective interventions to improve chances of reversing or retarding the disease process and reducing the adverse impact of complications.

natural immunity Immunity to pathogenic agents that is inherent and, often, species-specific. An example of natural immunity is human immunity to canine distemper. It is likely that some of the recently emergent pathogens responsible for human disease have circulated for prolonged periods in animal species that possess natural immunity to these pathogens.

natural law A system of rules of conduct based on a set of concepts about human nature; said to be the innate ways people behave toward one another under favorable circumstances. This includes cooperative mutual support, care, and protection of the vulnerable.

natural rate of increase A measure of the population GROWTH RATE, i.e., the difference between birth rates and death rates. In most nations throughout most of history this rate has been a positive number, but in several European nations since the 1950s, birth rates have fallen below death rates, so populations are declining in numbers or would be if there were no migration of newcomers to sustain the population, especially its working-age members who contribute to pension funds and old age security benefits. See also ZERO POPULATION GROWTH.

natural selection A central concept of evolutionary theory. CHARLES DARWIN'S original theory and its modern modifications hold that biological, behavioral, and environmental conditions determine which members of a species will survive and pass on their genes to the next generation. Darwin demonstrated this by his observations of varieties of finches, moths, etc, that "adapted" to environments in which specific adaptations, such as colors of the moths' wings, gave the best prospects for survival. A modern demonstration is the development of antibiotic-resistant strains of pathogenic microorganisms.

naturopathy An alternative health care system founded in 1902 by German-born Benedict Lust (1872–1945) based on the belief that disease is caused by violations of the laws of nature and can be prevented and treated by observing these laws. Lust stressed avoidance of bad habits, such as smoking, alcohol use, tea and coffee consumption, excesses of dietary intake and sexual indulgence, and cultivation of good habits, including exercise, sleep, and mental relaxation.

nearest neighbor method A method used mainly in veterinary epidemiology to assess the spatial distribution of disease and its relationship to geographical or topographical factors. The position of individuals is plotted, some are randomly selected, and their distance from nearest neighbors is measured in relation to their health status.

nebulizer A device to reduce a solid or liquid substance to fine airborne particles. Examples include aerosol sprays used to self-treat respiratory symptoms such as asthmatic bronchospasm.

necrosis Death of some or all cells in an organ or tissue while the rest of the organism remains alive, caused by interrupted blood supply by vascular thrombosis or embolism; burns; frostbite; chemical or physical injury; severe inflammation caused by pathogenic organisms; malignant neoplasm; or other causes of cell death.

needle exchange programs A system operated by public health authorities or voluntary agencies in many communities with the aim of reducing the risk of transmitting blood-borne infectious diseases, especially HIV/AIDS, by providing clean sterile hypodermic needles to illicit intravenous drug users on a no-questions-asked basis. This approach acknowledges the existence of illicit drug use, is not judgmental or punitive, and can provide a way to gain the confidence of illicit drug users as a preliminary step toward their rehabilitation.

needlestick injury Accidental penetration of the skin, usually of a health care worker such as a physician or nurse, by a needle that has been used to administer a drug to a patient and that could transmit a blood-borne infection (e.g., HIV/AIDS, hepatitis C) or by any other sharp object. Injuries caused by cutting instruments, needles, or other sharp objects such as broken glass (SHARPS) are a serious occupational hazard of the health care professions.

needs All things that are considered necessary or essential. The fundamental necessities of life are water, food, shelter, and clothing. Other concrete and abstract things that could be described as needs, including income, employment to provide access to these necessities of life, belonging to a family, a social support system, education, self-esteem, and access to health care of acceptable quality, are sometimes part of political platforms. See also MASLOW'S HIERARCHY OF NEEDS. Categorizing needs is essential in health care planning and is at least in part ideologically determined.

needs assessment A formal process conducted by health and social workers and others in health agencies to delineate the dimensions and severity of health and social problems of persons, families, and specified communities, especially those considered to be at high risk, so that resources can be deployed to manage them efficiently. Alternative approaches to needs assessment include the community-based survey and the CASE CONFERENCE. The latter is often used to compile an inventory of problems and resources available to deal with them; then the problems are prioritized and strategies and tactics developed to deal with them.

neglect Inability or failure to fulfill familial, occupational, or social responsibilities to care for self or others for whom there is a duty to care. There are several categories of neglect, e.g., child neglect, neglect of other dependent persons, medical neglect, or NEGLIGENCE.

negligence Willful neglect that is implicitly or explicitly considered to be dereliction of duty and that justifies calling the responsible person(s) to account for what was done or not done.

neighborhood A circumscribed locality in which appreciable proportions of the people can be expected to know one another if they have been residents for long enough to get acquainted, such as a "village within a city" or a suburban district.

neighborhood network The term usually applied to a SUPPORT GROUP comprising residents of dwellings in a circumscribed neighborhood.

nematode Any member of the phylum comprising roundworms, threadworms, with unsegmented bodies that taper at the head and tail ends. Many are parasitic, notably filarial worms, hookworms.

neonatal care Care of infants in the period immediately after their birth. The duration of the neonatal period is from birth to 28 days in vital statistics, but in clinical practice the period of neonatal care is flexible, dependent on the status of the infant.

neonatal tetanus Tetanus that occurs among newborns. This almost universally fatal condition has often been a prominent cause of early neonatal death because of inadequate hygiene during childbirth and remains so in some low-income countries. In the early 21st century, it causes about 2 million deaths annually. If contaminated by tetanus spores, the necrotizing tissue of the umbilical cord is an ideal medium for propagation of tetanus. The risk is aggravated by traditional customs, such as using a cow dung poultice or sprinkling ashes from the fire in a village hut on the cut end of the umbilical cord, as formerly practiced in Java. Immunization of girls in childhood or pregnant women considerably reduces the incidence of neonatal tetanus.

neonatology The study and specialized branch of health care devoted to newborns.

neoplasm Literally "new growth," with the implication that it is abnormal, either benign or, in the context in which the word is more often used, malignant, usually CANCER.

nephrotoxin A toxin that acts specifically on kidney tissues, e.g., a toxin that disrupts the action of the glomeruli or causes renal tubular necrosis. Nephrotoxins include certain drugs such as phenacetin; bacterial toxins include those produced by acute STREPTOCOCCAL INFECTION and septicemia.

nerve gases Gaseous or volatile liquid compounds, mostly organophosphorus compounds that are cholinesterase inhibitors. They act by paralyzing neuromuscular function. Some are derived from insecticides; some, such as sarin, were developed by the Nazis as chemical weapons and used in their death camps but not in warfare. Despite international agreements against the use of nerve gases, several nations are known to have research and development programs, ostensibly for defense purposes. Nerve gases are WEAPONS OF MASS DESTRUCTION. Sarin was used by terrorists in the Tokyo subway in 1995; the Iraqi dictator Saddam Hussein used nerve gases against his Kurdish and Iranian adversaries on several occasions in the 1980s and early 1990s.

nervous breakdown The lay term used to describe an episode of mental or emotional disorder causing disability or handicap without specifying the nature of the disorder, which might be anything referable to the mind or brain: a tendency to excessive tearfulness; acute alcoholism; onset of an episode of severe depression; schizophrenia, or a host of other possibilities.

nested case control study A CASE CONTROL STUDY that utilizes cases and control subjects already being studied for another purpose; often part of the larger population of a COHORT STUDY. The cases are those that arise in the larger population; the controls are other members of the same study population age- and sex-matched, but without the condition of interest. This is a nested portion of a larger group for all of whom some relevant information already exists.

net fertility rate Also called net reproduction rate, this is the average number of daughters that would be born to a birth cohort of women during their lifetime if they experienced a fixed pattern of age-specific fertility and mortality rates.

net rate The word "net" is used to describe a number or rate that has been adjusted to allow for inappropriate omissions, inclusions, etc. Thus, the net rate of increase of a population in a specified jurisdiction is the rate adjusted for the effects of migration into or out of the region.

network (n. and v.) 1. The social connections of individuals to one another; the act of connecting. Networks for most people are numerous, comprising family members, working colleagues, friends, neighbors, members of social groups for recreation, etc. There is usually a positive correlation between health and the richness and variety of a person's networks. 2. A group of two or more computers that share software, data.

networking The process of establishing and maintaining connections among individuals and agencies, organizations, either as an end in itself or to achieve some specific objective.

neural tube defects The brain and spinal cord are formed from the embryonic notochord, which normally closes early in embryonic life, leaving a narrow space for the cerebral ventricles. Failure of the neural tube to close leads to birth defects ranging from anencephaly and open spina bifida to relatively inconspicuous spina bifida occulta, which is usually associated with loss of some nerve function, such as loss of full control of bladder function and/or sexual function. Folic acid deficiency before and during pregnancy may cause this condition, and dietary supplements of folic acid can prevent it.

neuron The basic functional cellular unit of the nervous system, a cell with a nucleus and long fibrils, dendrites, that connect with other nerve cells at a synapse where nerve impulses are transmitted. The cell body and dendrites receive signals from other neurons via synapses, of which there may typically be 1,000 to 10,000 per neuron in the central nervous system; the neuron transmits and receives nerve impulses by an axon ranging in length from 3 mm to more than 1 meter, often splitting into many branches near its end, transmitting signals from the neuron to one or more other neurons, a muscle, or a gland.

neuropathy A pathological process affecting (peripheral) nerve cells and/or nervous tissue.

neurosis Syn: psychoneurosis. A distressing emotional or mental disorder, often chronic, in which there is no loss of contact with reality, in contrast to a PSYCHOSIS, in which the patient experiences delusions and/or hallucinations. Neurosis is a large, diffuse, rather loose diagnostic category, including anxiety and psychosomatic symptoms such as bowel, bladder, and sleep disorders and hysteria. Generally neuroses respond to pharmacological preparations and/or psychotherapy, but often they are chronic, recurrent, or intractable and consume a considerable proportion of personal and public health care expenditure.

neurotoxin A substance that impairs or disrupts nerve function, e.g., by interrupting neural transmission, impairing or destroying nerve cells, damaging myelin sheathes, etc. Many drugs, anesthetic agents, pesticides, and various by-products of petrochemical synthesis are neurotoxins.

neurotransmitter The molecular process and chemicals responsible for sending sensory or motor neural impulses from one nerve cell to another via the synapse connecting them.

neutron The component of the atomic nucleus that carries no electrical charge. Outside the nucleus, neutrons decay to produce a positively charged proton and negatively charged electron.

newton The SI unit of force, defined as the force that gives a mass of 1 kg an acceleration of 1 meter per 1/100th second. It is named for the British mathematician, natural scientist, and philosopher Isaac Newton (1642–1727).

NHS Health Technology Assessment Programme The program operated by the British National Health Service that is responsible for evaluating established and innovative equipment and technology used in all aspects of diagnostic and therapeutic health services in the United Kingdom, and also for assessing similar activities elsewhere in the European Union and other countries around the world. See http://www.ncchta.org for reports, current activities, research initiatives, etc.

niacin Vitamin B$_3$, also known as nicotinic acid. An essential dietary requirement. Niacin is synthesized in animal tissue, so deficiency occurs in people whose dietary intake of animal fat and protein is inadequate, e.g., VEGANS. In the body, niacin is required for the production of the enzyme nicotinamide-adenine dinucleotide, and deficiency causes PELLAGRA.

nickel (Ni) Metallic element with many industrial uses in both pure and alloy form, e.g., in vacuum tubes and electroplating with silver and as an alloy in coins. Nickel has several toxic effects and is a carcinogen, implicated in nasopharyngeal and lung cancer.

nicotine A toxic alkaloid derived from tobacco, responsible for the dependence of regular smokers on cigarettes. In small doses nicotine has a stimulating effect on the autonomic nervous system, causing raised blood pressure and pulse rate and impaired appetite. Large doses cause paralysis of the autonomic ganglia. As used in tobacco smoking, sniffing, or chewing, its effects are primarily stimulant and also calming, although not soporific or sedative. Nicotine may be the most powerfully addictive of all the drugs of addiction.

nicotinic acid See NIACIN.

nidus A focus or focal point. The word is most commonly applied to a nidus of infection, that is, to a situation or setting favorable to the initial propagation and spread of an infectious agent, but can also describe the anatomical site of origin of an infection or a neoplastic process.

night blindness Impaired or absent capacity to perceive visual stimuli in conditions of low illumination, such as twilight or near darkness, due to impaired function of the retinal cells called rods. This may be due to any of several causes, including deficiency of vitamin A, retinal degeneration, cataract, or optic atrophy. Impaired night vision commonly caused by cataract reduces the capacity of elderly car drivers to drive safely at night.

Nightingale, Florence (1820–1910) The British nurse and founder of modern nursing practice, emphasizing effective use of hospital hygiene, compassionate care, and, above all, a foundation in systematic statistical evaluation. She was a member of the Royal Statistical Society and the London Epidemiological Society, was proficient in compiling and analyzing hospital and health statistics, and designed the first HOSPITAL DISCHARGE ABSTRACT SYSTEM.

night soil A euphemism for human excreta that is collected in receptacles and disposed of by collection and/or used as fertilizer.

night sweats Profuse, drenching sweating, characteristically but not necessarily when in bed at night, associated with the resolving phase of recurrent fever and traditionally considered a symptom of tuberculosis.

NIH See NATIONAL INSTITUTES OF HEALTH.

NIMBY The initial letters of the words "not in my back yard," signifying resistance to proposals to establish an unsightly or distasteful industry or development, such as a halfway house for recovering drug addicts or a dump site, in the neighborhood. This resistance is often politically significant, so legislators and public health officials are obliged to take the sentiments seriously.

NIOSH See NATIONAL INSTITUTE FOR OCCUPATIONAL SAFETY AND HEALTH.

nitrates Salts of nitric acid containing the $-NO_3$ anion. They have many uses, for instance as basic ingredients of many chemical compounds. Ammonium nitrate is a fertilizer, used to add nitrogen to soil. Nitroglycerin and derivatives are used as vasodilators to treat angina pectoris.

nitrification The process of conversion of nitrogen compounds in the soil by oxidation of ammonia into nitrates, by the action of nitrifying bacteria, preceded by NITROGEN FIXATION.

nitrites Salts of nitrous acid containing the $-NO_2$ anion. They are used as meat preservatives, but if ingested they can cause methemoglobinemia, a condition of reduced capacity of the blood to carry oxygen that causes a bluish complexion.

nitrogen (N) The gaseous element that constitutes about 80% of the earth's atmosphere. It occurs in innumerable compounds as nitrates, nitrites, and in combination with carbon, hydrogen, and other elements (sulfur, phosphorus, etc.) in organic compounds that form proteins in all living creatures. Nitrogen moves through the living environment in the NITROGEN CYCLE that converts elemental nitrogen and nitrates and nitrites into organic compounds, including proteins in all land-based and marine ecosystems.

nitrogen cycle The biochemical process that transforms elemental NITROGEN and inorganic nitrogen compounds into organic compounds via synthesis of ammonia, amino acids, and proteins.

nitrogen fixation The process by which certain soil bacteria, especially those around the roots of plants such as clover, convert free atmospheric oxygen into ammonia as a preliminary to the other soil bacterial process of NITRIFICATION. The two processes, fixation and nitrification, are essential to the formation of plant proteins, so they are of great ecological importance.

nitrogen narcosis Syn: rapture of the deep. The state of impaired consciousness and reduced intellectual function due to excessive nitrogen in the blood that occurs when air at increased atmospheric pressure is respired. This soporific and intoxicating effect was first observed in deep sea divers, thus the name "rapture of the deep."

nitrogen oxides Nitrogen bonds with oxygen in several combinations, including nitrogen monoxide, which is manufactured and used industrially to make nitric acid, and nitrogen dioxide, a brownish irritant gas that is formed by the action of ultraviolet light on nitrogen monoxide and is the unpleasant ingredient in SMOG caused by the action of sunlight on automobile exhaust fumes.

nitroglycerine A pharmaceutical and an explosive, an oily liquid that the Swedish chemist Alfred Nobel (1833–1896) combined with either an absorbent clay or cotton to produce the stable explosives dynamite and guncotton. It is a powerful vasodilator used to treat angina pectoris, and because of this, occupational exposure can induce severe headaches of vascular origin. Chronic exposure can cause leukopenia, methemoglobinemia, and liver damage.

nitrosamines A group of chemicals formed by combinations of nitrites and amines that include several active carcinogens. Nitrosamines occur in many foodstuffs, including fish, meat, cheese, and products preserved with nitrites, and are formed when food protein reacts with nitrite salts in the stomach. They can also be formed by frying or smoking. Nitrosamines are responsible for many cancers associated with dietary factors.

nitroso compounds A class of chemical compounds of nitrogen, carbon, and hydrogen used as rocket fuels, in the manufacture of synthetic rubber compounds and pesticides, and for many other purposes. However, some, including NITROSAMINES, are animal and human carcinogens.

nits The common name for the eggs of HEAD LICE, the eggs adhere to hair by means of a sticky exudate secreted by the female louse as she lays and deposits the eggs.

Nobel Prizes The Swedish chemist Alfred Nobel (1833–1896), who invented dynamite, gelignite, and many other commercially profitable compounds, made a huge fortune from the manufacture of explosives and other chemicals. He bequeathed the greater part of his estate to establish the Nobel Prizes. These were first awarded in 1901. There are prizes for physiology or medicine, science, literature, and contributions to fraternity among nations, the Nobel Peace Prize. Many Nobel Prizes in physiology or medicine and Nobel Peace Prizes have been awarded to people and organizations that have advanced the causes connected with public health. These include RONALD ROSS; ROBERT KOCH; Charles Laveran; PAUL EHRLICH; Alexander Fleming,

Ernst Chain and Howard Florey; Macfarlane Burnett and Peter Medawar; Stanley Prusiner; the organizations include the International Red Cross, International Physicians for the Prevention of Nuclear War, and the United Nations Children's Fund (UNICEF).

noble gases The elements in group O of the periodic table that are gaseous and inert, i.e., do not readily combine with other elements or molecules. They include helium, neon, argon, krypton, xenon, and radon. Several have public health significance (e.g., helium, which is used to replace nitrogen in high-pressure breathing apparatus; argon, which is used as an insulating substance in double-glazing; and RADON, which seeps into houses from the foundations and is implicated in some cases of lung cancer).

no-fault insurance An insurance system in which, as the name states, no blame is attributed to any party in an insurance claim. Used mainly in automobile insurance, this system is also used by some public health authorities in claims for damages due to mishaps in preventive services, such as immunization programs.

noise 1. An unpleasant sound that is a nuisance and is sometimes intense enough to damage hearing. Noise ABATEMENT is sometimes available as a way to reduce this nuisance effect, for instance by erecting sound barriers at the ends of airport runways and along urban expressways. Noise is an occupational hazard in some occupations. See OCCUPATIONAL DEAFNESS. 2. In analysis of data, "noise" is a jargon word for unwanted extraneous information that can render analysis difficult or even impossible.

noise pollution Obtrusive, annoying, distracting, unpleasant persistent sounds that interfere with sleep or the ability to concentrate or enjoy life. It is one of the problems of high-density urban societies, with many possible causes, including unshielded machinery, heavy traffic, aircraft in flight paths above dwellings, and music amplified to broadcast far beyond the range of a nearby audience. It is a recognized public health problem, addressed in many jurisdictions by appropriate regulations, although these are often difficult to enforce.

nomads Roaming people, often groups, who have no fixed, permanent habitation. Some are vestiges of a hunter-gatherer way of life and are proficient at living off limited resources available to them in harsh environments. Examples are Australian Aborigines and the Inuit of northern Canada, who until recently subsisted by hunting and gathering. Many nomads do have temporary semifixed habitations; the animals they hunt or their herds of cattle, goats, or sheep wander, and the nomads wander with them. It is a harsh existence with precarious food supplies, and malnutrition frequently threatens health. Indigenous nomadic people in North America and Australia include many who have now settled in fixed homes.

nomenclature A system of names for specific entities. See also TAXONOMY.

nominal data Data that are identified in terms of their names (or numbers, used as labels rather than as numerical values) without regard for other qualities, such as rank or amount.

nominal scale A classification method (rather than a measurement scale) that organizes data according to specified qualitative criteria, such as country of birth, ethnic origin, without regard for any quantitative criteria, such as socioeconomic status.

nomogram Sets of line charts that are used to relate one set of variables to others that are displayed on a linear scale. The relationships are shown by drawing a line to connect the values of two known variables to a third, which is not known.

non-A non-B hepatitis An outmoded term formerly used to describe varieties of hepatitis that could be identified clinically and did not conform to the immunological pattern of hepatitis A or B. Most have now been reclassified as hepatitis C, D, E, F, or G.

noncommunicable conditions (diseases) A descriptive term for common and important conditions of public health importance that are not caused by infectious pathogens. Formerly some of these were classified as "chronic diseases," but this term is a misnomer when applied to cardiovascular disease such as acute myocardial infarction that causes sudden death. Even the adjective "noncommunicable" may be misleading when applied to cervical cancers caused by papilloma virus, some behavioral epidemics, or traffic-related injury and disability.

noncompliance Failure to adhere to or abide by the recommendations or instructions of health care professionals, such as failure to take prescribed medication or adhere to a dietary regimen.

nongovernmental organization (NGO) A generic name for not-for-profit organizations or agencies that are separate and independent from government. Many provide health and social services. Some are partially supported by government funds. Their independence renders them less susceptible to political pressures, and for this reason and others they often provide needed services that are low on governmental priority lists and sometimes engage in advocacy. Some NGOs may advocate a cultural, philosophical, or religious belief and seek to influence the communities to which they bring assistance, but most are impartial.

non-insulin-dependent   diabetes   mellitus (NIDDM) Syn: adult-onset diabetes, type 2 diabetes. This form of adult-onset diabetes is commonly associated with obesity and usually responds well to a strict dietary regimen; it does not usually require treatment with supplementary insulin. It is increasingly common at younger ages in wealthy countries and is associated with childhood obesity. In many low-income countries where undernutrition has long been common, NIDDM has become prevalent, perhaps because of a "thrifty gene" diathesis (see BARKER HYPOTHESIS).

nonionizing radiation Low-energy electromagnetic radiation that does not emit ions. It comprises visible light, infrared radiation, radar, microwaves, and long-wavelength radio waves. The biological effects of nonionizing radiation do not include mutagenesis or carcinogenesis, but, depending on the wavelength, there are other biological effects. For instance, microwaves and radar can cause dangerous heating of body tissues.

nonlinear relationship A relationship among variables that does not follow a mathematically predictable pattern.

nonmaleficence The ethical principle of doing no harm, expressed in the ancient medical maxim *primum non nocere* (first do no harm). Its approximate counterpart in population health is the PRECAUTIONARY PRINCIPLE.

nonparametric method Syn: distribution-free method. A statistical method that can be used regardless of the manner in which the data to be analyzed are distributed.

nonpoint source epidemic An epidemic that is demonstrably not emanating from a single focus of infection, over a brief time span; for example, a vector-borne epidemic or one spread by a polluted communal water supply that distributes water to multiple households.

nonprofit (not-for-profit) organization An organizational framework rather frequently used in the health and social sectors in which charges or fees generated for services rendered are either waived or returned to the operating budget of the organization.

nonresponders Individuals who fail to respond to questions in a survey or questionnaire. They are often qualitatively different from responders, and if they constitute a high proportion of the total population surveyed, efforts should be made to assess the nature of these differences; otherwise the findings of the survey will be distorted by various BIASES.

nonsense correlation Syn: spurious correlation. A statistically significant but otherwise meaningless association between variables that turns up in the course of analyzing a set of data but has no biological, social, or other significance.

nonspecific urethritis An inflammatory mucopurulent urethral discharge that is sterile on the usual culture media. It is commonly due to chlamydial infection, which may have other clinical manifestations such as conjunctivitis. It is usually a sexually transmitted disease.

nonsteroidal   anti-inflammatory   drugs (NSAIDs) A miscellaneous group of drugs that relieve the symptoms and signs of arthritis and soft-tissue inflammation. They work by inhibiting the production of prostaglandins and/or interfering with metabolic processes in synovial membranes. They include aspirin and its derivatives and the butazone family of drugs. Many are gastric irritants, and some suppress bone marrow. Some have other harmful effects.

nontraditional family A group of people living together in a mutually supportive relationship described as a "family" but not conforming to the usual definition, in that the group does not consist of two or more people united by genetic heritage, blood, or marital ties. Examples include COMMUNES and same-sex couples, especially if they are rearing child(ren).

no-observed-adverse-effect level (NOAEL) In occupational and environmental health, the highest dose at which no adverse effects are observed in an animal population that is challenged with graduated doses of a substance or agent that is known or suspected to be toxic or harmful. In setting safety standards for human exposure, it is usual to set the safety level two or more orders of magnitude above the NOAEL, i.e., 100 or 1,000 times higher.

norm 1. The usual value, customary behavior, method of practice. 2. In the sense of criteria and standards of behavior, desirable, which may not necessarily be customary or usual.

normal 1. In the context of health status, in good health, or physical findings and laboratory investigations indicative of good health. 2. In statistics, within the usual range of variation in a designated population or group. In more precise statistical terms for characteristics with a normal distribution, where less than about 5% of the values lie beyond two standard deviations from the mean for this population.

normal distribution In statistics, a distribution that is symmetrical about a midpoint, with the largest number of values clustered closest to this and diminishing further away, according to the mathematical formula proposed by the German mathematician Karl Friedrich Gauss (1777–1855), thus the alternative name GAUSSIAN DISTRIBUTION.

normalization 1. Establishment or return to "normal" or usual social, political, economic conditions after a period of upheaval. 2. Mathematical transformation of a set of data from log normal to normal.

normal limits The range, usually determined empirically, within which physiological variables such as height, weight, and blood pressure usually lie in a healthy person. This may be an arbitrary range or defined by a specified measurement, such as the 95% confidence limits. What is "normal" in one society may be abnormal in another, depending on the distribution of risk in the population.

normative data Data that conform to the expected or usual range of normal. Especially in psychology, test results that are normal and used as a baseline for assessing abnormal function.

noroviruses The viruses formerly designated Norwalk agents, first identified in Norwalk, Connecticut. They cause an indolent recurrent diarrhea that can occur also in explosive epidemics, e.g., among passengers on cruise ships when there is a carrier among the catering staff or the ship's water supply is infected. Prevention requires scrupulous handwashing and food hygiene.

Norplant See LEVONORGESTREL.

Norwalk agents See NOROVIRUSES.

nosocomial infection Syn: hospital-acquired infection. An infection that is acquired in a hospital or other health care setting. The ecology of nosocomial infections varies with time and from one institution to another. The most common pathogens recently have been multiple-resistant *Staphylococcus aureus* (MRSA); others include *Proteus* and *Pseudomonas* species. The most effective way to control all such pathogens is rigorous attention to aseptic precautions.

nosology Classification of sick persons into groups, using a systematic and agreed-on method and procedure for deciding which disease categories fit into each group. Assignment of names or diagnostic labels to each disease entity creates a

TAXONOMY and nomenclature of disease, also known as a nosography of disease.

notifiable disease A disease that by law or regulation must be reported to public health or other designated authorities because the community must be protected from harm to others that could result from contact with infected persons; because precautions such as vaccination are necessary to protect others from the disease; or because it is in the public interest to know how frequently the condition in question is occurring. There are several categories. 1. Contagious diseases for which INTERNATIONAL HEALTH REGULATIONS require a case report. These diseases are reportable to national public health authorities and to the World Health Organization. They include QUARANTINABLE DISEASES (plague, cholera, yellow fever), diseases under WHO surveillance (louse-borne typhus, relapsing fever, paralytic poliomyelitis, malaria, epidemic influenza A), and other diseases such as SEVERE ACUTE RESPIRATORY SYNDROME (SARS) and AVIAN INFLUENZA so designated. 2. Infectious diseases notifiable to local health authorities, for which national, regional, or local regulations exist. These are about 40 to 50 infectious diseases of public health importance, including SEXUALLY TRANSMITTED DISEASES. 3. Certain industrial, occupational, and environmental diseases are notifiable in many jurisdictions, including lead poisoning, asbestosis, and diseases caused by several toxic chemicals such as benzene and dioxin. 4. In many jurisdictions, all health workers are legally obliged to report suspected child abuse, whether physical or sexual, to child protection agencies. 5. In some jurisdictions, physicians must report to motor vehicle licensing authorities any patient they consider is no longer fit to drive a car for medical reason because to do so would endanger the lives of others on the roads. 6. Cancer and other malignant neoplasms are notifiable to CANCER REGISTRIES in many jurisdictions. See also QUARANTINE and REPORTABLE DISEASES.

nuclear family Two or more people related by blood, marital, or adoptive ties, or the common-law equivalent, comprising husband-wife or husband-wife-child(ren), usually living together and mutually supportive. A single-parent family is also a nuclear family.

nuclear fission Splitting or disintegration of the atomic nucleus with release of energy, the physical phenomenon by which nuclear reactors generate power.

nuclear fusion The process in which two atomic nuclei combine to produce the nucleus of a larger atom with release of energy. This can be used to make nuclear weapons and is advocated, but has not yet been successfully used, to generate energy in an environmentally friendly manner that would not generate radioactive by-products.

nuclear magnetic resonance imaging (NMRI) A diagnostic imaging technique. See MAGNETIC RESONANCE IMAGING.

nuclear medicine The specialized branch of medicine, the physical sciences, and engineering that uses ionizing radiation, radioactive isotopes, x-rays, etc., in diagnostic imaging and scanning and for the treatment of neoplastic conditions, etc.

nuclear power plants After the discovery of nuclear energy, nuclear power plants were an obvious industrial development to meet the world's increasing demand for energy, especially electric power. Nuclear power plants use the heat of nuclear reactions to make steam to drive turbines that generate electricity. In the United States, about 20% of electricity needs are met in this way. Worldwide the proportion is about 15% and rising, for instance in China. Enthusiasm for this source of "clean" (nonpolluting) energy ran high in 1950 when the first nuclear power plants were built, but it has waned in the light of accidents, e.g., at THREE MILE ISLAND, Pennsylvania, in 1979 and CHERNOBYL, near Kiev, in what was then the USSR, in 1986. There has been an increasingly serious, so far insolvable problem of disposing of "spent" nuclear fuel, much of which is highly radioactive and has a half-life of as long as several thousand years. There have also been persistent concerns about leakage of radiation from some plants, e.g., at Sellafield, United Kingdom. See also FAST BREEDER REACTOR.

nuclear reaction The reaction epitomized by the famous equation $E=MC^2$ discovered by the theoretical physicist and Nobel laureate Albert Einstein (1879–1955) associated with a change in the nucleus of an atom and release of energy in the form of ionizing radiation and particles, most of which are biologically active when they come into contact with living cells.

nuclear reactor An experimental or industrial installation to generate energy from nuclear material, i.e., radioactive substances that emit ionizing radiation. Nuclear reactors make use of the physics of radioactive material, in which the atomic structure changes with release of energy. In a nuclear reactor the energy is generated by a NUCLEAR FISSION chain reaction of fissile material such as uranium that can be used to generate electricity. By-products include radioactive isotopes, some of which are used in industry and in the health care system.

nuclear waste The residue of material left over from the production of nuclear energy. This includes some ores, mine tailings, and residual products of nuclear reactions that are radioactive with an extremely long half-life. Large quantities of nuclear waste are produced by nuclear reactors, and disposal of this waste is presenting serious problems.

nuclear weapon The most formidable of the WEAPONS OF MASS DESTRUCTION, which relies on the explosive power of NUCLEAR FISSION when radioactive material is suddenly compressed, as in atomic bombs, and a combination of fission and NUCLEAR FUSION in hydrogen bombs. Nuclear weapons explode with cataclysmic force in relation to their mass, causing MASS CASUALTIES from trauma and burns. RADIOACTIVE FALLOUT causes delayed death from malignant neoplasms. See ATOMIC BOMB.

nuclear winter A hypothetical scenario of the apocalyptic outcome of a large-scale nuclear war in which the earth's atmosphere would be filled with enough dust particles to obstruct solar radiation, precipitating a climatic catastrophe as the earth's surface would remain too cool for grain crops to germinate. Massive volcanic eruptions have had a similar effect, e.g., Krakatoa in 1883 and for several years afterward and, more briefly, Mount Pinatubo in the Philippines in 1991.

nucleic acid A complex organic compound consisting of chains of NUCLEOTIDES that conjugate with proteins in the nucleus and cytoplasm of somatic cells. In the cell nucleus they store and transmit the genetic code.

nucleotides Sugars such as ribose and deoxyribose that are the basic material from which nucleic acids (and therefore proteins) are formed.

nucleus 1. In biology, the component in the cell that contains genetic material and thereby controls the activity of the cell. 2. In physics, the central massive component of the atom.

nuclide A general term for radioactive nuclides, i.e., the ionized daughter atoms produced when a radioactive element or compound undergoes decay.

nuisance A source of annoyance, unpleasantness. In practice a nuisance is often defined as the source of unpleasant or noxious smells, such as a tannery or rendering plant, or a source of excessive noise. Local by-laws may provide ways to obtain relief from public health nuisances, which in some local health departments are a common cause of complaints.

null hypothesis The hypothesis that one set of variables is unrelated to another. Simply stated, the null hypothesis is that the relationship among distribution of variables in two or more representative samples is no different from what would be expected to occur by chance.

number needed to harm The number of patients who must receive a specified medication in routine therapeutic use to cause a specified adverse outcome in a patient. In the context in which the term is used, "adverse outcome" means death or significant impairment or disability that is attributable to the specified medication.

number needed to screen The number of people who must be given a SCREENING procedure to detect a case of the specified condition for which the screening procedure is conducted. The number varies widely according to the prevalence of the condition and whether the screening procedure is conducted in a general or a previously selected high-risk population subsample. The number can be calculated from available data on the incidence or prevalence of the condition.

number needed to treat In a clinical treatment regimen, the number of patients who must be treated to prevent the occurrence of a specified complication or adverse outcome of the condition under examination in a patient. This number is the difference between the occurrence rates of adverse outcomes in the treated and placebo groups in a clinical trial, which is the reciprocal of the ABSOLUTE RISK reduction. Details and descriptions of the method are available at http://www.jr2.ox.ac.uk/bandolier/band59/NNT1.html.

numerical taxonomy A system of naming entities in which each entity is assigned a unique number as well as a precise name. The INTERNATIONAL CLASSIFICATION OF DISEASES is an example of a numerical taxonomy.

Nuremberg Code The code of conduct for medical research involving human subjects that was composed after the Nuremberg trials of the Nazi war criminals in 1946–47. The central feature of the Nuremberg Code is contained in its first clause, which states that "The voluntary consent of the subject is absolutely essential." Other clauses deal with details, proxy consent, etc. See also HELSINKI, DECLARATION OF, and INFORMED CONSENT. The Nuremberg (Nürnberg) Code is frequently displayed in codes and guidelines on ethical conduct of research involving human subjects. It can be seen, for instance, at http://ohsr.od.nih.gov/guidelines/nuremberg.html.

nurse A person who has been trained to provide personal care of the sick, especially those who are confined to bed in a hospital. In most countries the training of nurses is a mixture of formal classroom teaching and clinical (bedside) instruction, is assessed by examinations, and is sanctioned by professional licensure. The specialized branches of nursing include intensive care nursing, pediatric nursing, maternal care (nurse-midwifery), and PUBLIC HEALTH NURSING.

nurse aide A nursing assistant, less qualified and trained than a nurse, but capable of providing simple nursing care, such as bed-baths.

nurse practitioner A health worker whose basic training is in nursing with additional training in clinical sciences that provides skills, including the ability to make basic diagnostic and therapeutic decisions; usually deployed in the community rather than in a hospital, to provide primary medical care that supplements and complements the care provided by family physicians. See also PHYSICIAN ASSISTANT.

nursing care Care, especially by nurses at the bedside of sick people. The modern nursing profession was established by the English woman FLORENCE NIGHTINGALE (1820–1910) first at the hospital of Scutari during the Crimean War, then in a formal training program at St. Thomas's Hospital in London. Nursing care focuses on the comfort of the patient, as well as meeting medical care needs as prescribed by the attending physician.

nursing home A residential facility for convalescent and/or long-term medical and nursing care, rather than acute, short-term care. Nursing homes provide accommodation and nursing care for patients convalescing from surgery or an acute illness, or provide long-term, even lifelong care for people with a wide range of physical or mental impairments, disabilities, and handicaps. There are many variations. At one extreme are well-financed facilities with a competent professional staff of nurses, nutritional advisers, physiotherapists, and visiting or attending physicians. Such facilities are often quite large and may be supported by insurance, charitable or private funds, or patients' charges for room and board. At the other extreme are small, inadequately staffed residences that may not even be in compliance with local regulations on quality standards. Regular inspection is a responsibility of local public health departments in many jurisdictions, and in some there are procedures for accreditation. In the United States, Medicare provides some support for nursing home care under certain conditions.

nutriceutical An invented portmanteau word combining "nutrient" and "pharmaceutical" to describe an enriched food preparation that is said to be pharmacologically active in some way. Examples include enriched protein foods and "muscle-building" foods containing steroids that have mostly been banned by sporting bodies such as the International Olympic Committee.

nutrient A substance that provides nourishment. Approximately 30 to 40 constituents of foods are classified as nutrients, and many other biologically active constituents are under investigation for their possible association with chronic diseases.

nutrient cycle The circulation of energy in nature in which cellulose from plants is converted into carbohydrates, and through the many phases of the FOOD CHAIN passes on through predators, and ultimately to the omnivorous animals at the top of the food chain.

nutrient medium A liquid or gelatin-based mixture of glucose or other sugars, protein, etc., in which micro-organisms can be cultured for diagnostic or identification purposes.

nutrition The field of science and technology that deals with the process by which an organism assimilates, digests, and uses food and liquids for normal function, growth, and development. Nutrition is concerned with the energy value (calories) and the content of carbohydrate, protein, fat, minerals, and vitamins in food items. Nutrition science also studies how nutritional intake relates to growth, development, and physiological function. Also included is the idea of an optimal balance of nutrients and whole foods, to enable the optimal performance of the body. This is an essential basic and applied science of public health practice.

nutritional assessment An assessment of nutritional needs in relation to age, sex, physiological status, height, and weight. A rational approach is to consider the observed BODY MASS INDEX in relation to the ideal or desired body mass index for that individual. Nutritional intake can then be prescribed rationally to achieve the ideal or desired body mass index. Wasting, stunting, weight for height, and height for age are convenient indicators in malnourished populations. In low-income countries—or anywhere during periods of scarcity—nutritional assessment can be used to target food relief programs.

nutritionist A health professional trained in nutrition science and practice.

nystagmus A rapid flickering or oscillatory movement of eye muscles, usually associated with inability to focus and indicative of impaired eyesight, e.g., miner's nystagmus, an occupational disease of underground miners.

O

O antigen 1. An antigen used to identify the serological classification of enteric bacteria, such as shigella, proteus, and some other organisms, such as rickettsia. 2. In blood typing, the absence of antigens for A or B blood groups.

obesity The presence of excessive body fat or adipose tissue in relation to lean body mass. The distribution and amount of body fat and the extent of ADIPOSITY are both clinically relevant, but precise measurement can be difficult. Measures of weight relative to height and a BODY MASS INDEX (BMI) above 30 are used to define clinical obesity, but some athletes with a lean body mass have a BMI above 30. Obesity is more loosely defined as being overweight in relation to height, age, and sex by two standard deviations or more above the mean in relation to data in national sample surveys. These vary with economic conditions, changing concepts of what constitutes a "healthy" diet, and especially in young females, what is fashionable. The changing shape of the "ideal" female form as portrayed in sculptures and paintings through the centuries makes clear that "ideal" standards and social values have varied, although the reasons for this are obscure. Increasingly prevalent obesity is a major public health problem in high- and middle-income nations, attributable to excess caloric intake and inadequate physical exercise. It is a risk factor for non-insulin-dependent diabetes and coronary heart disease. See also ADIPOSITY, OVERWEIGHT, PONDERAL INDEX, and QUETELET'S INDEX. A useful Web site with information about causes, prevention, and treatment is http://www.cdc.gov/nccdphp/dnpa/obesity/.

OB/GYN A common abbreviation for the medical specialty of obstetrics and gynecology.

objective A precise detailed statement of the aims toward which efforts are directed. The objectives of a program or service may be arranged in general or specific terms or hierarchically. See also TARGET for discussion of the distinctions between GOAL, objective, and target.

objectivity Syn: impartiality. The capacity to consider and decide among all points of view in issues and situations where alternatives exist. This is one of the criteria to be considered in resolving ethical problems in which EQUITY or JUSTICE is an issue.

obligate parasite An organism that cannot survive independently of a host species. Some pathogenic organisms, including the smallpox and poliomyelitis viruses, are obligate parasites.

observational study Any of several varieties of nonexperimental scientific investigation in which the investigator relies on direct or indirect observation of a situation or behavior, for example a NATURAL EXPERIMENT or an epidemiological study such as a CASE CONTROL or COHORT STUDY. There is only observation without intervention, and there is no EXPERIMENT in which an investigator manipulates or modifies conditions in some way.

observer bias The tendency of an observer to "see what is expected or wanted" rather than what is actually there. A common occurrence in everyday life and a problem sometimes encountered in science. Observer bias includes OBSERVER ERROR, which can be due to faulty instrumentation, as well as faulty interpretation of responses to interviews or self-administered questionnaires, but use of the word "bias" in this context implies existence of conscious or unconscious prejudice.

observer error An error of observation or measurement due to failure of the observer to identify, measure accurately, or interpret some aspect of the phenomena that are being observed. This can have many reasons and causes, including careless or hasty measurements, faulty instruments, erroneous or illogical interpretation, and/or any of many possible sources of BIAS. It erodes the credibility of science when it occurs.

observer variation This common phenomenon is not necessarily either OBSERVER ERROR or BIAS. There are two varieties. INTEROBSERVER VARIATION occurs when two or more observers observe the same phenomenon or situation and arrive at different conclusions. Examples include grading essay-type examination papers; assessing psychological symptoms; palpating tumors; and interpreting x-rays, notably chest x-rays where varying interpretation has been studied in detail, blood films, electrocardiograms, and almost every other kind of observational assessment in clinical medicine. Commonly no two experts agree completely on what they observe and how to interpret it. INTRAOBSERVER VARIATION occurs when the same observer repeats an observation, measurement, or assessment, especially of a complex phenomenon that is observed again after an interval during which other unrelated observations have been made or other tasks performed. The subsequent observation may lead to a conclusion that differs from the original one.

obsession A persistent, often troubling thought, or a ritualistic habitual behavior pattern that may or may not be rational. Obsessions can be productive but are frequently harmful to the affected individual and/or to others with whom that individual interacts.

obsessive compulsive disorder An anxiety disorder that affects 1% to 2% of the population, characterized by repetitive ritualized actions and disturbing thoughts about consequences of actions or departures from ritualized behavior. The condition is popularly believed to be compatible with normal life, but it is dysfunctional. It responds to anxiolytic drugs or behavior therapy.

obstetric care A specialized branch of health care provided by physicians, midwives, nurses, dietitians, and others that if properly conducted emphasizes health promotion and prevention of disease and complications during the process of pregnancy, labor, delivery, and PERINATAL CARE of mother and the newborn. An important aim of obstetric care is recognition of and effective management, including timely interventions, for high-risk pregnancies.

obstetrics The medical specialty concerned with the care of pregnant women, the management of their labor and delivery of infants, and their care during the postpartum period. Obstetrics should emphasize health promotion and prevention of untoward events in pregnancy, delivery, and the puerperal period, while also providing effective treatment of incidental diseases that may occur, so these, too, are the purview of obstetricians, and of general practitioners and others who supervise the conduct of labor, childbirth, and the puerperium. The high technology deployed in modern obstetrics practice may sometimes excessively "medicalize" labor and childbirth.

Occam's razor Syn: the principle of scientific parsimony. An important principle in logic and scientific reasoning, enunciated by the 14th century philosopher William of Occam. In his words, *Essentia non sunt multiplicanda praeter necessitatem*; i.e., the number of axioms or assumptions required to establish a truth or explain a phenomenon should be kept to the minimum possible.

occupancy rate The proportion or percentage of facilities in use, for instance, of hospital or other health care institutional beds or apartment units in a multiple-occupancy dwelling.

occupation The work that people do; the activity that fills most waking hours, and, for those who work for a financial or equivalent reward, a description of the nature of this activity. Occupation is a sociological criterion interrelated to the position of individuals in society and an important determinant of income and health. See also OCCUPATIONAL CLASSIFICATION.

occupational asthma Symptoms of wheezing, coughing, shortness of breath resembling those of asthma, attributable to occupational exposure to allergens that cause true asthma, or to dusts, fumes, or suspended atmospheric particles. Some types, for instance BYSSINOSIS, begin as a form of occupational asthma, but if untreated progress to chronic obstructive lung disease.

occupational classification An orderly way to arrange people into categories according to the nature of the work that they do. The simplest way to do this is to categorize two groups of occupations: manual and nonmanual (white-collar and blue-collar occupations). The British REGISTRAR GENERAL'S OCCUPATIONAL CLASSIFICATION, first used in 1910, recognized five broad occupational groups that equated approximately to SOCIAL CLASS. In the United States, the STANDARD OCCUPATIONAL CLASSIFICATION (SOC) lists 23 categories and more than 800 types of work. See http://www.bls.gov/soc/home.htm for an account of this.

occupational deafness A consequence of exposure of the sensitive end organs of hearing in the cochlea to very loud or high-intensity sound. Gunnery officers and workers in some occupations, including underground mining, blasting, metal foundry work, and popular music entertainment, are vulnerable. The popularity of personal sound systems and use of loud amplifiers in car radio receivers has led to occupational deafness of recreational origin among young people.

occupational diseases Disease that can be demonstrated to be attributable to an agent that was encountered in the workplace, such as a chemical toxin present in the workplace environment. Such diseases and the agents that cause them can be classified as occupational in origin, and in many industrial nations some are notifiable to relevant health protection agencies, and the costs of treating them are covered by workers' compensation insurance. Notifiable occupational diseases vary with the jurisdiction. Lead poisoning, coal worker's pneumoconiosis, asbestos disease, and certain varieties of cancer are notifiable in some jurisdictions.

occupational exposure assessment The process of determining whether workplace conditions are safe or harmful to health. In practice, this ranges from perfunctory review of workplace ambient temperature and humidity to detailed air quality studies, assessment of environmental contaminants, monitoring radiation exposure and dust and noise levels, etc., and periodic medical examination of workers exposed to toxic substances such as lead and PCBs. This may involve measurement of the body burden of contaminants by chemical analyses of blood, urine, and hair samples and genetic studies, sometimes repeated at specified intervals.

occupational hazards A general term covering all workplace hazards, i.e., attributable to all forms of environmental contamination and physical, ergonomic, psychological, and social stress.

occupational health/medicine The specialized branch of medicine, other health professions, and public health practice concerned with the health of workers, provision of healthy conditions in workplaces, and diseases related to occupational exposures. It has many aspects, including studies of the occupational environment; monitoring of working conditions and workers' health; identifying, preventing, and treating work-related diseases and injuries; and ensuring that workers are fit to carry out the tasks expected in specific occupations. An important aspect is identification, prevention, and control of chronic life-threatening diseases of occupational origin, such as cancer, chronic respiratory disease, and renal or hepatic failure. The "workplace environment" may include dwellings adjoining the workplace that may be affected by workplace conditions, as with exposure to asbestos, beryllium, and toxic emissions from factory smelter stacks. Specialists in this field require psychological skills because of the increasing importance and relevance of psychological problems in the working environment, and political skills because an important part of their work can include negotiations between labor and management about relationships between working conditions and health. Occupational and environmental medicine is a medical specialty of the American Board of Medical Specialists. See http://www.acoem.org/ for details. The British equivalent is the Faculty of Occupational Medicine of the UK Royal Colleges of Physicians; see http://www.facoccmed.ac.uk/. See also TOXICOLOGY and INDUSTRIAL HYGIENE.

occupational history An essential feature of every complete clinical assessment of healthy and sick individuals. This usually stops with the answer to a question about current work, but a truly comprehensive occupational history includes questions about past occupations, housework, and hobbies that might expose individuals to toxic substances or noxious conditions.

occupational hygiene See OCCUPATIONAL HEALTH/ MEDICINE and ENVIRONMENTAL HEALTH.

occupational safety and health The value of safety in the workplace is widely accepted. It has been an evolving concept since the earliest days of the industrial revolution, when public outrage at such practices as child labor and unsafe, unhealthy workplace conditions led to progressively more rigorous requirements, including prohibition of child labor, standards for ventilation and lighting in the workplace, protective clothing and equipment, and medical fitness for and permissible length of time at tasks where the safety of others, as well as the worker, is at stake.

Occupational Safety and Health Administration (OSHA) The US agency, within the US Department of Labor, that sets and enforces regulations to safeguard the safety and health of workers. The regulations include specific rules, recommendations, and guidelines about SAFETY STANDARDS and exposure limits for toxic substances, established by empirical observation and/or experimental animal studies. See http://www.osha.gov/ for details.

occupational stress This term usually is applied to the psychological tension that can occur in working environments, e.g., between senior management staff and industrial or office workers under their control and/or among workers competing for promotion or a bonus. Such "stress diseases" as peptic ulcer, hypertension, and skin eruptions are often attributed to this cause.

occupational therapist A relatively new profession focusing on ways to ensure integration of impaired, disabled, and handicapped persons into domestic and social as well as occupational settings where they can live as fulfilling a life as possible. Occupational therapists' training includes a wide range of skills, in aspects of physiotherapy, physiatry, ergonomics, biomechanics, applied psychology, sociology, etc.

occupational therapy A range of activities that has been a feature of long-stay hospitals for more than 100 years, occupation therapy consists of engaging hospital inpatients in some form of work. In the era of tuberculosis sanatoriums (early to mid-20th century) and in custodial mental hospitals, it mostly consisted of physical work making articles of light domestic furniture to distract patients and to provide pocket money. Occupational therapy as a formal feature of rehabilitation of patients with serious injuries became integral to orthopedic care during World War II. This is aimed mainly at re-education of muscles and joints but includes much else, notably social and psychological reintegration, vocational guidance, and, if necessary, retraining to prepare for new careers. Therefore, modern specialists in occupational therapy require a wide range of skills.

occurrence A word that can be used when the distinction is not clear between the incidence and prevalence and there is no defined time dimension of a condition being observed in a population.

octane rating Octane is the antiknock rating of petroleum fuels, i.e., an indicator of the efficiency of combustion. Pure iso-octane has a rating of 100, and commercially marketed gasoline is rated as a percentage of this. The harmful effects of gasoline sniffing increase with the octane rating, especially in places where tetra-ethyl lead additive, a powerful neurotoxin, is still used.

odds The statistical calculation of the number of events as a fraction of nonevents or as a fraction of all that are theoretically possible. For instance, in the roll of a six-sided die, the odds that a specific number will roll to the top are 1 in 6.

odds ratio Syn: cross-products ratio. Strictly speaking, the ratio of two odds, but as used in the analysis of data from a case control study, a simple calculation that yields an approximate value for the RELATIVE RISK of the exposure that has been examined in a CASE CONTROL STUDY. The odds ratio is best explained in a simple table.

	Exposed	Not exposed
Disease	a	b
No disease	c	d

The odds ratio is ad/bc. The odds ratio yields an approximation of relative risk that is valid for rare and uncommon diseases but not for diseases with an incidence rate greater than about 1/100.

odor A pervasive and usually unpleasant smell, sometimes one that falls in the category of a public health nuisance that can be dealt with under abatement regulations.

odorizer A substance with a powerful odor that overwhelms sensory input from other sources and is added to odorless dangerous toxic gases and volatile substances in order to warn those in the immediate environment of the presence of the dangerous substance. The device that adds this warning substance is also called an odorizer.

Oedipus complex In psychoanalytic theory, emotional attachment of a child to the parent of the opposite sex and antipathy to the parent of the same sex, said to occur roughly in the period from 3 to 7 years of age. An aberrant Oedipus complex is said to play a role in the etiology of NEUROSIS and some psychotic conditions, but evidence is tenuous; the concept is discredited. In the Greek myth, Oedipus killed his father and married his mother, a drama described in the trilogy of plays by Sophocles (c. 496–406 BCE).

offensive trade An official designation used in some countries to describe an industry or trade that damages the health and/or economic interests of significant numbers of people in the neighborhood or environment of that industry. The term is usually applied to an industry that produces unpleasant odors, such as a tannery or rendering plant, which in many jurisdictions is subject to public health regulations dealing with abatement of nuisances.

off-gassing The phenomenon observed when pressure is reduced on a liquid or solid substance in which gases are dissolved or absorbed, releasing the gas into the environment. When the gas is toxic, irritant, or flammable (e.g., methane in a coal mine) the consequences can be dangerous or catastrophic for anyone in the environment. The term also describes emissions of volatile organic hydrocarbons, such as formaldehyde. from carpet adhesives, building materials, etc.

Office for Human Research Protections The division of the US Department of Health and Human Services that is responsible for ensuring the maintenance and enforcement of rules and regulations that govern the ethical and legal conduct of research involving human subjects. See http://www.hhs.gov/ohrp/.

Office for National Statistics The UK government agency responsible for collecting, collating, analyzing, and disseminating statistics on demography and on vital events and health. It has replaced the former Office of Population, Census and Surveys and incorporates the General Register Office, which collects and collates information on registered births, marriages and divorces, and deaths. Its activities are shown at http://www.statistics.gov.uk/ and in divisions such as the former General Register Office, at http://www.gro.gov.uk/gro/content/.

Office of Alternative Medicine See NATIONAL CENTER FOR COMPLEMENTARY AND ALTERNATIVE MEDICINE (NCCAM).

Office of Disease Prevention and Health Promotion (ODPHP) The division of the US Office of Public Health and Science that has sponsored programs and initiatives in collaboration with professional academies and colleges in the health-related specialties, such as the work of the US PREVENTIVE

SERVICES TASK FORCE on screening and early detection protocols. This office also developed the 10-year health goals for the United States defined and discussed in *Healthy People 2000, Healthy People 2010*, etc. See http://odphp.osophs.dhhs.gov/.

Office of Homeland Security An influential agency of the US administration established after the terrorist attacks on New York and Washington in 2001, responsible for surveillance of persons and places regarded as potential security risks and for implementing measures aimed at preventing terrorism, including public health measures such as control of BIOTERRORISM. The agency has the difficult balancing act of ensuring public safety without infringing on human and civil rights. For details, see http://www.whitehouse.gov/homeland/.

Office of Public Health and Science The agency of the US DEPARTMENT OF HEALTH AND HUMAN SERVICES that includes many important divisions, e.g., the Office of the Surgeon General, Office of HIV/AIDS Policy, Office for Human Research Protections, Office of Research Integrity, Office of Minority Health, President's Council on Physical Fitness and Sports, and a number of others. For details and programs, see http://www.osophs.dhhs.gov/ophs/.

Office of Technology Assessment (OTA) The agency established by the US Congress in 1972 that existed until 1995 to assess existing and new technologies in all sectors and fields of activity. The OTA reviewed many technologies related to activities in the health sector, made recommendations, and published reports to assist decision making by health administrators. Other nations have similar government and private sector agencies. In the Netherlands, valuable work has been done on possible future technology developments as well as existing ones. Many other industrial nations have similar government agencies. The archives of the US Congressional Office of Technology Assessment are at http://www.access.gpo.gov/ota/.

office visit The technical term used for administrative and billing purposes for an encounter between a patient and a physician or other provider of health care services that occurs in the physician's consulting rooms ("surgery" in British terminology) or in a clinic or office. An encounter in a hospital is a HOSPITAL VISIT, and one in the patient's home is a house call or domiciliary visit when the details appear on claims for medical insurance benefits.

official statistics The statistics compiled and maintained by agencies of the nation, state, or local municipal authorities. These include economic and fiscal data, and VITAL STATISTICS, which deal with data on births, marriages, deaths, divorces and marital separations, as well as statistical data on activities in other sectors of society, such as the health, education, transport, and energy sectors. All usually appear in summary form in an annual yearbook or equivalent, as well as in greater detail in many specialized volumes, including those on vital and health statistics. In many nations, they are available on government Web sites. See, for example, http://www.cdc.gov/nchs.

oil 1. Petroleum oil is a viscous liquid hydrocarbon that has been the principal carbon-based fuel used worldwide for more than 100 years. It occurs in deposits in many parts of the world and is transported in pipelines and shipped in bulk tankers from the sites of deposits to refineries and markets in other countries. Petroleum oil and its many refined derivatives contain diverse toxic substances, but the benefits of an efficient, albeit polluting, fuel and its by-products are regarded in the 20th and 21st century petroleum-based industrial economies as more worthwhile than the harms they can cause. Combustion of oil in any form generates emissions of greenhouse gases and frequently atmospheric pollutants and smog. 2. Vegetable and animal oils, used in cooking, are triglyceride esters of fatty acids.

oil acne An unsightly folliculitis caused by prolonged exposure of the skin to petroleum oil, which blocks hair follicles, leading to inflammation and formation of pustules.

oil dispersants Chemicals that reduce surface tension between oil and water, used to help break up large aggregations of spilled oil that occur when heavily laden oil tankers encounter severe storms or suffer navigation errors, causing maritime disasters. The efficacy of dispersants is maximum with light oils that often disperse on their own, and some dispersants are toxic to birds, marine, and shore life.

oil spills Transporting huge quantities of petroleum fuel in supertankers that carry 100,000 tonnes over stormy seas and negotiating dangerous reefs and shoals inevitably has led to several massive oil spills that have caused great ecological damage. Even small spills can be harmful to fragile ecosystems. Evidence of direct harm to human health is more elusive, but some very large oil spills have been associated with symptoms of respiratory and gastrointestinal distress and vague transitory neurological symptoms among persons in the vicinity. However, the main effects on human health are indirect: disruption of commercial fisheries, oyster beds, etc.

old age An ill-defined age epoch for which euphemisms include retired persons, senior citizens, third age, and golden age. Vital statistics classify age-specific events in 10-year or larger categories,

commonly 0 to 14 years, 15 to 44 years, 45 to 64 years, and 65+ years, and in this system, 65+ years is old age. Some geriatricians classify patients into groups each of roughly a decade, in which the "young" old are persons as old as 65 to 70 years who are physically active, mentally alert, and either recently retired or still working; an intermediate group, aged 65 to 74 years, more often have minor impairments and/or disabilities requiring some medication and ongoing medical care; an older group is aged 75 to 84 years; and the final category, the OLDEST OLD, are those 85 years of age and older, a majority of whom have become or are becoming dependent on others for assistance with activities required for daily living. See also GERIATRICS and GERONTOLOGY.

old age assistance A tax-supported public assistance program for old people, i.e., retired, old age pensioners, etc., whose financial needs exceed their resources. In the United States it is administered by the states under the terms of Social Security legislation. Other Organization for Economic Cooperation and Development (OECD) nations have similar programs, many of which are more comprehensive and generous than those of the United States. See also SOCIAL SECURITY.

oldest old Loosely defined as those aged 85 years of age and older, many of whom have become dependent on others for assistance with activities of daily living (feeding, washing, bathing, dressing, shopping, etc.). Visual and hearing loss are common, and so is deterioration of mental function.

olestra A patented proprietary preparation of sucrose polyester, a synthetic fat substitute that is approved as a dietary ingredient in the United States. It resembles fat in appearance and taste but it is not digested or metabolized, so foods containing it can be consumed without contributing to obesity. Concerns about possible adverse effects have led several countries, including Canada, to refuse to license it as a food additive or substitute.

Omsk hemorrhagic fever A tick-borne viral hemorrhagic fever caused by a flavivirus that is prevalent in western Siberia, first described by physicians in Omsk, Russia. A similar or identical disease occurs elsewhere, for instance, in Kyasanur Forest in India.

onchocerciasis Syn: river blindness. A chronic filarial worm infection transmitted by the bite of a blackfly, *Simulium damnosum*, that is prevalent in rivers and streams in parts of Sub-Saharan Africa. The worm was introduced to Central America in African slaves, and the condition occurs in tropical regions of Mexico and Guatemala. The worm causes fibrous nodules in dermal tissue that ulcerate, allowing female worms to discharge microfilariae; it often invades the eyeballs, where it destroys the vitreous and aqueous, causing irreversible blindness. An elimination program sponsored by the World Bank, FAO, WHO, and UNDP is based on environmental vector control and use of larvicides to block transmission of microfilariae. Facts about the condition are available at http://www.cdc.gov/ncidod/dpd/parasites/onchocerciasis/default.htm and at http://www.who.int/tdr/diseases/oncho/default.htm.

oncogene A gene that normally directs cell growth. If altered, as by ionizing radiation or certain chemicals, some oncogenes can allow uncontrolled growth of cancer. Alterations can also be inherited. See http://ghr.nlm.nih.gov/ghr/glossary/oncogene.

oncologist A specialist, usually a physician, who cares for persons with malignant neoplastic conditions and may do research on aspects of cancer.

oncology The clinical specialty and scientific study of all aspects of malignant neoplasms, especially their pathogenesis, causes, prevention, and treatment.

one-tailed distribution A sequence of values of a variable extending from low to high with no diminishing values beyond the highest.

online A word for electronic communication between a computer and another at a remote location, which has become an inseparable component of modern commerce, industry, and all professional activities. Local health departments have online access to almost unlimited intellectual resources, as well as the ability to send and receive important health-related data and information virtually instantaneously, e.g., about relevant epidemic outbreaks elsewhere.

oocyst A cyst about 50 to 60 microns in diameter on the wall of the female anopheline mosquito's stomach that develops from the zygote of the PLASMODIUM (malaria parasite). The oocyst grows, and its contents divide to form SPOROZOITES, which are released into the body cavity of the mosquito when the oocyst bursts, then migrate to the mouth parts to be injected into a human host when the mosquito takes its next blood meal.

oocyte A cell from which an ovum develops in humans each month during a woman's reproductively active lifetime.

opacity The shadow of a substance or structure that obstructs the passage of visible light or electromagnetic radiation. The term is often applied to the appearance of a chest x-ray film in which an abnormal solid lesion is observed to be more dense than surrounding tissue.

opacity rating A measure of the quality and clarity of emissions from factory chimney stacks and coal- or oil-burning electric power-generating plants. Direct observation with a meter allows this rating to be recorded and reported on a numerical scale, called the RINGELMANN NUMBER.

open pit mining Also known as open cast or open cut mining. A method of extracting minerals in which the overburden of soil is removed to expose the mineral-bearing strata. This is safer than underground mining but disfigures the environment in ways that are sometimes difficult to repair.

open population A demographic term for a population that gains members by immigration and loses them by emigration, as well as gaining and losing by births and deaths, in contrast to a CLOSED POPULATION, which has no gains or losses attributable to migration.

open source Describes documents and computer programs that are in the public domain, accessible to all.

operating room Syn: operating theater (Britain). The location in a hospital where most surgical procedures are conducted. In modern hospitals, there is usually a suite of operating rooms in a secure area, with features that include positive air pressure to exclude airborne particles from other parts of the hospital, rigorous requirements for complete removal or covering of outdoor clothing, and a separate area for sterilizing surgical instruments and for scrubbing by operating personnel in preparation for surgery. These and other actions minimize the risk of infection, but despite all precautions infections still occur from infected wounds, endoscopies, or breakdown of aseptic procedures.

operational definition A definition that is used for convenience during the conduct of a study. It is intended to be practical and workable under the conditions of the study, although it may or may not be a legally or scientifically valid definition. For instance, an operational definition of a single-parent, mother-led family is operationally useful but may differ from a legal definition of the same family status.

operational research The systematic study of the way in which organizations function. This may be done by direct observation, a combination of observation and experiment, or statistical analysis of data from various aspects of the organization(s) under study. One form of operational research focuses on ways to improve performance, of both individuals and groups, and of their work setting and equipment. Other aspects deal with specific applications, e.g., in HEALTH SERVICES RESEARCH, where the aims include enhancing efficiency and reducing costs.

opiate A class of drugs containing opium or its derivatives. They are narcotic, often analgesic, often medically valuable, sometimes addictive, and sometimes illegal. They include opium, morphine, heroin, methadone, and codeine.

opinion leader An individual who helps to shape or set public opinion by virtue of prominence in public life, whether in a religious setting, politics, business or commerce, the mass media, the performing arts, or elsewhere. Opinion leaders may influence society and current affairs and events for good or ill, according to the nature of the message they seek to convey or the behavior they demonstrate for others to imitate. The words and actions of opinion leaders sometimes significantly affect public health, for instance, when media stars exhibit high-risk behavior.

opinion survey A survey by questionnaire or interview in which the opinions of selected persons are solicited. Such surveys vary greatly in quality and content. Market researchers, political pollsters, and media pundits conduct opinion surveys to inquire about everything from preferences for brands of breakfast cereals to the likelihood of the next world war. These frequently depart from accepted scientific methods of sampling, question design, and rigorous analysis of results and often are designed to solicit the opinions the survey designer wants to receive. Methodologically rigorous opinion surveys require skill and care in question selection, sequencing and design, the use of features such as the LIKERT SCALE, and the use of samples selected by random allocation. Examples of valid opinion surveys include family planning studies and the questionnaire-based portions of studies conducted by the National Center for Health Statistics, such as National Health and Nutrition Examination Survey (NHANES).

opium The active ingredient in the dried juice of certain species of poppy, comprising alkaloids with a bitter taste and characteristic sweet smell. Whether inhaled as smoke from combusted opium, ingested, or injected, the alkaloids have a powerful narcotic action. Both morphine and heroin are purified alkaloids of opium. These, especially morphine, are used medicinally, and in a lucrative illicit trade are estimated to generate several billion dollars annually for criminal cartels.

opportunistic infection An infection that occurs because the pathogenic organism(s) causing it have an opportunity to invade a susceptible host, usually when the host's immune system has been compromised by HIV infection, the use of immunosuppressive medication or radiation, or other factors, such as debility associated with advanced old age. Common opportunistic infections include mycoses such as *Candida albicans* and organisms such as *Pneumocystis carinii*. Latent tuberculosis can be reactivated by opportunistic infection.

opportunity cost The value of goods or services that could have been obtained for the same cost as that which has been expended on the provision of the specific goods/services for which the opportunity cost is being computed. For instance, the opportunity cost of facilities for intensive care of acute respiratory disease could include the cost of immunizations and other preventive measures aimed at preventing acute respiratory disease requiring intensive care.

oral contraceptive A medication that will prevent conception and that can be taken by mouth. The best known and most widely used is the oral contraceptive (OC) pill, a progesterone-estrogen combination colloquially known as "the pill" that has been used by millions of women worldwide since the 1950s. The American physician Gregory Pincus (1903–1967) led the team that developed and field-tested the contraceptive. Most women tolerate the OC pill without adverse or side effects, but a few experience menstrual irregularities. Thromboembolic events, including coronary thrombosis, retinal arterial thrombosis, venous thrombosis, and stroke, are rare complications. A potential oral contraceptive for men derived from an herb, GOSSYPOL, has been used with some success in China but has serious side effects. See also MORNING-AFTER PILL.

oral health Syn: stomatology. The aspect of health care that focuses on the condition of the teeth, gums, tongue, buccal mucosa, palate, and the upper pharyngeal region. Diseases that can occur in this region include inflammatory and neoplastic conditions, dental caries, post-traumatic lesions, etc. Dentists and family physicians are most often engaged in dealing with problems of oral health and dental hygienists and school nurses in preserving and protecting oral health.

oral hygiene Teeth cleaning and care of the gums, tongue, and mouth parts aimed at promoting a wholesome and pleasing appearance, freedom from unpleasant breath odors, and reducing the risk of dental caries. Cosmetic advantages are usually stressed because vanity makes this desirable, but the real benefit is improved dental and oral health. Dental hygiene is a specific aspect, for example, in New Zealand, where evaluation showed that dental hygienists significantly improved dental health.

oral rehydration therapy (ORT) A simple and effective way to replace fluid when infants have severe fluid and electrolyte loss due to diarrhea. It was invented in the 1960s and introduced in Asia and Africa by WHO, UNICEF, and other organizations and nongovernmental organizations. Some of these prepare and distribute a "dry pack," which reconstitutes with water to provide fluid, sodium, potassium, and glucose in biochemically appropriate amounts. The mixture contains 2.6 grams of sodium chloride, 2.5 grams of sodium bicarbonate, 1.5 grams of potassium chloride, and 213.5 grams of glucose in 1 liter of boiled fresh water. Oral rehydration fluid without potassium can be prepared at home with 1/2 teaspoonfuls of salt (3.5 grams) and 4 soup spoons of sugar (40 grams) per liter of freshly boiled water. This can be prepared and used easily by untrained parents of sick infants, and is life saving. Oral rehydration therapy is also used for adults, for instance in cases of cholera, and in many other conditions associated with dehydration. Oral rehydration therapy usually includes use of the supplement plus continued feeding (and breast feeding in the case of infants).

oral sex Stimulation of the external genitalia by the mouth and tongue of the sexual partner. This exposes sexual partners to each other's body fluids (semen, vaginal secretions, perhaps blood) and therefore risks transmission of sexually transmitted diseases, including HIV/AIDS, especially if there are open lesions in the mouth. It has become popular among adolescents in some contemporary Western societies and in this segment of the population it is sometimes not considered sexual intercourse, although it is a way to transmit sexually transmitted diseases.

order In TAXONOMY, an order is the division below class, and in turn is divided into families.

orderly A semiskilled worker in a hospital, responsible for conveying patients on stretchers or gurneys and other heavy manual nursing tasks. They may be trained in other tasks, such as applying and removing casts for limb fractures.

ordinal scale A system of classification into ordered categories, e.g., a socioeconomic grouping according to income and/or educational level. Contrast NOMINAL SCALE.

ordinance A law or regulation, commonly one enacted by a local or regional government.

ordinate The linear dimension of the vertical axis on a GRAPH.

orf A virus disease of sheep, goats, and wild ungulates, occasionally transmitted to humans who are in contact with infected animals. It causes indolent pustular lesions and is most serious if it affects the eyes.

organ donation The surgical procedure of transplanting vital organs into a recipient whose own organs are defective or have ceased to function as a result of disease. Transplantation of corneas from recently deceased donors was developed in the 1940s. Advances in immunology have made organ donation possible since the early 1960s, beginning with kidneys, then the heart, liver, lungs, pancreas, and segments of intestine. The donor of single vital organs, such as the heart, must of course be deceased, but one of a set of paired organs, typically kidneys, or part of a single organ, such as the liver, can come from a live donor. Essential steps in organ donation include ensuring an immunologically compatible match and the assurance that no life-threatening disease agent, such as HIV or prions of variant Creutzfeldt-Jakob disease, is transmitted to the recipient. Informed consent and speed in transfer of the donated organ or tissue are other requisites. In some low-income countries, an unconscionable trade has arisen to sell organs to surgeons and their patients in wealthy countries.

organic content The biologically derived component of sewage and other domestic waste that is of human or microbial origin, as assessed by tests, e.g., for volatile solids.

organic dusts Dusts of vegetable and sometimes animal origin, or with a large content thereof. Some organic dusts are highly allergenic and are capable of inducing or aggravating asthma, hay fever, and urticaria.

organic food All food is organic in origin. This term is applied to foods grown without using chemical fertilizers or pesticides, and/or not containing preservatives or genetically modified ingredients, such as in "organic" crops, foods, etc. These are said to be environmentally friendly and less likely to induce or help to determine human disease. However, there is no objective evaluation of these assertions, and the cost of organic foods is usually higher than that of comparable foods that are not labeled as "organic."

organic lead compounds Compounds of organic chemicals with lead include several of economic importance, e.g., alkyl compounds, tetra-ethyl, and tetramethyl lead. Like all lead compounds they are toxic, causing neurological and renal damage that can be permanent.

organic solvents A general term for any solvent of natural or synthetic organic origin. They are used as paint removers, degreasing agents, vehicles for glue and other adhesives, etc. These are volatile solvents, and some of them are highly toxic. Several are used as addictive inhalant substances, and these can cause brain damage and sometimes acute nephrotoxicity.

Organisation Mondial de la Santé (OMS) French for WORLD HEALTH ORGANIZATION.

Organization for Economic Cooperation and Development (OECD) An international agency based in Paris. Its members are 30 industrial nations. It aims to advance economic development in its own member states and in the less developed nations; to conduct studies of social and economic problems, such as youth unemployment; and seek solutions of these problems. For details, see http://www.oecd.org/home/.

Organization of American States (OAS) A grouping established in 1948 that includes all 35 nation states in the Western hemisphere, i.e., the Americas and the Caribbean. Its purpose is to promote social development and economic and political cooperation of the nation states of the region. It has a working relationship with the PAN AMERICAN HEALTH ORGANIZATION to deal with public health and social issues. See http://www.oas.org/.

organization theory The study of how and why organizations work or don't work. This has elements of SYSTEMS THEORY, anthropology, sociology, social psychology, and group dynamics and is an important set of concepts for public health administrators to comprehend and apply.

organochlorine compounds Several groups of hydrocarbon compounds include chlorine in their molecular structure, e.g., chloroform, carbon tetrachloride. Chlorinated hydrocarbons include DDT, hexachlorobenzene, and many others of commercial, industrial, and agricultural importance, and several are animal and/or human poisons.

organophosphate insecticides An ecologically and economically important class of chemical compounds that are acetyl cholinesterase inhibitors, i.e., inhibit neuromuscular transmission and cause death of insect pests by respiratory and autonomic system paralysis. Many, e.g., parathion, are also human poisons with effects similar to those of NERVE GASES.

ornithosis An acute generalized disease with fever, pulmonary congestion, and pneumonia caused by chlamydia and transmitted by birds, commonly parrots. See also PSITTACOSIS.

orphanage An institution for children who have no parents because their parent(s) have died or aban-

doned them and no other close relations are able to care for them. In modern societies, with well-organized social support systems, such children mostly receive FOSTER CARE, thereby avoiding the stigma of institutional custodial care and its somewhat Dickensian emotional associations from earlier generations. In Sub-Saharan Africa, millions of children have been orphaned by the death of their parents of AIDS. Some nongovernmental organizations and many informal groupings, mostly of grandparents, care for a modest proportion of these, but many are left to fend for themselves as best they can.

orphan diseases 1. Any rare disease for which no treatment has been developed. 2. Diseases for which no formal social organization or support network has been established, despite the fact that patients and their family members would find support and friendly advice helpful. Many orphan diseases are chronic, progressive, and ultimately fatal; others are chronic and recurrent. Examples include congenital deformities, some endocrine disorders, and some conditions of bones and joints.

orphan drug 1. A pharmacologically active therapeutic agent that is not chemically derived from or related to any previously known or widely used form of medication. 2. A drug that is used to treat one of the ORPHAN DISEASES. 3. A drug that may be useful in common diseases as well as rare ones, but that pharmaceutical manufacturers do not consider commercially profitable or for which the market is too small to interest profit-driven pharmaceutical manufacturers.

orthodontics The specialized branch of dentistry concerned with correcting the alignment and positioning of teeth, a protracted process in which children are treated by means of metal or plastic collars ("bands" or "braces") that are under tension and slowly move the teeth, improving their alignment. Children with bands on their teeth are a familiar sight in affluent suburban schools, and although a few may have had the procedure inflicted on them because it is fashionable or a status symbol, it can prevent the later occurrence of periodontal disease.

orthodox medicine See ALLOPATHIC MEDICINE.

orthomolecular medicine A term coined by the American molecular biologist and Nobel laureate Linus Pauling (1901–1994) to describe a regimen based on measured daily amounts of each of the essential vitamins and minerals that Pauling calculated were required to maintain the biochemical balance essential to good health. The regimen has been tried for learning disabilities, allergies, arthritis, depression, memory loss, etc. This contrasts with megavitamin therapy, another dietary regimen that Pauling also advocated for some of the same conditions. Evaluations have not provided convincing evidence for the efficacy of either therapeutic regimen or for efficacy of a specific application that Pauling called orthomolecular psychiatry, i.e., the application of this method to treat psychiatric illnesses such as schizophrenia.

orthopedics Etymology tells us this word means "straightening" or "correcting" (deformed) children, i.e., applying splints, extensions, and other devices to ameliorate or correct deformities such as a wasted limb due to nerve damage. In modern usage, the name applies to the surgical specialty that deals with fractures, dislocations, and other lesions of bones and joints, with emphasis on the aim of correcting bony deformities and minimizing residual disability.

orthopsychiatry A term used by some psychiatrists to describe the study and treatment of mental conditions known as borderline states, i.e., on the boundaries of normal-abnormal. The term also means an approach to mental health that emphasizes prevention, relying on one or more of several possible behavioral methods, including conditioning and group therapy. Others use the same word to describe orthomolecular medicine applied to psychiatric disorders.

orthoptics The specialty that deals with correction of defects of ocular muscles that cause squint and similar problems.

orthotics The science and technology of mechanical devices used to correct physical deformities, especially those associated with impaired mobility, particularly affecting the feet.

osmosis The process in colloid chemistry whereby a dilute solution becomes more concentrated as the solvent moves across a semipermeable membrane, i.e., tending to equalize the concentration on the two sides of the membrane.

osteoarthritis A degenerative age-related change in joints that often is attributable to heavy use of the affected joints, and therefore sometimes a condition associated with occupational exposure and/or attributed to the wear and tear of normal aging.

osteopathy An alternative medical system based on the capacity of the body to correct its own departures from normal, established by the American physician Andrew Still (1828–1917). Rather than using pharmaceutical preparations to treat disease, osteopathy relies on physical methods, heat and cold, massage, exercises, and manipulation and provides advice on other aspects of patients' lifestyles. Osteopathy has moved into the mainstream of medical practice in North America, although it is still regarded by many medical and public health organizations in Britain and parts of Europe as a "fringe" medical practice. Schools of osteopathic medicine in the United States undergo an accreditation process similar to that of medical schools and offer a curriculum that is essentially similar but has more emphasis on nonpharmacological methods of treatment.

osteoporosis Literally softening and reduced density of bones, due to insufficient intake or loss of calcium compounds, associated with aging, postmenopausal metabolic changes in women, and inactivity—less use of bones and joints that undergo atrophy from disuse.

Oswestry score A rating scale developed in 1980 at the Institute of Orthopaedics in Oswestry, Wales (UK), for assessment of disability associated with LOW BACK PAIN. The scale includes items on intensity of pain, self-care ability, lifting, walking, sitting, standing, sleeping, sex life, social life, and travel, each scored from 1 to 6, with highest scores indicating maximum disability.

otolaryngology The specialized branch of medical practice concerned with the prevention, diagnosis, and treatment of conditions affecting the ears, nose, throat, and larynx, often abbreviated as ENT. Variations of the specialty are otology and otorhinolaryngology.

Ottawa Charter for Health Promotion Syn: Ottawa Declaration. A statement of the principles of HEALTH PROMOTION drafted at meetings of experts from the European region of WHO with input by Canadian experts, ratified by representatives of member states of WHO at a conference in Ottawa, Canada, in 1986. The Ottawa Charter has a holistic view of the determinants of health and recognizes the importance of equity and human rights, the necessity of involving communities in priority setting and management of their environments, and people taking control of their own destiny. It sets out five action-oriented principles: build healthy public policy, create supportive environments, strengthen community action, develop personal skills, and reorient health services. The Charter stimulated the Healthy Cities and Healthy Communities movements and has had a significant influence on health policies in many nations. It can be seen at http://www.who.int/hpr/NPH/docs/ottawa_charter_hp.pdf. See also BANGKOK CHARTER.

outbreak A small localized cluster of cases of a condition, usually an infectious disease. The word is sometimes a euphemism used to downplay the seriousness of an epidemic.

outcome measures Quantifiable consequences of an action, set of actions, or procedure. In the health field, many outcome measures are used to assess and evaluate aspects of health care. A simple alliterative classification is death, disease, disability, and discomfort, which are measured by mortality and morbidity rates; functional ability; and responses to questions about pain, distress, sleeplessness, etc. Dissatisfaction with health care services is unobtrusively assessed by broken appointment rates and requests for transfer to an alternative service, but there are many confounding variables that raise questions about the validity of these measures.

outcomes All possible consequences of exposure to a risk, use of a therapeutic intervention, or the manner in which a health problem has been managed.

outcomes research Evaluative research aimed at determining the optimum therapeutic method for a condition, usually conducted by systematic comparative evaluation of the results of two or more alternative therapeutic regimens. See also OPERATIONAL RESEARCH.

outcome variable A variable with a value that varies according to the outcome of an intervention and that therefore can be used to assess or evaluate an intervention.

outdoor relief An obsolete term that was applied to the aspects of welfare assistance outside an almshouse, orphanage, or similar institute for the care of the destitute. Outdoor relief consisted of hot meals, provision of blankets for persons sleeping outdoors, etc., which remain necessary for homeless persons, although the term outdoor relief is no longer appropriate.

outgroup A sociological term for the population(s) not included in decision-making processes. Contrast INGROUP, those who participate in decision making.

outlier An observation that differs so much from the rest of the observations in a series that it appears not to belong in the same distribution. The numerical value of an outlier may differ so widely from others in a series that its inclusion can distort the entire analysis. Nevertheless, outliers should be considered for inclusion in statistical analysis of the series, or, if not, this should be clearly stated and the reasons given.

outpatient A patient who attends a hospital or clinic but does not occupy a bed.

outreach The work of staff in social and health agencies that is taken outside the office into the community, and the publicizing of available services so those who need them become aware that the services exist.

outsourcing Contracting services from a public agency such as a health department to private individuals, agencies, or corporations because the public agency responsible for the services lacks the financial resources and/or salaried staff to provide this service. Outsourcing is a common consequence of reduced budgets caused by tax cuts. It is usually more costly, less efficient, and less personal than the same services would be if they were provided by a public agency.

overcrowding Although sometimes a subjective judgment, overcrowding, which means dense occupation of living and especially of sleeping space, can be measured objectively using an index of overcrowding, such as one developed in the United Kingdom by the Office of Population, Censuses and Surveys (now the Office for National Statistics), that counts the number of persons in households at a density of greater than one per room, as a proportion of all persons in private households. Respiratory infections, including tuberculosis and childhood respiratory infections, are associated with overcrowding, which promotes dissemination of airborne pathogens. Overcrowding has adverse effects on health and educational performance of school children in Britain, where it has been extensively studied. The Web site http://www.odpm.gov.uk/stellent/groups/odpm_control/documents/contentservertemplate/odpm_index.hcst?n=4625&l=3 gives details of current British findings. In animals, as well as humans, overcrowding induces stress and increases the frequency of stress-related disorders. See also TOWNSEND SCORE.

overdose A deliberate or accidental excessive intake of medication. The term is usually applied to a drug overdose, and it may be a euphemism for an attempted suicide or a suicidal gesture by means of ingested narcotic or analgesic drugs.

overload capacity The extent to which a facility, such as a sewage treatment plant, is able to deal effectively and safely with demand in excess of the amount for which it was designed. Most well-designed facilities have inbuilt capacity in excess of the expected load, but capacity to perform safely and effectively is the criterion by which true overload capacity should be judged.

overrepresentation In sampling surveys, the deliberate selection of a larger proportion of subjects in one or more strata than in others, with specific aims, such as attempting to ensure that relatively uncommon events or conditions are not overlooked if a suspicion exists that these might occur more often in such strata than in others. In surveys, overrepresentation can help to ensure that if there is substantial loss to followup enough subjects remain to permit valid analysis.

over-the-counter drug A drug such as aspirin, laxatives, and cough suppressants that can be purchased direct from the attendant at the counter of a pharmacy, chemist's shop, or drugstore without a physician's prescription.

overview See META-ANALYSIS and SYSTEMATIC REVIEW.

overweight A body mass index (BMI) above "normal" (25) but below 30, i.e., not sufficient to be defined clinically as OBESITY. The "normal" is defined in national surveys such as NHANES.

overwintering The capability of a species to survive through cold winter seasons and to revive and resume its usual activities when warmer weather returns. The term usually applies to this capability in insects and is in some ways akin to hibernation in certain mammals but differs in that it is a complete cessation, rather than merely a slowing, of metabolic activity.

oviparous Descriptive of animals (including insects such as mosquitoes) that lay eggs.

ovulation Release of an egg, or ovum, from the ovary so it can pass down the fallopian tube to the uterus. This process happens in all oviparous animals. In women, it occurs approximately every 28 days, about 14 days after the beginning of the previous menstrual period.

OXFAM An acronym for the Oxford Committee for Famine Relief, the nongovernmental organization founded in Oxford, United Kingdom, in 1942 to cope with wartime famines. OXFAM is now a major worldwide nongovernmental organization dedicated to providing food relief, medical services, and supplies to distressed populations, whether the cause of their predicament is a natural disaster, such as drought, earthquake, or flood, or a manmade disaster, such as local or regional warfare. The activities of the original agency are at http://www.oxfam.org.uk/. OXFAM's worldwide activities can be reviewed at http://www.oxfam.org/.

oxidant A substance or chemical compound that causes OXIDATION.

oxidant smog Syn: photochemical smog. The type of smog produced by oxidation of exhaust gases from internal combustion engines, caused by the interaction of nitrogen oxides and VOLATILE ORGANIC COMPOUNDS (VOCs) with ionized solar radiation, i.e., ultraviolet radiation. This kind of smog is a serious upper respiratory irritant. If exposure is prolonged and/or frequently repeated, it can cause permanent respiratory damage.

oxidation The process of absorbing or chemical bonding with oxygen.

oxides of nitrogen Nitrogen combines with oxygen in several compounds, three of which are harmful atmospheric contaminants. Nitrous oxide, N_2O, a colorless gas, plays a role in the NITROGEN CYCLE but is not an atmospheric pollutant. Nitrogen oxide (NO) is a colorless poisonous gas that reacts with oxygen and ozone to form nitrogen dioxide, NO_2, which is a brownish toxic gas, the principal constituent of PHOTOCHEMICAL SMOG. Another compound in smog is dinitrogen tetroxide, N_2O_4. Mixtures of these toxic oxides of nitrogen are collectively called NO_x.

oxygen Syn: O_2. The element that constitutes about 20% of the earth's atmosphere and is essential to the metabolism of all air-breathing animals, such as vertebrates, and of course including humans.

ozone Syn: O_3. An isotope of oxygen in which three atoms, rather than the usual two, are bonded. It is a toxic, irritant gas. See OZONE, TROPOSPHERIC.

ozone attenuation (depletion) The biosphere's protective ionized OZONE LAYER is vulnerable to destruction by several varieties of ozone-destroying substances that convert ozone to oxygen. The best known of these are the chlorofluorocarbon compounds (CFCs) that were widely used as refrigerants, industrial solvents, and cleansing agents and were believed to be inert but decompose to chlorine monoxide, which degrades stratospheric ozone molecules to oxygen. Bromine and other halogen compounds, e.g., used as fertilizers for rice crops, have a similar action, and so do additives for supersonic aircraft fuel.

ozone layer A stratospheric region at an altitude of approximately 20 to 24 km above the earth's surface, where ionized solar radiation converts oxygen to ozone. Ozone acts as a filter that helps to reduce the intensity of short-wave ultraviolet (UV) flux that penetrates to the lower levels of the biosphere, and in this way provides protection to all living things from the potentially lethal damage that would be done if larger concentrations of UV radiation reached the earth's surface.

ozone, tropospheric Ozone forms in the lower atmosphere (troposphere) when solar radiation splits nitrogen dioxide into nitrous oxide and an oxygen radical, which combines with oxygen to form ozone. This occurs mainly in urban regions with heavy motor traffic on warm summer days with intense sunlight. It is a toxic, irritant gas, a constituent of PHOTOCHEMICAL SMOG.

P

p, P 1. The abbreviation for the estimated probability of a result equal to or more extreme than that observed in a study, usually appearing in publications together with the symbol < for "less than" and familiar to all who read articles containing statistical analyses. Conventionally, a probability of less than 1 in 20, i.e., $p < 0.05$, is considered unlikely to have occurred by chance in many situations arising in medicine, e.g., results of clinical trials. CONFIDENCE INTERVALS usually convey more information about the uncertainty attaching to an estimate than do p values, and are therefore a preferable way to express results of a study. 2. When used to refer to the probability of an adverse outcome, as in physical sciences, engineering, and many biomedical sciences, a far smaller probability, e.g., $p < 0.001$ or $p < 0.0001$ is conventionally required. For instance, in RISK rating of situations in environmental health, such as drinking water quality, a risk of less than 1 in 1,000 of infection due to water contamination is unacceptable; a risk of less than 1 in 100,000 is mandatory. Likewise for VACCINE EFFICACY AND SAFETY, the risk of serious adverse reactions should be less than 1 in 100,000. However, all such probability levels are arbitrary. Confidence intervals are often a preferable way to state results and statistical and clinical or public health significance.

PAH compounds See POLYCYCLIC AROMATIC HYDRO-CARBONS.

pain A distress signal transmitted by sensory nerves to warn that all is not well with some aspect of bodily function or structure. Pain can be caused by stimulation of exposed nerve endings, as in lacerations, abrasions, burns, toothache; buildup of pressure in a body cavity or tube that is obstructed, giving rise to reflexive smooth muscle contractions that cause abdominal, renal, and gallbladder colic; histamine and certain toxic chemicals that cause the ischemic pain of muscle cramps and myocardial infarction; stimulation of nerve endings and plexuses by inflammation or neoplastic change; and inflammation or irritation of nerve roots, as in the pain of herpes zoster.

pain and suffering A phrase that covers the non-monetary costs of illness or injury for which the victim(s) and/or family seek financial compensation. A proportion of the monetary compensation sought by plaintiffs in tort cases is almost always a financial claim for pain and suffering, which law courts attempt to estimate in dollars.

pain management Prolonged or chronic pain requires effective relief to permit patients to sleep, and the specialty of pain management has evolved to deal with this. Specialists in this field seek effective psychological measures as well as effective analgesics, and also aim to minimize the risk of addiction to strong analgesics and narcotics. It can be a difficult balancing act with decisions differing according to prognosis, for instance, more attention to total pain relief in terminally ill patients than in those with relatively short-term conditions for which powerful medications carry the risk of inducing addiction.

paleoclimatology The scientific study of climates in previous eras, which can be indirectly inferred from evidence of distribution of vegetation, tree rings, air bubbles trapped in ancient ice, etc. Facts on ancient climates are relevant to modern public health because the world has entered an era of accelerated climate change, and by looking far enough back, it becomes easier to prepare and plan for likely future environmental conditions, e.g., distribution of insect vectors.

paleoepidemiology The use of epidemiological methods to infer how certain diseases might have been distributed in ancient times and how, why, and where they originated, and armed with this information, predict possible futures of communicable and other diseases, possible trends in the emergence of new diseases, and re-emergence of old ones. Evidence comes from contemporary accounts and archeological studies of bones, teeth, stomach contents, etc. Much can be inferred about past infections and epidemics, such as smallpox or tuberculosis, famines, or severe food shortages and their effect on ancient populations, often with applications relevant to the present.

paleopathology The study of pathological processes using fossils, bones, the analysis of fossilized intestinal contents, etc., to infer the nature of diseases that afflicted these individuals while they lived. Many interesting results have emerged, e.g., about the antiquity of tuberculosis and healing around trepanning holes in the cranial vault, which indicates that this heroic procedure (perhaps performed to let out evil spirits from the brain) was not always fatal.

palliative care Medical, nursing, and other supportive care that aims to provide comfort, pain abatement, and other symptomatic relief, but not cure, for conditions considered incurable.

Pan American Health Organization (PAHO) The autonomous division of the World Health Organization (WHO) that deals with the health affairs and disease problems of North, Central, and South America. In practice, this means mainly diseases and health problems in Central and South America, but PAHO also deals with circumpolar health problems in the high Arctic. PAHO evolved from the PAN AMERICAN SANITARY BUREAU when the WHO was established in 1948. See http://www .paho.org for details of current activities.

Pan American Sanitary Bureau The oldest international health agency, established in 1902 by the ORGANIZATION OF AMERICAN STATES (OAS). It dealt with problems such as malaria, yellow fever, hookworm, pellagra, and other deficiency diseases. It had a distinguished record of research on and control of yellow fever, Chagas disease, and other serious public health problems before it also took on the role of Regional Office for WHO for the Americas and has continued its work in the years since WHO was founded.

pancreatic cancer Malignant neoplasm in the parenchyma of the pancreas, often symptomless unless or until the common bile duct is obstructed, whereupon severe progressive jaundice occurs. It may be an extremely painful cancer. The prognosis is always poor, and fatal outcome is common within months of diagnosis. There is often a history of cigarette smoking, and in many cases this appears to be a tobacco-related cancer.

pandemic An epidemic, usually caused by an infectious pathogen, that transcends national boundaries and extends over much or all of the world, attacking people in all affected regions. The most dramatic recent examples have been worldwide INFLUENZA pandemics in 1918–1919 and 1957–1958. The seventh CHOLERA pandemic began in 1961 and reached the Americas in 1991. Historically, the pandemic of the BLACK DEATH in 1347–1350 was among the most lethal, with a case fatality rate as great as 30% in Europe. The current pandemic of AIDS had infected more than 40 million people and killed about 12 million as of 2005. Some modern pandemics are due not to infectious pathogens but to changes in behavior, diet, etc., for example pandemic tobacco addiction and tobacco-induced diseases, traffic injuries, and adult-onset diabetes.

panel study Cross-sectional studies conducted periodically on members of a population that is also being studied longitudinally, i.e., a cohort study population. This has the advantages of being able to adjust for biases and confounding variables while the data from the cross-sectional studies add power to the eventual findings of the cohort study. The small size of the panels permits in-depth assessment of aspects such as physiological and molecular processes that may be part of the pathogenesis of the disease(s) that are being studied.

Panum, Peter Ludwig (1820–1885) A Danish physician who in 1846 observed an epidemic of measles in the Faroe Islands, from which measles had been absent for many years, so herd immunity was low. Panum's clinical observations provided the first accurate account of the natural history of measles, including incubation period, prodromal symptoms, clinical course, period of infectivity, occurrence rates of serious complications, case fatality rates, and the greater risk of severe disease among older people never exposed to measles.

papilloma virus Syn: human papilloma virus (HPV). The virus that causes warts. There are many varieties, some of which cause common warts, others cause venereal warts. Two strains, HPV16 and HPV18, are confirmed human carcinogens for carcinoma of the cervix. These are candidates for vaccines. See http://www.cie.iarc.fr/htdocs/mono graphs/vol64/hpv.htm.

Pap (Papanicolaou) test The cytological examination of epithelial cells from the uterine cervix that was developed by the Greek gynecologist George Papanicolaou (1883–1962) and is used as a reliable way to detect dysplastic and other abnormal cells that are usually early evidence of cancer of the cervix. See also SCREENING.

papule A small raised, red, pimple-like skin lesion that may be solitary or occur in a skin rash as part of a generalized systemic or skin disease, e.g., as in secondary syphilis.

Paracelsus The Latinized name, by which he was and is universally known, of Theophrastus Bombastus von Hohenheim (1493–1541), a colorful pioneer in medical chemistry. He described miner's silicosis; recognized the relationship between goiter and cretinism; used morphine, sulfur, and lead medicinally; and realized that common mental disorders were diseases rather than manifestations of "possession by the devil." He was a founding figure of environmental and occupational medicine and a contributor to the transition from alchemy to modern chemistry, but drunkenness, a habit of insulting respected scholars, and blasphemous language led to his disgrace and exile.

paracusis A general term for any condition that impairs hearing.

paradigm A way of thinking or conceptualizing a body of knowledge and ideas that encompass a field of scholarly activity. A paradigm determines whether innovative ideas or new discoveries are coherent with what is already known and understood. If the new knowledge can be confirmed by irrefutable observations and/or experiments and is at odds with what has previously been believed to be true in a field of science, the field undergoes a paradigm shift, as described and discussed by the American historian and philosopher of science Thomas Kuhn (1922–1996) in *The Structure of Scientific Revolutions*. Throughout the latter part of the 20th century, scientific reasoning in the biomedical sciences including epidemiology was influenced by the new paradigm in methods of scientific reasoning enunciated by the Austrian-British philosopher of science, Karl Popper (1902–1994) in *Logik der Forschung* (1935), translated as *The Logic of Scientific Discovery* (1959). Toward the end of the 20th century, a new paradigm of scientific thinking based on TRANSDISCIPLINARITY and COMPLEXITY THEORY emerged.

paraffins Syn: alkenes. A class of aliphatic hydrocarbons with a double carbon bond that are relatively stable when mixed with other chemicals. Their main uses are as fuels and solvents.

paralysis Loss of muscle function, usually due to disrupted signal transmission from nerve to muscle. The causes include neurological conditions, such as spinal cord or nerve trauma; infections such as polio; neuromuscular poisons; and idiopathic and degenerative diseases, such as multiple sclerosis, motor neuron disease, and muscular dystrophy.

paralytic shellfish poisoning A dramatic potentially fatal food poisoning that usually begins within minutes of ingesting bivalve shellfish such as oysters that have fed on dinoflagellates lower in the food chain that proliferate during certain types of algal blooms, known as "red tide." The cause is the presence in the shellfish of the powerful toxins saxitoxin and gonyautoxin. The condition is seasonal and regional and occurs along the northeast coastal regions of North America.

paramedical personnel A general term for medical assistants. A specific type with specialized training in cardiopulmonary resuscitation, use of parenteral therapy, and other emergency tasks and procedures work as ambulance attendants, in hospital emergency rooms, and in combat zones in many armed forces. Their professional name is often abbreviated to "paramedics."

parameter A measurable entity that in the biomedical sciences is often estimated by means of suitable statistical methods. Examples include mean, standard deviation, correlation coefficient.

parametric method A statistical method based on the assumption that the distribution being analyzed has predictable dimensions, for instance, that it is normally distributed.

paranoia A psychotic disturbance characterized by isolation from and suspicion of others and, in more severe forms, delusions of persecution and/or grandeur not amenable to reason and often resistant to all forms of psychiatric treatment. Persons with paranoid psychosis may have normal or above-average intelligence. World history has occasionally been punctuated by the rise to power of a paranoid national leader who has wreaked great suffering on his own people and those of other nations. Acute paranoia occasionally causes murder-suicide tragedies.

paraplegia Paralysis of all voluntary muscles below the level of the lesion in the spinal cord or chorda equina that has disrupted neuromuscular transmission. When the lesion is high enough to paralyze the arms as well as the legs, it is called quadriplegia. With rare exceptions, such as GUILLAIN-BARRÉ SYNDROME, spinal cord lesions cause permanent paralysis. Control of bladder and bowel function is disrupted, and pressure sores can develop on the skin unless care is taken to avoid them. Many paraplegics are able to live full lives despite their disability. Improved social arrangements, wheelchair accessible buildings, and increased awareness of the needs of the disabled have made life less onerous for paraplegics since the middle of the 20th century.

paraprofessional A trained health worker specialized in a narrow range of skills, such as acute emergency (PARAMEDICAL PERSONNEL) care, venipuncture, operating imaging equipment, etc.

paraquat A bipyridyl broad-leaf herbicide that is quick acting and nonselective, destroying green plant tissue on contact. It is used as a crop desiccant and defoliant and as an aquatic herbicide. It has a field half-life of 2 to 3 years. It has been used, among other things, to destroy plantations of MARIJUANA. Paraquat is highly toxic: ingestion or inhalation causes pulmonary necrosis.

parasite An organism that cannot survive independently of a host species from which it derives nourishment. An obligate parasite cannot survive independently of a host; a facultative parasite is capable of either independent or parasitic existence. Parasitism in humans is usually associated with disease, which is often prolonged and debilitating, as with intestinal worms. It is not in the parasite's survival interests to kill the host unless the survival of its own species has already been assured. Many parasites have complex LIFE CYCLES involving dependence on two or sometimes three other species: humans and anopheline mosquitoes, humans and freshwater snails, humans, freshwater crustaceans, fish, etc. See also SYMBIOSIS.

parasitemia Invasion of the bloodstream by parasites, e.g., the plasmodial parasites of malaria.

parasitism A relationship between organisms in which the parasite derives sustenance solely from and to the detriment of the host. Many parasitic relationships must have originated when free-living species became dependent on unrelated species for sustenance. Some have evolved complex interrelationships over past millennia. For example, plasmodia (malaria parasites) are parasitic on two unrelated species, mosquitoes and vertebrates, including humans, and schistosomes are parasitic on freshwater snails and vertebrates, including humans. Some parasites can survive in alternative hosts that shelter them but play no active part in their life cycle, called paratenic hosts. The origins of these parasitic relationships are of great interest to evolutionary biologists.

parasitology The scientific study of parasitic organisms and of the diseases that they cause. This science flourished in the 19th and early 20th centuries when many previously mysterious diseases caused by tropical and temperate-zone parasites were clarified and, in many cases, methods of control were developed, although not very well for schistosomiasis and only partially for malaria. Parasitology continues to be an important basic and applied science of human and animal disease control. It is an essential public health science.

parasuicide A suicidal attempt or gesture that does not terminate fatally, providing opportunities to initiate psychiatric treatment and/or social support aimed at preventing the completion or accomplishment of suicide.

parasympathetic nervous system The component of the AUTONOMIC NERVOUS SYSTEM that controls involuntary activities such as respiratory and cardiac rate and rhythm and intestinal muscle contraction. Its activity, using acetylcholine as transmission agent, is concerned with conserving and restoring energy. It reduces heart rate and blood pressure and facilitates digestion and absorption of nutrients and excretion of waste. See also SYMPATHETIC NERVOUS SYSTEM.

paratenic host A species that acts as a secondary or subsequent intermediate host for a parasite with a complex life cycle that usually involves two or more species. The parasite does not undergo developmental stages in the paratenic host but exists in a quiescent or encysted state until it has an opportunity to move to a definitive host species. This occurs, for instance, at the intermediate host stage of some nematode parasites. See also PARASITISM.

parathion A highly toxic organophosphorus insecticide. Like other insecticides in this chemical family, it is a nerve poison absorbed through the skin. Exposure can cause respiratory paralysis and death. It is essential for those who work with parathion to wear protective clothing to avoid the risk of lethal poisoning.

parent A mother or father of offspring. A biological parent is one who has passed on genes to offspring. An adoptive parent is one who has children by adoption rather than as a biological parent. A surrogate parent is one who has had a child using genetic material (sperm or ovum) from someone other than the officially or legally designated parents of a child. A foster parent provides long-term family care for child(ren) of parents who are unable or unfit to care for them. A stepparent assumes a parental role when married to a solo parent with dependent child(ren).

parental leave Provision of time off from work to care for a newborn. This is a statutory provision for women and sometimes for men in some countries, e.g., the Scandinavian nations, and a fringe benefit of employment in some commercial and industrial organizations in other industrial nations.

parent education program A program provided by MATERNAL AND CHILD HEALTH services, or by child protection services, sometimes both, that aims to enhance the ability of persons who lack adequate skills to care for a child or children. The emphasis is usually on basic skills required to ensure that infants and children receive the necessities of life, i.e., adequate food, clothing, and shelter; that washing, toilet-training, disciplinary measures, etc., are sensibly conducted; and overall that family resources are deployed with economy and efficiency in the child's interests.

parenteral medication Medication that is administered by infusion into the bloodstream or by injection into tissue, usually muscle, to facilitate more efficient or effective absorption than that provided by way of the gastrointestinal tract.

parenting skills The set of behaviors of mothers, fathers, and other close family members who care for children that are considered essential ingredients for healthy childrearing. These include providing for physical, social, psychological, educational, and spiritual needs, ensuring time for mutually enjoyable activities, family fun, training in problem solving, discipline, conflict resolution, appropriate use of rewards and punishments, consistency of responses to child behavior, and provision of suitable role models. Some parents, especially from broken or disturbed homes, require formal training in parenting skills. This training is provided by some public health and social service departments, usually in collaboration with educational services.

Parents Without Partners A US self-help organization that has become international, providing social and emotional support and practical advice to single, divorced, and widowed parents who are raising children. See http://www.parentswithoutpartners.org for details.

parity The status of a woman who has given birth to viable child(ren). A nullipara is a woman who has not borne children, a multipara is a woman who has borne more than one live-borne child.

Parkinson's disease A progressive neurological disease first described by the British physician James Parkinson (1755–1824) that affects specific cells in the midbrain, causing tremors, gait disorders, and loss of facial mobility due to increasing muscular rigidity; leading, in late stages, to deteriorating intellectual function. It can be a late sequela of viral diseases, such as epidemic encephalitis lethargica or an idiopathic degenerative disease.

partial pressure In atmospheric physics, the law of partial pressure, enunciated by the British scientist John Dalton (1766–1844), states that in a mixture of gases, e.g., oxygen, nitrogen, and carbon dioxide, the pressure of a gas is the same as if that gas alone occupied the same space. This becomes physiologically important at high altitudes or under increased atmospheric pressure when the sea level balance of oxygen and nitrogen is disrupted.

participant observation A method of study used mainly in the social and behavioral sciences in which the investigator is a member of the group or organization that is the subject of study. This is a useful way to gather information, sometimes in quite intimate detail, that would be impossible to obtain in any other way, but it may be difficult to maintain scientific objectivity. Ethical concerns may arise about this and conflicts of interests.

participatory action research A common form of ACTION RESEARCH in which the researcher(s) belong to the system or the team providing the service that is the subject of the research. It is an economically viable method, but inevitably it is subject to observational biases. It may have the advantage of relatively easy linkage to interventions.

particle A discrete object that can be physically defined by its size, composition, etc. In subatomic physics, an array of particles (protons, neutrons, mesons, muons, etc.) comprise the nucleus of atoms. Particles between 1 and 10 microns in size that can be inhaled and lodge in the lungs concern specialists in environmental and occupational health.

particularization In logic, the method of reasoning in which a general rule is applied to a specific set of facts and circumstances, minimizing assumptions and axioms (the principle of scientific parsimony, or OCCAM'S RAZOR) and making the most logical conclusion.

particulate matter See SUSPENDED PARTICULATE MATTER.

partner notification A procedure for formally advising a potential or actual sexual partner that the other party to the act of sexual intercourse has a sexually transmitted disease. This procedure is mandatory in some jurisdictions in cases of HIV infection, but it is more often voluntary and not always observed.

parts per million (ppm), parts per billion (ppb) The units of measurement commonly used to record trace amounts of substances, such as environmental contaminants, fluoride concentration in drinking water, etc. It is not always clear whether the measurement refers to parts by weight or parts by volume, but at the low concentrations concerned, this seldom matters.

parturition Syn: labor. The process of giving birth. The process has three stages. The first is the onset of strong rhythmic contractions of uterine muscle, with dilation of the cervix and, usually at this stage, rupture of the membranes comprising the amniotic sac ("breaking the waters"); this leads to descent of the fetal head into the birth canal, full dilation of the cervix, appearance of the fetal head at the vulva, and birth of the neonate. The third stage is separation and delivery of the placenta. The entire process may take anything from a few minutes to a few days. Usually the process is normal, but it can be complicated and go wrong in many ways, including malposition, malproportion of fetal head and maternal pelvis, infection, hemorrhage, shock, and eclampsia.

pascal The SYSTÈME INTERNATIONAL (SI) D'UNITÉS unit of pressure, equal to 1 NEWTON per square meter. The name honors the French mathematician, physicist, and philosopher Blaise Pascal (1623–1662).

passage In microbiology and infectious disease investigation and control, this is the process of culturing and subculturing microorganisms to refine the bacterial strain and to attenuate virulent strains from which attenuated vaccines can be prepared.

passenger variable A variable that varies systematically with the dependent variable under study but is not causally related to it. Although it is epidemiologically irrelevant, a passenger variable may be useful in that it may be easier to identify and assess than the dependent variable that is the subject of the study.

passive immunity Immunity that is conferred on an individual by an antibody produced in another host. Natural passive immunity is conferred on an infant by transfer of maternal antibodies from the mother. Artificial passive immunity is provided by parenteral injection of antiserum or immune globulin.

passive (involuntary) smoking Exposure to the tobacco smoke of other people. Environmental tobacco smoke consists mainly of SIDESTREAM SMOKE containing harmful ingredients, carcinogens, irritants, and toxic substances, and lesser amounts of exhaled smoke. The concentration of toxicants including known carcinogens is higher in sidestream than inhaled smoke because the burning tip of an idling cigarette has a lower temperature and therefore less complete combustion of tobacco and increased formation of many toxicants. Advocates of smoke-free workplaces, restaurants, public transport, etc., prefer the term "involuntary" to "passive" when describing this environmental health hazard because exposure is involuntary but not necessarily passively accepted; indeed, it is often resisted.

Pasteur, Louis (1822–1895) The French chemist who became the greatest bacteriologist of his time with a series of brilliant investigations, discoveries, and trials of innovative preventive regimens that included pasteurization, identification of pathogenic microorganisms, and preparation of vaccines derived from attenuated strains of pathogenic microorganisms, including chicken cholera, anthrax, and rabies. PASTEURIZATION of milk has saved innumerable lives from premature death caused by bacterial contamination. He founded the Pasteur Institutes, which specialize in the treatment and prevention of infectious diseases.

Pasteur effect Inhibition of certain metabolic pathways when oxygen concentration rises, leading to decreased lactic acid accumulation and reduced tendency to muscle cramps. The Pasteur point is the oxygen concentration at which this process takes effect.

pasteurization Heat treatment of milk, dairy products, and other foodstuffs to kill potentially harmful microorganisms, including especially pathogenic organisms and organisms that cause spoilage and bad odors and tastes. The process was invented by the French bacteriologist LOUIS PASTEUR and first used to treat beer that had been contaminated during fermentation. Several methods of pasteurizing milk can be used, e.g., high-temperature-short-time (HTST) and ultra-high-temperature (UHT)-very-short-time, which interferes less with the appearance and flavor of milk and dairy products.

pastoral counseling The work of priests, ministers of religion, rabbis, lay preachers, etc., in advising members of their flock about personal, family, and social problems. Some of these problems have relevance in preventive medicine and public health.

pastoralist A person who derives livelihood from grazing animals on pasture. The term applies to peasant herdsmen and wealthy landowners alike. Pastoralists may be permanently settled or, as in parts of Africa and Asia, migratory, moving from one locality to another as seasons change. Health risks, for example of zoonoses, vary with the locality.

patch test A skin test for sensitivity to a specific antigen that is administered in the form of a solution or suspension impregnated on an absorbent patch in contact with the skin for a period of hours or days to elicit a reaction such as localized swelling and inflammation.

patent The official legal document that confers ownership of intellectual property and the right to claim royalties for an invention, a modified version of an existing device, or a scientific or technical process. The WORLD TRADE ORGANIZATION (WTO) recognizes patents for a wide range of intellectual property, including pharmaceuticals and synthetic organic compounds that simulate naturally occurring derivatives of living organisms. US patent law has allowed patents for genetically modified (GM) organisms such as strains of rice "created" in a laboratory. US patents have been approved for naturally occurring genes associated with high breast cancer risk, and royalties claimed for screening tests that use the patented genes. Other nations that have ratified the UN Convention on Biodiversity (which the United States has not done) do not all recognize "ownership" of genetic characteristics and decline to pay royalties. Patent law and WTO rules notwithstanding, many people believe it is morally wrong to patent parts of living organisms and claim royalties, especially when their use can save lives. Drug patents enforced usually for 20 years can inhibit manufacture and sale at low cost in low-income countries of generic versions of the same drugs. This often deprives people in low-income countries of effective treatment for their diseases. These issues are a current topic of international discussion.

patent medicine 1. A class of medications made under a patent, often advertised, and available without a prescription. They include analgesics, antiseptics, many cough remedies, indigestion remedies, laxatives, skin ointments, and some sedatives. In the United States, the Food and Drug Administration regulates their sale and tests their safety and efficacy. See also ALTERNATIVE MEDICINE. 2. Compounds flamboyantly promoted as tonics and treatments. Most were of dubious efficacy and occasionally harmful—some contained ingredients that caused addiction, paralysis, or abortion. They also caused harm if taking them masked symptoms of serious disease. Patent medicines flourished during the 19th century, but the 1906 Pure Food and Drug Act regulated their claims, and the 1936 Act banned them altogether.

paternalism An attitude to others based on the belief that these others are not able or equipped by intellect, training, or experience to make decisions for themselves. Paternalism was a common attitude among physicians and administrators in colonial public services and still exists among some public health administrators and their professional staffs. See also AUTONOMY.

paternity Fatherhood, the process of fathering a child. DNA analyses permit identification of paternity with virtually 100% precision; without DNA analysis, there is sometimes uncertainty. On the other hand, maternity, the act and process of becoming a mother, can be established beyond doubt by observation. However, SURROGATE motherhood has complicated the legal, if not the genetic, aspects of deciding who should be identified as the mother of an infant born to a surrogate mother from an implanted fertilized ovum donated by another woman.

path analysis A method of analysis that emphasizes the sequencing and directionality of the associations between variables, or steps in a sequenced procedure. These are displayed in flow charts or path diagrams. When several alternatives are compared, a critical path analysis (review) can determine which is most credible and efficient. Path

analysis is often used in OPERATIONAL RESEARCH and sometimes in forward planning. See also ALGORITHM.

pathogen An organism that causes disease (*patho,* disease; *gen,* cause).

pathogenesis The process by which a disease originates. This seeks to account for the way a disease agent induces the pathological transformation from normal to diseased state, preferably considered at the molecular, cellular, tissue, and organ level, so that the disease is explained and the symptoms, signs, course, and prognosis can be understood.

pathology The scientific study of the gross and microscopic changes in body tissues and organs associated with the occurrence and progression of diseases. Divisions include systemic, gross, and microscopic pathology, and, in the health care system, laboratory medicine, clinical, general, and forensic pathology. Pathologists diagnose disease, notably cancer, from biopsy material, cervical (Pap) smears, blood films, etc.

patient management The formal statement of the prescribed treatment regimen for a patient. This is preferably a written document, as it may sometimes become medicolegally important.

Patients' Bill of Rights A statement prepared by the American Hospital Association in 1973, setting out rights, e.g., preserving personal dignity, the right to privacy, and the right to participate in decisions about aspects of health care. Although intended for hospital patients, evolving values have made infringement of rights by public health professionals unacceptable or hard to justify. There have been many modifications by advocates for particular groups, such as retired persons, minorities, and patients with cancer. In 2001, a modification was suggested in the bipartisan McCain-Edwards-Kennedy bill in the US Senate. The provisions of this bill of rights are available at http://democrats.senate.gov/pbr/summary.html.

patriarchy A social system determined by tradition and culture in which the most senior male member of the extended family or clan is recognized as the leader and principal decision maker, sometimes responsible for making decisions affecting the family or clan as a whole. In some cultures matriarchy prevails: the most senior female is head of the family and principal decision maker. INFORMED CONSENT in patriarchal and matriarchal cultures begins with the family head, but ethics guidelines require that it be followed by obtaining individual consent also.

pauper Literally a poor, usually a destitute, person. In the health care system, the term is applied occasionally to someone who has been rendered destitute by the combination of disabling illness or injury and medical expenses greater than available financial resources.

PBB See POLYBROMINATED BIPHENYL.

PCB See POLYCHLORINATED BIPHENYL.

PCP See PHENCYCLIDINE HYDROCHLORIDE.

PCR See POLYMERASE CHAIN REACTION.

Peace Corps A US government-funded organization founded in 1961 by the administration of President John F. Kennedy that sends small teams of young volunteers to low-income nations to provide training for local people in skills relevant in agriculture, resource management, administration, and public health, among other fields. See http://www.peacecorps.gov/ for details and current activities of the program.

peace movement A loose coalition of organizations that seek nonviolent solutions to disputes causing violent armed conflicts. International public health and WHO are engaged in the peace movement by way of the initiative called HEALTH AS A BRIDGE FOR PEACE.

peak flow meter A device to measure respiratory function and vital capacity by measuring the maximum rate at which lungs can be emptied of inspired air, using an anemometer.

pecking order In social psychology, a hierarchy in which individuals in an organization are ranked in order of importance, influence, authority, by fellow members and sometimes by others outside the group. The term derives from observations of wild birds and domesticated poultry. A pecking order helps to determine the relationship of hierarchical position and health risks of individuals in large organizations, such as government departments.

pectin Hemicellulose polymer ingredient of plant tissue, an ingredient in fruits and the agent that causes jelly to set. It is a nonstarchy food ingredient useful in low-carbohydrate diets.

pediatrics The medical specialty concerned with prevention, diagnosis, and treatment of diseases of children. Pediatricians emphasize health protection, health promotion, and disease prevention to a considerable extent, often more so than clinicians in most other specialties.

pediculosis Infestation with lice. This condition comes in several forms: infestation with the body louse, *Pediculus corporis*, the only louse that can be a vector of disease (typhus, relapsing fever); with the pubic louse, *Pthirus pubis* (colloquially known as "the crabs"); or with the head louse, *Pediculus capitis*. This last one is common among school children. See also NITS.

pedigree The record of ancestry of animals and people in which their parentage and that of their forebears is traced back for as many generations as possible. Short generation time and the value of purebred stock make this relatively commonplace and easy with racehorses, dogs, roses, etc., but it is more difficult with people. One characteristic of the noble households of Europe is their ability to provide genealogical records maintained over many generations (albeit with occasional blemishes), whereas most people of more humble parentage have difficulty tracing their ancestry for even half a dozen generations. Members of the Church of Jesus Christ of Latter-Day Saints, the MORMONS, believe they can ensure the eternal salvation of their ancestors by retroactively baptizing them into the faith. The importance of exploring family pedigrees led the Mormons to establish a large genealogical institute in Salt Lake City, Utah. See also GENEALOGY.

peer group Any group in which individuals perceive one another as sharing values, have about equal social standing and educational level, and share activities that define the group. Perception of peer group members and nonmembers is often flexible, and membership may be fluid. Peer groups sometimes have a hierarchical structure, an acknowledged leader, a policy of exclusion of outsiders, and codes of conduct or unwritten rules that may have implications for health. For example, adolescent peer groups may reject adult values about harmful behavior, such as drug use, or have hazardous initiation rites.

peer pressure The psychological and social influence exerted on individual members by the peer group to encourage conformity to the group's behavioral norms. This process may work by coercion, modeling, or mimicking behavior of an admired peer group leader or conformity to the peer group norm. It is particularly important in shaping adolescent conduct with respect to adoption of tobacco, alcohol, illicit drug use, sexual promiscuity, and other hazardous behavior.

peer review The process in which the activities of professional workers are assessed by others with comparable qualifications and experience, who are not close colleagues and preferably are not known to those being assessed. It is the customary and usual way to evaluate the quality of scientific endeavors in all fields of science. Peer review is used to assess research projects and programs, manuscripts submitted to scientific journals, and applicants for promotion and tenure. Peer review may be conducted by an appointed expert committee, a peer review committee, or by one or more individuals acting at the invitation, for instance, of a medical or science journal editor. After scientific work has been published or posted on a WEB SITE, it may be subjected to the most rigorous peer review of all by the authors' scientific peers all over the world who scrutinize the work at leisure. Peer review is imperfect if it discriminates against unorthodox innovative ideas but is widely accepted as the best way to ensure that the quality of science reaches the highest level attainable. See also INSTITUTIONAL REVIEW BOARD (IRB).

peer support The form of social bonding and group solidarity whereby peer group members assist one another in adversity.

PEL See PERMISSIBLE EXPOSURE LIMITS.

pellagra A disease due to dietary deficiency of NIACIN, vitamin B$_3$. In its full-blown form, it is typically characterized by dermatitis, diarrhea, and dementia. Usually it occurs in mild form with dermatitis and loose stools. Until the American public health physician JOSEPH GOLDBERGER (1874–1929) identified the cause and dietary regimens were developed to prevent it, it was a common seasonal disorder in communities where people subsist on a diet of corn and maize, such as formerly in the US southern rural states in late winter and spring, before the new crops matured and replaced the previous year's stored corn, which was deficient in niacin.

pelvic examination A euphemism for vaginal examination that is seldom performed to delineate the dimensions of the pelvis but usually to seek evidence of disease of the vagina, uterus, and adjacent organs, or to ascertain the progress and stage of labor during childbirth.

pelvic inflammatory disease A miscellaneous group of diseases of the vagina, uterus, fallopian tubes, and adnexum, caused by various pathogenic organisms, including some sexually transmitted diseases. Other causes such as ENDOMETRIOSIS may be associated with hormonal disorders. The sequelae include painful sexual intercourse, increased risk of miscarriage, and infertility.

penetrance The proportion of individuals of specific genotype exhibiting the phenotype under specified environmental conditions.

penicillin The first effective ANTIBIOTIC derived from a fungus or mold, a serendipitous discovery made in 1928 by the British microbiologist Alexander Fleming (1881–1955). Techniques to refine and purify penicillin were developed during World War II by Howard Florey (1898–1968), Ernst Chain (1906–1979), and others. Fleming, Florey, and Chain received the Nobel Prize for their work on penicillin. Unlike other lifesaving antibiotics, penicillin has remained in the public domain, not protected by a patent conferring ownership on a profit-making corporation. For more than a decade, penicillin transformed the never-ending war between humans and pathogenic bacteria, then penicillin-resistant pathogens proliferated and its efficacy declined. Many people became acutely allergic after being treated with penicillin.

penicillinase An enzyme produced by staphylococci, gonococci, and other microorganisms that can inactivate penicillin, rendering these organisms penicillin-resistant. Resistance is transmitted not only to bacteria of the same species but also to other species of bacteria.

pennyroyal An aromatic herb traditionally used to treat menstrual disorders, abdominal pains, and respiratory symptoms. It is toxic, causes uterine cramps, and can induce miscarriages.

pentachlorophenol A chlorinated phenolic compound, a white crystalline solid used mainly as a wood preservative, also as a molluscicide for the intermediate snail hosts of schistosomiasis and an herbicide. Commercial-grade pentachlorophenol usually contains dioxin and other highly toxic organochlorine contaminants. It is absorbed cutaneously and is toxic and irritant, causing mucosal irritation and severe systemic effects, including cardiovascular collapse that can be fatal. It is a potential human carcinogen.

People for the Ethical Treatment of Animals (PETA) An international organization that aims to protect domestic animals from cruelty and abuse. It sometimes adopts militant and destructive tactics, notably in attacks on animal laboratory facilities used in biomedical research, and on some scientists who work with animals on vaccine production and diagnostic services.

pepper spray Oleoresin capsicum in an aerosol suspension, an incapacitating irritant used to subdue violent persons without harming them, e.g., in riots and civil disturbances. Occasionally it causes severe and even fatal idiosyncratic reactions.

percolation The process of passing or forcing a liquid through a porous solid in order to extract ingredient(s) from the solid to produce a solution or suspension containing the ingredient(s) in the percolate (also called LEACHATE). Percolation can be used to purify solid particles, to extract toxic substances, or, as with coffee, to make a beverage.

performance indicator Data, or sets of data, that demonstrate the process(es) by which a specific task has been conducted and the outcomes, e.g., the way a physician has conducted routinely required actions involved in patient care: taking a medical history, performing a routine physical examination and necessary ancillary investigations, and providing appropriate treatment. In public health, "process" performance indicators include immunization uptake rates, proportions of eligible populations covered by maternal and child care services, and smoking prevention programs. Notifications of vaccine-preventable diseases are an indicator of inadequate population coverage by immunization programs.

performance standards The criteria, often determined in advance, e.g., by an expert committee, by which the performance of health professionals is assessed. Alternatively, the empirically observed or theoretically determined capacity of machinery, e.g., the specified increments by which an aircraft can exceed the speed of sound.

perinatal care Medical and nursing care of a woman and her offspring "around" the natal period, i.e., preceding, during, and for a short time after childbirth. The perinatal period is loosely defined for this purpose, although not for statistical purposes.

perinatal mortality Perinatal mortality, according to the *International Statistical Classification of Diseases and Related Health Problems* (ICD-10), includes death of the fetus any time after 22 weeks' gestation, stillbirth, and death of infants born alive who die during the first week of life. There is some debate about the definition of fetal viability. Advances in medical care of very immature infants have led some perinatologists to propose an earlier beginning of the perinatal period. Others assert that extremely immature fetuses have imperfectly formed brains and, although technically alive, they are likely to be severely brain damaged.

perinatal mortality rate The numerator of this rate is the number of fetal deaths of 22 weeks' gestation and later, deaths during labor, and deaths during the first week of life. The denominator is the total of all live births and fetal deaths after 22 weeks' gestation, plus stillbirths.

perinatal period Technically, the period from the onset of labor to restoration to normal of the maternal uterus and adnexum after delivery of the infant. For statistical purposes, e.g., calculation of perinatal mortality rates, the perinatal period lasts from the 28th week of pregnancy until the end of the first week of life of the infant.

perinatal transmission The usual form of VERTICAL TRANSMISSION of pathogenic agents, e.g., hepatitis B and HIV, from mother to infant.

perinatology The discipline concerned with protecting health and treating departures from health during the PERINATAL PERIOD. It has become a high-technology specialty at the boundary between obstetrics and pediatrics, including the prenatal diagnosis and treatment of malformations of the heart, using diagnostic imaging techniques and microsurgery.

periodic health examination A systematic assessment of apparently healthy individuals that is customarily conducted at specific age epochs, including soon after birth, at weaning, beginning of grade school and secondary school, or at puberty, at the beginning of adult life or military recruitment, before employment, before marriage, during and after pregnancy, around the time of menopause and at about the same age for men, about retirement age, and then more often with advancing years. The questions asked and tests performed are tailored to specific risks associated with age epochs. The concepts and practice of age-appropriate health examinations follow evidence-based guidelines and replace the former "routine physicals" that were often an inefficient and cost-ineffective approach. Although periodic health examinations may reveal evidence of serious disease, their efficacy and cost-effectiveness are matters of debate. Periodic reassessment of patients with known chronic diseases is not usually included in this definition. The current guidelines are at http://www.guideline.gov/summary/summary.aspx. See also CANADIAN TASK FORCE ON PREVENTIVE HEALTH CARE and PREVENTIVE SERVICES TASK FORCE.

periodic table The orderly arrangement of the elements according to their atomic numbers, in which elements with similar properties are arranged in the same families in vertical columns. This table was the insight of the Russian chemist Dmitri Ivanovich Mendeleyev (1834–1907).

periodontal disease Inflammation of the gums, specifically at the junction between gums and teeth, the condition sometimes known as periodontitis. Commonly associated with malpositioned teeth, and with inflammation caused by tobacco smoke, alcohol, highly seasoned foods, and trauma. Other periodontal diseases include neoplasms.

peripheral neuropathy A general term for inflammatory or degenerative diseases of the peripheral nerves. The causes include vitamin B_1 deficiency, leprosy, and conditions leading to destruction of myelin sheaths, a group of demyelinating diseases of toxic or idiopathic origin.

peritoneal dialysis The use of the endothelial lining of the peritoneum as a site for exchange of metabolites in cases of renal failure. It is a hazardous procedure because of the risk of infection leading to peritonitis, and because it cannot be repeated frequently, it is unsuitable for chronic renal failure.

peritonitis Inflammation of the peritoneum, the endothelial lining of the abdominal cavity, an acute life-threatening condition, most often a complication of acute appendicitis, occasionally a more chronic condition associated with tuberculosis.

permafrost The layer of permanently frozen soil at the surface of the ground at high latitudes. The prefix "perma" implies permanency, but permafrost is dynamic: it moves, thaws, and refreezes. Infected cadavers and toxic substances buried in it can come to the surface and contaminate the environment. This health risk could increase as global climate change leads to thawing of extensive zones of permafrost. Waste disposal is a serious challenge in permafrost regions. Another risk is that some permafrost regions have a high content of frozen rotting organic matter, and as this thaws, methane is released. If this were to happen over wide regions because of global warming, the released methane would contribute to greenhouse gas buildup and aggravate the warming trend.

permeability The extent to which a solid membrane permits liquids to pass through it. This varies considerably. A semipermeable membrane is a plasma membrane that permits the passage of small molecules but blocks the passage of large ones. This is the essential quality in DIALYSIS.

permissible exposure limit (PEL) An occupational and environmental safety standard set by the highest safe level of a toxic substance that can be encountered in the workplace environment. The PEL is set by empirical observation and/or animal tests and is usually expressed as a concentration such as parts per million of a gaseous toxin, either as a TIME-WEIGHTED AVERAGE during a 6- or 8-hour work day or as a MAXIMUM ALLOWABLE CONCENTRATION.

pernicious anemia Syn: megaloblastic anemia. A chronic disease of the blood-forming bone marrow tissue due to deficiency of vitamin B_{12} that was invariably fatal until the essential enzymes responsible for erythrocyte maturation were discovered and treatment with liver extract was initiated, then later replaced by vitamin B_{12} supplements.

persistent organic pollutants (POPs) A class of substances, mainly chlorinated hydrocarbons, resistant to chemical, biological, or physical decomposition or transformation into less harmful substances, and therefore environmentally persistent. They include substances that can have several serious adverse effects on the nervous system, the immune system, and the endocrine system, and some that increase the risk of cancer. POPs include organochlorine pesticides, dioxins, furans, and PCBs. A conference convened by the United Nations Environmental Programme (UNEP) established the Stockholm Convention on Persistent Organic Pollutants in 2004. See http://www.pops.int/ for details. As of 2005, it has been ratified by more than 50 nations and is being implemented in these and others.

persistent vegetative state A condition in which consciousness and intellectual functions have been lost or destroyed but brain activity as detected by electroencephalography and heart beats under autonomic control continue if LIFE SUPPORT SYSTEMS can maintain respiration, provide nourishment, and control fluid and electrolyte balance. Patients rarely recover consciousness and intellectual capacity after prolonged periods, but this has happened, so there is an ethical responsibilty to continue intensive care as long as there is a reasonable hope of eventual recovery.

personal health services The range of health and medical care functions involving encounters between individuals and the physicians, nurses, and other health service professional workers who provide preventive, curative, and palliative care on a one-to-one basis in clinics, offices, or the homes of patients or clients in the community.

personality The combination of intellectual, emotional and other psychological, cultural, and social characteristics, some inherent, some shaped by familial, educational, and other experience, that make each human unique.

personality disorders Psychosocial or psychiatric conditions that impair the ability to form and maintain normal healthy relationships with others. They include antisocial personality disorder (psychopathic personality), mild paranoid or schizoid symptoms, antisocial personality disorder, narcissism, and dependent personality disorders. See also BORDERLINE PSYCHOSIS.

personality test Any of several established, field-tested, and validated survey instruments, e.g., the MINNESOTA MULTIPHASIC PERSONALITY INVENTORY (MMPI), used to assess aspects of personality, i.e., introversion, extroversion, passivity, and aggression, and to sort people into personality types such as TYPE A BEHAVIOR, TYPE B BEHAVIOR. All such tests should be used and interpreted with caution because, even though they have been validated, they can yield misleading results.

personal monitoring device A device worn by workers in occupational environments where they are exposed to hazards such as ionizing radiation or toxic inhaled substances. A well-known example is the badge containing a radiation-sensitive film used by x-ray technicians.

personal protective equipment This term covers a wide range of protective clothing, face shields, respirators, gloves, ear protectors, and other equipment used to provide protection from specific exposure hazards in the workplace. Occupational safety and health laws make the use of personal protective equipment mandatory in many jurisdictions.

persons living with HIV/AIDS (PLWHA) During the first decade of the HIV/AIDS pandemic, the usual term was persons living with AIDS (PLWA), but for surveillance purposes PLWHA is preferable because this describes people infected with HIV who are not overtly ill and are able to live a more or less normal life with their symptoms controlled by antiviral medication, as well as persons with overt AIDS. The term puts a positive emphasis on the person's life rather than on the sickness.

person-time A combined measurement of persons and time in the denominator to calculate incidence, mortality, and other rates when individuals enter a study at varying intervals of time and their collective experience is being calculated. It is the sum of the periods of time that each individual in the study has been at risk. It is most often expressed as person-years. Related or similar expressions, such as person-dose, are sometimes used.

pertussis Syn: whooping cough. A debilitating bacterial respiratory disease of children that is often prolonged, can be complicated by bronchopneumonia, and can cause emphysema. It can be fatal, especially in children younger than 1 year of age. It can be prevented by pertussis vaccine, which is most efficacious if commenced before infants are 6 months old.

pertussis vaccine A suspension of killed *Bordetella pertussis* administered in three doses in the first 6 months of life provides a high degree of protection against pertussis. The vaccine has some adverse effects, but the risks of these are considerably less than the risks of death or dangerous complications associated with pertussis, especially in infants. For international recommendations, see http://www.who.int/vaccines/en/pertussis.shtml; the US recommendations are similar.

pest An insect, animal, or plant that is a nuisance. In public health the word is usually applied to insects and animals that not only are annoying but also compete for nourishment and habitat with humans, food crops, or domestic animals, and/or can carry disease agents to humans.

PEST analysis Systematic analysis of an organization such as a public corporation that considers the political, economic, social, and technological characteristics of the organization.

pesticide A solid, liquid, or gaseous substance that kills pests. There are many varieties, almost all of which act by poisoning the pest against which they are directed. Unfortunately, some also poison people, so they must be used with care. Pesticides include herbicides that kill weeds, larvicides that kill aquatic mosquito larvae, insecticides that kill insects, fungicides that kill fungi, biocides that kill most pests, and various other substances.

pesticide poisoning A diagnostic label applied to any form of poisoning attributable to exposure to pesticides. As these include neurotoxins, compounds of arsenic, mercury, lead, etc., and diverse other chemicals, it is a vague label, useful only in relating a condition to an occupational or environmental origin.

pestilence A biblical word for a widespread plague that kills many people. In the popular imagination, shaped by the associations evoked by the use of the word in the Bible, the kind of epidemic or pandemic, e.g., plague, epidemic typhus, or insect or animal infestation, associated with the presence of pests such as locusts or rats.

pest management The set of technologies and professional expertise required to control the various kinds of domestic, agricultural, and industrial pests. These include entomology, ecology, toxicology, and environmental sciences. Pest control officers in health departments usually possess at least a technical qualification in one or more of these fields.

petrochemicals A general term for all organic chemical derivatives of petroleum, covering a very wide range of compounds that include many of great economic importance, such as fuels and plastics, as well as many that are toxic.

petrol The word used in the United Kingdom and many other countries of the Commonwealth of Nations for GASOLINE.

petroleum fuels A large class of carbon-based fuels derived from petroleum, which is mostly obtained from oil wells and refined into gasoline (petrol), diesel oil, and paraffin.

peyote A cactus that grows in Mexico and the southwestern United States containing the psychoactive alkaloid MESCALINE, which induces hallucinations and a euphoric trance-like state when ingested. It was used in rituals by pre-Columbian people and in most circumstances is now an illicit substance in the United States. However, its use is legal in traditional peyote religious ceremonies.

pH The hydrogen ion concentration of a substance, a logarithmic scale, a measure of its acidity or alkalinity. A pH of 7 is neutral; anything below is acid and anything above is alkaline.

phage See BACTERIOPHAGE.

phagocytes The scavenger cells responsible for consuming foreign organisms and dead or diseased tissue, and for contributing to immune responses. Microphages are polymorphonuclear leukocytes that consume and destroy foreign cells such as bacteria; macrophages are mononuclear monocytes that ingest dead tissue and degenerating body cells as well as bacteria.

pharmaceutical industry A large industry responsible for development and manufacture of drugs, medications, pesticides, etc., for human and veterinary use. The pharmaceutical industry conducts and sponsors research on pharmacology and therapeutics, seeking new remedies and improved modifications of existing drugs for human and animal diseases. This industry has accomplished much that is good but may be slow to develop drugs to prevent and treat prevalent diseases of low-income countries (malaria, schistosomiasis, tuberculosis) and to make available at low cost some essential drugs in low-income countries. It has lobbied to extend the duration of patent protection of drugs, thus delaying manufacture of cheaper generic preparations with pharmacologically identical properties. Generic drug manufacturers in Brazil, India, and Thailand have partially relieved this situation. The industry has responded to the demand for lucrative drugs to enhance sexual potency, modify moods, and reduce weight. It is accused of influencing decisions about licensing of certain drugs by suppressing publication of scientific studies that question the safety or efficacy of drugs, and by demanding representation on government advisory bodies responsible for decisions about such drugs.

pharmaceuticals Syn: drugs. A class of manufactured chemicals with medicinal properties. Some, including digitalis, quinine, morphine, are purified chemical extracts of naturally occurring traditional herbal remedies. Others, such as aspirin, are artificially manufactured chemicals that replicate ingredients of traditional remedies. An increasing number are synthetic chemicals designed to mimic or enhance known pharmacological actions of other substances. Some of these are designed to bind to specific sites on target molecules, thereby activating or inhibiting them.

pharmacist A professional person trained in preparing, mixing, and dispensing drugs and medicinal preparations and advising the public in their use. Pharmacists play an important role in primary health care, providing advice and suggesting appropriate medication for many complaints for which people turn first to their neighborhood drugstore.

pharmacoepidemiology The application of epidemiological methods to the study of actions and adverse reactions to drugs. The study includes the use of specific drugs in population groups and the study of drug costs and outcomes of their use.

pharmacogenetics The study of how genetic makeup influences reactions to specific drugs. Genetically based enzyme differences, such as acetylator genes, influence drug metabolism.

pharmacokinetics The study of how drugs act and interact, including details such as routes and manner of absorption, metabolic pathways, and routes and times for decomposition and excretion.

pharmacology The scientific study of pharmaceutical preparations and how they work, a science that evolved out of and is closely related to biochemistry and physiology.

pharmacy 1. Syn: chemist's shop, drugstore. A shop, store front, or hospital department where prescribed drugs are prepared and dispensed and where over-the-counter drugs are sold. 2. The name for the profession practiced by pharmacists.

pharynx The anatomical region behind the nose and mouth at the upper end of the respiratory and gastrointestinal tracts.

phase I, II, III clinical trials CLINICAL TRIALS of new drugs and vaccines begin with a phase I trial on a small number, typically fewer than 50, of healthy volunteers to study pharmacological properties, mode of action, and safety. A phase I trial also can test routes of administration and doses. A phase II trial is the initial trial of efficacy, a small randomized trial (perhaps 200 to 300 participants) to compare the safety and efficacy of the new drug with existing alternatives. A phase III trial is a larger study, with perhaps thousands of volunteer participants with random allocation and sometimes multiple study centers. All phases require ETHICAL REVIEW and an assurance that INFORMED CONSENT requirements have been met.

phencyclidine hydrochloride (PCP) Street named ANGEL DUST, it is an easily synthesized DESIGNER DRUG popular among young people at parties known as "raves." It has a euphoric effect at low doses but it is very dangerous because it causes delirium, convulsions, and death in higher doses.

phenols A class of hydrocarbon compounds with one or more hydroxy (OH) groups bound directly to benzene rings. The simplest compound in the group is hydroxybenzene or carbolic acid, an antiseptic and disinfectant, used as the basic ingredient for many drugs, dyestuffs, etc. JOSEPH LISTER (1827–1912) used carbolic acid spray as an antiseptic that made surgical operations comparatively safe, greatly reducing the high risk of postoperative infection.

phenotype The physical appearance and functional characteristics of a person (or organism) that develop from the GENOTYPE under the influence of environmental factors.

phenoxy herbicides These derivatives of phenoxyaliphatic acids include two economically important broad-leaf herbicides, 2,4,5-T and 2,4-D, that were developed in the 1940s and used widely ever since. Until the 1990s, 2,4,5-T usually contained dioxin contaminants, including 2,3,7.8-TCDD, a dangerous dioxin contaminant that is a mutagen, teratogen, and carcinogen. 2,4-D is also a suspected carcinogen, implicated in several epidemiological studies as a possible cause of non-Hodgkin lymphoma.

phenylalanine One of the essential amino acids. It has a benzene ring structure, and its rather complex metabolism is controlled by a hepatic enzyme that is deficient or absent in the recessive genetic disorder of PHENYLKETONURIA.

phenylketonuria (PKU) A metabolic abnormality inherited as an autosomal recessive condition, caused by deficiency of a hepatic enzyme that converts phenylalanine to tyrosine. Phenylalanine accumulates in the body in the absence of the enzyme and causes irreversible brain damage. A simple screening test for the presence of phenylketones in the urine of newborns can detect this metabolic abnormality, which can be prevented from exerting damaging effects on cerebral function by a special dietary regimen that restricts intake of foods containing phenylalanine. To prevent deterioration, this dietary regimen must begin soon after birth.

pheromone Complex organic substances with properties resembling those of sex hormones that act via the olfactory nerves. Pheromones have been studied mainly in insects and animals that have seasonal sexual activity. They are released into the environment by an insect or animal and elicit a physiological and/or behavioral response in another individual of the same species, usually related to sexual activity or response. In human females, pheromones may account for the phenomenon of synchrony of the menstrual cycles of women in an institution. The role of pheromones in human sexual responses is not known.

philanthropic foundations Organizations that derive their capital from large bequests and/or donations and disburse funds to causes that fit within their terms of reference. Philanthropic FOUNDATIONS have been great benefactors of the health sector. The Rockefeller Foundation provided funds to establish many schools of public health in the United States and elsewhere and supported research and development of prevention and control measures against tropical diseases. The Ford Foundation, the Commonwealth Fund, the Josiah Macy, Jr. Foundation, the Milbank Memorial Fund, the Carnegie Corporation, the Wellcome Trust, the Nuffield Trust, the Wolfson Trust, the Bill & Melinda Gates Foundation, and others in the United States, United Kingdom, Japan, and western Europe have been important major contributors to health research and development, often in low-income countries.

phocomelia Intrauterine failure of long bones in the arms and/or legs to develop, so the hands and/or feet are attached to the trunk by a stump. It occurs as an adverse reaction to THALIDOMIDE taken early in pregnancy, and extremely rarely apart from this.

phosgene Carbonyl chloride, $COCl_2$, one of the poisonous gases deployed during World War I. It is used in the manufacture of isocyanates, such as toluene, in pesticides, dyestuffs, and pharmaceuticals. It is a powerful respiratory irritant that can cause fatal pulmonary edema.

phosphorus (P) A nonmetallic element that combines with carbon, hydrogen, and other elements in several organic compounds essential to life, e.g., in the process of phosphorylation, which is the central feature of energy transfer in all living organisms.

photochemical reaction A chemical reaction that is activated by visible or ultraviolet (solar) radiation. The most important reaction of this type is PHOTOSYNTHESIS. It is also the basis for photography, photocopying, and many other industrial processes. This reaction is also the basis for the formation of photochemical smog. Another manifestation is photosensitivity, a condition in which exposure to sunlight induces a skin reaction, typically a maculopapular eruption or generalized erythema, such as in sunburn but occurring after minimal, rather than prolonged, exposure. Some drugs can induce this condition.

photochemical smog A brownish gaseous haze in which the most important irritants are ozone, aldehydes, and nitrogen dioxide. This is formed from VOLATILE ORGANIC COMPOUNDS (VOCs), mainly from motor vehicle emissions and nitrogen dioxide in a series of reactions catalyzed by solar ultraviolet radiation. Photochemical smog is a troublesome problem in large cities with heavy automobile traffic, long hours of sunlight, and climatic conditions favoring stagnation of air. Los Angeles is well known for its smog, but the problem occurs in many other motorized cities all over the world, such as Houston, Mexico City, São Paulo, Cairo, Delhi, Shanghai, and Beijing.

photoelectric effect The phenomenon that occurs when some metals and related compounds emit energized electrons, i.e., an electric current, on being struck by photons, i.e., bathed in visible radiation (or radiation of wavelengths close to the visible spectrum).

photometer An instrument for measuring the intensity of light.

photon Light is composed of photons, defined as the unit of energy in visible electromagnetic radiation, specified as hv, where h is Planck's constant and v is the frequency of the radiation.

photosensitivity An erythematous reaction to solar radiation in the wavelengths of visible, ultraviolet, and shorter wavelengths with flushing, tanning, and, in severe cases, blistering and desquamation. Fair-complexioned people are more photosensitive than are those with plentiful protective melanin pigment. Some diseases and drugs cause enhanced photosensitivity.

photosynthesis The conversion of carbon dioxide and water into organic compounds under the influence of chlorophyll in all green plants from phytoplankton to the largest trees. The organic compounds include carbohydrates and plant proteins that are the direct or indirect source of the food consumed by herbivores.

phototropism A TROPISM, i.e., biologically mediated attraction to light. Plants containing chlorophyll exhibit phototropism. Many mammals, including humans, are also attracted to the light, although the attraction is believed to be a behavioral, rather than a biological, imperative. One manifestation of phototropism might be SEASONAL AFFECTIVE DISORDER (SAD), a reaction to low light levels and/or brief hours of daylight.

phthalate compounds These chemicals are used as plasticizers in polyvinyl chloride products, including building materials, blood bags, and children's toys, and as additives in consumer products such as cosmetics, personal care products, wood finishes, and insecticides. Some are used as herbicides for ground crops such as strawberries. They are cutaneous irritants and intense gastrointestinal irritants, and also can cause asthma-like symptoms. In experimental animals their toxic effects include testicular atrophy and malignant neoplasms after prolonged exposure.

phylum A group of organisms descended from a common origin, distinguished by possession of an important characteristic that all share. The taxonomy of life forms places the phylum (plural: phyla) at the top of a hierarchy, below which there are divisions into classes, genera (singular: genus), and species. Animals with backbones belong to the phylum Vertebrata (vertebrates); all with exoskeletons are in the phylum Arthropoda. Above the level of phyla are two great kingdoms: plants and animals. The phylum location of some organisms, for example lichens, has not been definitively determined.

physiatry The medical specialty dealing with PHYSICAL MEDICINE and rehabilitation.

physical activity level (PAL) A physiologically based measure of the level of physical activity, defined as total energy expenditure divided by basal metabolic rate. Average PALs in high-income countries are in the range 1.55 to 1.60. To prevent widespread obesity, it is estimated that mean PALs should be raised to 1.75 or greater, an increase that would require a considerable increase in daily energy expenditure. The adverse effects on health of low PALs and increased body fat (to which high dietary fat intake contributes) are an important unresolved public health problem in high-income countries and increasingly in middle- and low-income countries, too.

physical culture A term that describes a regimen of vigorous calisthenics, breathing exercises, dietary guidelines, and life habits, including rest and plentiful hours for sleep, primarily aimed at school children and young adults.

physical examination ("physical") At its simplest, a cursory inspection of heart rate (pulse) and respiratory function by listening to the breath sounds with a stethoscope. A thorough physical examination includes meticulous inspection, palpation, auscultation of the functions of respiratory, cardiovascular, gastrointestinal, neurological, genitourinary, hematological, musculoskeletal, and epidermal systems, reinforced with relevant laboratory and radiological investigations.

physical fitness See FITNESS.

physically handicapped Although the terminology has been superseded, this term is still used to describe persons whose impairment or disability affects their capacity to function in a way expected in the society in which they live. For instance, a person who cannot speak (a disability) cannot readily communicate with others (a handicap). Impaired vision and hearing are common and important forms of physical handicap. As a label, the word "handicapped" is opposed by many people with impairments or disabilities because they feel it reflects societal expectations rather than their actual capacity to function effectively in society.

physical medicine The medical specialty dealing with prevention, diagnosis, and treatment of chronic disabling disorders, especially those affecting the bones and joints but also cardiovascular, neurological, and respiratory disorders, often with emphasis on REHABILITATION.

physician Syn: medical doctor. A professionally qualified person who has had medical school education and supervised training, has passed the necessary qualifying examinations, and is legally licensed to practice medicine, that is, to diagnose, treat, and prevent disease. The period from entering medical school to completion of education and training varies from 6 to 10 years. Most physicians now specialize in a particular field or discipline. There are many recognized specialties, including public health, preventive medicine, and occupational medicine, which have advanced training programs, are assessed by examinations or comparable procedures, and in many instances are periodically reassessed to maintain specialty certification.

physician assistant A trained person who conducts a usually rather narrow range of specific specialized tasks in a physician's office or hospital, with or without supervision by a licensed physician. These tasks include medical history taking using a prepared questionnaire; measuring and recording blood pressure, visual acuity, or results of other clinical tests; and specialized procedures, such as setting up and monitoring intravenous fluid infusions. In public health, a comparable level of training equips field workers for many tasks, especially in low-income nations, e.g., the feldshers of Eastern Europe and the BAREFOOT DOCTORS of China,

now mostly superseded. Physician assistant training and prior background vary considerably. One important category in some jurisdictions is the NURSE PRACTITIONER, a qualified nurse who has had additional training in diagnostic and treatment methods and procedures, although in other jurisdictions nurse practitioners are autonomous, independent health professionals.

physician-assisted suicide A form of euthanasia conducted with the active collaboration of a physician, a procedure that is illegal and unethical in almost all nations but is legal and ethical in the Netherlands, within the terms of very strict guidelines that include written informed consent, the agreement of at least two physicians, and a waiting period between the patient's request and the initiation of the procedure.

Physicians for Social Responsibility (PSR) An international organization of physicians, formerly International Physicians for the Prevention of Nuclear War (IPPNW), which won the Nobel Peace Prize in 1985. Whereas IPPNW was a single-issue organization, PSR has three aims: preserving and protecting the environment and health, promoting human security, and preventing violence, especially violent armed conflict. See http://www.psr.org/.

physics The science dealing with the properties of matter, energy, and radiation, and the laws governing their interactions. Physics is an essential basic science of public health. It is linked to astronomy and mathematics and concerned with answering questions about the nature of matter and energy. The English scientist Isaac Newton (1642–1727) clarified the fundamental laws of motion. In the 20th century, understanding of the nature of matter and of physical laws was transformed by theoretical physicists. The German-Swiss, later American, Nobel laureate Albert Einstein (1879–1955) conceived theories of relativity, and the German physicist Max Planck (1858–1947) conceived the quantum theory. Others who followed them included the teams that developed nuclear weapons and those who discovered the properties of subatomic particles and waves. Several aspects of public health science, notably environmental health, require understanding of physics.

physiology The science concerned with the way the body and its organs and tissues function and with processes that maintain the equilibrium of bodily systems. Many of the advances of medical science from early in the 19th century onward had their roots in physiology or the closely related science of biochemistry, led by the French pioneer CLAUDE BERNARD (1813–1878), Ernest Starling (1866–1927) in England, and others. There are many specialized fields, dealing for instance with the physiology of body systems, cellular physiology, etc.

physiotherapy Syn: physical therapy. The use of physical methods, such as massage, passive movement, heat, etc., to treat conditions that impair physical function. These methods are applied by a physiotherapist, a professionally trained person who is licensed to provide this form of treatment.

phytoplankton Microscopic aquatic organisms relying on chlorophyll-based metabolic systems, plants rather than animals, that are at the base of marine ecosystems and food chains. They have an important role in absorbing atmospheric carbon dioxide. Phytoplankton are sensitive to some widely distributed toxic pollutants and to solar ultraviolet radiation, which can impair their capacity to absorb atmospheric carbon dioxide.

phytotoxin A general term for any toxin of plant origin. The word also describes substances that are toxic to plants.

pica The behavioral aberration of eating dirt, sometimes a symptom of severe mental disorder, a relatively normal behavior of small children who explore and experiment with many new taste sensations. Among toddlers and older children, a dangerous form of pica consists of eating flakes of lead-based paint, which tastes sweet, from peeling walls. This can cause severe, even fatal, lead poisoning.

piece work Work on designated tasks with payment per unit of work completed, often part-time or done in the worker's own home on an informal contractual basis. When piece work consists of cooking batches of food for sale in stores, there may be concerns about standards of hygiene, and many public health departments have local ordinances that address these concerns or alternatively prohibit the practice. Other concerns include health and safety issues of unsupervised work.

pie chart A useful method for the visual display of numerical data by a circular figure in which segments represent the proportions of the total number of entities in each of two or more groups.

pill (the Pill) An ORAL CONTRACEPTIVE (OC), a combination of progesterone and estrogen. The OC pill was developed and field-tested in the early 1950s by the American biologist Gregory Pincus (1903–1967) and colleagues, with financial backing from MARGARET SANGER and others. It has been available throughout most of the world since the early 1960s and has been used by hundreds of millions of women, liberating them from unwanted pregnancies without the inconvenience of contraceptive devices. Epidemiological studies suggest that, if anything, the contraceptive pill is associated with reduced risk of breast cancer, but there is an increased risk of thromboembolic phenomena, especially among smokers and women approaching the end of their reproductive years.

pilot study A small-scale trial or field test to evaluate methods and procedures that will be used in a larger-scale project if the methods work satisfactorily and without adverse consequences.

pineal gland A midline gland at the base of the brain that developmentally resembles the "third eye" of some primitive lizards. It is responsible for production of melatonin, so it plays a role in control of circadian rhythm.

pink disease Syn: acrodynia. A condition of weanling children characterized by limb pain, red scaly skin, irritability, etc. It was so common in the first half of the 20th century that children's hospitals sometimes had whole wards devoted to the care of affected infants. The cause was eventually discovered to be mercury poisoning caused by the use of mercury compounds in teething powders used to soothe children with the symptoms of irritable gums and erupting primary teeth.

pink eye See CONJUNCTIVITIS.

pit privy A safe and simple method to dispose of human excreta, a pit privy is an excavated pit about 2 meters deep beneath a toilet seat, with the whole enclosed in a small shed for privacy and to exclude flies. Lime or ashes may be sprinkled on the contents from time to time to reduce the odor, but disinfectant is not used because it could interfere with the natural biological processes that digest the contents and can make a well-designed pit privy virtually everlasting.

pituitary gland disorders The pituitary gland at the midline base of the skull is sometimes called the leader of the endocrine orchestra because it activates several other endocrine glands: the gonads, the thyroid, the suprarenals. Pituitary tumors may cause overproduction of growth hormone, producing acromegaly or giantism. Inadequate production of growth hormone in childhood causes dwarfism. Hypopituitarism may cause diabetes insipidus due to insufficient production of antidiuretic hormone. Various disorders of reproductive activity may be caused by malfunction of follicle-stimulating hormone or lead to lactation of male breasts. Pituitary gland disorders often disrupt other endocrine gland functions. They may be due to genetic anomalies.

placebo An inert preparation with no pharmacological effect that is used for comparison with an active regimen in a CLINICAL TRIAL to study the outcome of interventions with an experimental drug or innovative regimen. Placebos may have a "placebo effect," a physiological or emotional action attributable to the power of suggestion. The ethical requirement of INFORMED CONSENT obliges investigators to inform participants in placebo-controlled trials that they may receive a placebo rather than the active medication being investigated.

placenta The organ that develops in the lining of the uterus in mammals during pregnancy. It is the vehicle for transfer of oxygen and nutriments to the fetus and carbon dioxide and metabolic waste products from fetus to mother. The placenta blocks transfer of some, but not all, pathogens and toxins to the fetus. It is also an endocrine organ, producing gonadotrophin, estrogen, and progesterone, all essential for maintenance of pregnancy. It is discharged from the uterus after birth of the neonate (and colloquially called the afterbirth) during the third stage of labor. Incomplete separation of the placenta during labor can cause life-threatening hemorrhage. In very early pregnancy, before about the 10th week but after the placenta has formed, it is possible by CHORIONIC VILLUS SAMPLING to test for fetal chromosomal abnormalities.

plagiarism Theft of intellectual property, ideas, or written material composed by someone else and represented as the work of the thief. It is not uncommon in science. It is a serious offense, but it is not always taken seriously because brief quotations of the work of others are acceptable, provided these are acknowledged. It is a fine judgment call to decide what is a "brief" quotation and the firmness of the rules about attribution to the source.

plague A ZOONOSIS (or anthropozoonosis) primarily affecting rats and other rodents that is one of the most dangerous contagious diseases. It is caused by a rod-shaped bacterium, *Yersinia pestis*, transmitted to humans by the bites of rat fleas. The flea bites introduce the pathogen that causes BUBONIC PLAGUE, characterized by acutely painful swellings of lymph glands (buboes); without treatment this has a case fatality rate of 50% to 60%. Plague bacilli are directly transmissible from person to person and can cause pneumonic or septicemic plague, which untreated have case fatality rates of 85% to 95%. There is an effective vaccine, and most cases respond to broad-spectrum antibiotics if immediate treatment is given. Plague is one of the possible candidate diseases of BIOLOGICAL WARFARE, a so-called weapon of mass destruction. See also BLACK DEATH. For more information, see http://www.cdc.gov/ncidod/dvbid/plague/.

plankton A general name for the living creatures at the base of aquatic food chains, comprising PHYTOPLANKTON (plants) and ZOOPLANKTON (animals). Plankton metabolize toxic chemicals such as PCBs, which are further concentrated higher in the food chain. Phytoplankton at the base of the food chain and the plant kingdom is an important component of the global CARBON SINK, metabolizing carbon dioxide.

planned parenthood See FAMILY PLANNING.

Planned Parenthood Federation A private voluntary agency established in 1921 by MARGARET SANGER (1883–1966). Originally called the American Birth Control League, the name was changed in 1939, when the organization became the International Planned Parenthood Federation. There are many national chapters of IPPF. See http://www.ippf.org for details.

plaque A region of discontinuity, a patch or eruption, e.g., atheromatous plaques in large arteries, patches of accreted bacterial deposits on dental enamel.

plasma 1. The liquid component of blood, from which all cells have been removed. It can be used to replace blood loss in an emergency when the blood group is unknown and as the vehicle for injection of antibody. 2. In nuclear physics, a mixture of electrons and positive ions.

plasmid A small particle of genetic material that is separate from a chromosome, can replicate itself, and can confer specific properties on daughter cells.

plasmodium (Plural: plasmodia) The protozoan parasite that lives in human red blood cells and liver cells. It is the causative organism of MALARIA. Plasmodia have an asexual developmental phase in humans and a sexual phase in anopheles mosquitoes.

plaster of Paris A compound of calcium hydrate that sets hard when mixed with water and dried. It was used for more than 100 years to immobilize bones after fractures had been corrected; it is now largely superseded by fiberglass casts, which are lighter and remain rigid when wet.

plasticizers Additives to paint, varnish, and cement that facilitate their application. They include PHTHALATE COMPOUNDS that are reproductive toxins and carcinogens in experimental animals.

platelets The smallest of the three cell types in blood, round or oval non-nucleated cells (about 150,000 to 400,000 per mm^3). Platelets liberate thrombokinase required for blood clotting.

pleura The serous endothelial lining between the lungs and the ribs.

pleurisy Inflammation of the pleura, a condition that sometimes complicates pneumonia and causes severe pain on breathing and coughing.

plumbism The clinical syndrome of chronic LEAD POISONING with colicky abdominal pains, constipation, intellectual dullness, peripheral neuropathy, reticulocytosis, and, among women in the reproductive years, inability to conceive or a history of miscarriages. It is an occupational disease of lead workers, e.g., those exposed to batteries at recycling centers and workers with lead paints, and an environmental disease, e.g., of children and others exposed to flaking lead paint.

plume The trail of smoke, vapor, or other material emanating from a source, such as a smelter stack, and carried by prevailing winds in a particular direction. The term also describes the nuclear fallout zone that follows nuclear explosions or accidents, such as at CHERNOBYL in 1986.

pluralism Cultural and social diversity, and the political climate favoring this trend.

plutonium (Pu) A radioactive element produced from uranium in a NUCLEAR REACTOR. It is the active ingredient in nuclear weapons. By nuclear fission, it produces isotopes, some of which have a half-life of as long as 75 million years and are among the most poisonous substances known.

PM10, PM2.5 Particulate matter that is 10 microns in size or smaller or 2.5 microns or smaller, respectively. Particles of less than 10 microns can be inhaled, and particles of less than 2.5 microns can penetrate to and lodge in alveolar spaces when inhaled.

pneumococcus vaccine A vaccine prepared from purified polysaccharides of *Streptococcus pneumoniae* that has been useful in elderly people to provide some protection against this form of pneumonia. A vaccine that confers longer-lasting immunity is prepared from polysaccharides that have been conjugated with protein and can be given to infants and children. For more information, see http://www.who.int/vaccines/en/pneumo coccus.shtml.

pneumoconiosis A general term for a fibrotic lung disease induced by inhaling particles of dust. The principal varieties are ANTHRACOSIS, ASBESTOSIS, and SILICOSIS, caused by inhaling coal dust, asbestos fibers, and silica dust, respectively.

Pneumocystis carinii A common and usually innocuous microorganism that causes a serious, often ultimately fatal, disease described as OPPORTUNISTIC INFECTION in immunocompromised individuals, typically persons infected with HIV, in whom *Pneumocystis carinii* pneumonia is common. See http://www.cdc.gov/ncidod/dpd/parasites/pneumocystis/default.htm for details.

pneumonia An inflammatory disease of lung tissue caused by bacteria or viruses in which the alveolar spaces fill with fluid and impair the ability to exchange air efficiently. Classic pneumonia causes consolidation, in which the alveolar fluid turns to a jelly-like solid substance that is lethal if extensive, but antibiotics have made this uncommon. Pneumonia is a common terminal illness among the elderly and in debilitated patients. Pathological changes resembling those caused by pneumonia can also occur after inhalation of smoke and toxic fumes.

pneumonic plague See PLAGUE.

pneumonitis A general term for an inflammatory disease of the lungs that does not cause the alveoli and bronchi to become consolidated with fluid, i.e., is usually less serious than pneumonia.

podiatry The specialty concerned with diagnosis and treatment of disorders of the feet, also known in Britain as CHIROPODY.

point prevalence See PREVALENCE.

point source A single identifiable person or place and time that is the origin of an EPIDEMIC.

poison A substance that causes life-threatening disruption of essential physiological functions when ingested, inhaled, injected, or absorbed through the skin. Usage is loose, but the usual distinction between a poison and a TOXIN is that toxins are derived from living organisms and they usually do not have life-threatening effects unless ignored, untreated, or neglected. Poisons may be of organic or inorganic origin. Many varieties are recognized, e.g., corrosive, metabolic, genetic, neurotoxic, carcinogenic, mutagenic, teratogenic, fast-acting, slow-acting.

poison control center An agency, usually at a state, municipal, or other large regional level, that is a clearinghouse for reporting cases of acute, subacute, and chronic poisoning, staffed by physicians trained in toxicology or by toxicologists who are available on call on a 24-hour, 7-day-a-week basis to provide detailed information and advice about emergency treatment, antidotes, aftercare, and prevention and control regimens, including public education.

Poisson distribution A distribution function to describe rare events, or the sampling distribution of isolated counts in a continuum of space or time, such as cases of uncommon diseases. The name is that of the French mathematician Siméon Denis Poisson (1781–1840), who adapted an earlier version by Abraham de Moivre (1667–1754), who first described it.

polarization 1. Aligning electric and magnetic fields of electromagnetic waves, as in polarized light, which oscillates in only one plane. This is accomplished by passing light through a polarizer consisting of a prism or crystal plate that separates light waves into planes. 2. A sharp, extreme divergence of emotional, social, and political opinions about an issue, for example about a woman's right to choose when and whether to become and remain pregnant.

polarized light Light waves, i.e., electromagnetic radiation in the visible spectrum, in which all light waves oscillate in the same plane rather than as light waves usually do, in all 360 degrees. This has advantages that include reduced glare.

police power The authority conferred on public health officials by laws and local regulations to take action to protect the health of the public. It includes the power to detain persons diagnosed with contagious diseases that endanger others and has in the past included the authority to enter and search premises to seize persons who have or are in contact with certain contagious diseases. Overzealous use of police powers in the early 20th century, to search homes and seize healthy child contacts of cases of diphtheria, typhoid, or poliomyelitis, received unfavorable publicity that sometimes gave public health authorities an unsavory reputation. Police power is seldom invoked today but has been used occasionally to restrain irresponsible promiscuous individuals with diagnosed HIV disease.

policy A course or principle of action adopted or proposed by a government, party, business, or individual; the written or unwritten aims, OBJECTIVES, TARGETS, STRATEGY, tactics, and plans that guide the actions of a government or an organization. Policies have three interconnected and ideally continually evolving stages: development, implementation, and evaluation. Policy development is the creative process of identifying and establishing a policy to meet a particular need or situation. Policy implementation consists of the actions taken to set up or modify a policy, and evaluation is assessment of how, and how well, the policy works in practice.

policy statement A written statement recording the policies of an organization. Such statements aim to summarize policies concisely and clearly. They often present the consensus of a group or committee with diverse views, but those who draft them have a duty to make them as clear and unequivocal as possible. Policy statements are intended to guide those within an organization and sometimes to inform others about the aims, purposes, and methods of the organization.

poliomyelitis Syn: infantile paralysis. A contagious virus disease transmitted by the fecal-oral route that usually is associated with symptomless development of antibodies but can cause acute inflammation and disruption of function of the anterior horns of spinal nerves, causing paralysis of the muscles controlled by these nerves. Three varieties of the polio virus, designated types 1, 2, and 3, can cause paralytic poliomyelitis. Paralytic poliomyelitis can be prevented by vaccination with killed organisms in the SALK VACCINE or ingestion of live attenuated SABIN VACCINE.

poliomyelitis eradication The polio virus is an obligate human parasite. Therefore, it can be eradicated from the population by mass vaccination of all susceptible individuals. Campaigns to accomplish this have been successful in the Americas, Europe, Australasia, and in most countries in Africa and Asia. In 2002, only seven countries (Afghanistan, Egypt, India, Niger, Nigeria, Pakistan, and Somalia) reported indigenous cases. Unfortunately, political factors disrupted the polio vaccination campaign in Nigeria after 2002 and led to return of paralytic poliomyelitis in 18 countries (Yemen, Indonesia, and 16 African nations). A WHO/UNICEF/CDC initiative aims to eradicate polio worldwide. See http://www.polioeradication.org/.

polio virus vaccines See SABIN VACCINE and SALK VACCINE.

political correctness Careful choice of words in spoken and written communications and actions, intended to avoid giving offense to ethnic, racial, cultural, or sexually oriented groups, disabled persons, and other designated groups that may be stigmatized. The aim is worthy, but implementing it can lead to circumlocution or mealy-mouthed utterances and subtle shifts in the meaning of words. An example is replacement of the suffix "man" in genderless words, such as chairman or alderman, by neologisms, such as chairperson, often abbreviated to chair.

political economy The aspect of government concerned with the systematic study of the nature and causes of the wealth of nations. The term is often used loosely to describe political aspects of economic policy making and the economic implications that should be considered in public policy and decision making, but often without actual economic analysis. Public health policy and resource allocation for health systems are integral parts of policy making, so the political economy of public health systems is an important aspect of public health planning.

politics A set of activities associated with governance, organization, and running of public affairs at local, regional, national, and international levels. It is essential for public health professionals to comprehend health-related political factors because health and politics are entwined. Politics is the art of getting things done, but what is done is not always rational or just. It may be the action that is most expedient, least costly, or most agreeable to the dominant political party or an influential pressure group. It is a field of human endeavor that is often full of sound and fury, signifying nothing. In *The Devil's Dictionary* (1906), the American writer Ambrose Bierce (1842–1914?) described politics as "a strife of interests masquerading as a contest of principles; the conduct of public affairs for private advantage." The last phrase describes how politics is sometimes conducted, and this can have unfortunate consequences for health and social policy that it is in the public interest to pursue.

pollen Plant spores mainly of microscopic size carried long distances by wind. As they are plant protein, they are usually antigenic in action, and some induce severe allergies. In communities where high proportions of people experience these allergies, weather forecasts often include the pollen count during relevant seasons.

pollutant An undesirable solid, liquid, or gaseous substance that contaminates soil, food, water, clothing, or the atmosphere with a toxic or noxious substance or agent. Common pollutants include human and animal waste; toxic industrial waste products and by-products, notably many from the petrochemical industry; and heavy metals (lead, mercury) and their compounds.

polluter pays principle The principle that the industrial corporation or persons responsible for causing environmental contamination must pay the costs of cleaning up, controlling the cause, and preventing further fouling of the environment. While this is desirable, it is not always possible to identify the source, and many polluting industries are able to evade responsibility.

pollution Contamination or undesirable modification of soil, food, water, clothing, or the atmosphere by a noxious or toxic substance. Any form of pollution can have adverse effects on health. The varieties with the most widespread adverse effects are outdoor air pollution, drinking water pollution, and INDOOR AIR POLLUTION.

Pollution Prevention and Control (PPC) A system of integrated pollution management for certain industrial activities that is taking effect in the United Kingdom during the period 2000 to 2007. It has introduced the concept of "best available techniques" to environmental regulations and replaces the previous system of integrated pollution control. For details of this system, see http://www.defra.gov.uk/environment/ppc/.

polybrominated biphenyls (PBBs) PBBs were used as fire retardants to impregnate fabrics to render them less flammable but were found to be carcinogenic to animals and banned. The chemicals were responsible for a regional episode of animal poisoning in Michigan in 1978, when a batch of PBB-contaminated cattle feed caused a bizarre wasting disease in cattle and equally bizarre neuropsychiatric symptoms in people who drank milk or ate meat from the affected cattle.

polychlorinated biphenyls (PCBs) A class of complex chlorinated hydrocarbons that includes several of considerable commercial and industrial importance. They have been widely used as insulators, wood sealants, and plasticizers, and in carbonless copying paper and many other applications. Although the evidence is controversial, they are suspected human carcinogens and also implicated in birth deformities. Acute exposure causes skin eruptions called CHLORACNE, neurological symptoms, and endocrine disorders. They are environmentally persistent and can be destroyed only by high-temperature incineration.

polychlorinated dibenzo-p-dioxin See DIOXINS.

polycyclic aromatic hydrocarbons (PAHs) A miscellaneous group of complex hydrocarbon compounds that are ingredients of emission of biomass fuels and combusted tobacco. They include several confirmed carcinogens.

polygenic A pattern of inheritance, also called multifactorial inheritance, involving multiple interacting genes. Some important individual characteristics, including height, eye color, and extent of skin pigmentation, are determined not by a single gene but by many genes, each having a small effect individually. Characteristics controlled in this way show continuous variation.

polymer A long-chain molecule comprising several or many smaller molecules, or monomers.

polymerase chain reaction (PCR) A laboratory technique to copy strands of DNA molecules in order to magnify the amount present through multiple replications and thereby achieve concentrations high enough to permit testing for specific DNA molecules.

polymer fume fever An occupational disease that occurs among workers with polymers, causing asthma and intermittent fever.

polymorphism 1. Occurrence of an organism in different forms at different stages of its life cycle. 2. Occurrence of naturally occurring variations in the DNA sequence of a gene, which sometimes contributes to varying susceptibility to pathogens, chemical toxins, or other hazards.

polysaccharides Carbohydrates with high molecular weight, such as starches and cellulose, that metabolize to monosaccharides, such as simple sugars.

polyunsaturated fats A dietary ingredient, polyunsaturated fats have two or more double bonds and are inherently unstable, therefore liable to rancidity in the absence of antioxidants. They occur mainly in vegetable fats, and consuming them in place of saturated fats tends to have a favorable effect on blood cholesterol concentrations. The process of "hardening" of vegetable oils, as formerly done in the manufacture of margarine, reduced the proportion of double bonds, saturating the fats and making them more likely to have an adverse effect on blood lipids.

polyvinyl chloride (PVC) A widely used clear plastic compound derived from VINYL CHLORIDE. PVC is inert and not readily biodegradable, but its manufacture exposes workers to the hazards of hemangiosarcoma, acroosteolysis, and POLYMER FUME FEVER.

ponderal index An anthropometric measure of body mass, defined as height divided by the cube root of weight. This is regarded as less satisfactory than the BODY MASS INDEX.

Pontiac fever An acute nonpulmonary form of LEGIONNAIRES DISEASE (legionellosis) caused by infection with *Legionella pneumophila*. It is usually a self-limited disease lasting 3 to 5 days. It is named for the town in Michigan where it was first identified as a distinct disease.

pooling Aggregation of data and/or results from two or more sources or studies.

poorhouse Syn: almshouse, homeless shelter (obsolete). An institutional system of shelter for the destitute funded by private charities or from local or regional government sources. The term is obsolete, but the need for this system of subsidized shelter remains considerable in nations with widening gaps between rich and poor and the increasing prevalence of HOMELESSNESS.

poor laws (obsolete) Originally a series of harsh laws that punished poor people by incarcerating them in debtors' prisons; this term is now applied to any legislative measure aimed at providing relief and social care for people in severe poverty, such as WELFARE laws.

poppers A slang expression for amyl nitrate inhalants that are used to induce euphoria. They cause respiratory irritation and are said to impair the immune system. Their use is mainly confined to circumscribed groups, such as members of the gay community. They are also used by some drug addicts.

popular culture The entertainments, media, that are believed to appeal to most people. Television is the popular cultural medium in the early 21st century, and its star performers are often OPINION LEADERS. Public health workers who seek to communicate important messages to the general public, e.g., about the wisdom of refraining from tobacco use, are wise to identify and recruit opinion leaders of popular culture to convey their message.

population All the inhabitants of a country or other designated region. In public health sciences, especially in epidemiology, many subsets of the entire population are identified and selected for intervention and study. Such a group is called a TARGET POPULATION.

population at risk In epidemiological studies, the actual group of people that can be precisely defined in numbers, and preferably also in regard to other characteristics, in which the occurrence of specified events is studied.

population attributable risk The risk of a specified disease or other outcome of interest in a defined population that can be attributed to an exposure of interest. The term implies a risk, i.e., a probability, but attributable risk is often expressed loosely as a proportion or fraction of the total risk of interest that can be attributed to the exposure of interest.

population control A term for FAMILY PLANNING that is preferably avoided because it implies an authoritarian approach and an emphasis on discouraging unrestrained human reproduction.

population density A measure of the number of people in a defined jurisdiction in relation to the size of the jurisdiction. For instance, Singapore has a population density of 6,400 persons per 1,000 hectares, which is very high; Australia has a low population density of 24 persons per 1,000 hectares.

population dynamics The process by which changes occur in the composition of a population through births, deaths, migrations, and related observable social and economic changes.

population explosion A surge in the natural rate of increase in numbers of people caused by reduction in infant and child death rates and an increase in the proportion of the population in reproductive age groups. The increased numbers of reproductively active couples combines with behavioral factors, such as optimism about the future or attitudes regarding desired family size, to increase the fertility rates of populations. An example was the postwar BABY BOOM that began in 1946. Similar surges in numbers of births had less favorable outcomes in Sub-Saharan Africa, where population growth outstripped available resources. See DEMOGRAPHIC TRAP.

population genetics The study of the genetic composition of populations; studies of gene frequencies and selective factors that influence them are the main aims.

population health The health of the population, measured by health status indicators. Population health is influenced by physical, biological, behavioral, social, cultural, economic, and other factors. The term is also used to refer to the prevailing health level of the population, or a specified subset of the population, or the level to which the population aspires. Population health describes the state of health, and PUBLIC HEALTH is the range of practices, procedures, methods, institutions, and disciplines required to achieve it. The term also is used to describe the academic disciplines involved in studies of determinants and dynamics of health status of the population.

population laboratory A community that has been identified, delineated, its numbers counted, and its characteristics documented in order that it can be used as the setting for genetic, biological, behavioral, epidemiological, or other studies, usually over a period of years or even decades. Examples include Framingham, Massachusetts; Tecumseh, Michigan; and Peckham, England.

population medicine An alternative term proposed as a replacement for PUBLIC HEALTH that, like several others, including "community medicine," "social medicine," and "public health medicine," may be as much an indication of insecurity of medically qualified public health professionals about their roles and responsibilities as an attempt to find a phrase that describes the nature of the work of public health specialists. It is sometimes linked to the concept of "population as patient" or to the practice of clinical preventive medicine with a combination of formal screening programs and ad hoc or opportunistic screening tests to detect early evidence of treatable conditions such as high blood pressure, diabetes, and cancer of the breast.

population prevented risk The proportion of the total risk of an exposure of interest that would exist in a specified population if that population were not protected by the exposure of interest. An example is the proportion of heart attacks expected in a population that does not consume alcohol that are prevented by exposure of a proportion of the population to moderate alcohol drinking.

population pyramid A diagrammatic representation of the age and sex composition of a population, e.g., of a country at a particular period of time. The diagram shows the proportions or the actual numbers in each age and sex division, conventionally with males on the left, females on the right. The shape of the "pyramid" (or profile) varies with the age composition of the population. When birth rates are high and death rates at all ages are also high, the shape is pyramidal. When birth rates are low and death rates in infancy and childhood are low, higher proportions survive to old age, producing a shape that is not pyramidal but tends toward, and in extreme instances becomes, top heavy.

porphyria The name of several disorders affecting the synthesis of the hemoglobin molecule characterized by excessive secretion of porphyrins or their precursors. The causes may be an inherited genetic defect or biochemical disruption of porphyrin metabolism caused by exposure to specific chemicals such as hexachlorobenzene.

porphyrins A class of pigmented organic compounds that include chlorophyll, heme (from which comes hemoglobin), and cytochrome. Disruptions of porphyrin metabolism include inheritable and acquired disorders with generalized effects. e.g., periodic psychosis.

positron A positively charged subatomic beta (β) particle with mass and charge equal to but opposite from that of an electron.

positron emission tomography Syn: PET scan. A diagnostic imaging technique using streams of positrons, which are passed through tissue into which radioactive trace amounts of biochemically active compounds have been infused. This produces images that reveal the metabolic activity of the tissue during the very brief half-life of the radioactive compound. It is a useful diagnostic technique that is claimed to be free of any risk of exposure to excessive ionizing radiation.

postmortem Syn: autopsy. 1. A pathological examination of a dead body that aims to discover the exact cause of death. The emphasis is on gross anatomical changes and on the microscopic appearance of tissues and organs that have been affected by disease. In cases where foul play is suspected, a wide range of investigations in the field of forensic pathology are also conducted; such investigations are the topic of many popular television series. See also FORENSIC MEDICINE, PATHOLOGY, and VERBAL AUTOPSY. 2. Any inquiry conducted after the fact to determine what happened.

postnatal, postpartum Descriptive of the state of having recently given birth to a child or of having recently been born.

post-traumatic stress disorder Syn: battle neurosis. A psychiatric disorder characterized by symptoms including sleeplessness, nightmares, depression, emotional lability, and behavioral aberrations. It not uncommonly occurs among soldiers and others who have been directly involved in violent armed conflicts, and among other people who have had direct personal experience of violent events involving death and serious injury of other people, as in disasters, or who have been subjected to TORTURE. Information is available at several Web sites, such as one offered by the US Veterans Administration at http://www.ncptsd.va.gov/ and one by the National Mental Health Association at http://www.nmha.org/reassurance/ptsd.cfm.

postulate A proposition that has been demonstrated to be true by empirical observation or that is assumed to be true without need for further proof.

potable The quality of water that is safe to drink without danger of bacterial or chemical contamination.

potassium (K) An extremely reactive silvery metallic element that combines readily with many other elements and compounds, e.g., exploding on contact with water to produce potassium hydroxide. It is the body's principal cation, an essential nutrient, and an essential trace element in metabolism of vertebrates, including humans, and in nerve and muscle function.

potential years of life lost (PYLL) A measure of the effect of diseases and injuries in reducing the life span below national or a hypothetical ideal (COUNTERFACTUAL) life expectancy. The PYLL is computed for specific causes of death by summing the expected years of life remaining (according to a reference table) for each individual age at death for the cause of interest. The effect is greatest for causes operating strongly at young ages, such as AIDS, fatal vehicular injuries, and homicides in young black males in the United States. PYLL do not take disability into account and, to that extent, are a less useful measure than DISABILITY-ADJUSTED LIFE YEARS (DALYs).

potentiation Enhancing the power or efficacy of a substance, especially in neurophysiology and in relation to actions of a drug, by combining it with another with which it has a synergistic action. A process required to consolidate memory, promoted by opiates, norepinephrine, and dopamine. More generally, the synergistic interaction of two substances or events to produce an effect that is greater than the effect of either in its own.

poverty The condition of having insufficient resources to obtain or provide the necessities of life. People afflicted with poverty are especially vulnerable to adverse events they cannot control and often lack political influence and access to needed health and social services. The World Bank defines poverty in low-income nations as an income of US $1 per day or less. In the Organization for Economic Cooperation and Development (OECD) nations, poverty is arbitrarily defined as financial income below a specific level, which varies from one nation to another and from year to year, depending on the cost of living. This is useful for administrative and statistical purposes, but it falls short of explaining frequently associated misfortunes, particularly poor health, which may be either a cause or a consequence of poverty of financial resources. Useful sources are http://www.undp.org/poverty/ and the World Bank's *World Development Report* 2000–2001. See also POVERTY CLASSIFICATION AND MEASUREMENT.

poverty classification and measurement Social workers and others involved in supporting persons and families in poverty find classification according to income level inadequate. Income poverty is only one dimension of the problem and may be a consequence as often as a cause of the underlying problem, which may be unemployment, physical or mental impairment and handicap, environmental conditions such as severe prolonged drought, or disruption of or dispossession from customary habitat, e.g., by violent conflict. Behavioral scientists further distinguish features that include social and cultural poverty, i.e., lack of connectedness to society and community, and moral poverty, i.e., absence of moral values, such as attachment to family and others. Disparity across income groups, as measured by the GINI COEFFICIENT, is used with the classification system.

poverty reduction strategies A range of actions available to public health and other agencies to alleviate poverty. These include provision of educational services and facilities, empowering poor people in ways that enable them to gain greater control over their own destiny, enhance their self-esteem, and achieve greater success in finding work. In low-income countries, the provision of small interest-free or low-interest loans, i.e., microcredit schemes, to impoverished people to enable them to make modest capital investments, to purchase a bicycle to get to work or a sewing machine for a woman to make clothes, is an effective strategy, as shown by the Grameen Bank in Bangladesh and similar programs. See http://www. grameen-info.org/.

poverty threshold An income level below which it is deemed impossible in a specified setting to meet basic human needs for food, shelter, clothing, and support of dependent family members. This is a relative term with considerable variation from one locality to another.

poverty trap The condition in which poor families cannot escape from poverty because they lack the financial resources, intellectual ability, social skills, or guidance from community agencies that might enable them to do so. This is a sadly common fate of single-parent, mother-led families subsisting on WELFARE, one condition of which is that the welfare payments cease if there is any other source of income.

power 1. In statistics, the capacity of a scientific study to demonstrate the strength of statistical association between variables. 2. Energy, derived from combustion of carbon-based or other fuel or from hydroelectric or nuclear generation. 3. Political power is the exercise of authority by whatever means is possible in a political system.

poxvirus A family of viruses (Poxviridae), of which the most common is the poxvirus that causes molluscum contagiosum, a direct-contact disease that is often, but not always, sexually transmitted.

practice guidelines See CLINICAL PRACTICE GUIDELINES.

precautionary principle In management of health risks, shaping of health policy, and all public policy decisions, this is the conservative, "better safe than sorry" approach that wisdom dictates should be the rule when there is any doubt about long-term consequences of irreversible decisions affecting control of the environment or a situation. It is a variation on the theme of the ethical principle of nonmaleficence, *primum non nocere*, or first do no harm.

PRECEDE-PROCEED model These acronyms spell out in summary form five steps in planning and evaluating a health promotion program. The letters PRECEDE stand for predisposing, reinforcing, and enabling constructs in educational diagnosis and evaluation; PROCEED stands for policy, regulatory, and organizational constructs in educational and environmental development. This is a conceptual model for assessing health and quality-of-life needs and for designing, implementing, and evaluating health promotion and other public health programs to meet these needs, described by Lawrence Green and others in *Health Education Planning* (1980).

precipitate The solid matter that descends to the bottom of a liquid when dissolved solids come out of solution in the process of precipitation.

precision In measurements, the quality of being exact or sharply defined. A measurement of length to decimal places of millimeters is more precise than a measurement to the nearest meter. Precision or exactness must be distinguished from ACCURACY, i.e., conformity to the true or real value.

preclinical sciences Syn: basic medical sciences. In medical education, this term is applied to the disciplines that traditionally have been studied before students are introduced to patient care, comprising the natural and biological sciences, gross and microscopic anatomy, biochemistry, cell biology, genetics, physiology, microbiology, and sciences at the interface with clinical studies, pathology, pharmacology, and epidemiology. In medical education by problem-based learning, traditional divisions are blurred. Students learn by coordinated studies of basic and clinical sciences, along with social and behavioral sciences and, in some schools, humanities.

precursor In the natural history of disease, a precursor is an anatomical, physiological, or biochemical state that precedes the onset of identifiable pathological changes. For example, elevated serum cholesterol levels are a precursor of atheromatous arterial changes.

predictive value In diagnostic and screening tests, the predictive value of a positive test is the probability that person whose test result is positive actually has the disease or condition for which the test was done. The predictive value of a negative test result is the probability that a person with a negative test result does not have the disease or condition for which the test was done. Predictive value is influenced by the prevalence of the condition or trait being investigated.

preferred provider organization (PPO) A prepaid health insurance plan that designates the physicians, other health professionals, clinics, and hospitals for which it will reimburse charges for services rendered.

pregnancy The physiological condition in which a fertilized ovum implants in the uterine mucosa and grows into a fetus and placenta that are expelled from the uterus after the gestational period has ended. For most women, pregnancy is a normal physiological process, but there are many ways in which the process can go wrong and that justify emphasis on antenatal care.

premature birth A loose term to describe a birth that occurs before the normal duration of pregnancy has been reached. Birth weight is preferred as an indicator of a neonatal infant's survival potential. Infants of LOW BIRTH WEIGHT often have a poor prognosis.

premature death Theoretically any death that occurs before average life expectancy is achieved could be called "premature," but because that would not allow for a range around the average, the term is usually reserved for deaths that occur a considerable but undefined number of years before average life expectancy is achieved. Thus, death in childhood falls in the category of premature death. The term is usually applied to death in relatively early adult life, such as violent death from accident, suicide, homicide; death caused by cancer, heart disease, stroke before the average age at which such deaths occur; and death caused by infection, such as HIV/AIDS. In calculating DALYs, the LIFE EXPECTANCY in Japan is taken as the benchmark by which life expectancy in other countries is lower, so premature death is more likely.

premenstrual tension A syndrome characterized by emotional lability, depression, loss of interest in usual activities, and other mood or personality changes, sometimes with physical discomfort. Some women experience it after ovulation and before the onset of the menstrual period. Rarely, this condition can impair judgment and interfere with fitness for work.

prenatal period The period (months or weeks) preceding the birth of a neonate, not precisely defined either statistically or biologically but often assumed to be from about 28 weeks' gestation until the onset of labor.

prepatent period The period in a parasitic infection analogous to the incubation period of a bacterial infection, when the parasite has invaded the human host but has not yet caused pathological changes that reveal its presence by causing symptoms.

presbyopia Long-sightedness, a common condition in middle age, caused by loss of the ability to accommodate the shape of the lenses of the eyes for close vision, usually requiring corrective spectacles and gradually progressive with increasing age.

prescription Strictly speaking, a written directive from a physician to a pharmacist, describing the medication that the physician wants the patient to take, along with its dose and frequency of use.

prescription drug Medication that is usually available from a pharmacy only on presentation of a prescription signed by a licensed physician or other health care professional. Generally, these cost more than over-the-counter drugs, and prices are higher for proprietary than generic drugs.

preservative A substance, such as a chemical additive, that prolongs the period during which a food item will remain free from deterioration, putrefaction, etc., and therefore will be safe to eat. Traditional preservatives include salt (strong saline solution) and syrup (strong sugar solution). Both alter the flavor, appearance, and nutritional value of preserved foods.

pressure group An organization or association of people, commonly large and well organized, that exerts or attempts to exert influence over democratically elected officials in order to bring about a desired political decision. Many pressure groups seek to influence the outcome of political decisions about matters affecting the health sector. An American example was the campaign orchestrated by a coalition of several interest groups that successfully obstructed the passage of legislation to provide comprehensive health insurance coverage in the United States in the early years of the Clinton administration.

prevalence The total number of designated conditions, such as cases of a disease or patterns of behavior, that are present in a population at a point in time, regardless of the duration of time for which the condition or disease has been experienced by individuals in the population. This is often called point prevalence, in contrast to period prevalence, which describes the total number that are present for at least part of a designated period of time, usually a calendar year. See also INCIDENCE and CUMULATIVE INCIDENCE RATE.

prevented risk in the exposed The additional risk of a disease or other outcome of interest that would have occurred among exposed persons in a defined population if they had not been protected by the protective exposure of interest. See also POPULATION PREVENTED RISK.

prevention Policies and actions to eliminate a disease or minimize its effect; to reduce the incidence and/or prevalence of disease, disability, and premature death; to reduce the prevalence of disease precursors and risk factors in the population; and, if none of these is feasible, to retard the progress of incurable disease. Several levels or categories of prevention are defined, but in some situations the distinction is more artificial than real. PRIMORDIAL PREVENTION includes elimination of predisposing risk factors, such as environmental control of disease vectors, and predisposing factors, such as illiteracy and maternal deprivation. PRIMARY PREVENTION includes protection from effects of exposure to a disease agent, e.g., vaccination against infectious pathogens. Secondary prevention includes the use of SCREENING TESTS or other suitable procedures to detect serious disease as early as possible so that its progress can be arrested and, if possible, the disease eradicated. An example is the PAP TEST to screen for cancer of the cervix. TERTIARY prevention includes interventions aimed at arresting the progress of established disease.

prevention paradox A term coined by the British epidemiologist Geoffrey Rose (1926–1993) to refer to the fact that while public health measures such as smoking cessation and more exercise demonstrably improve population health, they may have little or no effect on a specific individual's health. See also ECOLOGICAL FALLACY.

preventive medicine The specialized branch of clinical medical practice devoted to promoting health and preventing disease and premature disability. Activities aimed at promoting health may operate at the personal level and at the level of communities and populations. The clinical specialty practice of preventive medicine requires competence in biostatistics; epidemiology; administration, including planning, organization, management, financing, and evaluation of health programs; environmental health; and understanding and application of knowledge about social and behavioral factors in health and disease, food and nutrition, workplace hazards, and the application of primary, secondary, and tertiary prevention measures in clinical medicine. The AMERICAN COLLEGE OF PREVENTIVE MEDICINE provides a definition and information about the specialty at its Web site, http://www.acpm.org.

Preventive Services Task Force The US Public Health Service's expert committee that was established in 1984, following the lead of the CANADIAN TASK FORCE ON THE PERIODIC HEALTH EXAMINATION. The task force of some 20 experts studied and made recommendations about a wide range of strategies, tactics, methods, and procedures to promote health and prevent disease, injury, and premature death, with emphasis on the role of clinicians. In 1989, its first large report described 169 preventive interventions, providing evidence on the efficacy of each. There have since been many additional recommendations. See http://www.ahrq .gov/clinic/uspstfix.htm.

preventive strategies Approaches to elimination or control of disease, injury, and premature death based on the concept of primordial, primary, secondary, and tertiary prevention, i.e., on the removal or reduction of predisposing and precipitating causes, detection at the earliest possible stage in the natural development and evolution of disease, and, when these fail, provision of the best possible therapeutic regimens to minimize the risk of deterioration or complications.

prickly heat An urticarial skin rash mainly affecting infants, associated with hot, poorly ventilated conditions, and wearing damp clothes, diapers, etc.

primary health care 1. The WHO defines primary health care as essential health care made accessible at a cost that the country can afford, with methods that are practical, scientifically sound, and socially acceptable. Everyone should have access to it and be involved in it, as should other sectors of society. It should include community participation and education on prevalent health problems, health promotion and disease prevention, provision of adequate food and nutrition, safe water, basic sanitation, maternal and child care, family planning, prevention and control of endemic diseases, immunization against vaccine-preventable diseases, appropriate treatment of common diseases and injuries, and provision of essential drugs. 2. Health care, or medical care, that begins at the time of the first contact between a physician or other health professional and a person seeking advice or treatment for an illness or injury. It is provided by nonspecialized physicians and other health workers. In upper-income countries, it may be mainly a GATEKEEPER role with referral to specialists for high proportions of those seen, but for most of the world's population it is the only available health care, often called primary medical care.

primary prevention Strategies, tactics, and procedures that prevent the occurrence of disease. Examples include provision of safe drinking water; sanitation and hygiene; the use of immunizations or vaccinations that confer immunity against certain communicable diseases; and mass medication, such as use of iodized salt to prevent the occurrence of cretinism and goiter in iodine-deficient regions.

primordial prevention Strategies and tactics that eliminate exposure to significant risk factors of disease, e.g., genetic counseling to avoid unions of partners carrying lethal recessive genes. The distinction between primordial prevention and primary prevention is ill-defined, and many people consider the term "primordial prevention" to be an unnecessary addition to the language.

principle of scientific parsimony See OCCAM'S RAZOR.

prion Infectious proteinaceous particle, a protein molecule discovered by the American neurologist Stanley Prusiner (b. 1942), who coined the word and in 1997 received a Nobel Prize for his work on it. Prions have some of the properties of viruses and are the agents of several deadly forms of TRANSMISSIBLE SPONGIFORM ENCEPHALOPATHIES, including kuru, BOVINE SPONGIFORM ENCEPHALOPATHY (BSE), and CREUTZFELDT-JAKOB DISEASE.

Pritikin diet A dietary regimen rich in complex carbohydrates, such as whole grains, fruit, and vegetables, with restricted fat, protein, salt, sugar, and coffee, devised by the American scientist Nathan Pritikin (1917–1985) in 1958 to treat his own coronary heart disease by reducing cholesterol intake. Its efficacy is uncertain as few systematic evaluations have been conducted.

privacy The condition of freedom from public attention or scrutiny, one of the basic rights specified in the UNIVERSAL DECLARATION OF HUMAN RIGHTS. Privacy is sometimes threatened or violated by public health measures, and some essential measures are resented, such as partner notification in cases of sexually transmitted diseases, which is often perceived as excessively intrusive and inadequately limited by legal or ethical constraints.

private sector A general term for those aspects of the economy that function by means of the purchase and sale of goods and services to generate the income required for subsistence (or better than mere subsistence), as contrasted with the PUBLIC SECTOR, which requires financial support from collective, i.e., government, resources. It is a central tenet of capitalist philosophy and ideology that the private, implicitly profit-making, sector is more efficient than the public sector, but this is manifestly not universally true, notably in the financial and administrative structure of health services, and has not been adequately tested by controlled experiment in educational services, where publicly funded systems are generally more equitable than the private sector.

privatization The process of moving an agency, service, or entire sector of society from public or governmental ownership into the private sector, where it usually becomes a profit-oriented activity. The process is often ideologically driven at the political level, rather than based on objective analysis of the fiscal, economic, and social facts, which may demonstrate greater efficiency and more favorable outcomes of public rather than private ownership and administration of health and education sectors of society.

privileged communication A term that is intended to mean much the same as "personal and confidential" or "protected," i.e., that a document is intended only for certain persons who are privileged to see it because of the position they occupy.

probability A measure that ranges from zero to 1 of the likelihood that a random event will occur or the degree to which a statement or assumption is true. This must lie between 0 and 1: the probability is 0 if the event is certain not to occur, 1 if it is certain to occur. Predictions such as disease prognosis in clinical medicine are derived from past experience. In public health, the future course of an epidemic can sometimes be expressed in terms of probability in a similar way or how frequently events of this type have occurred, or projected from theoretical models. The design and interpretation of results of clinical trials use statistical tests to assess the probability that observed differences between study and control groups might have occurred by chance. Case control and cohort studies likewise apply probability theory to interpret results and derive inferences about conclusions from such studies. See also NULL HYPOTHESIS and RANDOM.

probability distribution A mathematical function that states the probabilities of a random variable having each of a sequence of possible values. Examples include the NORMAL, BINOMIAL, and POISSON DISTRIBUTIONS.

probability sample Synonym for RANDOM SAMPLE.

proband Syn: PROPOSITUS. The person in a family PEDIGREE whose condition first draws attention to the existence in that pedigree of a genetic trait that may affect other members of the same pedigree.

problem-based learning An educational method that has become increasingly popular in medical and some other health professional training programs since the 1980s. It departs from conventional systematic study of separate disciplines and subjects and is based on presentation to students of problems resembling those encountered in practice. Students integrate knowledge and skills from all disciplines that are relevant to the problem, to arrive at diagnostic decisions and formulate therapeutic regimens. The method is claimed to be more enjoyable and interesting than conventional teaching. The end results, as judged by objective examinations, are about the same. It is claimed that the method encourages the habit of lifelong learning by recourse to reference material in current medical journals. There is insufficient long-term followup to establish whether the claim is valid.

problem oriented medical record A method of clinical record keeping devised in the late 1950s by the American physician Lawrence Weed (b. 1924) that bases treatment decisions on the problems that the patient identifies and creation of a hierarchical problem list. It is a useful pragmatic approach to patient care, but it is sometimes difficult to reconcile problem lists and rubrics of conventional diagnostic categories.

PROCEED See PRECEDE-PROCEED MODEL.

process research A term occasionally used to describe studies of the way a service or system is functioning. It is the third element of the triad of health services research when this is considered under headings of structure, process, and outcome. For instance, in studying an outpatient hospital service, process research would focus on the way patients enter, interact with staff in component parts of the service, and emerge at the end of their experience, without necessarily considering OUTCOMES.

pro-choice movement The advocacy groups, organizations, and individuals who uphold the rights of women to make their own free choices about reproduction, their right to decide for themselves whether to become and to remain pregnant. It uses political action and education about human sexuality, reproduction, and contraceptive methods, and advocates access to and provision of facilities for contraception and, when necessary, access to safe abortion facilities. The pro-choice movement is generally more political than educational. See also PRO-LIFE MOVEMENT.

prodroma The premonitory or precursor symptoms of a disease, especially a communicable disease. In the case of communicable diseases that present clinically with a skin rash, prodromal symptoms are those usually preceding the appearance of the rash. For example, the characteristic skin rash of measles is preceded by prodromal symptoms that include fever, cough, inflamed conjunctivae, and Koplik spots. The prodromal period varies widely according to the natural history of the particular disease, from a few hours or less to many months.

productive efficiency The actions that minimize costs, such as loss, economic penalty, for a given outcome. See EFFICIENCY.

profession An occupation that requires specialized education and/or training that is often available only in a college or university and is usually assessed by a sequence of examinations. Professions are characterized sociologically as self-regulating, having a group identity, and being internally hierarchical. There is an informal British ranking of professions in which judges, physicians, bishops, and senior officers in the armed forces are accorded higher status than school teachers, stockbrokers, and bankers. Tradition and snobbishness play a role in this rank order, but professional status and health measured by longevity may be associated.

Professional Activity Study The original hospital discharge abstract system, developed and implemented by the COMMISSION ON PROFESSIONAL AND HOSPITAL ACTIVITIES in 1955, and adopted by many hospitals in the United States, Canada, and other countries. It tabulates data on diagnoses, procedures, length of hospital stay, and outcomes, yielding profiles of performance by hospitals, services, and individual attending physicians. It has been superseded by computerized medical records.

professionalism The combination of qualities and conduct regarded as essential to professional practice. These include knowledge, skills, relevant competence, behavioral qualities, and values of honesty, integrity, ethical probity, and capability of working well with patients or clients, colleagues, and representatives of the public. See also MEDICAL PROFESSIONALISM.

Professional Review Organization (PRO) The name since 1987 of what was previously called the Professional Standards Review Organization. The name change was made after legislative and fiscal changes following the introduction of DIAGNOSIS-RELATED GROUPS (DRGs) of conditions, which led to greater rigor in setting standards for treatment and management of conditions according to standardized treatment protocols.

Professional Standards Review Organization (PSRO) A US federally mandated program to review the need, suitability, and quality of medical and surgical services provided to beneficiaries of the MEDICARE and MEDICAID programs. It was established as a result of the Social Security

Amendments of 1972 to promote the effective, efficient, and economical delivery of health care services of proper quality for which payment may be made under the Act. The amendments call for creation of local or statewide organizations of physicians to monitor services to ensure that the services conform to professional standards and are provided only when medically necessary and in the most economical and medically appropriate settings. Legislative and fiscal changes led to a name change of the program to PROFESSIONAL REVIEW ORGANIZATION in the late 1980s.

progesterone The female sex hormone secreted by the corpus luteum of the ovary that prepares the uterus for implantation of a fertilized ovum, inhibits ovulation during pregnancy, and prepares the breasts for lactation.

prognosis A prediction of the likely future course of a disease. The term is often generalized to apply to prediction of the future course of events in other situations and systems.

program A description or plan of action for an event or sequence of actions or events over a short or prolonged period. More formally, an outline of the way a system or service will function, with specifics such as roles and responsibilities, expected expenditures, outcomes, etc. A health program is generally long term and often multifaceted, whereas a health project is a short-term and usually narrowly focused activity.

program evaluation and review techniques (PERT) A work-scheduling procedure that uses algorithms and states the principles, methods, resource allocation details, specific tasks, costs, expected outcomes, etc., and specifies what will be evaluated and how this will be done.

progressive massive fibrosis A pathological condition of the lungs usually caused by inhalation of coal dust that causes emphysema, fibrotic changes, and emphysema. It is often compounded by chronic infection, notably tuberculosis.

Project Gutenberg An expanding library of electronic books, prepared by scanning volumes in reference libraries. Information is available at http://www.gutenberg.org/. The aim ultimately is to make available the entire collections of some of the world's principal reference libraries. As of June 2005, some 17,000 books are freely available on line. See WORLD WIDE WEB.

projection Extrapolation of data along a trend line to predict what might happen in the future.

pro-life movement A politically influential coalition that advocates putting the rights of the fetus on an equal footing with the rights of the mother. Its members include devout Christians and members of other religious faiths, and a small, militant fringe who sometimes bomb clinics that perform abortions and provide family planning advice, and even maim or murder the physicians and nurses who staff them. It is opposed to the PRO-CHOICE MOVEMENT.

propaganda A range of oral and written communications and film and television presentations designed to promote a political cause. The word usually has negative connotations, implying that the cause is not a desirable one, so it is most often used pejoratively. Health education programs aimed at elimination or reduction of tobacco smoking could be described as propaganda but are usually called health promotion or health education.

propellant A gas under high pressure in a small closed container, used with aerosols to expel a fine atmospheric suspension of droplets, mist, or occasionally solid particles.

prophylaxis The preventive management of disease in individuals and populations.

proportion A RATIO in which the numerator is included in the denominator, that is, the ratio of a part to the whole. It may be expressed as a fraction, a decimal fraction, or a percentage, and it must, by definition, lie between zero and 1. Numerator and denominator have the same dimensions so these cancel out; a proportion is a dimensionless entity. See also RATE.

proportional mortality ratio (PMR) A useful, frequently used but often poorly understood indicator of aspects of population health. The PMR is the number of observed deaths from a specified cause in a defined population divided by the number of deaths that would be expected in a standard population, with both numbers expressed as a proportion of all deaths. PMR does not require data on the age composition of the population (unlike the STANDARDIZED MORTALITY RATIO). The "standard population" can be any arbitrarily selected suitable one. The PMRs of specific occupational groups are sometimes used to determine whether their mortality experience differs significantly from that of the general population, justifying further investigation.

propositus The clinically affected family member whose condition first draws attention to the occurrence of a genetic trait. The word is occasionally used to refer to a diagnosed case of a condition that is not of genetic origin when others in the family may also be affected.

proprietary Pertaining to the ownership of and benefits derived from property, including intellectual property and a commercial or industrial enterprise.

proscriptive A prohibitive or condemnatory order or edict.

prospective study A general term for a study in which data are collected from a starting date until some future time. The term was formerly loosely used by some to describe a COHORT STUDY, but many randomized controlled trials and some case control studies also collect cases (and controls) prospectively, and for this reason the term is preferably avoided.

prostaglandins Unsaturated fatty acid molecules occurring in all human tissue, with the highest concentration in semen. Prostaglandins are secreted and act locally, rather than having distant hormone-like properties, but they have significant actions on the nervous system, circulation, metabolism, and female reproduction; e.g., they can induce miscarriage.

prostate cancer Among the most common cancers of men, prostate cancer is often an indolent disease that has not had time to kill old men before they die of other causes, but it can be a rapidly developing and lethal cancer in younger men. It is more common in men who have had many sex partners than in celibate or monogamous men, suggesting a sexually transmissible agent. It can be detected by the presence of a high titer of PROSTATE SPECIFIC ANTIGEN (PSA), but the test has a high false-positive rate and a modest false-negative rate, so screening is unreliable and has not been shown to confer benefit in appropriate trials.

prostate specific antigen (PSA) An antigen that rises in concentration when prostatic disease, especially cancer, occurs and is therefore used as a screening test, although its specificity and sensitivity have been called into question.

prosthesis An artificial replacement for a limb, organ, or other body part.

prostitution The purveying of sexual services for money or equivalent. The "oldest profession," now called the SEX INDUSTRY, is indeed ancient. Buying sexual services of girls and women is common, of boys and men less so. Those of either sex engaged in prostitution are called SEX WORKERS. In most societies, their prevalence indicates economic stress, high unemployment, and social inequality, and often reflects the inequitable status of women in society. Prostitutes are often condemned as the source of

sexually transmitted diseases, but their clients who infect them are more guilty. Legalizing prostitution facilitates improved surveillance and control of sexually transmitted diseases and protection of sex workers from aggressive clients and abusive pimps. When the law and regulations include medical supervision, the health and social problems associated with prostitution usually are much reduced.

protective clothing, equipment A wide range of apparel and devices, such as coveralls resistant to corrosive liquids or toxic chemicals; respirators; goggles, gloves, and face shields to prevent exposure to workplace hazards; steel-toed shoes; and many other varieties of clothing and equipment, to enhance safety.

protective factor A factor the presence of which reduces the likelihood that a particular disease or adverse health outcome will occur. The opposite of a RISK FACTOR.

protein One of the essential dietary ingredients, proteins are composed of various amino acids, important components of meat, legumes, and grains, metabolized in the body to other proteins that build and repair body tissues, provide energy, and perform essential physiological functions. Proteins are essential to the structure and function of all cells. Many are enzymes, others have a structural role in body cells, and others are components in immune responses.

protein deficiency Dietary deficiency, especially during growth phases of early childhood, has some pronounced and obvious effects, including stunting of growth in infancy and childhood and impaired development, as seen in KWASHIORKOR. In adults, protein deficiency causes metabolic disruption, impaired immune response, edema, and diverse other clinical manifestations.

protocol The formal plan or set of procedures to be followed in implementing a plan, such as the sequence of steps in a research design, or the reduction and elimination of a health hazard, such as the effects of ozone-destroying substances on the stratospheric ozone layer under the terms of the MONTREAL PROTOCOL.

proton 1. A positively charged subatomic particle. 2. An undifferentiated embryonic body part or organ, or the rudimentary remnant of this that persists into adult life.

protoplasm The parenchyma of a cell, i.e., the cellular material other than the nucleus.

protozoa A large phylum of single-cell organisms. Some have plant-like metabolism, i.e., using chlorophyll. Others feed on living or dead tissue, i.e., behave more like animals. These include disease agents such as the amebae that cause dysentery, the plasmodial malaria parasites, trypanosomes, and the protozoa that cause leishmaniasis.

proximal risk factors The risk factor(s) in the causal chain that actually precipitate disease, as distinguished from predisposing or DISTAL RISK FACTORS. See RISK FACTOR for further discussion.

pseudoscience A derogatory term for studies and their results based on dubious or spurious science; slipshod methods; false premises, axioms, and assumptions; sensational presentation of findings; predetermined outcomes; and various combinations of the above. Examples include claims for cures of incurable conditions, such as muscular dystrophy and advanced cancer, for human cloning, etc. Sometimes the term is an ad hominem defense of the indefensible, as when industry spokesmen use it as a label in attempts to discredit evidence on the harmful effects of environmental chemical pollution. See also JUNK SCIENCE.

psittacosis An acute generalized disease with pulmonary congestion, transmitted to humans by birds. This is sometimes an endemic infection of bird colonies, especially parrots, budgerigars, canaries, finches, pigeons, and poultry. The causal organism is an intracellular bacterium *Chlamydia psittaci*. The birds are often asymptomatic carriers. The infection is transmitted to humans by inhalation from handling the birds or by contact with feathers, feces, or cage dust, but person-to-person transmission also occurs. The symptoms include fever, dry cough, severe muscle pain, and headache; occasionally, a severe generalized systemic illness results. The condition is indolent, can be fatal, and usually responds to tetracycline or erythromycin.

psychiatry The specialized branch of medicine dealing with the diagnosis, classification, treatment, and prevention of mental disorders, diseases affecting the emotions, mind, and brain. Although mental diseases have always existed, psychiatry did not exist as a specialty until the 19th century, when it evolved from empirical studies of hysteria and innovative (albeit now not generally accepted) psychoanalytic theories of Freud, Jung, and others. The word "psychiatry" was first used by the German anatomist J. C. Reil (1759–1813). Discovery of mood-modifying drugs and innovative therapeutic methods such as psychotherapy led in and after the 1960s to a revolution in care of the mentally disturbed, which no longer relied on custodial care in mental hospitals.

psychoactive drugs Drugs that alter moods, modify emotional states, and sometimes alter states of consciousness. They include narcotics, tranquilizers, and illicit substances used to induce euphoria.

psychoanalysis The therapeutic method developed by the Viennese school of psychiatric thought in the 1920s and 1930s under the leadership of the Austrian psychiatrist Sigmund Freud (1856–1939) based on the belief that emotional disturbances are linked to disordered subconscious thoughts, repressed ideas, and emotional trauma in early childhood and that emotionally disturbed individuals could be helped by discussing their thoughts in a series of lengthy monologues or dialogues with a psychoanalyst. Although there is little evidence in support of these concepts and no convincing evaluations of efficacy (because randomized trials are not feasible), this method of treatment remained popular until at least the late 20th century. It has been mostly superseded by PSYCHOTHERAPY and use of PSYCHOACTIVE DRUGS.

psychogeriatrics Psychiatry and geriatrics join forces in this field, concerned with management of mental disorders, principally dementia in elderly people, often in an institutional setting.

psychology The field of scholarly activity concerned with the scientific study of the human mind, including intelligence and its determinants, moods, emotions and their expression, and with behavior.

psychometric tests A term to describe tests of intellectual ability, emotional state, personality types, etc. Examples of validated tests of proven reliability are the Binet-Simon and Wechsler intelligence tests, the Minnesota and Maudsley multiphasic personality tests.

psychoneuroimmunology Syn: mind-body medicine. A branch of medical science that studies interrelationships of emotional, psychological, neurological, endocrine, and immune systems in health and disease. The main emphasis is on the study of how states of mind and emotional stress influence immune reactions, hormone-mediated systems, and stress-related conditions.

psychopathic personality Syn: antisocial personality, moral defective. A psychiatric disorder in which the affected individual lacks insight into the distinction between right and wrong, has little or no moral restraint, and has no concern about consequences of actions for others.

psychosis A mental disorder in which the affected person has such severe disorder of thoughts and emotions as to lose contact with reality. Persons with psychoses may have delusions or hallucinations, or their intellectual function may be disrupted to an extent that makes rational thought and judgment impossible. Psychoses may be acute short term or chronic and progressive. The causes include dementia, schizophrenia, paranoia, and acute mania.

psychosomatic disorders Conditions affecting the mind and emotions that induce somatic symptoms. Examples include many so-called stress diseases, such as many cases of hypertension. Some somatic disorders, e.g.,eczema, asthma, psoriasis, are aggravated by emotional states, such as anxiety and depression.

psychotherapy A specialized formal treatment regimen based on communication between and the development of trust between the patient and a therapist, psychiatrist, psychologist, or social worker; usually a long-term relationship, in which treatment consists mainly of a dialogue between patient and therapist.

PsycINFO A database of abstracts and a search engine for information about psychology that is maintained by the American Psychological Association. It contains summary information as well as abstracts dating back to the 1800s. See http://www.apa.org/psycinfo/ for details.

puberty The epoch marking transition from child to adolescent and then to adult. The onset of puberty in females is marked by MENARCHE, the first menstrual period; male puberty is less precisely defined, e.g., by growth of axillary and pubic hair, beginning of seminal emissions, and descent and enlargement of testes. In both sexes, puberty is usually preceded by a prepubertal growth spurt.

public domain The setting in which written work or visual displays are accessible to everyone without hindrance or financial barriers to access, not protected by copyright or patent.

public health An organized activity of society to promote, protect, improve, and, when necessary, restore the health of individuals, specified groups, or the entire population. It is a combination of sciences, skills, and values that function through collective societal activities and involve programs, services, and institutions aimed at protecting and improving the health of all the people. The term "public health" can describe a concept, a social institution, a set of scientific and professional disciplines and technologies, and a form of practice. It encompasses a wide range of services, institutions, professional groups, trades, and unskilled occupations. It is a way of thinking, a set of disciplines, an institution of society, and a

manner of practice. It has an increasing number and variety of specialized domains, and it demands of its practitioners an increasing array of skills and expertise. Discerning political leaders, including Otto von Bismarck, Benjamin Disraeli, Lloyd George, Franklin D. Roosevelt, and John F. Kennedy, have recognized and stated for more than 150 years that protecting and improving the health of their nation's people is their most important responsibility.

Public Health Agency of Canada (PHAC) Established in 2004, the PHAC aims to help protect the health and safety of all Canadians. Its activities focus on preventing chronic diseases, including cancer and heart disease; preventing injuries; and responding to public health emergencies and infectious disease outbreaks. The emphasis has been mainly on the last of these activities, notably protection from pandemic disease. Details are available at http://www.hc-sc.gc.ca/ahc-asc/branch-dirgen/phac-aspc/index_e.html.

public health associations There are public health associations, societies, academies, etc., in many nations and some regional aggregates of nations. Most are dedicated to advancing the public health in their nation and region. Membership is usually open to persons in all professions engaged in public health practice and research and sometimes also to members of the general public as individuals or representatives of consumer organizations, etc. They include the American Public Health Association (http://www.apha.org), the Canadian Public Health Association (http://www.cpha.ca), the Public Health Association of Australia, the European Public Health Association (http://www.eupha.org), and many others. Most arrange annual meetings of their members, and many belong to regional and worldwide networks of public health organizations, notably the WORLD FEDERATION OF PUBLIC HEALTH ASSOCIATIONS (WFPHA). Almost all are listed on the WFPHA Web site, http://www.wfpha.org, with links to the organizations' Web sites.

public health competencies The set of skills required of public health practitioners and assessed in examinations such as those of the AMERICAN BOARD OF PREVENTIVE MEDICINE. These include proficiency in epidemiology and biostatistics, public health aspects of genetics, microbiology and environmental health, communicable and noncommunicable disease control, hygiene and sanitary sciences, public health law, health promotion and health education, and administration and management of health services. Some important domains of public health require additional competence, for instance in maternal and child health, occupational health, environmental toxicology, and mental health care and services. A competency not usually assessed by examinations is the ability to marshal political arguments and present these eloquently and effectively when they are needed. The range of competencies has been much discussed, especially in the United States since the Institute of Medicine's report *The Future of Public Health* was published (1988). These competencies are used to set the curriculum in many schools of public health. See http://www.phf.org/link.htm.

public health dentist A dentist specially trained in aspects of public health, e.g., epidemiology, oral hygiene, preventive dentistry, and dental health promotion.

public health impact assessment An assessment of the implications for public health of changes in an environment that accompany arrival of new industries, housing developments, construction of hydroelectric dams, influx of large numbers of immigrants, etc.

public health laws Laws enacted by national, regional, or local governments on matters affecting the public's health. The principal laws in this category are concerned with protection from the risk of contagious diseases and life-threatening environmental hazards. The laws are reinforced by enabling regulations and ordinances. During the past 150 years there have been progressive improvements and modifications of the laws as the pattern of contagious and environmentally related diseases has changed. There has often been resistance from commercial and industrial groups who think stronger laws and regulations threaten their economic interests.

public health nurse A member of the nursing profession with specialized training in the theories and practices of public health. Public health nurses play a major role in provision of local public health services, e.g., maternal infant and early child care, health education, contact tracing in communicable disease surveillance and control, and home visits to elderly and infirm housebound residents in the community, and various other specialized roles.

public health physician A physician with specialized training in the theories and practices of public health, usually one who has passed examinations and obtained specialist registration.

Public Health Practice Program Office The division of the CENTERS FOR DISEASE CONTROL AND PREVENTION that is concerned, as its name indicates, with enhancing the practice of public health. It focuses on a strong community public health presence, the public health workforce, organizational

effectiveness, scientific capacity of public health laboratories, and systems to manage public health information. See http://www.phppo.cdc.gov/.

public health sciences A collective name for the scholarly activities that form the scientific base for public health practice, services, and systems. Until the early 19th century, scholarly activities were limited to natural and biological sciences sometimes enlightened by empirical logic. The scientific base has broadened to include vital statistics, epidemiology, environmental sciences, biostatistics, microbiology, social and behavioral sciences, genetics, nutrition, molecular biology, and more. Scholars in the domain of public health have embraced new concepts of disease and its causes and control, and have developed generalizations and axioms to explain observations and to enhance control measures. Occasional misguided beliefs, such as those about race and eugenics, remind us of our fallibility. Schools of public health are focal points for many studies of public health sciences, and this has become a popular title for university departments.

public health sentinels See SENTINELS.

public health workforce The numbers and variety of skilled specialized workers in the public health services reflect its importance to society. This is seldom appreciated when tax cuts are on the agenda and public health services are a target for staff reductions, although reduced funding may be justified when there is insufficient objective evidence of program success. Public health specialists require lengthy training, so financial cuts in training programs that lead to reduced output of trained professionals can take as long as a decade to produce critical shortages as those in existing posts retire or die, and equally long to correct when funding is restored. Formerly called "public health manpower," the accurate and politically correct term "public health workforce" recognizes that females are in the majority in most branches of public health services.

public policy This includes planning, decisions, resource allocation, and actions in every sector of society, often in a hierarchical order of perceived national importance. Public policy is shaped by elected governments and their scientific and technical advisers, by public opinion, and by pressure groups. Health issues and concerns are high in the hierarchy in affluent nations, but priorities within the health sector are often oriented toward glamorous or emotionally appealing aspects, such as high-technology diagnostic and treatment facilities, children's hospitals, and the like, whereas most aspects of public health are unappreciated and receive less than 5% of the portion of national budgets allocated to "health." In most low-income countries, health and social policies have low funding priority and the gap is partially closed by nongovernmental organizations (NGOs).

public-private partnerships (PPP) A method used by some governments in affluent nations to reduce expenses and the need for increased taxes by forming alliances with private sector groups to cover the capital cost of investment in buildings, equipment, and/or other infrastructure. Toll roads are an example, and private clinics to provide costly diagnostic services such as imaging equipment are another. The costs are passed on as user fees. The ultimate costs are higher than if the same service is provided entirely in the public sector because of the private sector's need to generate profits.

public relations The measures adopted to enhance or preserve the image of individuals, organizations, and governments, e.g., by means of advertising, lobbying, appearances on television, interviews, press releases. Representatives of public health seldom excel in public relations and are often less successful than private interest groups, who are often their adversaries.

public sector In political economy, the portion of the nation's services, goods, capital resources, etc., that is financed from taxation and administered and staffed by people who are paid from the public purse. Usually public sector personnel, especially at the professional level, are publicly accountable, but in nations where senior staff members are political appointees, accountability is often less, and so sometimes is competence.

PubMed One of the most useful online bibliographic resources of the NATIONAL LIBRARY OF MEDICINE, PubMed is a searchable data base of authors' names, article subjects, abstracts, etc., that can be used to identify and retrieve original contributions on subjects in the biomedical field. It is accessed at http://www.ncbi.nlm.nih.gov/entrez/query.fcgi?DB=pubmed or at http://www.pubmedcentral.nih.gov/.

puerperal sepsis A formerly lethal septicemia that occurs when infection is introduced into the uterus by the birth attendant. It was epidemic from the 18th to the late 19th century in western Europe and the United States, when childbirth was conducted by obstetricians who did not wash their hands before performing obstetric maneuvers. In Boston, Oliver Wendell Holmes (1809–1894) and in Vienna, IGNAZ PHILIPP SEMMELWEIS (1818–1865) independently discovered that it could be prevented by hand-washing. Semmelweis published a detailed

statistical analysis to prove his point. Unfortunately, their peers rejected the findings and advice, and another generation of parturient women fell victim to puerperal sepsis before JOSEPH LISTER introduced ANTISEPSIS into surgery in 1865, and the method was adopted also in obstetrics.

pulmonary edema Accumulation of fluid in the lungs, usually caused by heart failure, or by inhaling irritant fumes.

pulmonary function tests These are tests of VITAL CAPACITY, spirometry, forced expiratory flow, lung volume, etc., and specialized tests such as flow volume, used to assess the progress of chronic respiratory disease and to evaluate treatment.

punch card A data storage and sorting system based on sequences of holes that are made in cards that are then sorted according to the positions of the holes. This method of processing large data files by means of card-sorting machines was widely used until the advent of electronic computers rendered them obsolete. Varieties included hand-held and machine-sortable punch cards.

pupa The stage in metamorphosis of insects that follows larval development and precedes the imago and adult stages.

pure culture A laboratory culture of a single strain of a microorganism.

purine A nitrogenous base compound precursor of adenine and guanine. A genetically determined defect in purine metabolism renders some people susceptible to gout.

putative father The presumed or reputed father of a child.

putrefaction Anaerobic decomposition of organic matter by bacteria, fungi, or other organisms. Putrefied organic matter provides a suitable culture medium for many pathogens, including anaerobic bacteria that generate methane and hydrogen sulfide, so it is malodorous.

pyogenic Productive of pus or purulent material.

pyrethrin insecticides Insecticides prepared from the natural alkaloid pyrethrum found in chrysanthemums and related plants. They are effective against many insects, less toxic than many synthetically produced insecticides, but more expensive to manufacture than synthetics.

pyridoxine The basic chemical constituent of vitamin B_6, a white crystalline solid.

Q fever An acute zoonotic rickettsial infection caused by *Coxiella burnetii*, with cattle and sheep as primary hosts and airborne spread to humans. The bacterium was named for the Australian microbiologist Macfarlane Burnet (1899–1985), who first isolated it. Q may stand for Queensland, Australia, where the disease was first identified, or for "query," because at first the origin of the disease was unknown. It is an occupational disease of people who work with cattle and sheep, e.g., stockmen, veterinarians.

qualitative analysis Analysis that relies on descriptive accounts of behavior, beliefs, feelings, or values, with few or no numerical data available for statistical analysis. The qualitative method consists of critical scrutiny of all the available descriptive material, somewhat in the manner used by lawyers and judges in the courts when they weigh the evidence and arrive at a decision. The method is sometimes criticized on the grounds that it relies on subjective judgments rather than objective measurement, but if observational evidence is assessed without emotional value judgments, it can be a useful, reproducible method. It is sometimes a preliminary to or may lead to quantitative research or alternatively may help to make sense of statistical associations.

quality-adjusted life expectancy (QALE) A model for clinical decision making in which estimates of impairment or disability are factored into calculation of life expectancy. It is also a method of adjusting life expectancy to allow for reduced quality of life caused by chronic conditions. Many chronic conditions shorten life on average by predictable amounts. These expected amounts can be estimated from available sources, such as hospital discharge data and health survey data, and used to produce a QALE for individuals or subsets of the population. At the individual level, the QALE is based on clinical judgment and subjective opinions of patients about their quality of life, preferably arrived at by consensus between clinicians and patients.

quality-adjusted life years (QALYs) An adjustment of life expectancy to allow for the fact that chronic diseases, disabilities, and handicaps often shorten life by predictable amounts. In practice, numerical weights are assigned to represent the severity of disabilities, just as with calculation of DISABILITY-ADJUSTED LIFE YEARS (DALYs) and BURDEN OF DISEASE, to calculate QALYs. More precisely, QALY is a unit of health gain attributable to an intervention typically used in cost-utility analysis. It is the product of the absolute change in survival and the quality of life experienced during that period, e.g., a year of life gained at a level half as good as perfect health would be 0.5 QALY. It is logically similar to but distinct from DISABILITY-ADJUSTED LIFE YEARS (DALYs).

quality assurance The procedures, methods such as audits, and corrective action taken to ensure that preventive and therapeutic practices are conducted in conformity with best practices and standard operating procedure aimed at achieving the highest attainable level of outcomes in institutional and community-based health care. The Armenian-American Avedis Donabedian (1921–2000) stated that the determinants of health care quality are science, technology, and their appropriate application by qualified health care professionals.

quality circle Syn: quality control circle. A small, voluntary group of individuals who work together as a unit, consider together the problems they encounter in their work, identify possible solutions for these problems, test the solutions, and, if they work, implement them. The aim is to enhance efficiency and effectiveness, i.e., quality, of the work for which the unit is responsible.

quality control SURVEILLANCE and/or MONITORING of the human and mechanical activities involved in production of goods, e.g., pharmaceutical drugs, or provision of a service, to detect deviations from acceptable standards and take pertinent corrective action.

quality of life (QOL) An essentially subjective judgment of the way people perceive themselves as contented and happy or otherwise, and able to function physically, emotionally, and socially. Others, including health workers, can make a relatively objective judgment of some of these aspects of a person's way of living, but the affected individual is the ultimate judge.

quality-of-life scales Several alternative measurement scales or survey instruments have been used to arrive at numerical scores for quality of life. These include the ACTIVITY STATUS INDEX developed at Duke University (Durham, North Carolina), which assesses physical function; the London School of Hygiene and Tropical Medicine questionnaires for angina and dyspnea; the Medical Outcomes Study short form general health questionnaire; the Quality of Well-being Scale; the SICKNESS IMPACT PROFILE; and several others. Most are variations on the theme of asking specific questions about what people can do and how they feel about it, in relation to the presence or absence of specific symptoms. See also HEALTH-RELATED QUALITY OF LIFE.

quantal effect Syn: all-or-none effect. An effect expressible only in binary terms, e.g., as occurring/not occurring.

quantile One of a number of equal divisions of an ordered sequence of values. A decile is a tenth, a centile is a hundredth, and a quintile is a fifth equal part of the total.

quarantinable diseases Contagious diseases of humans, animals, or plants that by law and international health regulations are subject to quarantine. Under revised INTERNATIONAL HEALTH REGULATIONS (2005), member states of the WHO are required to report cases of cholera, plague and yellow fever, paralytic poliomyelitis, epidemic influenza, and other diseases as specified from time to time, for instance, severe acute respiratory syndrome (SARS) and avian influenza. In the United States, the list is expanded to include other contagious diseases: cholera, diphtheria, infectious tuberculosis, plague, smallpox, yellow fever, and viral hemorrhagic fevers. By executive order in 2003, SARS was added to the list..

quarantine Isolation of an animal or person who is a known contact of a case of a contagious disease for the duration of the period of communicability of the disease in order to prevent transmission of the disease, which might otherwise occur during the incubation period if the contact has been infected. Quarantine may be absolute or modified. Absolute quarantine is strict limitation of freedom to move and in the past was often implemented by incarcerating contacts in a quarantine hospital or station, typically located at a port of entry for overseas shipping. Animal quarantine for diseases transmissible to humans or other animals, such as rabies, after a prolonged incubation period may last several months. Modified quarantine is selective or partial limitation of movement. A common form is voluntary quarantine, in which contacts of known cases of a contagious disease isolate themselves in their own homes for the duration of the incubation period of the contagious disease, e.g., when children stay away from school because a family member has a contagious disease. Quarantine presents public health professionals with an ethical problem when the decision to impose it causes drastic restriction of freedom of movement, which is regarded as a fundamental human right. In this situation public health officials must make individ-

ual rights subservient to the public safety, i.e., the need for the community to be protected from harm, the contagious disease for which quarantine is imposed. Imposition of quarantine is a legal process and procedure within which public health officials must confine their actions. The word *quarantine* derives from Italian *quaranta dies* (40 days); the practice originated in 15th century Venice and was used to protect the citizens from plague that might otherwise have been introduced by returning merchants.

quartan fever The fever that characteristically occurs in *Plasmodium malariae* malarial infection with recurrent bouts of fever every 72 hours or every fourth day.

quartile Division of a quantity into four equal parts, each of which is a quarter of the whole.

quasi-autonomous nongovernmental organization (QUANGO) A semipublic body that is at least partly supported by government funds and has both elected and appointed members, the latter generally government-appointed but at arm's length from the government and able to make decisions and take action independently of government. This method of organizing public affairs in health and social services is often used in the United Kingdom but less so in Europe and almost never anywhere else.

quasi-experiment A situation in which the investigator lacks full control over the number and nature of subjects, and/or the variables that are to be studied in an observation or intervention, and/or the times at which changes occur but is able to record and measure all relevant variables and make usable inferences based on these.

questionnaire A set of written questions, preferably carefully designed so those who answer must choose from a limited range of responses (such as "yes" or "no") to each of a series of specific questions. Questionnaires may be given or mailed to respondents for them to complete and return, or the questions may be read aloud to respondents and their answers recorded by an interviewer. The latter method of inquiry is usually called an INTERVIEW SCHEDULE.

Quetelet, Lambert Adolphe Jacques (1796–1874) A Belgian polymath, astronomer, social scientist, mathematician, and statistician, eponymously remembered in the health sciences for Quetelet's index (the BODY MASS INDEX) and for his contributions to social science theory and practice.

Quetelet's index See BODY MASS INDEX.

queueing theory A theory that uses mathematical models to simulate the movement or processing of people through a system, such as a hospital emergency room or public health clinic.

quick and dirty method A method of investigation that can be done rapidly and inexpensively, although it may not necessarily be accurate or reliable. It is often the first step in investigating an epidemic. It may take any of several forms, e.g., a hastily mounted case control study or the use of powerful antibiotics without awaiting the results of laboratory tests to identify the responsible pathogenic organism. See also RAPID EPIDEMIOLOGICAL ASSESSMENT.

quickening The traditional name for a pregnant woman's first perception of fetal movements, which happens at about 16 weeks' gestational age. Muslims call this the stage of ensoulment, when the fetus becomes a person. In Islam, termination of pregnancy before ensoulment, or quickening, is morally acceptable to devout Muslims; after ensoulment, it is not.

quinine An alkaloid derived from the bark of the South American indigenous cinchona tree that was used by the pre-Columbian inhabitants of Central and South America to treat the symptoms of malaria and as a way to provide some protection against malarial infection. Quinine acts by inhibiting the growth and reproduction of plasmodia and was the most widely used antimalarial until after World War II. Most strains of plasmodia are now resistant to quinine.

Quinlan case A medicolegal case in 1975–1976 that tested US law regarding the rights of a person in a PERSISTENT VEGETATIVE STATE or that person's next of kin to decline treatment to prolong life. This was the first of several cases to challenge a hospital's right to continue treatment when the patient's next of kin do not wish treatment to be prolonged. In 1975, Karen Ann Quinlan lost consciousness after ingesting alcohol and tranquilizers. After she had spent nearly a year in a persistent vegetative state, her parents obtained the New Jersey Supreme Court's permission to turn off her respirator.

quinolones A family of antimicrobial agents taken by mouth or applied topically that initially were efficacious against a wide range of pathogenic microorganisms, but, as with other antibiotics, resistance has evolved. Details about indications, efficacy, toxicity, etc., are at http://www.cdc.gov/ncidod/hip/Lab/FactSheet/quinlolones.htm.

quinsy An old word for severe swelling of the throat and neck, usually caused by peritonsillar abscess and sometimes by other causes of swollen lymph glands, such as lymphoma.

quota sampling A sampling method in which the proportions vary in designated subgroups according to such criteria as age group, occupation, social class, etc.

quotient The result obtained when one number is divided by another.

R

rabies An almost invariably fatal zoonosis caused by a bullet-shaped neurotropic virus that is transmitted in saliva by the bite of an infected animal. In humans, a long incubation period may precede symptoms of apprehension, followed by delirium, fever, convulsions, and death. Rabies occurs in wild dogs, raccoons, skunks, etc., and domestic animals, e.g., cattle. It is fatal for most of these but can be an innocuous disease in bats, which may act as a natural reservoir for the virus.

rabies virus vaccines The French bacteriologist Louis Pasteur (1822–1895) began experimenting with attenuated vaccines, including one against rabies, in about 1880 and in 1885 had the opportunity to test his vaccine on a young boy, Joseph Meister.

Pasteur's achievement was remarkable, conducted half a century before the virus was isolated and visualized by electron microscopic analysis. His attenuated vaccine regimen required multiple subcutaneous abdominal injections, a prolonged and painful experience. Human diploid cell vaccines were introduced in 1967 and are safer but more costly. No one dared to attempt a randomized trial of alternative regimens until the development in the early 1990s of genetically engineered vaccines (human diploid cell vaccine). Both postexposure and prophylactic vaccines are available.

race In biology, vital statistics, epidemiology, and several other disciplines, this word designates identifiable groups for classification purposes. Social scientists challenge the biological concept of race, asserting that it reflects ideological and culturally determined values rather than verifiable or classifiable criteria. In the United States, the word has an emotive connotation that make its use politically volatile in some contexts. The dictionary definition "a major division of humankind having distinct physical characteristics" is generally valid and useful for simple statistical classification. A "racial" classification of humans is difficult, if not meaningless, because of genetic overlaps, but some risk factors are so strongly correlated with characteristics (mainly socioeconomic factors) customarily identified as "racial" that it would be foolish not to use them in statistical analyses.

racial profiling The practice of generalizing about the presumed behavior of population groups that may be loosely associated with their appearance, skin color, hair texture, and mode of dress. It is reprehensible because it is often accompanied by negative or hostile attitudes and aggressive conduct toward members of the profiled group.

racial segregation Separation of people into presumed racial groups for purposes that include housing, education, and access to public transport and other services, including health care. It was common in European ghettos until the early 20th century and written into laws and regulations in the southern United States until the 1960s and in South Africa until the 1990s. It is now unconstitutional in these jurisdictions, but vestiges of the practice persist there and elsewhere. Where it exists, its consequences include inequitable access to health care services.

racism Attitudes and behaviors based on a belief that people in a particular group or class are inherently different from and inferior to others and that it is therefore justifiable to discriminate against them; to stigmatize, persecute, and victimize them; deny them access to services available to others; and, at the most extreme, to torture and murder them. Racism may be overt and individual or covert and institutionalized. Racism always has adverse health consequences for the group that is stigmatized and discriminated against, even in the absence of overt violence, and has adverse psychological consequences for the group that discriminates.

rad Abbreviation for radiation absorbed dose, the unit of measurement of the absorbed dose of ionizing radiation, equivalent to 100 ergs per gram of absorbing tissue or material, now replaced by the GRAY (GY): 1 Gy = 100 rads.

radar Acronym for radio detection and ranging, a system that uses microwaves to identify and delineate objects such as aircraft from the patterns of radiation reflected from them. In the early days of this technology, radar operators experienced health problems, such as sleeplessness and headaches, that were attributed to exposure to microwave radiation, but effective shielding of equipment appears to have eliminated these. The tissue-heating effect of microwave radar remains but can be prevented by shielding the equipment.

radiant heat Energy in the form of infrared electromagnetic radiation that is transmitted from a source such as hot coals in a fire or any object that emits heat.

radiation A general term for all forms of electromagnetic energy transmitted as waves and subatomic particles. This includes ionized, shortwave, solar, and long wave radiation. Radiation is transmitted at the speed of light and is absorbed by body tissue with penetration that varies inversely with wavelength. In order of increasing wavelength, electromagnetic radiation consists of very short wavelength gamma (γ) rays, x-rays, ultraviolet, visible, and infrared radiation (radiant heat). The least penetrating ionized rays are α waves, which are emitted by radioactive matter (radium, uranium, etc.); β radiation is made up of electrons and is more penetrating; the γ short-wavelength electromagnetic radiation is highly penetrating. All three varieties of ionized radiation are carcinogenic, and gamma radiation is mutagenic and teratogenic.

radiation sickness Generalized systemic illness caused by exposure to large doses of radiation that kill body cells and tissue and impair or destroy the immune defenses. With very high doses of radiation, digestive glands in the gastrointestinal tract are among those disrupted, aggravating the symptoms. A total body radiation dose exceeding 250 to 350 rads causes death in 1 to 3 weeks in 50% of those exposed; exposure to as much as 200 rads causes symptoms persisting for days to weeks and increased risk of leukemia and brain and kidney cancer after a latency period of as long as 20 years.

radioactive fallout Suspended particulate matter from a nuclear explosion or nuclear power plant accident that disseminates radioactive material. The fallout is greatest along the path of prevailing winds, producing what is known as a radioactive PLUME.

radioactive waste The residue of spent nuclear fuel. Some of this is highly radioactive and includes ingredients with an extremely long half-life, as long as several million years. Disposal has been tackled in various ways. Some radioactive waste can be reprocessed to generate more fuel, but most cannot. The solutions have included dumping in deep ocean canyons and burial in disused deep mine shafts. Humans many generations hence may unearth this material, or it might surface after tectonic plate movement at even more remote future times. If so, our descendents may have reason to berate us for causing such damage to the environment and to ecosystems. Low-level radioactive waste, such as that from radioisotopes, has a brief half-life and is seldom a serious problem.

radioactivity The process of disintegration of atomic nuclei with release of ionizing radiation as gamma rays and emission of radioactive alpha and beta particles. This occurs naturally with high atomic weight elements such as radium and with natural or artificially produced radioactive isotopes of elements of almost any atomic weight. The process is called radioactive decay and is associated with release of energy that may be fluorescent or luminescent and is biologically active and capable of inducing mutations, fetal malformations, and malignant changes. Exposure to radioactivity can cause RADIATION SICKNESS. It is used in diagnostic imaging and therapeutic devices. Calibrated doses can be used to treat cancer and other conditions.

radio frequency fields Electromagnetic radiation on wavelengths used for radio transmission, as in cell phones, is believed not to have harmful biological effects. The possibility that this form of radiation may cause cancer, for instance of the brain, became the topic of epidemiological study in the late 20th century.

radiographer A person who has been professionally trained to operate x-ray machines and other equipment that emits ionizing radiation as used in the diagnosis and treatment of many conditions. Radiographers are occupationally exposed to ionized radiation. Modern equipment and shielding against exposure are generally effective in preventing excessive occupational exposure, and occupational risks are further reduced by strict guidelines on working conditions.

radioimmunoassay An immunological test that uses a radioactive isotope to track molecular changes involved in immune reactions and uses these reactions to determine the composition of biological specimens.

radioisotope A radioactive ISOTOPE. Some radioisotopes are used in medical diagnostic and therapeutic procedures, some have industrial uses, and some are useful in studies in other fields; for instance, radioactive carbon dating is much used in paleontology.

radiologist A physician who is trained and specialized in the use of x-rays and other equipment, such as diagnostic imaging to diagnose and treat disease. Formerly this was a specialty in which there was a high risk of disease and premature death caused by excessive exposure to ionizing radiation, but radiologists are now almost always effectively shielded from these risks.

radionuclide The nucleus of a specific isotope of a radioactive element or compound.

radiosensitivity The extent to which body tissues react to ionized radiation. Germinal cells in the testes and ovaries are very sensitive, and so is lymphoid and hemopoietic tissue. Highly differentiated cells (muscle, bone, peripheral nerves) are relatively radioresistant.

radiotherapy The treatment of disease by means of ionizing radiation, using directed beams of high-energy beta and gamma particles, radioactive isotopes, e.g., implanted at the site of a lesion such as a malignant neoplasm, or injected or ingested. Radiotherapy is used mainly to treat malignant neoplasms, leukemia, etc., but also has been used to treat other conditions, e.g., severe ringworm of the scalp (tinea capitis) and paronychia caused by fungus infection, occasionally with adverse effects, such as malignant neoplasms many years later.

radium (Ra) A metallic element with very high density that has several radioactive isotopes with a half-life as long as 1,600 years, used in radiotherapy and to make luminous paint. Workers in radium mines have a high risk of cancer from exposure to ionized radiation, as did workers with radium salts (used to make luminous paint) until protective measures were applied. The properties of radium were investigated by the French physicist Pierre Curie (1859–1906) and his Polish wife, Marie Sklodowska Curie (1867–1934). She received two Nobel Prizes for her work but ultimately died of radiation-induced cancer.

radix The root or base of a numbering system. Specifically, the number of the hypothetical birth cohort in life tables, usually 100,000.

radon (Rn) A radioactive element that is a decay product of radium and uranium. It exists as a gas in trace amounts with a half-life of 3.8 days and emits α and γ radiation. It is occasionally an environmental health problem in localities where there is a high naturally occurring level of radium as a trace contaminant in rocks or soil, and it often occurs as a trace contaminant in modern buildings. It is associated with increased risk of childhood leukemia, adult lung cancer, and other malignancies. See http://www.epa.gov/iaq/radon/index.html.

ragweed A common weed that grows profusely, especially in the northeastern region of North America. Its pollen is one of the most common causes of acute allergenic rhinitis, i.e., hay fever, and asthma. It is often difficult to desensitize susceptible individuals.

Ramazzini, Bernardino (1633–1714) An Italian physician renowned as the "father of occupational medicine," who observed and classified workers in many occupations and reported his conclusions about the diseases to which each of these was vulnerable in *De Morbis Artificum Diatriba* (*Diseases of Workers*, 1713). He was the first physician to recognize the relationships of specific occupations to disease risk.

random Events and phenomena governed by the laws of probability or chance, rather than predictably determined by deliberate actions or controllable processes. Many biological processes, notably specific gene frequencies passed from parents to offspring, are random. Gene–environment interactions subsequently influence survival prospects.

random allocation Allocation of persons or entities, such as therapeutic regimens, by a formal process using an accepted method of random sampling, such as a table of random numbers.

random error The portion of the variations of measurements and other observations that is due to the operation of chance alone. Random error increases in size and importance if sampling methods are poorly chosen and response rates are low.

randomized controlled trial (RCT) The optimal experimental method used to determine which of two or more preventive or therapeutic regimens or other interventions has the most favorable outcome. The essential features are: 1. Genuine uncertainty about the relative merits of two or more alternatives, a situation known as EQUIPOISE. 2. RANDOM ALLOCATION of persons to test and control groups, and/of interventions to study subjects, by means that are scientifically valid, e.g., by using a table of random numbers in the allocation process. 3. Properly INFORMED CONSENT of the study participants, or subjects, to take part in the study. Information supplied to participants must include the facts that there is uncertainty about the best regimen and that the regimen for particular study participants is determined by chance. 4. Steps to minimize the influence of BIAS due to factors such as expectations of physicians and patients that one regimen may be superior to another, for instance, the additional step of withholding from both physicians and patients the identity of the regimen

that a particular patient is receiving, a procedure described as MASKING or a DOUBLE-BLIND STUDY.

random sample Syn: probability sample. A sample drawn by a process of RANDOM ALLOCATION from a UNIVERSE population in a manner aimed at ensuring representativeness. A simple random sample is one in which each member of the universe population has an equal chance of being selected or not selected into the sample for study. Common variations on this process include a stratified random sample, in which the universe population is first divided into strata, for instance, on the basis of age distribution, occupation, or other criteria intended to ensure that a particular group is adequately represented in the sample.

random walk The sequence of steps in a process when each step is determined by chance in direction, magnitude, or both, without regard to the direction or magnitude of the preceding step. Random walks occur in the migratory behavior of insects and the location of self-sown seeds, so they are of more than theoretical interest.

rank The process of arranging in a meaninkgful order; the position of entities after ranking.

rape crisis center A community service agency usually staffed by volunteers, perhaps a social worker, a psychologist, and a nurse, with facilities for the care and treatment of victims of rape and sexual assault. They may function primarily as hotline telephone access crisis centers with referrals to relevant specialists but preferably have on-site staff constantly available, and some also have OUTREACH services.

rapid epidemiological assessment Inherently speedy and usually inexpensive method(s) that can yield enough information about a health situation to facilitate immediate control measures, e.g., in the aftermath of a natural or manmade disaster, or when a major life-threatening epidemic has struck a community. The details of assessment methods vary according to the nature of the epidemic or relevant emergency. The emphasis is mainly on clinical findings. For example, in earthquakes and floods, the focus is on evidence of fecal-oral transmission. When there are large numbers of refugees, the emphasis is on diarrhea and acute respiratory disease, especially among infants and children. See also EPIDEMIC INVESTIGATION.

rare earths Syn: lanthanoids. A group of silvery, highly reactive elements, some of which, e.g., cerium and ytterbium, are commercially important. Some produce compounds that are toxic to humans by ingestion, inhalation, or skin contact.

rat A small, hardy rodent that commonly nests in or close to human dwellings and lives largely on kitchen waste. It is implicated as a carrier of fleas, lice, or mites in two of the great scourges of humankind, bubonic plague and typhus, and in some lesser ones, including TRICHINOSIS, Weil's disease (leptospirosis), and RAT BITE FEVER. Two important varieties are the black rat, *Rattus rattus*, which prefers to nest and forage inside dwellings, and the Norway brown rat, *Rattus norvegicus*, which forages and nests mainly out of doors. In the 16th century, the more aggressive Norway rats displaced black rats from the ecological niche they had long occupied in Europe, and this probably contributed to the decline of the devastating pandemic PLAGUE at that time. Rats are notorious pests and are also widely used in laboratory studies of disease, genetic studies, studies of animal behavior, and toxicology and pharmacological testing.

rat bite fever The name for two different bacterial diseases associated with rats and possibly with being bitten by one. The rat bite fever caused by a streptobacillus occurs worldwide and can be spread by laboratory rats. Rat bite fever caused by spirillum organisms is confined to Asia.

rate 1. In vital statistics, demography, and epidemiology, a rate is a measure of the frequency with which specified events occur in a defined population in a designated period of time. In general terms, a rate is a measure of the frequency of occurrence of any phenomenon. Rates, rather than raw numbers, must be used in order to ensure that comparisons are meaningful. It is good practice to indicate the numerical values of the numerators and denominators on which rates are based. Rates have three components: a numerator, the number of events, a denominator, the numbers in the population at risk of experiencing the event, and a time dimension, the period over which the events occur.

Rate =

$$\frac{\text{number of events in a specified period}}{\text{number in population at risk of the event}} \times 10^n$$

The denominator can be expressed as PERSON-TIME. Statisticians prefer to calculate an instantaneous incidence rate, the rate at which an event occurs in an instant of time. This is a theoretical concept and is rarely used in VITAL STATISTICS. The word "rate" is loosely used in terms such as PREVALENCE rate and SURVIVAL RATE. Point prevalence, the prevalence of a condition at a point in time, has no time dimension. The term "annual prevalence" can be confusing because conditions such as acute respiratory infection often occur more than once in a year. Survival rates are usually proportions, although they are often expressed with a time dimen-

sion, e.g., 5-year survival rates for breast cancer. CASE FATALITY RATE, an important indicator of the severity of a condition, is sometimes stated without a clear definition of the time dimension, merely with the numerator (number of deaths) and denominator (the population that has been exposed to the risk of dying). 2. The charge for a service is also called a rate, such as municipal rates, the charge for services such as street sweeping or collection of domestic waste.

rating, rating scale A method of classifying entities that involves measuring variable aspect(s) that can be ranked, usually on an ordinal or interval MEASUREMENT SCALE. Rating scales are most often used to score the responses in interviews and self-completed questionnaires, but they have many other applications, e.g., to score the strength of muscular contractions such as handgrip (although there are ways to do this with calibrated instruments).

ratio The result of dividing one quantity by another without regard for details such as a time dimension. Rates, proportions, and percentages are all types of ratios. The distinction between a proportion and a ratio is that, whereas the numerator of a proportion is included in the population defined by the denominator, this is not necessarily so for a ratio, which expresses the relationship of two separate and distinct quantities, neither of which is included in the other. See also PROPORTION and RATE.

rationing A method for allocating limited quantities of an article, commodity, or service that is intended to ensure equity in allocation. FOOD RATIONING has been used in times of scarcity, as in Britain and most of Europe during World War II, where it had the unexpected benefit of leading to improved early child development because previously deprived children received adequate nutritional intake. Scarce health care resources, such as the services provided by diagnostic imaging equipment, are rationed in some countries, mainly by the cost of the service, and in others by time, such as lengthy waiting times for the test. See also RESOURCE ALLOCATION.

rauwolfia A plant native to India that contains an alkaloid, reserpine, long used in Ayurvedic medicine to treat fever, anxiety, and depression and as an antidote to snake poisoning. In the 1950s, Western physicians learned about its efficacy, and it had a vogue in the treatment of hypertension.

raw food Hominid precursors of humans discovered almost a million years ago that meat placed in or near a fire to cook improved in flavor, was easier to digest, and did not go bad as rapidly, but it has been only about 150 years since humans discovered that raw meat, fish, and milk can cause disease because they contain or are good culture media for pathogenic organisms. Even so, many people enjoy raw foods, such as oysters, sushi, and uncooked vegetables. Provided raw foods are fresh and food hygiene is satisfactory, the risk of food poisoning is small.

Raynaud's disease, syndrome A peripheral vascular disease, first described by the French physician Maurice Raynaud (1834–1881), that causes vasospasm and ischemia in the affected blood vessel distribution, i.e., fingers, toes, sometimes more proximal regions of the limbs, especially after exposure to cold environments. Preventable causes include vasospasm due to the action of nicotine that occurs as a consequence of heavy smoking and use of vibrating machinery, such as pneumatic drills.

rayon See VISCOSE RAYON.

reaction time The time taken to respond to a neural stimulus. The term usually applies to the response time for sensory stimuli such as the brake lights of the car ahead of a highway driver or a warning signal of trouble on a factory production line. The same term is used to describe reaction to reflexes, but that usage is discouraged. Reaction time varies with age, health status, and training, and is adversely affected by narcotics, sedatives, and alcohol intoxication.

reason for encounter A phrase used mainly by family physicians to describe and explain why patients choose to see them. This reason may be recorded as a diagnostic label, a problem list, an administrative procedure, etc. The term has the advantage of flexibility but the disadvantage of some difficulty when classifying and measuring activity in the physician's office.

recall bias A systematic error that is caused by differing degrees of accuracy in remembering past events, including previous medical history. This bias often arises when people's past history includes events that they have forgotten or not mentioned because they consider them irrelevant, embarrassing, or shameful, e.g., details of premarital or extramarital sexual activity, or because their memory of unpleasant experiences has been suppressed.

receiver operating characteristic (ROC) curve A term based on studies of radar operators that assessed their ability to detect faint signals. It is a graphical method to display data used to assess the value of a screening test as a way to distinguish healthy from potentially sick people.

receptors, receptor cells In sense organs, the cells that are specially adapted to receive and react to relevant stimuli, which may be mechanical (pressure, pain), chemical, or "electrical" or response to electromagnetic radiation. Examples include the rods and cones in the RETINA, the "taste buds" or chemoreceptor cells on the tongue, and pain receptors in the dermis.

recertification A method adopted by physician specialty boards in the United States and comparable bodies in other nations, following the lead of the UK Royal College of General Practitioners in the 1970s, to reassess physicians' professional competence at intervals. This is established as a routine procedure for physicians throughout the English-speaking world. In the United States it is used by all specialty boards, including the AMERICAN BOARD OF PREVENTIVE MEDICINE, with specified requirements, e.g., credits for continuing medical education. Formal examinations are seldom part of the process, but peer reviews of performance sometimes are. Details of methods used in recertification by the various specialty boards are available on their Web sites. See also AMERICAN BOARDS.

recessive trait A genetic trait that is expressed as the phenotype in an offspring only when present in both parents.

recidivism Reversion to an undesirable behavior pattern, such as committing another criminal offense after punishment or becoming drug-dependent again after an apparent cure of addiction. Recidivism rates are measured by recording the proportion of persons who must return to a custodial institution or a treatment clinic after having been declared "cured."

reciprocity A formal or informal arrangement that allows exchange of items or entities with the assumption that they are of equal value. Reciprocity of professional qualifications means that these are accepted in a jurisdiction other than that in which the qualifications were obtained.

recombinant DNA A type of DNA that has been artificially modified by having genes from another organism inserted into it, as in the process of GENETIC ENGINEERING. Recombinant DNA has an increasing number of uses in clinical and preventive medicine, e.g., in the manufacture of vaccines devoid of protein to which people might have adverse reactions.

recommended daily intake A term for a vaguely defined concept that often appears on the labels of proprietary foods and dietary supplements. The problem that frequently arises is failure to specify by whom the recommendation is made. It may be a respected national government agency, such as the US Food and Drug Administration; a designated committee of specialists, for instance, in nutrition; a self-appointed group; or a team or individual selected by the manufacturer of the proprietary food or dietary supplement in question.

recommended dietary allowance (RDA) Guidelines based on calorie, vitamin, and mineral intake in studies that assess ingested food in relation to nutritional and general health status, thereby leading to empirical decisions about daily needs in relation to age, sex, height, and weight. Details of US RDAs are available at http://www.nal.usda.gov/fnic/etext/000105.html.

recommended exposure level (REL) The maximum safe concentration of a substance to which occupational or environmental exposure can occur. The RELs of more than 600 substances have been identified by the US National Institute for Occupational Safety and Health. Similar, usually lower, safety levels are specified by the criteria of the European Union.

record See MEDICAL RECORD.

record linkage A method for relating a set of information about an individual to one or more other sets, collected at different times and often different places, with the aim of demonstrating a connection, such as effects that are remote in time and place from their underlying causes, e.g., cancer with long latency between exposure and onset of disease. An essential prerequisite is a reliable and consistent way to identify individuals, using tested and proven methods to do so. One method that works with very high reliability is to use a sequence of numbers and letters for the individual's birth date, sex, birth place, birth order in cases of multiple births, personal name, and mother's family name at the time of her birth. The odds of repeating the same sequence for two individuals, and thus confusing their identities, are less than one in a trillion if this system is adhered to. In some nations, record linkage studies are conducted in a national census office, where the officials (statisticians, epidemiologists) have taken an oath of secrecy to preserve personal privacy and confidentiality. In some nations, record linkage studies require the informed consent of the individuals to be studied, which is obviously impossible when the individuals are deceased.

recreational drug A mood-altering drug that is taken for reasons other than prevention or treatment of disease, i.e., for pleasure rather than need. CANNABIS (MARIJUANA) is an example.

recreational water A body of water, such as a swimming pool, hot springs, or spa, that is used for sport, exercise, or pleasure. Monitoring the safety and purity of recreational water to ensure that it does not carry pathogenic organisms is an important routine task for sanitarians. Public health authorities sometimes must close small lakes to swimmers during severe heat waves or after heavy rainstorms that introduce runoff contaminated by animal waste because it is not feasible to eliminate potential pathogenic microorganisms that expose to risk a large number of people who swim in water that is not circulating and cannot be purified or chlorinated.

recrudescence A flare-up of the symptoms of a disease after a temporary remission, such as a recurrence of fever that had previously subsided. The word also describes a surge in new cases of an epidemic that had begun to subside.

recycling Methods and procedures to recover useful and/or scarce ingredients from discarded domestic and industrial products and materials in order to use them again in similar products and to conserve scarce resources. Increasing numbers and varieties of recycling are practiced, but it is not always risk-free. Breaking used car batteries to reuse the lead carries a high risk of lead poisoning and environmental contamination with lead dust. Recycled food containers must, of course, be thoroughly cleansed and disinfected before reuse. Water from rivers such as the Mississippi, the Danube, and the Rhine may be recycled, or purified for drinking, many times during its progress from the source to the sea.

red blood corpuscles See ERYTHROCYTES.

Red Cross An international nonpartisan organization founded by the Swiss philanthropist Jean Henri Dunant (1828–1910), initially to provide emergency medical and surgical care for those injured in violent armed conflicts. Dunant was the first recipient of the Nobel Peace Prize in 1901. The organization was later broadened and became the INTERNATIONAL COMMITTEE OF RED CROSS AND RED CRESCENT SOCIETIES. In addition to wartime medical relief, it provides public health, medical, and social relief for people afflicted by natural disasters such as earthquakes. Although it aims to be strictly neutral, the organization has increasingly been drawn into violent conflicts in the sense that it is viewed as partisan by one or both sides, as in Palestine/Israel and more recently in Iraq. It receives about a quarter of its financial support from the United Nations. Because of religious symbolism associated with both the cross and the crescent, there has been some recent discussion about another symbol devoid of any associations of this nature (a diamond shape has been suggested). See http://www.ifrc.org/who/emblem.asp.

red eye See CONJUNCTIVITIS.

red light district A locality identified as an occupational site for prostitution, whether legalized and regulated, unregulated and illegal, or on the fringe of local laws and regulations. Red light districts are often the setting for other criminal activity, such as drug trafficking. In jurisdictions where prostitution is legal and regulated, medical examinations of sex workers and patrolling by police to enhance their safety from harm by violent clients may help to ensure that this otherwise marginal occupation is less hazardous and unhealthy than in the absence of legality.

red tide Reddish discoloration of tidal waters by dinoflagellates. These are toxic, and if they are ingested by filter-feeding shellfish that are then eaten by humans, severe and sometimes fatal PARALYTIC SHELLFISH POISONING can occur.

reductionism The method of studying complex systems by studying their component parts, a time-honored approach based on the philosophical concepts of Francis Bacon, René Descartes, and others, that the whole can be considered as the sum of its parts. The biomedical sciences address problems at the population, individual, organ, tissue, cellular, and molecular levels, and by proceeding in this way have made tremendous progress during the past few centuries. However, reductionism encourages increasing specialization and fails as a way to solve problems when the whole is qualitatively or quantitatively different from the sum of its parts. SYSTEMS THEORY and COMPLEXITY THEORY are alternative conceptual models that recognize ways in which the whole can differ from the sum of its parts and encourage other approaches, such as TRANSDISCIPLINARITY or integrative research.

Reed, Walter (1851–1902) The American public health physician and tropical disease specialist who discovered that the culicine mosquito *Aedes aegypti* is the vector for yellow fever. The US Armed Forces hospital in Washington DC is named in his honor.

reference group A group that is used as a standard for comparison with others being studied.

refinery An industrial installation where raw material is treated to extract valuable or needed ingredients or to concentrate them. Many refineries use industrial processes that generate toxic emissions and polluting substances that require surveillance or monitoring and control by various means, often strengthened by legislation and regulation. A furnace is required to refine metals, and emissions often contain trace amounts of toxic compounds made up of other metals, such as arsenic or lead, that may create a serious environmental health danger.

reform school The section of the law enforcement services that provides disciplinary custodial care for juvenile offenders. Formerly harsh penal institutions, reform schools now mostly attempt to educate and rehabilitate youthful offenders. Some of these offenders have psychiatric problems, substance abuse, or other health problems that require specialized care.

refraction In physics, this is the process of a change in the direction of light or sound waves as they pass from one medium or region of density to another. It is the process responsible for the focusing function of a lens. In ophthalmology and optometry, it is the process of testing the ability of the eyes to accommodate for close and distant vision, and fitting corrective lenses to overcome or minimize refractive errors of vision.

refugee Person who has been forced to leave his or her home and usual habitat by natural or human-induced disasters to move to another country. The UNITED NATIONS HIGH COMMISSIONER FOR REFUGEES (UNHCR) distinguishes refugees from INTERNALLY DISPLACED PERSONS, who have been forced out of their home and habitat but have not had to cross an international border. Refugees often have serious health problems, and refugee community health care is an important field for public health practice and community medicine. The total number of refugees in the world fluctuates from 16 to 20 million. In June 2005, it was 19 million. Some, such as the Palestinians, have been living in refugee communities for many years with little or no hope of a better way of life. For details see http://www.unhcr.ch/cgi-bin/texis/vtx/home.

refugee camp A temporary place of sanctuary for people who have been displaced from their usual home and habitat by natural or manmade disaster, typically violent armed conflict. Strictly speaking, refugees are people who leave their own country; those who do not leave are described as INTERNALLY DISPLACED PERSONS. Camps are often primitive, with makeshift facilities that may be improved by the intervention of UN agencies, the Red Cross, and nongovernmental organizations, with weatherproof tents, safe clean water supplies, toilet facilities, provision of medical and nursing care, and social support to reunite family members and organize permanent resettlement. At this stage, the temporary holding camp often evolves into a REFUGEE COMMUNITY. The common health problems include respiratory and gastroenteric infections, post-traumatic stress disorder (especially when families have been fragmented), and often trauma.

refugee community A long-term settlement of REFUGEES, which may become a semipermanent or permanent home, such as Palestinian refugee communities in the remnants of their former habitat in Palestine and the neighboring nations or Lebanon, Jordan, and Syria. Diasporas of ethnic groups, Armenians, Ukrainians, Jews, and others fleeing persecution and conflicts in Europe throughout the 20th century led to many physically fragmented, but culturally cohesive, communities in the United States and other countries.

refuse Syn: garbage, trash. Solid waste, regardless of how it is generated. It is differentiated into domestic, industrial, and street refuse. All contain material harmful or hazardous to health and require sanitary methods of disposal.

refutation Demonstration that an observation or a belief is false or based on false premises. The Austrian-British philosopher of science Karl Popper (1902–1994) analyzed how science advances and pointed out in *Logik der Forschung* (1935), translated as *The Logic of Scientific Discovery* (1959), that verification may merely help to per petuate false beliefs about incompletely studied problems, whereas suitable study may refute previously held false beliefs. According to Popper, the only valid way to uphold a scientific truth is failure of refutation.

regimen An organized plan of action, e.g., a therapeutic regimen that specifies aspects of a treatment plan, including details about matters such as diet, exercise, rest, and medications.

regionalization Organization of services for several sectors of society on a regional basis, rather than either nationally or locally. The aims include enhancing efficiency while, as far as feasible, preserving personalized services in health care, education, and social services.

regional planning Formal administration and organization of infrastructure, services, facilities, physical plant and equipment, workforce numbers and needs, and staffing structure, on a regional basis, preferably dealing with facilities and services for several sectors, for instance, the integration of health, education, and social services to minimize overhead costs.

register, registry A data file containing information about all the identified cases of a condition, such as cancer, ideally in a region (state, province, or nation) with a defined population. The information should include age, sex, other pertinent identifying data such as occupation and place of residence, and precise diagnosis. The publicly accessible data consist only of tables, graphs, perhaps choropleth maps, but no personal identifying information. Registries are used in many studies of cancer, in which incidence rates can be related to environmental, occupational, and other factors, survival rates can be related to methods of treatment, etc. Registries are used for other conditions also, e.g., twin registries, birth defect registries. Preferably a registry should provide statistically compiled data on all identified cases in a specified jurisdiction with a defined population, so that rates and prevalence can be calculated, but registries are useful even without a defined population because case fatality and survival rates can be calculated for the populations in specified diagnostic categories.

registered nurse (RN) A professional person who is licensed to practice as a nurse, after formal education and practical training in nursing care and passing a licensure examination. In the United States and Canada, RNs take a university degree and get supervised clinical experience in hospitals and often in community clinics in a course lasting 3 or more years. Registered nurses are equipped by training and expertise to take responsibility for many aspects of patient care, including drug dosage supervision, monitoring of vital signs, immediate emergency bedside intervention, and assessment of needs for a physician's more specialized services. Contrast LICENSED PRACTICAL NURSE, who has not had such rigorous training. See also PUBLIC HEALTH NURSE.

Registrar General's Occupational Classification The British medical statistician T. H. C. Stevenson (1870–1932), who worked in the Registry Office for England and Wales in the late 19th and early 20th centuries and designed an occupational classification that categorized employed persons into five "social classes," conventionally designated by Roman numerals I to V. Class I is professional occupations, typically requiring university-level education, such as physicians, lawyers, ministers of religion, etc.; Class II is described as intermediate professional and managerial occupations, such as bank managers and school teachers; Class III, skilled workers, is divided into skilled clerical and skilled manual workers; Class IV is semiskilled workers, such as bank clerks, farm laborers, and factory assembly line workers; and Class V is unskilled workers, e.g., shop assistants and food servers in fast food establishments. This classification, first used in the 1911 census, was routinely used until the 1980s and remains a useful tool for many sociological, epidemiological, and economic analyses. Social class correlates closely with many causes of death, disease, and disability. See also SOCIOECONOMIC CLASSIFICATIONS.

registration The process of recording details such as personal identifying data in a REGISTRY.

registration system A systematic, comprehensive method and procedures to record essential details about particular events or phenomena in a specified population. Well-known examples are registration systems for births, marriages and divorces, and deaths, so-called vital events that are registered in official statistics for various statutory purposes. DISEASE REGISTERS, such as cancer registries, function by means of overlapping automatic notification procedures to ensure that the information about all pathological and other diagnostic reports, surgical operations for cancer, autopsies, and death certificates in the region covered by the registration system are reported. Relevant recorded information includes personal identifying data, diagnostic details, and, in the case of cancer registries, information about treatment methods, survival time after diagnosis, and other analyses.

regression The British geneticist Francis Galton (1822–1911) coined the term "regression to the mean" to describe the tendency for extreme qualities such as tall or short stature, high or low intelligence, to move closer to the average in successive generations. The term entered the language and often appears in articles and books as "regression" without qualification, but with the implication that it refers to a decline or deterioration, which was not Galton's meaning: he used the term to refer equally to improvement or deterioration of inherited qualities.

regression analysis A statistical procedure that is used to find the best "fit" between a dependent variable y and one or more independent variables, x_1, x_2, etc., so their relationship conforms to a mathematical model. The best known, most commonly used, model is for linear regression, which is defined by a regression line.

regulations A written set of rules and procedures governing the conduct of individuals or groups, such as members of the public in relation to a social institution or a service. Typically, regulations provide details intended to implement a more general law. Regulations are usually drafted by a committee; for instance, public servants write regulations to cover details about ways to adhere to or comply with actions specified in laws enacted by an elected representative assembly, such as a congress or parliament. Regulations are usually public documents, whereas BYLAWS often relate mainly to the approved and proscribed conduct of members of a specific organization.

rehabilitation Efforts by qualified health professionals to assist persons with impairments or disabilities to achieve optimum levels of function, restore them to normal or as near normal as possible, and to reduce the problems they face in daily living because of impairment, disability, or handicap. This is an important aspect of health care for many people with chronic disabling illnesses or injuries. In tertiary care hospitals, departments of rehabilitation medicine are staffed by physicians, physiotherapists, occupational therapists, social workers, prosthetics makers, psychologists, and other technically qualified specialists. See also PHYSICAL MEDICINE.

relapsing fever A contagious louse-borne or tick-borne spirochete infection due to *Borrelia* that causes intermittent fever and prostration and has a 10% to 20% case fatality rate if untreated. Wild rodents are the natural reservoir. This was formerly one of the QUARANTINABLE DISEASES, but it is now rare and no longer subject to strict isolation because it responds readily to antibiotics.

relative humidity The ratio of observed atmospheric water vapor pressure to expected water vapor pressure if the atmosphere were saturated at the same temperature. High relative humidity reduces the evaporative cooling effect of sweating and is the basis for the HUMIDEX reading, i.e., an adjustment of ambient temperature to allow for humidity.

relative risk 1. Syn: risk ratio. The ratio of the risk of disease or death or other exposure-related outcome among those exposed to a risk to the risk among those not exposed. 2. The ratio of the cumulative incidence rate in those exposed to the cumulative incidence rate in those not exposed. 3. In the analysis of results of a case control study, the ODDS RATIO is usually considered to be an approximation of the relative risk.

relaxation techniques A general term for methods of reducing emotional tension in medical procedures, work, sport, daily life, interpersonal relationships, etc. Many methods rely on a form of meditation, e.g., YOGA or Zen. Some sports psychologists employ conditioning, using the power of suggestion to maximize the will to win and minimize apprehension. Least desirable and not very effective are methods that rely on use of mood-modifying substances.

reliability Syn: reproducibility. The characteristic by which a measuring instrument or procedure yields a series of identical or closely similar measurements of the same variable that is repeatedly measured by the same observer using the same instrument or procedure. See also REPLICATION and REPRODUCIBILITY.

relief 1. Provision of material and financial aid for victims of natural or manmade disasters. In the United States and many other countries, disaster relief is made available under provisions of federally mandated laws. 2. A traditional term for several outmoded methods of assisting needy people with monetary support, food supplies, clothing, etc.

religion A system of belief in a higher power than humans, usually with rites, traditions, values, and customs that govern aspects of behavior, including many with implications for health and human rights, such as marital customs, rights of women, childbearing and human reproduction, permitted and proscribed foods, methods for disposal of the dead, and attitudes toward others with different beliefs and/or practices. Religious leaders, missionaries, and other believers in particular faiths have brought great benefit to others, especially in the health and education sectors, and religious faith can provide solace to people at times of stress, such as bereavement. Critics of religion object to its reliance on unverifiable faith over the objective facts of science, to its occasional manifestations of intolerance and attempts to enforce compliance with its practices on people outside that belief system, and the reluctance of some faiths to accept certain scientific discoveries. The three monotheist religions—Judaism, Christianity, and Islam—share many beliefs, values, and customs. However, intolerance by individuals proclaiming each of these religions for those proclaiming the others, and for Hinduism and Buddhism, has led to hostility, hatred, and violence, with much suffering, death, and social devastation.

religious diets Members of many religious faiths adhere to specific diets and dietary customs, some of which have important implications for health. There is persuasive evidence, for instance, that vegetarian diets are often associated with longevity and with low incidence of and mortality rates from coronary heart disease and many varieties of cancer.

rem Abbreviation for roentgen equivalent man, the quantity of ionizing radiation that delivers the energy of one roentgen per gram to living tissue.

remote sensing Collection, analysis, and interpretation of information at a distance from the location of the phenomenon under observation, now mainly by satellite observation. Remote sensing provides information about changing environmental and ecological conditions, such as altered distribution of vegetation due to climate change. This is an indicator of ecosystem change, with implications for distribution and abundance of insect vectors, such as mosquitoes.

renal calculi Syn: kidney stones. A condition in which some salts excreted by the renal system, e.g., calcium oxalate, crystallize out in urine, often because of inadequate fluid intake. This causes the acutely painful condition of renal colic and sometimes leads to renal damage, renal hypertension, and renal failure with uremia, i.e., metabolic poisoning.

renewable resources Resources derived from natural systems that are not finite, such as solar, tidal, and wind energy, or from living organisms, such as trees that can be replaced by others as they are used. The term is used mainly in referring to energy resources; renewable energy resources are those derived from sun, wind, tides, or vegetable or animal sources. These include BIOMASS FUELS, ethanol (alcohol derived from fermentation, e.g., of corn), METHANE generated by fermentation of manure or human waste, and, technically, power generation using solar, wind, and tidal energy. See also GREEN ENERGY.

repeatability The quality of a test whereby repetition of the same protocol and procedures yields the same or closely similar results or responses each time. This is an important criterion of tests used in clinical diagnosis. The distinction between repeatability and RELIABILITY is that the latter is a property of the measuring instrument, whereas repeatability is determined by interaction of the observer, the subject, and the instrument. See also REPLICATION and REPRODUCIBILITY, which are similar but not identical concepts.

repetitive strain injury (RSI) Also called repetition strain injury and cumulative trauma disorder. A common soft-tissue disorder that may affect the arms from shoulder to wrist and fingers and may also affect the neck, causing pain that may be severe and even debilitating. The pain may persist and may interfere with sleep. It is an occupational disorder of keyboard operators that causes sufficient lost time from work to be described as a public health problem. It can usually be prevented by correct positioning of the computer keyboard in relation to wrists and fingers and attention to other relevant ergonomic factors, such as seating and position of computer screen. As well as the physical circumstances, the power of suggestion may play a role, e.g., in inducing "behavioral epidemics" of the condition in office workers. "Tennis elbow," "housemaid's knee," and several other occupational soft-tissue disorders are variations.

replication 1. The process of repeating an experiment or observation, perhaps many times, by different observers, to confirm or refute findings of original experiments or observations. It is an important property of all sound science that experiments and observations can be replicated, to help establish validity of observations and conclusions, conforming to the scientific criterion of REPRODUCIBILITY. It is a sine qua non of good scientific practice to make full details of research protocols readily available, to facilitate replication by other scientists. 2. In virology, replication is the multiplication of organisms.

reportable disease See NOTIFIABLE DISEASE.

repression 1. A psychological defense mechanism in which memories and ideas are expelled from consciousness into subconscious thought because they cause anxiety, emotional conflict. One of the aims of psychotherapy is sometimes to uncover repressed emotions and deal with them at the conscious, rational level. 2. In politics, the attempt to expunge political beliefs at odds with those of an authoritarian regime, e.g., by police or state-sponsored paramilitary forces.

reproducibility The quality of an experiment or test wherein repetition under identical or similar circumstances gives the same or a closely similar result to that achieved on the first occasion. See also RELIABILITY and REPEATABILITY.

reproductive care See MATERNAL AND CHILD HEALTH (MCH).

reproductive disorders A wide range of conditions affecting spermatozoa and/or ova, the process of fertilization, implantation, and early fetal development. These include anatomical anomalies, sexually transmitted and other diseases of the genital tract, systemic conditions that impair capacity to become pregnant, and some psychosomatic conditions.

reproductive fitness Syn: genetic fitness. The capacity of members of a species to reproduce and leave descendents of their genetic lineage to follow in their footsteps. This is the quality referred to as "survival of the fittest" by evolutionary biologists.

reproductive freedom See REPRODUCTIVE RIGHTS.

reproductive health Aspects of health that affect reproductive performance. Factors that enhance reproductive performance include physical fitness, adequate nutritional status, and good health. Issues of concern to specialists in reproductive health include adolescent development, the status and societal roles of girls and young women, efficient physiological function of endocrine and reproductive organs, adequacy of the pelvis for vaginal delivery, and monitoring of maternal health and fetal development. See http://www.who.int/reproductive-health/ for World Health Organization initiatives and actions regarding reproductive health.

reproductive rights This means respect for female autonomy, the right of women to make decisions for themselves about whether to become and to remain pregnant. This right and the accompanying freedom are severely infringed in many societies and traditional cultures and are under threat in others, including some democracies. See CAIRO DECLARATION.

reproductive technology This term describes methods of investigation and treatment for couples who desire to have a child and have failed to conceive one. Most methods were developed in the last third of the 20th century. They include the use of artificial insemination, in vitro fertilization, fertility-enhancing drugs, embryo freezing, and, theoretically, human use of cloning comparable to cloning that has been successfully used with animals, albeit with many failed attempts. Almost all new reproductive technologies present challenging moral and ethical problems.

reproductive toxicology The specialized application of toxicology to research, prevention, and treatment of impaired reproductive fitness attributable to, for example, industrial chemicals that cause impaired spermatogenesis, fetotoxicity, miscarriage, birth defects, etc.

research Activities designed to develop or contribute to generalizable knowledge, i.e., theories, principles, relationships, or the information on which these are based, that can be confirmed or refuted by recognized methods of observation, experiment, and inference. Research may be conducted simply by observation and inference, or by the use of experiment, in which the research worker alters or manipulates conditions in order to observe and study the consequences of doing so. When humans are the subjects of research, it is mandatory to submit the research proposal for ethical review and to obtain the informed consent of the subjects. In public health, there is an ill-defined distinction between research and routine surveillance, case finding, etc.

research design The method and procedures employed in a specified research project or program. This is an integral part of the research PROTOCOL, a mandatory requirement when a research proposal is submitted to a funding agency. It should be sufficiently detailed and explicit for other research workers to replicate the design.

reservoir A receptacle for storage. The word describes water collection and storage for drinking and irrigation. Water reservoirs have important public health implications relating to the purity, safety, freedom from pathogens, essential mineral content, etc. Another context of the word is "reservoir of infection," which refers to human or animal hosts of infectious pathogens.

residential care This term can mean either home (i.e., domiciliary) care or care in a specialized residential setting, such as a long-stay care institution or a hospice. Because of its ambiguity, the term is preferably avoided.

resistance 1. Opposition, for instance by the people of a country to an invading foreign army. 2. The resistance of a host to an invading pathogen, which is mediated by the immunological defenses of the host. 3. The phenomenon of antibiotic resistance that develops in pathogenic organisms is living proof that evolution is a biological fact, not a theory. This most often occurs because of the selective survival and reproduction of strains of an organism that have an inherent metabolic capacity to survive exposure to the antibiotic. It is facilitated and aggravated by overuse of antibiotics in health care and in animal husbandry.

resistant organism Unqualified, the term means an organism resistant to all antibiotics, but usually it is qualified to designate the antibiotic(s) to which an organism is resistant.

resolving power The capacity of a system or measuring instrument to distinguish between truly distinct entities that are very close together or closely resemble one another. Resolving power or resolution differs from "precision" in being concerned mainly with distinguishing differing entities.

resource allocation The process of deciding how to distribute limited quantities of goods and services, numbers of qualified staff, specialized facilities, and available funds among competing claims for them. Ideally, it is evidence based, with supporting data from demographic, epidemiological, sociological, and economic sources and takes due account of ethical and political concerns. Sometimes, when it involves allocation of financial resources, it is entangled in political and emotional considerations that overwhelm rational debate. When it involves RATIONING of costly life-saving equipment and specialized technology, as for long-term renal dialysis, difficult ethical decisions are often required.

respirable particle A particle of matter that is small enough to be inhaled into the respiratory tract. Generally this is a particle 10 microns in size or less. Particles 2.5 microns or smaller can penetrate to and lodge in alveoli.

respirator A device or piece of equipment to facilitate respiration. The word is used to describe a device to filter air or remove toxic and poisonous gases and fumes, i.e., a gas mask, or a machine to assist or replace the action of respiratory muscles, e.g., an IRON LUNG or Drinker respirator, or the machine used in anesthesia when respiratory muscles are deliberately paralyzed during surgical procedures.

respiratory diseases a large group of inflammatory, environmental, neoplastic, and degenerative conditions affecting the respiratory system. They include acute, subacute, and chronic conditions that may affect any or all parts of the respiratory tract from the nasopharynx to the bronchioles and alveoli. Many can be prevented or treated. Chronic respiratory diseases, mainly emphysema and bronchitis, and pulmonary fibrosis, are among the leading causes of death.

respiratory distress syndrome A serious, sometimes fatal, condition of newborns, usually caused by hyaline membrane disease, sometimes by acute respiratory infection. In adults, this was manifest in the epidemic of SEVERE ACUTE RESPIRATORY SYNDROME (SARS) in 2003.

respite care Short-term care of long-term sick person(s) in order to give regular caregiver(s) a brief rest or respite, for example for a vacation.

response rate The proportion, percentage, or fraction of individuals who reply to inquiries that have been directed to all the individuals in a population, or a representative sample of them. The validity of findings or results and conclusions derived from them is dependent on the response rate. If the response rate is low, i.e., if there are large proportions of nonresponders, the validity of the results is dubious, even if impeccable sampling methods have been used, because of the magnitude of random error.

response time In neuroscience, psychology, social sciences, etc., the time that elapses between a stimulus and a specific response to this stimulus.

restaurant A place that sells meals prepared and served on the premises. Restaurant types include diners, bistros, and trattorias, all of which are usually small and modest. The size, volume of business, clientele, and gastronomic quality of restaurants vary enormously, but all have in common the fact that, because they serve meals to members of the public, they must comply with public health laws and regulations about food handling and hygiene. Routine restaurant inspection is an essential public health function.

restaurant hygiene Sanitarians (health inspectors) monitor restaurant hygiene to safeguard the public from harm caused by food poisoning. Routine inspections seek evidence of cleanliness, good housekeeping, kitchen hygiene, and whole someness and freshness of food, with emphasis on safe handling of food items with brief shelf life, hygienic disposal of kitchen waste, absence of infestation with pests, hygienic behavior and absence of contagious diseases of workers (food handlers, cooks, and waiters), and various other criteria, e.g., acceptable occupancy levels.

rest home A facility for long-term care of people who are infirm because of physical or mental impairment, disability, or handicap. A rest home usually offers shelter and meals but little or no nursing care and only episodic medical care.

restorative dentistry The branch of dentistry concerned with repairing and filling carious teeth and with other ways to restore the efficiency of painless mastication.

restructuring A term used by administrators and planners to describe arrangements for the reorganization of a workforce

resuscitation Emergency measures to restore breathing and heart beat, as in CARDIOPULMONARY RESUSCITATION (CPR) and artificial respiration, when only respiratory function is disrupted. For guidelines, methods, etc., see http://www.resus.org.uk/siteindx.htm.

retardation Syn: mental deficiency. Subnormal mental or intellectual function, usually originating in infancy or childhood. There are several levels, based on scores on the WECHSLER SCALES. Mildly retarded persons are educable; moderately retarded persons can be trained to use the toilet, dress, and feed themselves; severe and profoundly retarded persons require varying degrees of personal care and supervision. See MENTAL IMPAIRMENT.

retina The tissue at the back of the eyeballs that contains the rods and cones, the sensory cells that are the end organs of sight.

retirement The phase of life that follows the end of the regular working lifetime. For most people in affluent nations, this comes in the seventh decade, usually around age 60 to 65 years. It is a major milestone for many people, often a time when nascent chronic disabling diseases declare themselves because their natural history determines their overt onset, or emotional stresses associated with declining income and loss of self-esteem precipitate their onset. In an ideal world, it would be the epochal milestone when the expertise of preventive geriatrics would be deployed to minimize the impact of age-related impairments and disability.

retrospective study 1. Any descriptive study in the social sciences or epidemiology that considers how the past history of a group of persons has influenced their present status. 2. An undesirable synonym for CASE CONTROL STUDY.

retrovirus A virus that has the ability to replicate itself by copying its genome, i.e., all its DNA, into cells of a host organism. HIV is a retrovirus. Other lymphotropic retroviruses, such as human T-cell lymphotropic virus type II (HTLV-II), can cause leukemia.

reverse osmosis See DESALINATION.

reverse transcription The process of viral replication used by retroviruses such as HIV, in which the viral RNA genome is inserted into host cells where the viral DNA is then produced. The process is facilitated by an enzyme, reverse transcriptase.

Reye syndrome An acute, potentially fatal childhood disease with encephalopathy and hepatic necrosis. Its presumed cause is the use of aspirin to control fever in acute febrile infections. Mild forms that pass unnoticed may be relatively common. Named for Australian pathologist Ralph Reye (1912–1978), who first described the syndrome and identified its relationship to aspirin use.

Rhazes (c. 850–c. 923 CE) The Westernized name of Abu Bakr Muhammad ibn Zakariya al-Razi, a Persian scientist, physician, and Platonist philosopher in the Islamic age of enlightenment. He fostered the expansion of empirical medical knowledge and practical procedures for treatment, rather than theoretical reflections on illness and health. His contributions to public health included a recommended behavioral regimen to preserve good health and, in the field of clinical communicable disease control, criteria to distinguish smallpox from measles and much else.

Rhesus factor (Rh factor) An antigen on the membrane of red blood corpuscles, so named because it was first identified in rhesus monkeys, occurs in 80% to 85% of humans of European origin. Those lacking this factor develop antibodies on exposure, either by transfusion or when a pregnant woman who is Rh negative has an Rh-positive fetus; in a subsequent pregnancy, maternal Rh antibodies cause grave fetal damage, the extreme form of which is fatal erythroblastosis fetalis.

rheumatic fever An acute inflammatory disease of joints and endocardial tissue that occurs as an autoimmune response to infection with hemolytic streptococcus. A pharyngitis or scarlet fever. It was a common childhood disease until the advent of sulfonamides and penicillin, to which the hemolytic streptococcus was sensitive. A very high proportion of children with rheumatic fever developed chronic valvular heart disease, typically mitral stenosis, which usually shortened their lives by causing heart failure in early or middle adult years. The disease still occurs in some low-income nations and among marginalized populations in rich nations.

rheumatism An all-purpose name for painful, stiff, perhaps swollen joints. The common types of rheumatism are: 1. Osteoarthritis, a degenerative disease of joints, especially weight-bearing and other joints that have been worked hard throughout life; 2. Rheumatoid arthritis, an inflammatory disease affecting young adults that often begins in small joints of the hands, is accompanied by systemic illness probably of autoimmune origin, and often causes progressive disability and crippling deformities; 3. Gout, a metabolic disease that usually begins in middle age; and 4. Miscellaneous other conditions, including fibromyalgia, soft-tissue inflammatory and post-traumatic lesions, etc. All forms combined are the leading cause of disability and lost time from work and among the leading reasons for physician visits and for obtaining and using both prescribed and over-the-counter medications, as well as visits to alternative healers.

rheumatoid arthritis A chronic inflammatory autoimmune disease affecting mainly the small joints of the hands and feet, typically beginning in late adolescence or early adult life, more often in females than males, causing chronic pain, debility, progressive deformity, and disability.

rheumatology The medical specialty that deals with inflammatory and degenerative diseases of joints and their soft-tissue adnexa.

Rh factor See RHESUS FACTOR.

rhinitis Inflammation of the nasal mucosa. Infectious rhinitis is the stage of the common cold when there is acute rhinitis and a profuse seropurulent nasal discharge. Allergic rhinitis is hay fever. Rhinitis can also be caused by irritant or toxic fumes.

rhythm method The method of reducing the risk of pregnancy by restricting penetrative sexual intercourse with ejaculation to times when fertility is believed to be minimal because of the phase of the menstrual cycle. In theory, a woman is least likely to conceive during her menstrual period or shortly before and after her period. The critical word is the adverb "shortly" because ovulation can occur late or early rather than in the middle of the menstrual cycle, and it is believed that some women ovulate under the stimulus of orgasm. A refinement of the rhythm method is to record temperature fluctuations because a slight rise may accompany rupture of the Graafian follicle and release of an ovum from the ovary. However, even with this refinement, the rhythm method, advocated as the only acceptable method for Roman Catholics who adhere to papal pronouncements, is unreliable.

riboflavin Syn: vitamin B_2. A water-soluble member of the vitamin B complex that is essential for cellular, tissue, and organ growth. Foodstuffs rich in riboflavin include nuts, eggs, and vegetables.

riboflavin deficiency See VITAMIN B_2 (RIBOFLAVIN) DEFICIENCY.

ribonucleic acid (RNA) One of the two forms of nucleic acid in cell nuclei, comprising ribose nucleotides, adenine, guanine, cytosine, and uracil. MESSENGER RNA transcribes (copies) the genetic code from a DNA template, so it is essential for cell reproduction. Transfer RNA and ribosomal RNA are involved in protein synthesis.

Richter scale A method invented by the American geophysicist C. F. Richter (1900–1985) to record on a logarithmic scale the magnitude of earthquakes from 1 to a theoretical maximum of 10, indicating the amplitude and duration of the shock wave in the ground that is produced by shifting tectonic plates. An earthquake measuring 2 on the Richter scale produces a perceptible tremor. At Richter scale 6 and above, there is damage and destruction of buildings. The most violent earthquakes ever recorded, the Chilean earthquake of 1960, measured more than 9.5 on the Richter scale. The earthquake that produced the Indian Ocean tsunami in December 2004 measured 9.15 on the Richter scale.

rickets A condition caused by vitamin D deficiency that produces softening and deformity of weight-bearing and other bones. It was a common disease of deprived children in dark and gloomy environments, such as tenement housing in 19th century industrial cities where smoke obstructed sunlight (which synthesizes vitamin D in the skin). One consequence was often obstructed labor and death in childbirth, when affected girls with a deformed pelvis grew up and became pregnant. It can be prevented and its progress halted by daily ingestion of vitamin D, an oil-soluble vitamin contained in fish oils and routinely added to milk.

rickettsiae A family of organisms of size and biological characteristics between bacteria and viruses, responsible for various infections of humans and other mammals. Most are transmitted by arthropod-borne vectors, such as ticks, mites, lice, etc., and many are dangerous. The diseases include epidemic louse-borne TYPHUS, ROCKY MOUNTAIN SPOTTED FEVER, and many others. The name commemorates the American pathologist Howard Ricketts (1871–1910).

Rift Valley fever A mosquito-borne arbovirus infection of cattle, causing fatal hepatitis, that occasionally affects humans, in whom it causes a dengue-like illness that is directly transmissible person to person. Severe human cases with hemorrhagic fever or encephalitis can be fatal.

right to die The ultimate autonomy, the freedom of individuals to choose to end their own life. The right to die movement provides emotional and sometimes social, but rarely political, support for the right of incurably ill individuals to end their lives and shorten a period of unbearable suffering. It is a position that entails morally and ethically difficult choices.

right to life The UN Universal Declaration of Human Rights asserts that everyone has the right to life. The phrase often refers to a movement driven by religious belief in the sanctity of life and especially aims to preserve the right to life for the human fetus.

Right to Life (pro-life) An activist religious movement based in the United States that believes human life begins at conception, that all fetuses have a right to life, and that opposes interference with or termination of pregnancy.

rinderpest An acute, highly fatal cattle disease caused by a rhinovirus transmitted by droplet or the fecal-oral route. It does not affect humans, but humans who depend on cattle for livelihood or food suffer when an epidemic wipes out their herds. The disease occurs mainly in Africa, the Middle East, and south Asia.

Ringelmann number A colorimetric scale for atmospheric opacity that measures emissions from furnaces, incinerators, etc. A Ringelmann number of 0 is clear air, 5 is totally opaque. The system was developed by the French engineer (1861–1931). It is a subjective measure although still used, despite that better techniques for measuring emissions are now widely available.

ringworm Syn: dermatophytosis. A fungus infection of the skin of humans and domestic animals such as dogs, cats, and horses. In addition to the circular skin lesions that give it its name, the infection causes other related conditions, including ATHLETE'S FOOT.

Rio Declaration The declaration that summarized the deliberations of the delegates to the World Summit on Sustainable Development in Rio de Janiero, Brazil, in 1992 (the Rio Summit). These were expressed in 27 principles, focusing on ways to strike a balance between economic development and protection of global life support systems, application of the PRECAUTIONARY PRINCIPLE, and an agenda for action to enhance prospects for improved quality of life while safeguarding essential ecosystems, known as Agenda 21. The full text is available at http://www.unep.org/Documents.multilingual/Default.asp?DocumentID=78&ArticleID=1163.

riparian rights The ancient right of access to a source of fresh water for drinking and irrigation, sanctioned by tradition rather than formal law, possessed by people living along the banks of a river or lake. Encroachment on riparian rights, such as by diversion of water sources, can cause wars.

risk The probability that an event will occur. In a nontechnical sense, the word covers several meanings and measures of probability, and these often obscure the technical meaning, confusing risk with HAZARD, which can mean any harmful or potentially harmful agent or factor. In technical discussions, as in actuarial estimates and environmental risk assessments, use of the word "risk" is best confined to contexts in which a probability of an event can be estimated or calculated.

risk analysis The process of assembling, categorizing, measuring, and analyzing all the evidence related to a particular risk or group of risks, as well as any protective factors that may occur in the same setting.

risk assessment Quantitative and/or qualitative estimation of the likelihood that an outcome, such as an adverse effect, will result from exposure to a specified hazard or hazards, or from the absence of protective or beneficial factors. Risk assessment is an integral part of health policy. It makes use of clinical, toxicological, epidemiological, environmental, and other data. There are four steps in risk assessment: 1. Hazard identification, which is identifying agents responsible for adverse effects and outcomes, delineating the exposed population, and describing exposure circumstances; 2. Risk characterization, i.e., describing potential effects of exposure, quantifying dose-effect and dose-response relationships; 3. Exposure assessment, which is assessing and measuring exposure and dose in specified populations on the basis of measurements of environmental and individual levels of toxic substances and pollutants, biological monitoring, etc.; and 4. Risk estimation, which means assembling the relevant data to quantify the risk level in a specific population, the end result of which is estimates of the numbers affected by defined and specified outcomes.

risk-benefit analysis Strictly speaking, an economic analysis in which the direct and INDIRECT COSTS of an action or intervention are set out in a balance sheet with the economic benefits in the opposing columns, but in practice more often a qualitative comparison of predictable risks and expected benefits or, if done after the fact, pairs of lists setting out the benefits that have followed actions or interventions for which the identifiable risks (or harms) were also known. See also COST-BENEFIT ANALYSIS.

risk characterization The process of describing all relevant aspects of a specified risk, including its qualitative and quantitative dimensions.

risk communication The process of informing and educating all persons exposed or potentially exposed to a specified risk about the qualitative and quantitative dimensions of the specified risk. This can be a complex process, particularly because many people have difficulty with the concept of probabilities, which involves Bayesian statistics — the fact that one person in a million may be struck by lightning does not help a golfer carrying steel-shafted golf clubs calculate the risk that he may be struck by lightning if he plays during a thunderstorm. See BAYESIAN INFERENCE.

risk evaluation A combination of risk analysis and risk assessment.

risk factor A term first used in the 1950s in reports of results from the FRAMINGHAM STUDY of heart disease, meaning an aspect of behavior or way of living, such as habitual patterns of diet, exercise, use of cigarettes and alcohol, etc., or a biological characteristic, genetic trait, or a health-related condition or environmental exposure with predictable effects on the risk of disease due to a specific cause, including in particular increased likelihood of an unfavorable outcome. Other meanings have been given to this term, such as a DETERMINANT of disease that can be modified by specific actions, behaviors, or treatment regimens. Risk factors may be divided into those directly related to disease outcomes (proximal risk factors), such as nonuse of seat belts and risk of injury in automobile crashes, and those with indirect effect on outcomes (distal risk factors). An example of the latter is the influence of ozone-destroying substances, such as CFCs, on the risk of malignant melanoma, mediated by increased exposure to solar ultraviolet radiation because of depletion of protective stratospheric ozone.

risk identification As the term makes clear, this means identifying a risk, often one that involves situations and circumstances that previously had been accepted as harmless.

risk management Actions and policies aimed at reducing the levels of risk to which persons and populations are exposed. These actions proceed in several stages involving investigation, monitoring, management, and politics. 1. Risk evaluation, i.e., comparing calculated risks of impact of known environmental exposures with other risks, and expected costs and benefits of actions taken to reduce risks, using all these sets of information to decide what is an acceptable risk level. 2. Exposure control, i.e., actions taken to maintain exposure below the maximum acceptable level. 3. Risk monitoring, i.e., observation, assessment, measurements to determine efficacy of actions to control exposure, and, if necessary, surveillance of indicators that the risk may recur.

risk marker Syn: risk indicator. An attribute associated with increased probability of disease occurrence caused by exposure.

risk monitoring The act of monitoring an identified risk.

risk reduction Specific action that is taken to reduce and then preferably, if feasible, to eliminate a specified risk.

risk-taking behavior Actions ranging from ignorance and foolishness to recklessness that are sometimes regarded as adventurous or brave. For example, rock climbing, whitewater rafting, and sky diving can endanger life if conducted without prior training or adequate supervision, so they are extreme forms of risk-taking behavior, but less extreme for those who have had training. Other types of risk-taking behavior include gambling for high stakes at long odds and crossing busy roads in the midst of heavy, fast-moving traffic. Cigarette smoking and unprotected sexual intercourse with strangers are types of risk-taking behavior. In short, the term is vaguely defined but describes many kinds of conduct that are generally known to be harmful to life, limb, and health. Health workers must take into account the psychological makeup and defenses of persons who engage in such conduct and must avoid blaming victims of risk-taking behavior when this has adverse health outcomes.

river blindness See ONCHOCERCIASIS.

road rage Displays of anger and violence by automobile drivers, associated with frustration caused by traffic delays and perceived bad behavior of other road users. Studies of factors leading to traffic crashes have demonstrated that as many as 20% to 30% may be associated with road rage.

Robertson-Berger meter An electronic instrument used to measure ultraviolet radiation flux, which is a component of solar radiation. Originally designed in Australia by D. R. Robertson (1914–1989) in the 1950s, the meters were modified by D. S. Berger (b. 1923) in the United States. Robertson-Berger meters are used to assess the potential risk to humans and other organisms from solar ultraviolet radiation. Alternative measuring instruments for UV radiation flux are described; some employ biological monitoring.

Rocky Mountain spotted fever Syn: North American tick typhus. A rickettsial infection due to *Rickettsia rickettsii*, transmitted from dogs, rodents, and other mammals to humans by the bite of an infected tick in which it is maintained by transovarial and transstadial passage. It is not transmissible person to person. It causes fever, a papillomacular rash on the limbs, muscle pains, and malaise and has a case fatality rate of 10% to 25% if untreated. It responds to chloramphenicol and other broad-spectrum antibiotics. See http://www.cdc.gov/ncidod/dvrd/rmsf/ for details.

rodenticides Poisons that kill rats. The most effective until a few decades ago was a witch's brew of arsenic phosphate, which was also extremely poisonous to people, especially children. It has been superseded by warfarin derivatives, which work by preventing blood clotting and encouraging internal hemorrhages. These have the advantage that the dead rats are relatively odorless and innocuous to domestic pets, such as cats and dogs, and that death takes enough time after ingestion for the rats not to be suspicious about the bait.

rodents The mammalian order Rodentia, characterized by sharp incisor teeth with which they cut and chew their food, and which grow continuously as the edges wear away. Many rodents carry diseases that affect humans, and some are economically important, e.g., rats and mice that infest grain stores.

rodent ulcer Syn: basal cell skin cancer. A variety of skin cancer that invades locally but rarely metastasizes. If untreated, it can invade local tissues, including cartilage and bone, causing great disfigurement. It is causally related to exposure to solar radiation and responds to treatment with radiotherapy as well as surgical removal.

roentgen The unit formerly used to measure radiation dose (x-rays or gamma rays), named for the German physician Wilhelm Röntgen (1845–1923); his name is anglicized to Roentgen. It has been replaced by the SI unit SIEVERT (Sv).

Roe v. Wade The landmark case in the US Supreme Court in 1973 that led to liberalizing of previously punitive abortion laws, making it legal for women to obtain a medically induced and supervised termination of an early pregnancy. One consequence has been that illegal back street abortions with their high morbidity and mortality rates became a thing of the past. Those who oppose abortion under any circumstances, even incest or rape, have waged campaigns ever since, seeking to overturn this decision and have made inroads that undermine some aspects of the original protections provided for women in the Roe decision.

role playing An educational and training method that places learners in the imagined situations they would occupy if performing in real life the tasks they are learning to perform. The method is increasingly and effectively used in educating health professionals.

Roll Back Malaria A WHO campaign to control, and where possible eliminate, malaria from endemic regions. It relies mainly on preventing access of mosquitoes to susceptible persons by the use of bed-nets, environmental control, and larvicides. See http://www.who.int/malaria.

Rose questionnaire A questionnaire developed by the British epidemiologist Geoffrey Rose (1926–1993) to screen for symptoms of cardiovascular disease, especially for evidence of ischemic heart disease. The questions, which deal with ischemic pain on exertion and difficulty breathing, have been validated in many trials.

Ross, Ronald (1857–1932) An Indian-born British physician, mathematician, tropical disease specialist, entomologist, and poet, Ross is remembered mainly for his discovery of the role of the anopheline mosquito as the vector and intermediate host of the malaria parasite. He also worked out the first mathematical model of malaria epidemiology. He received the Nobel Prize in Physiology or Medicine in 1902 for his work on malaria.

rotator cuff injury Painful limitation of shoulder movements in which rotation of the shaft of the humerus is especially affected. It is due to injury and/or inflammation of the muscular and ligamentous tissue that holds the ball-and-socket shoulder joint in place. It is often caused by a sports injury or by repetitive occupational movements, such as operating a lever under tension.

rotavirus A genus of virus responsible for some severe gastrointestinal infections. In infants and small children, the severe dehydration it causes can be life threatening. This is a double-stranded RNA-containing virus, so named because of its wheel-like appearance under the electron microscope. It is most often transmitted by the fecal-oral route.

roundworms A family of helminths that includes several ubiquitous intestinal parasites, notably the lumbricoid worms, pinworms, etc.

Royal Institute of Public Health An independent society for sanitary inspectors and others in all aspects of public health practice and for the organizations in which they work. It offers training programs and certification in such fields as food inspection. It evolved from beginnings in the late 19th century. For more information, see http://www.riph.org.uk.

Royal Society The British academic association founded in 1660 by King Charles II to which natural, physical, biological, and social and behavioral scientists are elected on the basis of their contributions to their field of scientific and scholarly activity. It serves as an advisory body to the British government and publishes original articles of major importance on scholarly studies in its journals, which include the Proceedings of the Royal Society. See http://www.royalsoc.ac.uk.

Royal Society for Promotion of Health A British charitable health advocacy organization founded in 1876 following the Public Health Act in 1875, in a period of great advances in public health provision and sanitary reform, to which it contributed significantly. It became a leading authority, often consulted by governments and the media on health-related issues. Since the 1970s, it has focused on examinations, certification, and the *Journal of the Royal Society for the Promotion of Health*. For more information, see http://www.rsph.org.

RU 486 See MIFEPRISTONE.

rubella Syn: German measles. A childhood infectious disease that causes a fine macular rash, mild fever, and conjunctivitis. It is usually innocuous, but in the early 1940s the Australian ophthalmologist Norman Gregg (1892–1966) observed that patients with congenital cataract had a history of prenatal exposure to maternal rubella, which had occurred in a widespread epidemic some months earlier. Subsequently, rubella during early pregnancy was found to increase the risk of other abnormalities if rubella infected the fetus, i.e.,

congenital rubella. Vaccination against rubella protects girls and women of child-bearing age and their offspring against this risk.

rubric The term used to describe a chapter heading or section in a classification system, such as the International Classification of Diseases.

rules and regulations Regulations are formal statements of permitted and proscribed conduct, drawn up by an official body, such as a standing or ad hoc committee; rules are sets of statements about procedures to be followed in specific circumstances or conditions.

rumor Unsubstantiated, often false stories that spread through a community person to person by word of mouth in a manner rather similar to the spread of communicable diseases. Rumor can affect the behavior of crowds for good or ill—unfortunately often for ill, e.g., by provoking riots.

runaway A dependent child who runs away from home, or from a foster home, often to escape physical, emotional, or sexual abuse. Runaways tend to become homeless street children and are vulnerable to pedophile predators, substance abuse, prostitution, and sexually transmitted diseases.

runoff The direction of flow taken by precipitation down slopes toward lower levels, where it collects in streams, rivers, lakes, etc., on its way, usually, to the sea. Along the way it dissolves all sorts of contaminating or polluting substances, including many that are environmentally harmful and some that are toxic. It may also erode productive topsoil.

rural health The health of people living in rural regions. Because of their relative distance from a wide range of health services, isolation, and perhaps a restricted gene pool, the health of rural people is often different from and usually inferior to that of comparable people in urban and suburban regions of the same country. However, the absence of crowding and the stress associated with urban living reduces some health risks in rural populations.

rural health services The range of health (and social) services provided for rural populations. On a per capita basis these services are seldom equitably distributed in comparison with urban regions. In the United States, rural health services are coordinated by the Health Resources and Services Administration from the Office of Rural Health Policy within the Department of Health and Human Services. See http://ruralhealth.hrsa.gov/.

Rush, Benjamin (1745–1813) American physician, statesman, reformer, and one of the signers of the Declaration of Independence. He campaigned for free education and religious tolerance and against alcohol abuse. He was a pioneer in enlightened understanding of mental disorders and used occupational therapy to treat it.

rust 1. Oxidized iron, i.e., the brown coating that forms on the surface of articles made of iron and of steel that has not been alloyed to render it stainless. 2. The name of several plant diseases, especially the contagious fungus disease that attacks wheat.

S

Sabin vaccine The oral POLIOMYELITIS vaccine developed by the Russian-born American microbiologist Albert Sabin (1906–1993). This includes all three polio virus types. It is given by mouth to infants aged 6 to 18 months in a dropper that delivers a measured dose directly onto the back of the tongue. This vaccine induces a good humoral antibody and mucosal intestinal response and is cheaper to administer than inactivated poliovirus vaccine (Salk vaccine). It has been used widely throughout the world in regional poliomyelitis eradication campaigns. It is heat-labile, so an essential feature of the campaign in rural regions is to preserve the COLD CHAIN. Wild polio virus entering a person already immunized with oral polio virus vaccine cannot multiply, so this is a preferred vaccine for containment of outbreaks in countries where polio remains a risk. In countries where polio does not occur, such as those in western Europe, SALK VACCINE should be used in the event that a case is reported and others are believed to be at risk.

saccharin Benzoic sulfimide, an artificial sweetener discovered in 1879. It is 500 times sweeter than sucrose and contains no calories, so it is used by people seeking to lose weight and those with diabetes. At high doses, saccharin is an animal carcinogen. There is no evidence of increased cancer risk in humans, although it was briefly a suspected cause of bladder cancer.

Safe Drinking Water Act Most upper-income nations and some others have legislated standards for safe drinking water with which all purveyors of potable water must comply. The current US law was enacted in 1972. Federal Water Pollution Control Act amendments are enacted from time to time, almost always strengthening existing requirements.

safe period The part of the menstrual cycle between the previous period and a few days before ovulation, during which unprotected sexual intercourse is less likely to lead to fertilization than intercourse at other times. It is the basis for the RHYTHM METHOD of family planning, but its safety is only relative. Ovulation is sometimes stimulated by sexual intercourse, and spermatozoa may survive long enough in the uterus to fertilize an ovum released more than a week later.

safe sex Sexual activity that is free from the risk of pregnancy and SEXUALLY TRANSMITTED DISEASES (STDs), or at least minimizes the risk of infection. *Dr. Ruth's Encyclopedia of Sex* (1994) asserts that solitary masturbation is the only truly safe sexual activity. Sexual intercourse using a correctly fitting CONDOM provides a high degree of protection from the risk of pregnancy and moderately effective protection against many STDs, probably including HIV, but condoms do not provide protection from genital herpes or pubic lice.

safety factor Strictly speaking, the opposite of a RISK FACTOR, but in practice the term applies to specific protective measures in industry and when working with moving machinery, including driving a vehicle. Safety factors include adequate illumination; clean, dust-free, tidy work sites; barriers to shield workers from moving machinery and other hazards; accessible showers if chemical spills could occur; fire extinguishers; use of hard hats, steel-capped shoes, protective goggles, and seat belts or equivalent safety harness when driving a vehicle; and warning notices about hazards. Some are mandated by traffic laws or occupational safety regulations, some are voluntary, with the incentive of favorable insurance rates to encourage their use.

safety inspection A routine or ad hoc examination and assessment of conditions, circumstances, equipment, food production, ships, automobiles, or aircraft, often conducted by experts qualified in the field in which they inspect, concerning environmental and occupational health and safety of power tools, materials, and the like. Safety inspections are often mandated by laws and regulations.

safety net The concept that persons, families, and social and cultural groups have access to a range of publicly or privately funded services to help them deal with physical or mental health and social problems they cannot solve on their own, for economic, social, or psychological reasons.

safety standards A set of requirements on MAXIMUM ALLOWABLE CONCENTRATIONS, TIME-WEIGHTED AVERAGES, etc., arrived at by a combination of animal testing, empirical observations, laboratory studies, and administrative fiat. In the United States, occupational safety and health standards are established under the Occupational Safety and Health Act, by either national consensus or federal regulation. In the European Union, safety standards are mostly more rigorous and less susceptible to modification through political pressure than in the United States.

Saint John's wort A floral essence containing flavonoids, glycosides, volatile oils alleged to enhance consciousness and to have antibacterial, anti-inflammatory, expectorant, and sedative properties. It is a traditional remedy for a wide range of complaints, including arthritis, bronchitis, bedwetting, anxiety, depression, and menstrual pain. Its efficacy has not been critically evaluated, although favorable reports from methodologically valid randomized trials on its use appeared in the medical press in 2005. See http://nccam.nih.gov/health/stjohnswort/ for details.

saline A solution of salt, sodium chloride (NaCl), in water. The concentration of the solution is referred to as its salinity. Sea water contains an average 3% solution of NaCl, but enclosed bodies of shallow sea water and lakes in hot regions with high levels of solar evaporation concentrate to 10% or more, as in the Dead Sea and the Great Salt Lake in Utah. Saline solutions with the osmotic pressure of body fluids are used in transfusions and with added glucose are used in ORAL REHYDRATION THERAPY (ORT).

saliva tests Saliva consists of watery secretions from salivary glands that can be used in tests for various chemicals, e.g., COTININE, which is a metabolic product of nicotine and is a sensitive test for the presence of nicotine, useful therefore to validate smoking/nonsmoking status, and for the presence of drugs. Saliva can also be used to test for the presence of antibodies such as HIV or other infectious disease agents, including *Helicobacter pylori*, and for DNA by extracting buccal cells that are suspended in saliva.

Salk vaccine The killed, inactivated POLIOMYELITIS vaccine developed by the American microbiologist Jonas Salk (1914–1995) and successfully tested in the late 1950s and early 1960s. It induces excellent humoral response but only minimal intestinal mucosal response. It was widely used until superseded

in many jurisdictions by the orally administered and much less costly SABIN VACCINE.

salmonella A genus of Gram-negative, rod-shaped aerobic bacteria. Many are motile, and many cause human and/or animal diseases. The most common is gastroenteric infection. Members of this genus include *Salmonella typhi*, now renamed *S. enterica* subspecies enterica serovar *Typhi*, the causative organism of TYPHOID.

salmonellosis An acute bacterial disease with sudden onset of acute diarrhea, malaise, colicky pains, sometimes vomiting, fever, generalized toxemia, and other systemic manifestations. It is most commonly introduced into the body in contaminated or spoiled food. Many varieties of salmonella organisms are pathogenic, including *Salmonella typhi, S. typhimurium, S. enterica*, and many others. Most infections are due to nontyphoidal species. Salmonellosis can be life threatening, but disease due to *S. typhi* and *S. paratyphi* can be partially prevented by immunization, and all are preventable by effective sanitary and hygienic practices. For details, see http://www.cdc.gov/ncidod/dbmd/diseaseinfo/salment_g.htm.

salt Sodium chloride. Sodium is an essential dietary ingredient. Daily sodium requirements can be met by the amount normally present in food. Substantial extra salt is used in traditional methods of food preparation, and modern food processing methods add even more, so diets often contain 10 g/day or more. This contributes to hypertension and may have other harmful effects. National dietary guidelines typically recommend keeping mean daily salt intake below 6 g, i.e., about 2.4 g sodium/day. A "salt-free diet" is really a salt-restricted diet, e.g., as used in medical regimens to treat hypertension and congestive heart failure.

salvarsan Arsphenamine, the original "magic bullet," the compound of mercury and arsenic invented by the German microbiologist Paul Ehrlich (1854–1915). This was the first effective medication for treating syphilis. Ehrlich received a Nobel Prize for this discovery in 1908.

Salvation Army A Christian religious denomination and charitable organization derived from Methodism, founded in Britain in 1878 by William Booth (1829–1912). It is active in more than 100 countries and provides preventive and therapeutic care for conditions such as leprosy in endemic regions. It is an important force against poverty and its health impact. Members wear uniforms and have a quasimilitary rank system. They run clinics, hospitals, community centers, shelters for the homeless, SOUP KITCHENS, disaster relief services, and alcohol and drug rehabilitation centers.

For details of its national and international operations, see http://www.salvationarmy.org.

Samaritan services The word Samaritan implies ALTRUISM, so Samaritan services could apply to a wide range of community and outreach services run by volunteers to assist those in need. Usually the term applies particularly to SUICIDE PREVENTION services, which often function through a telephone HOTLINE. Most Samaritan services offer assistance to many other distressed individuals to help alleviate psychological and social problems.

same sex partners A stable union with bonds of affection between two people of the same sex, a union of two gay men or two lesbians. In some jurisdictions and with the blessing of churches of certain denominations, such unions are called marriage, with recognition of survivor benefits. Same sex marriage has been legalized in Holland, Belgium, Spain, and Canada.

sample 1. A selected subset of a larger group or population (the "universe" population). Samples may be selected in several ways, only a few of which are acceptable for scientific purposes. The probability or RANDOM sample is selected by an approved random sampling method, such as the use of a table of random numbers. Its most important feature is that each individual in the universe population has a known, usually equal, chance of selection into the sample. Random samples are sometimes stratified (STRATIFICATION), e.g., to ensure that sufficient numbers of individuals are selected from classes that are not numerically large or to ensure that sufficient numbers possessing some characteristic of interest are selected. A CLUSTER sample or an area sample, such as a selection of dwellings in particular localities or city blocks, can be randomly selected at the level of clusters or areas selected from all those available, and then individuals in each cluster or area can be selected at random. Nonrandom samples include systematic samples, such as every tenth name on an alphabetical list, convenience samples, and grab samples, which are arbitrary collections of individuals who happen to be handy or available. These are scientifically unsatisfactory because there is no way of knowing whether those selected or excluded are in any predictable way "representative" of anything in particular. 2. A portion of air, water, or other material collected for laboratory or other testing. 3. Biological material (blood, urine, hair, mucosal swab, etc.) collected for laboratory testing.

sampler A device for obtaining and measuring samples. An air sampler, which may be small enough to be carried or worn on clothing or a larger instrument mounted on a building or in an open space, collects environmental air in a known ratio in order to assess its quality, the presence of pollutants, etc. A water sampler performs a similar function in rivers and lakes. A radiation badge measures cumulative exposure to ionizing radiation of workers exposed to this hazard.

sample registration system A method and procedure for estimating vital rates in national and regional populations by intensively registering and verifying vital events in population samples. For instance, in India more than 4,000 rural and 2,000 urban sample units, with a total of more than 6 million persons, i.e., less than 1% of the total national population, are included in a sample registration system that provides a reasonably reliable picture of the national pattern of vital events at a cost that is feasible and reasonable.

sampling The process of selecting a sample. In scientific studies this utilizes a formal, acceptable, explicit sampling method, such as the use of a table of random numbers to allocate individuals, entities, or definable units to be included in or excluded from a sample.

sampling error All samples embody an element of chance. Sampling error is that part of the error in an estimate that is due solely to the operation of chance.

sanction A word used with two diametrically opposite meanings that are clear only from the context. One meaning is to confer the official approval of a course of action. The other meaning is to prohibit or punish noncompliance with designated acts or behaviors.

sandblasting The use of an abrasive granular material, such as sea sand, blown under very high pressure over a surface, such as the rough stone fabric of a building, in order to clean, polish, or smooth it. Sandblasting exposes workers to a high risk of pneumoconiosis, especially silicosis, and the high-intensity noise is harmful to hearing. Since these dangers have been appreciated and worker safety laws enforced, sandblasters wear both respirators and ear protectors. Water-based sandblasting considerably reduces exposure to hazardous inhalable particles.

sandfly A species of small blood-sucking biting flies whose usual habitat is sandy soil. They are vectors of some important diseases, including LEISHMANIASIS, several arthropod-borne virus diseases, bartonellosis, and sandfly fever.

Sanger, Margaret (1883–1966) American public health nurse, champion of women's rights and social reformer prosecuted for educating working-class women about contraception, author of books and pamphlets such as *What Every Girl Should Know* (1913). Although vilified for her discussion of taboo subjects such as masturbation, she and her ideas were eventually triumphant.

sanitarian A person who is knowledgeable about sanitary sciences. In the United States, this is the usual name for a SANITARY INSPECTOR. In many jurisdictions, a technical college or university training program and qualifying examinations provide quality assurance and a recognized diploma as a registered sanitarian.

Sanitary Commission A name applied to several high-level, government-appointed expert groups of public health specialists, including the Pan American Sanitary Commission, which gave birth to the Pan American Sanitary Bureau.

sanitary engineer A professionally trained engineer specializing in sanitary disposal of sewage, design and working of sewage treatment plants, and/or provision of pure, safe drinking water through a reticulated water-supply system, other aspects of environmental surveillance and control, including air quality and solid waste disposal.

sanitary inspector Syn: health inspector, sanitarian. A technically trained specialist who is qualified to detect environmental risks to health due to such causes as deficiencies in sanitation, ventilation, food handling, restaurant hygiene, pest control, etc. Sanitary inspectors are very important members of staff in local health departments, and in large health departments may be specialized, e.g., to inspect meat, restaurants, hotels and rooming-houses, etc. They are qualified to inspect premises, identify actual and potential dangers to public health, and recommend necessary corrective action. Public health laws can be used to enforce their recommendations.

sanitary landfill A widely used method of garbage disposal. Areas of wasteland, such as worked-out quarries, are selected for dumping garbage, which is sometimes compacted. When the site has been used for some years and the contents have fully decomposed, the area is landscaped and converted into playing fields or for other public-use purposes. It may not be used as a site for dwellings in most jurisdictions. Swamps and tidal marshlands were popular landfill sites until their ecological importance was recognized, so they are now spared from official garbage disposal in many jurisdictions although sometimes still used for illegal dumping.

sanitary revolution The term commonly applied to the set of policies and actions implemented in western Europe and North America, beginning in the last third of the 19th century after several severe cholera epidemics and as knowledge accumulated about polluted water as the causes of this and other FILTH DISEASES transmitted in dirty water or food. Provision of safe drinking water, sanitary disposal of human and animal waste, and hygienic food handling led directly to a spectacular decline in death rates from all the diarrheal diseases, notably among infants and young children.

sanitation A set of public health policies and actions to provide safe drinking water and hygienic disposal of human, animal, domestic, and industrial waste, thus minimizing the risks of transmitting fecal-oral disease and other conditions attributable to poor community hygiene and lack of sanitation. The essential features include sanitary engineering to provide a safe water supply piped directly to each household, water-carried disposal of sewage, collection of kitchen and other domestic waste and industrial waste, and sanitary inspection. Food safety is another feature of sanitation, implemented by food inspection. Education of the public about safe disposal of domestic and industrial waste, especially toxic waste, is another aspect of sanitation, which is an essential feature of all organized public health services.

saponifier A chemical compound that forms a soap or a soapy solution capable of dissolving or loosening greasy substances impregnated on cloth or cooking utensils. Saponifiers act on grease in the skin but may cause an irritating rash or allergy. Soap and water produce better personal hygiene than water alone, but wastewater disposal may be a challenge. See GRAY WATER.

saprophyte An organism that feeds on dead or decaying organic matter.

sarcoid Syn: sarcoidosis. A granulomatous neoplasm affecting many parts of the body, not a malignant neoplasm in the conventional sense, in that it neither invades nor metastasizes. It often occurs in immunocompromised individuals.

sarcoma A malignant neoplasm of mesothelial origin, that is, arising from the lining of the pleural, peritoneal, or pericardial cavities.

SARS See SEVERE ACUTE RESPIRATORY SYNDROME (SARS).

sauna A Nordic system of steam bathing, consisting of a small enclosed space maintained at a temperature of about 40°C with hot coals, over which water is sprinkled to maintain humidity at 100% so those within the enclosure sweat profusely. In Finland, Sweden, and other nations where sauna bathing is a cultural custom, the ritual ends with a swim in a cold lake. Aficionados assert that the experience enhances their health and well-being. The steamy environment of an enclosed sauna creates a microclimate and ecological conditions that increase the risk of fungal infections, such as DERMATOPHYTOSIS, and of LEGIONNAIRES DISEASE.

Save the Children Fund A social service organization founded in the United Kingdom in 1919 that became international with similar organizations in many countries from 1920. It began in the United States in 1932 to help children affected by the DEPRESSION. Its mission is to provide financial and material support for deprived families, with a primary concern for the welfare of families with small children. Since the late 1940s, the Save the Children Fund (Alliance) has assisted development and child health in many low-income nations. Details of its operations are available at http://www.savethechildren.net/alliance/index.html.

scabies A parasitic infection of the skin caused by a mite, *Sarcoptes scabei*, that burrows into the deeper layers of the epidermis and causes intense itching. It is transmissible from person to person and occasionally occurs in epidemic form among classes of school children. It responds to topical application of lotion or cream containing antiscabies compounds, such as permethrin or benzene hexachloride. Transmission is prevented by a combination of cleanliness, personal hygiene, and education. All affected members of a closed community or household must be treated at the same time to avoid reinfestation.

scale 1. A device for measuring portions of a total entity or the value of a specific quantity within a range covered by the measuring device. The measurement scale may be ordered, i.e., zero to infinity, or relative proportional. Many entities are measurable in biology, medicine, and public health (length, mass, pressure, time, radiation dose, etc.), and the instruments used to measure them all have some sort of scale. See also MEASUREMENT SCALE for discussion of categories of scale. 2. The deposit of solid matter on the inside of boilers, kettles, etc. 3. Skin lesions with dried seborrheic exudate and/or horny excrescences on the skin. 4. The deposit of tartar compounds that collects on the teeth.

scarlet fever Syn: scarlatina. A contagious disease formerly common among children and young adults, caused by hemolytic streptococcus A infection, with acute pharyngitis and an erythematous rash on the face, trunk, and limbs. Without treatment, it was often serious, even fatal, and often followed by acute nephritis or rheumatic fever. Since the advent of sulfonamides and penicillin, it has become rare and mostly innocuous. See STREPTOCOCCAL INFECTION.

scatter diagram A visual display of data points indicating the distribution of two variables in relationship to each other. It is often a good way to identify relationships of two variables.

scavenger An organism, person, or substance that consumes or cleans up waste products. Scavenger species include rats, carrion birds, and bacteria. The word describes people who sort garbage, a dirty and hazardous occupation. In industrial processes, scavenging is the removal of polluting substances from factory furnace emissions or removal of impurities from molten metals.

scenario A plausible description of situations or sets of variables that could operate in a complex system at future times, usually based on possible variations in each of many variable determinants that could influence the way the system as a whole might behave. Scenarios have been used to good effect in health planning, e.g., to plan ways that technological innovations and advances could influence future needs for expensive specialized services, and in modeling future patterns of climatic variables, including both "normal" climates and climatic extremes. See also HEALTH PLANNING and VISIONING.

schistosomiasis Syn: bilharziasis. Human and animal infection with blood flukes, also called schistosomes. A tropical disease affecting about 200 million people. The larvae develop in freshwater snails and burst free from the snails as free-swimming cercarial larvae that penetrate the skin of the human or mammalian hosts when they wade in freshwater lagoons or paddy fields. In the human host, the cercarial larvae develop into mature blood flukes that reside in blood vessels surrounding the bladder or rectum, releasing eggs that enter water when the host urinates or defecates. The flukes of *Schistosoma haematobium* (African schistosomiasis) settle around the bladder, causing hematuria and ultimately sclerotic lesions, sometimes bladder cancer; those of Asian or intestinal schistosomiasis, mainly due to *S. mansoni* or *S. japonicum*, settle around the rectum, where they can cause cancer of the rectum and hepatic cirrhosis. They slowly destroy the target organ and can cause prolonged debility and ultimately death from complications. The old name, bilharziasis, honors the German parasitologist Theodor Bilharz (1825–1862), who identified the cause and natural history of the condition in 1852. See also SWIMMER'S ITCH.

schizogony See MALARIA LIFE CYCLE.

schizophrenia A psychosis, a serious form of mental disorder characterized by loss of contact with the real world, flat affect or emotional status, and delusions and/or hallucinations. It was formerly dealt with usually by incarceration in a long-stay custodial mental hospital but now is often treated by medication and ambulatory care services. Unfortunately, cost cutting that followed the political drive to reduce taxes has stripped mental health services of resources to cope with this serious mental disorder, so there are large numbers of HOMELESS MENTALLY ILL people with schizophrenia in some countries.

school health services Monitoring the health of children at school, treating incidental conditions such as head lice, and providing education on nutrition, human sexuality, and harmful habits such as use of tobacco, alcohol, and mood-altering substances are all part of well-run school health services that are provided in many communities, mainly by nurses, with financing usually from local taxes. See also STUDENT HEALTH SERVICES.

school of public health An institution for advanced education and research in all aspects of public health science and practice, including environmental sciences, microbiology, epidemiology, biostatistics, behavioral and social sciences, health administration, etc. Some are affiliated with a medical school in the same university; some are freestanding. For information about distribution, governance, curricula, courses of study, and other details in the United States, see http://www.asph .org or http://www.ceph.org.

science A way of examining, explaining, reflecting on, and predicting natural phenomena that employs systematic observation, experiment, and logical inference to formulate and test hypotheses with the aims of establishing, enlarging, and confirming knowledge and the laws of nature. Science advances through conjecture or intuition, hypothesis, refutation of deductions from previous and imperfect hypotheses, and ultimately verification of hypothesis by induction. Occasionally, science undergoes a PARADIGM shift as long-established principles and laws are overturned by new discoveries.

Science Citation Index A serial publication of the Institute for Scientific Information (ISI) that provides bibliographic information, abstracts, and references from more than 3,700 scientific journals in more than 100 disciplines. It is a valuable resource for searches of specific scientific topics and one of the sources for bibliometric studies of scientific output. The *Social Science Citation Index* performs a similar function for social and behavioral sciences, and the Web of Science covers about 8,700 high-impact journals containing original articles in all scholarly fields. They

are published by Thomson Scientific. See http:// scientific.thomson.com/products/sci.

scientific method Conventionally, and in graduate programs throughout the world, the scientific method has followed a standard pattern, although with variations and flexibility at several levels, as follows: define the problem; if possible, frame the problem as a hypothesis; select in advance a valid and proven method and specify procedures to study the problem; conduct all observations according to a stated protocol that is or will be available for examination by peers; include all observations in the stated results; and, if any observations or measurements are discarded or disqualified, the reason must be stated and explained. Little or none of this formal approach was taken with some of the most important scientific advances ever made. Newton's insight into gravity and Darwin's insight into evolution relied on INTUITION, and Einstein relied on THOUGHT EXPERIMENTS rather than on adherence to a stereotypical scientific method.

scientific misconduct A term for several varieties of crimes against the truth that can be perpetrated by dishonest or corrupt scientists, including public health scientists. Some varieties of scientific misconduct include undeclared CONFLICTS OF INTEREST, PLAGIARISM or theft of intellectual property, FABRICATION OF DATA, FRAUD, and some common lesser misdemeanors, such as fictitious authorship and multiple publication of the same information, which spuriously inflates an author's publication list and wastefully clutters libraries and electronic search and retrieval systems with repetitive material.

scientism The belief that scientific methods can be applied to all problems, with the consequent application of inappropriate scientific methods in unsuitable circumstances.

Scientology A belief system founded by L. Ron Hubbard (1911–1986) that is described as a religion, the Church of Scientology. Its leaders assert that their teachings and practices enhance mental health and physical vitality, and expect their followers to adhere to somewhat rigid conduct.

scientometrics Measurement of the scientific productivity and output of scientists. This is a concern of auditors for grant-giving public agencies and private foundations that want to ensure that their investments of funds in research grants are delivering value for the funds invested. A simple and crude measure is the number of original publications in peer-reviewed publications, presentations and abstracts in peer-reviewed scientific congresses, and patents applied for and granted. The "citation index"—the number and frequency of citation by others in subsequent publications—is an approximate measure. A more sensitive measure is the IMPACT FACTOR. A difficult criterion to assess is the frequency and timeliness with which original scientific work is applied successfully and with benefit by others.

scintillation counter An electronic device that counts pulses of gamma radiation emissions. It is the most sensitive method of detecting ionized radiation. See also GEIGER COUNTER.

scombroid fish poisoning A form of histamine poisoning caused by eating certain species of fish with high levels of free histamine as a consequence of partial bacterial decomposition. See also CIGUATERA FISH POISONING.

scrapie A SPONGIFORM ENCEPHALOPATHY of sheep. It is caused by a PRION that produces progressive neurological deterioration, one symptom of which is to make the sheep scrape their fleece against posts, tree trunks, etc., apparently to relieve itching, thus the name of the disease. The prion that causes scrapie appears to have "jumped species" from sheep to cattle, where it causes mad cow disease or BOVINE SPONGIFORM ENCEPHALOPATHY.

screening Identification of previously unrecognized disease or a disease precursor, using procedures or tests that can be conducted rapidly and economically on large numbers of people with the aim of sorting them into those who may have the condition(s) for which the screening procedures have been carried out and those who are free from evidence of the condition(s). The UK Screening Committee defines screening as a "public health service in which members of a defined population, who do not necessarily perceive they are at risk of, or are already affected by, a disease or its complications, are asked a question or offered a test, to identify those individuals who are more likely to be helped than harmed by further tests or treatment to reduce the risk of a disease or its complications." When screening for noncommunicable conditions, the benefits for the individual should exceed the costs or risks. With communicable diseases such as tuberculosis or chlamydia, the primary aim is to protect population health by preventing transmission of the infectious pathogen to susceptible persons, but of course the infected individual benefits too. Screening may be conducted for a single condition, e.g., mass miniature radiography screening to detect pulmonary tuberculosis, or may consist of a battery of tests, as in multiple or multiphasic screening programs. Much information about screening is available at several Web sites. See, for example, http://www.cancerscreening.nhs.uk/http://www.nsc.nhs.uk/ and http://www.ahrq.gov/clinic/cps3dix.htm. See also SENSITIVITY, SPECIFICITY, and PREDICTIVE VALUE.

screening test A screening test is a preliminary to more specific diagnostic tests. Ideally it should have high SENSITIVITY, i.e., be able to detect all who might have the disease even at the cost of a relatively high proportion of false-positive test results. Screening tests can be applied easily and inexpensively to large populations, aiming to sort people into those who can be reassured that they do not have the disease or condition of interest and others whose disease or health status can be definitely demonstrated by further, perhaps more costly and time-consuming, diagnostic tests. Thus, a good screening test should be sensitive, but it need not necessarily be very specific. Above all, it should not miss true cases of the disease of interest; i.e., it must have a very low rate of FALSE NEGATIVES. Wilson and Jungner's criteria, formulated for WHO in 1968 and revised by others since then, include rapidity, simplicity, low cost, high sensitivity, and prognostic value; i.e., the detected condition(s) should be amenable to effective treatment. Widely used screening tests include analysis of urine in neonates for abnormal metabolites, Pap smears to detect dysplasia of the cervix, and mammography to detect breast cancer.

scrubber A general name for any of several types of device to separate solid particulate matter from gases in the emissions from a furnace, electric power generating plant, etc. Scrubbers may be operated by water sprays, centrifugal force, inertia, electrostatic forces, or a series of filters.

scrub typhus Syn: Tsutsugamushi disease. The rickettsial infection caused by *Rickettsia tsutsugamushi*, an acute febrile illness transmitted to humans by the bite of a trombiculid mite that occurs in south and southeast Asia and the western Pacific region. It can occur in epidemics but is usually sporadic. See also TYPHUS FEVER.

scurvy A systemic disease caused by deficiency of VITAMIN C, ascorbic acid. The symptoms include anemia and petechial, subperiosteal, and intracranial hemorrhages. The cause—dietary lack of fresh fruit and vegetables—and the cure—daily intake of citrus fruit—were empirically proved by the Scottish naval surgeon James Lind (1716–1794). Ascorbic acid was identified and isolated about 200 years later in 1928, and synthesized in 1933.

seafoods A generic name for fish, crustacea, and mollusks, mainly from the sea but often loosely interpreted to include freshwater fish, etc. Seafoods tend to deteriorate by putrefaction more rapidly than does animal meat and sometimes harbor toxic contaminants.

search engine An Internet-based indexing system to search for and retrieve information from the

World Wide Web, specifically from libraries and other reference sources, such as the US National Library of Medicine. In the health field, this is probably the most widely used source, but for general searches several powerful tools are available. The best known probably is Google, which is accessed at http://www.google.com.

seasonal affective disorder (SAD) A syndrome of irritability and depression said to be caused by the short spells of sunshine and the dull, gloomy days of high-latitude winters and to be cured by exposure to artificial or "white" light.

seat belts A safety device installed in cars initially on a voluntary basis in the late 1950s, then as a mandatory requirement at varying times in many jurisdictions when their efficacy as a way to save lives in serious traffic crashes had been proved beyond doubt. In the United States, a mandatory requirement to use seat belts was seen by some as an infringement of liberty, so AIR BAGS were developed as an alternative safety device. Epidemiological evidence demonstrates the superiority of seat belts compared with air bags. The combination of seat belts and air bags is most effective.

secondary prevention See PREVENTION.

second generation surveillance A term used in HIV/AIDS control programs to describe the regular, systematic collection, analysis, and interpretation of information to track and describe trends in the HIV/AIDS epidemic. Second generation surveillance also gathers information on risk behaviors, using these to warn of or explain changes in levels of infection, and includes sexually transmitted infection (STI) surveillance and behavioral surveillance to monitor trends in risk behaviors. For more information, see http://www.who.int/hiv/topics/surveillance/2ndgen/en/.

second-hand smoke Tobacco smoke that accumulates in confined or poorly ventilated spaces that usually comprises a mixture of exhaled and SIDESTREAM SMOKE.

sect A group of people who share a belief system, such as a particular set of religious beliefs. In this context, the use of the term is usually confined to a subset of believers who adhere to specific and sometimes somewhat different, even deviant, views from those of the mainstream of the religion.

sector 1. A segment of a circle. 2. In the language of UN agencies and everyday speech, a social institution, as in the education, health, financial, transport, and communication sectors, etc. 3. In political economy, public or private sectors are distinguished.

sedimentation The process by which solid matter suspended in a liquid medium of lower density slowly settles to the bottom to form a sediment as it obeys the law of gravity.

seepage Penetration of water or other liquid through a porous material, usually soil or the foundations or basements of buildings. Seepage can permit the contents of a PIT PRIVY or SEPTIC TANK to penetrate to aquifers, springs, and wells that are sources of drinking water.

SEER Acronym for Surveillance Epidemiology and End Results, a program of the US NATIONAL CANCER INSTITUTE that uses cancer registry data to calculate incidence and survival rates in relation to treatment regimens for all common and some rare cancers in the registration regions of the United States.

segregation 1. The process of sorting individuals or entities such as bacterial cultures or chemical compounds into groups according to some predetermined system. Applied to the process of sorting individuals and families according to "racial" characteristics, such as the color of their skin, i.e., as RACIAL SEGREGATION, this was widespread in some societies, including the United States and the Republic of South Africa until the latter part of the 20th century. It is condemned now as a violation of human rights, although some subtle forms still survive, e.g., club memberships segregated by sex or color. 2. In genetics, the separation of genetic factors during gamete formation and their random reunification

selection The process of sorting entities into groups. It is a fundamental to the theory and fact of evolution by natural selection, and at a very different level is used in selection of entities for study by some established sampling method.

selection bias Systematic error due to differences between those selected for study and those not selected. For instance, if a study relies on volunteers, these tend to be qualitatively different from those who do not volunteer for whatever reason, such as being able to attend a clinic because they are mobile. Hospital patients are a selected sample of persons with a condition, such as coronary heart disease, from which those at either end of the continuum from sudden death to silent infarct are excluded.

selenium (Se) A nonmetallic element used in photoelectric cells, as a hardening agent, and in ceramics and cosmetics. It is a skin irritant and is toxic on ingestion. Severe selenium deficiency can cause cardiovascular disease, as seen in parts of rural western China.

self-care Provision of medical or other necessary care by the individual needing it. This may be adequate for minor illness and injury, and it can have a role in chronic disease management, but without expert care, it is almost always a bad idea for persons with chronic or serious disease, unless it is part of a regimen under medical and/or nursing supervision.

self-examination Individuals are encouraged as part of health-promotion and disease-prevention programs to perform breast self-examination, testicular self-examination, self-examination for evidence of skin cancers insofar as it affects visible parts of the body, etc. Ideally, this should be preceded by education about how to do it and accompanied by professional confirmation that self-detected lesions are actually present. Unfortunately, there is no reliable way, other than confirmatory medical tests, to detect false-negative examination, i.e., failure of a person to find lesions that are actually present. The efficacy of breast self-examination is considered limited, at best.

self-help organizations These are organizations that offer guidance to people with certain specified problems that enable affected individuals and families to help themselves. Several validated self-help programs exist in many countries. Some are part of the SOCIAL SAFETY NET. Examples include ALCOHOLICS ANONYMOUS (AA) and many organizations for families in which there are psychiatric problems or someone with Alzheimer's disease, hemophilia, or cystic fibrosis.

self-regulation Voluntary adherence to accepted standards, e.g., as applied by physicians to the provision of medical care. This method is advocated by conservative governments for industries to police themselves, e.g., to monitor and control their own environmental pollution. This rarely works as well as professional self-regulation because corporations and industries have agendas and goals but seldom have codes of conduct or sanctions for violation of codes.

semen The viscous fluid produced by the testes, which contribute spermatozoa, combined with secretions from the prostate, accessory sex glands, and the seminal vesicles in which it is stored. From 2 to 5 mL are ejaculated during orgasm, with at least 20 million spermatozoa per cubic milliliter. Impaired male fertility can be detected by low sperm counts and/or high proportions of deformed or nonmotile sperm. Semen can be a vehicle for many SEXUALLY TRANSMITTED DISEASES.

semicircular canals The bilateral sense organs of balance and orientation of the body in space. MOTION SICKNESS is the consequence of dissonance between the sensory input about position in space and input of other senses, especially vision.

Semmelweis, Ignaz Philipp (1818–1865) The Austro-Hungarian physician and obstetrician who made the connection between childbed fever (puerperal sepsis) and poor hygiene in obstetrics. He recorded the survival rates of women after childbirth, when their obstetric attendants adhered to his regimen of hand-washing before attending women in labor, proving that washing hands in a disinfectant solution prevented PUERPERAL SEPSIS. But his ideas were rejected by his colleagues; he experienced a paranoid psychosis and ended his life in a mental hospital.

senescence The consequences of the aging process as body cells and tissues in various organs progressively fail to adapt efficiently to external stressors. The biological explanation of this is not altogether clear. One theory is that clones of some cell types are programmed for a finite number of descendent cells. Senescence affects different persons and organs in varying ways, with varying consequences for personal and population health. With aging populations, smaller family size, and shrinking social support systems, the challenge of providing and paying for the care of increasingly large senescent populations is becoming formidable.

senile dementias An obsolete term for a group of conditions causing memory loss and other defects of mental and intellectual function among old people. They include Alzheimer's disease, arteriosclerosis causing cortical dysfunction, and depression. Sensory deficiency, especially hearing loss, can mimic dementia.

senior citizen Syn: elderly, older, retired person. A person past retirement age (the "third age"), which is not precisely defined but is often 65 years. The incidence of cancer, heart disease, degenerative joint changes (arthritis), and mental deterioration all rise in this age range.

seniors center A community-based setting for provision of a range of social support services to meet the needs of senior citizens, i.e., members of the population loosely defined as "elderly," i.e., older than 60 or 65 years.

sensitivity In SCREENING and diagnostic testing, sensitivity of a test is the property of testing positive for the highest possible proportion of individuals who have, or might be suspected of having, the condition for which the test is performed. A sensitive test should have a very low or zero proportion of false-negative results, i.e., negative test result when the disease is actually present. However, it might have a rather high proportion of false-positive results, i.e., positive test result when the disease is actually not present. See also SPECIFICITY.

sensitization Development of physiological or pathological reactions to repeated stimuli or antigen challenges, e.g., the occurrence and recurrence of asthmatic reactions to cotton dust. See also DESENSITIZATION and HORMESIS.

sensor A mechanical, chemical, or electronic device or system to detect, measure, and react to the presence of environmental factors that could affect health. Biological sensors include the 19th century canary in the mine shaft; sniffer dogs to detect alive or dead people in earthquake ruins; drugs or explosives; and microbiological and ultraviolet radiation sensors for blood stains, semen, feces, etc.

sentinel The word means a lookout. In public health, it is the process of systematic surveillance for a sentinel event, such as the first case of a contagious disease that may (or may not) be expected to occur. In primary care or family medical practice, a sentinel physician is one who maintains special surveillance among the practice population for the first patient who presents with clinical evidence of diseases of interest. See also SENTINEL SURVEILLANCE.

sentinel event An event, such as the first detected case of an unusual condition or a sudden and otherwise unexplainable surge in sickness absences from work, that presages the onset of an epidemic or the occurrence of other trends or changes in the level of population health. The event may be detected retrospectively; e.g., analysis of mortality statistics may reveal a cluster of cases of birth defects or an uncommon malignant condition.

sentinel surveillance A surveillance system based on selected population groups that are chosen because they are representative of relevant experience of these groups, sometimes backed up by relevant professional organizations such as local physicians. Standard case definitions and formal protocols are used to ensure validity of comparisons.

separation anxiety A phenomenon in which children fear that parent(s) have abandoned them, leading to stress expressed as behavioral disturbances, such as refusal of food, screaming, etc. Rarely, separation anxiety persists into later life or returns in adult life, e.g., projected on a spouse.

separation (from hospital) The administrative term used in analysis of hospital discharge statistics to describe the termination of a period as an inpatient, without distinguishing whether the patient was discharged alive or was deceased.

separator A device or equipment that can separate ingredients in a mixture. Mechanical methods include agitating platforms to separate mineral ore from mining waste, which can be a noisy, dusty operation, and centrifugal separators used for many purposes. Chemical separation uses reagents to dissolve or fix some components and separate these from others. Some reagents used for this purpose are extremely toxic.

septicemia A serious, potentially fatal condition in which products of bacterial infection or their toxins circulate in the bloodstream, where they can be detected by suitable tests. Bacteremia is circulation of bacteria, toxemia is circulation of toxins, and viremia is circulation of viruses.

septic tank A method of water-carried sewage disposal for domestic use. The contents of the toilet bowl are conveyed by flushing into a receiving tank, where settling, digestion, and bacterial decomposition of feces occur, leaving a liquid residue that can be drained into adjacent soil. Because the process relies on biological decomposition, antiseptics must not be used, as these would disrupt the bacterial decomposition.

sequencing The term used to describe the process of isolating and defining sequences of DNA in biological material.

sequential sampling and analysis A statistical method that is based on random allocation of study and control subjects in such a way as to permit ending an experiment as soon as ongoing analysis shows that results have achieved a predetermined level of statistical significance.

serendipity Discovery of new information by a happy accident when actually seeking something altogether different. A famous example was the discovery by the British medical scientist Alexander Fleming (1881–1955) of the antibiotic property of penicillin mold.

serial interval The period that elapses between the comparable phases, such as appearance of a rash or onset of fever, in two successive cycles of an epidemic that spreads via person-to-person contact.

seroepidemiology A precursor of MOLECULAR EPIDEMIOLOGY, in which inferences about the past course of infectious disease in a population, and current levels of herd immunity, were based on the distribution of antibodies in the population. The method was used to elucidate details of the epidemiology of important communicable diseases, such as diphtheria and poliomyelitis, and is still widely used, e.g., to assess prevalence of WEST NILE VIRUS infection.

serology Examination of serum to determine its ingredients and detect the presence of circulating antibodies, etc.

seroprevalence Prevalence of antibodies in a population as determined by serological surveys, a useful method of assessing levels of resistance and susceptibility to infectious pathogens. In the past, seroprevalence surveys were used to assess levels of susceptibility or resistance to common infectious diseases, such as poliomyelitis. Now a frequent use is in unlinked ANONYMOUS HIV TESTING.

serotonin A compound derived from tryptophan that occurs in the blood and is secreted by platelets and nerve cells in the cerebral cortex. It is a neurotransmitter and vasoconstrictor, interacts with various receptors, excites some nerves, inhibits others, and affects mood and emotional state. Low serotonin levels are associated with depression and high levels with excitement or mania.

serum The liquid components of blood plasma containing all except fibrinogen.

serum hepatitis A name formerly used to describe the variety of hepatitis that occurred after receiving a parenteral injection of serum. This is most often caused by HEPATITIS B or C.

set and setting A sociological term; a set is a small close-knit group of people, e.g., a teenage gang, who behave similarly, have similar values, and mutually reinforce one another to maintain these values and behavior. A setting is the social milieu in the context of which particular behaviors are observed. The combination of set and setting is a determinant of many aspects of social conduct, especially in adolescence, including health-related customs and behavior.

settlement tank Syn: settling chamber. A container in which liquids containing suspended solids are maintained at rest for a sufficient period for the suspended solids to settle in a layer of sediment at the bottom, or if lighter, a layer of supernatant ("scum") on the surface of the liquid. Settlement tanks are an essential feature of sewage treatment plants and are widely used in industrial processes, e.g., to allow settlement of solid particulate matter in furnace emissions.

Seven Countries Study An epidemiological and dietary investigation of factors associated with the morbidity and mortality attributable to heart disease in the United States, Netherlands, Italy, Greece, Finland, Yugoslavia, and Japan, conducted by a team based at the University of Minnesota, led by the American nutritional physiologist

Ancel Keys (1904–2004), whose own longevity supports his belief in the important role of nutrition in maintaining good health.

Seventh Day Adventists A Christian religious denomination that is epidemiologically interesting because many of its members are vegetarian and abstain from use of alcohol, tobacco, coffee, and tea, and are unusually "health-conscious," engaging in healthful habits such as regular exercise and use of screening tests. Predictably, they have life expectancies above average compared with others in the same community and have low incidence and mortality rates associated with coronary heart disease and tobacco-related cancers. Other groups with similar life habits have similar health experience.

severe acute respiratory syndrome (SARS) A newly emerged infectious disease with fever, prostration, cough, and dyspnea that caused epidemics with high case fatality rates in China, other Asian nations, and Canada in 2003. It is caused by a coronavirus that appears to have jumped species from animals sold in markets, such as civet cats. It is highly infectious for humans by direct contact and droplet spread. In the 2003 epidemics, cases were common among nursing and medical attendants caring for patients until the high infectivity of the SARS virus was recognized and rigorous infection control measures, including protective face visors and goggles as well as masks, gloves, and personal hygiene, were adopted. Sporadic cases were reported again in China in 2004.

severity score A numerical way to record information about the severity of a condition. There are many examples, e.g., the APGAR SCORE used in neonatology, scoring systems for cancer, etc.

sewage Solid or semisolid human waste, which is disposed of in a SEWERAGE system. Other animal waste is called MANURE.

sewage gas Gas, mainly or entirely consisting of methane, generated by bacterial decomposition of sewage.

sewage sludge The accumulated solid waste that settles as sediment in a sewage treatment plant. Once rendered free of pathogens, it can be used as fertilizer, and in some jurisdictions it is converted to sludge cakes that are marketed as fertilizer.

sewage treatment The process of disposing of sewage, i.e., human waste. The waste travels through sewerage pipes to a sewage treatment plant, where it undergoes a series of processes, including moving through settlement tanks where suspended solids are separated from supernatant fluid, then aeration, filtration, a second stage of settlement, sludge digestion and drying into sludge cakes, disinfection of waste water by chlorination, ozonation, or other means, release of pathogen-free water (assessed by the COLIFORM COUNT below a predetermined safety standard), and disposal of the dried sludge, which can be disposed of as fertilizer.

sewerage The system of toilets, pipes, collection, and sedimentation tanks, etc., for disposal of sewage.

sex Differentiation into females and males, which depends ultimately on possession of XX or XY chromosomes, ovaries or testes, and primary and secondary sexual characteristics to match. Sex and the emotions it generates are pivotal for human reproduction and the stimulus for much of the world's great art, literature, pleasure, pain, joys, and sorrows. See also GENDER.

sex discrimination Differential conduct toward or treatment of members of one sex over the other. This may be part of a consciously implemented policy, an ingrained social custom, or the result of imprinting and cultural conditioning by parents, school teachers, and others in society. In this way, school girls may be steered toward traditionally "female" occupations, such as office work, school teaching, and nursing, and away from physical sciences, engineering, and medicine. A more sinister aspect of this is differential infanticide of infant girls.

sex education A program for school children, sometimes for adults, with instruction on the anatomy and physiology of sex and discussion of human sexuality, SEXUALLY TRANSMITTED DISEASES, and pregnancy and how to avoid it when it is unwanted. Depending on cultural sensitivity and other considerations, classes may or may not be segregated into boys and girls. Education about human sexuality, as well as about human reproduction and the risks and harms caused by promiscuous sexual conduct, are widely recognized as important aspects of health promotion and prevention of unwanted pregnancy, HIV/AIDS, and other sexually transmitted diseases. Some groups assert that sex education encourages promiscuity, but there is no evidence to support this assertion.

sex hormones The steroid hormones estrogen and progesterone, and testosterone and anabolic steroids. Estrogen and progesterone, secreted by the ovaries, are responsible for feminine sex characteristics, regulation of the menstrual cycle, and the metabolic and other physiological changes that occur in pregnancy. Testosterone and anabolic steroids are secreted mainly by the testes, also by the

suprarenal glands. They are responsible for masculine sex characteristics, hair distribution, and muscle development.

sex industry, sex trade The large, lucrative, commercial activity dealing with manufacture, marketing, and distribution of pornography, sex toys, and purveying sexual services by and for persons of either male or female sex. Sex workers themselves seldom make much money, but those who run the trade (frequently on the edge of the law) can become very rich. The trade in sexual services is a vehicle for transmission of many SEXUALLY TRANSMITTED DISEASES. It is rare for sex trade workers to collaborate with public health authorities, but in places where they do, such as in Australia, the sex trade workers benefit from improved health and safety.

sex linkage Inheritance of characteristics by way of genes in the sex chromosomes. Genes on the Y chromosome can be inherited only by male offspring; genes on the X chromosome may be recessive or dominant.

sex ratio A demographic term for the ratio of males to females at birth and at later ages. At birth, the ratio is about 1.05:1. It approaches unity around adolescence in most industrial nations, and falls thereafter until it reaches about 0.5 by age 75 to 80 years. In nations in which boys are valued more than girls, the availability of ultrasound to determine the sex of an early fetus and selective abortion of female fetuses has drastically altered the sex ratio at birth, and higher losses of females from infancy onward due to neglect, female infanticide, and chronic malnutrition further distort the ratio. Recent census data from India reveal a sex ratio in children younger than 10 years to be approximately 120 boys to 100 girls; in rural China, the ratio is similarly distorted.

sex roles The assigned social roles associated with being male or female, commonly transmitted to children by imitating the behavior of male and female adults, especially their parents.

sexual abuse A crime perpetrated by a person in a position of trust against a vulnerable person or persons, using force or persuasion, commonly a crime against children and minors.

sexual customs and practices Much has been said and written about the ways people seek to enhance their sexual attractiveness. Many have implications for public and personal health. For instance, women in many cultures since antiquity have worn high-heeled shoes, which alter their carriage and distort and may cripple weight-bearing bones in the feet. Corsets were popular to alter women's shape, and taken to extremes these also were unhealthy. In some African communities, women use astringent herbs to dry out the vagina, to enhance the pleasurable friction of sexual intercourse; this causes abrasions that increase the risk of sexually transmitted diseases, including HIV/AIDS. FEMALE GENITAL MUTILATION is a more pernicious traditional custom in parts of north Africa and the Middle East. Male circumcision has been widely practiced in the United Kingdom, the United States, and Australia since the early 20th century among populations without a religious or ritual reason for the practice.

sexual deviation A pattern of sexual behavior that departs from the generally accepted norm by projecting eroticism to an object rather than a partner of the opposite sex, such as homoeroticism or paraphilia.

sexual dysfunction A condition in which one or more of the sex organs does not work correctly. Examples include premature ejaculation and loss of potency in men and vaginal muscle spasms and severe pain on intercourse in women.

sexual harassment Psychological, occasionally also physical, pressure, often by a senior person in an organization on persons of lower rank, with the intent to obtain sexual favors. Sometimes the purpose is to intimidate women who have entered traditionally male occupations.

sexually transmitted disease (STD) Syn: sexually transmitted infection (STI); venereal disease (obsolete). About 25 miscellaneous diseases with a variety of causal agents, having in common the fact that all of them are transmitted from person to person by direct contact, and the responsible pathogen usually resides in the genital tract and/or in blood and other body fluids. The epidemiologically important STDs in North America and Europe include syphilis, gonorrhea, genital herpes, chlamydia, human papilloma virus infection, and HIV/AIDS. Further information is at http://www.cdc.gov/nchstp/dstd/disease_info.htm, which has links to several other relevant Web sites with more details about each of the important STDs.

sexual misconduct A variety of misdeeds involving offenses such as nonconsenting sexual touching, genital fondling, and sexual intercourse; a term usually applied to offenses committed by persons in a position of trust, such as school teachers, physicians, or priests. The term is not applied to violent sex crimes such as rape and murder.

sexual orientation The direction taken by erotic impulses, usually toward an attractive person of the opposite sex but sometimes toward a person of the same sex.

sexual stereotyping The assumption that certain occupations, social roles, and behaviors ought to be confined to members of one gender; e.g., chief executive officers, firefighters, and underground miners should be male, and nurses, grade-school teachers, office workers, and filing clerks should be female. Some attitudes linked to stereotyping, if not the assumptions, persist.

sex worker A person who derives income or subsistence from the SEX INDUSTRY, usually a person who provides sexual services for money, but in low-income countries it can be a person who provides sexual services merely for subsistence.

SF36 A 36-item set of questions about health status and health behavior derived from the longer questionnaire used in the National Health Surveys conducted by the US National Center for Health Statistics. The SF36 assesses eight sets of variables: physical function, social function, role limitation, mental health, energy, vitality, pain, and self-perceived general health status.

shaken baby syndrome A serious, sometimes fatal neurological trauma caused by violently shaking an infant or small child and thereby inducing petechial or larger hemorrhages in the brain. It happens when a caregiver shakes the child out of frustration, e.g., trying to stop crying.

shaman A tribal medicine man in traditional cultures who derives healing powers from inducing trance-like states, sometimes augmented by traditional herbal remedies. Transplanted to literate industrial societies, the word has come to mean anyone wise in the nontechnical ways of healing and helping to solve difficult problems in or related to the health sector.

shantytown A form of slum housing consisting of makeshift and/or dilapidated dwellings, often lacking sanitation, safe water supplies, and other services, such as electric power supplies. These are the periurban slums surrounding many large cities in Latin America and are the main form of housing in many cities in South and Southeast Asia. Until the 1960s, they were common in the segregated cities of the southern United States, and many vestiges of these survive. They are often infested with vermin and harbor or potentially harbor many endemic diseases. See also INTERNALLY DISPLACED PERSONS, REFUGEES, and SQUATTER SETTLEMENT.

sharps Any sharp object encountered in a health care setting that is capable of penetrating the skin, commonly hypodermic needles, scalpel blades, broken glass vials, etc. A jargon term.

shellfish poisoning Shellfish feed by filtering water through their bodies, so they tend to collect a variety of toxic substances not necessarily harmful to themselves but harmful to anyone who eats the shellfish. The best known form is caused by toxic algae, but it can also be caused by toxic chemicals, such as mercury, as was the case with MINAMATA DISEASE. Shellfish such as oysters that feed on water contaminated by human sewage can transmit hepatitis A, typhoid, etc.

shelter A place of refuge for homeless people, refugees, victims of natural or manmade disasters, or victims of domestic violence. Shelters may be permanently established for the last of these or temporarily set up during emergencies. Provision of health care, including preventive services, is a high priority in shelters.

sheltered workshop A program to provide employment for people with mild mental retardation and sometimes physical disabilities, such as cerebral palsy or severe epilepsy, where the affected individuals can work safely and productively under supervision, often with medical assistance readily available. See also THERAPEUTIC COMMUNITY.

shift work A work scheduling system to maintain production without loss of time at night and weekends. Shift work is required in essential services (police, ambulance, fire brigades, hospital emergency departments, etc.) and is an economic imperative in many industries. The health risks are greater than for comparable workers in occupations with normal hours on and off the job because disrupted sleep patterns impair concentration, leading to high rates of industrial injury.

shigellosis Syn: bacillary dysentery. An acute bloody diarrhea caused by *Shigella* organisms of four distinct species: *S. dysenteriae, S. flexneri, S. boydii,* and *S. sonnei.* Transmission is fecal-oral, e.g., linked to poor food hygiene and/or infected or carrier food handlers, or water-borne. This can be a prostrating and debilitating illness, although it is seldom life threatening, except in infants, small children, and persons already debilitated and dehydrated by other disease.

shingles See HERPES ZOSTER.

shoe-leather epidemiology Collection of epidemiological and other pertinent data relevant to an epidemiological investigation by painstaking direct inquiry among all or a representative sample of the affected people, for example by walking door to door (wearing out shoe leather in the process, hence the term) to ask direct questions. JOHN SNOW used this method in his investigations of cholera in the 1850s, and it was refined in the United States by the field officers of the EPIDEMIC INTELLIGENCE SERVICE (EIS).

shooting gallery The colloquial name for a place frequented by illicit intravenous drug users to inject drugs and buy supplies from street vendors. This may be an abandoned building in a decayed slum neighborhood or a secluded city park. In some European cities, for instance in Switzerland, and in Australia, such places are maintained in hygienic conditions by municipal or other public authorities, who also offer rehabilitation. In the United States, those who use them may be targets for punitive law enforcement with no attempts at rehabilitation.

Shope papilloma virus The human papilloma virus causing malignant papilloma of the cervix, identified by the American virologist Richard Shope (1902–1966). See PAPILLOMA VIRUS.

shut-in A person who is confined to home, often to a bedroom, because of impaired mobility, commonly an elderly person who, because of confinement, may experience nutritional deficiencies and other health problems caused by progressive reductions in mobility from housebound to chairbound to bed-bound, a natural history that ends with bedsores, urinary infections, hypostatic pneumonia, and death, unless active intervention arrests the process.

SI See SYSTÈME INTERNATIONAL (SI) D'UNITÉS.

sick building syndrome A condition arising in a multiple-unit, high-rise apartment dwelling or office tower that is insulated against fluctuating environmental temperatures but inadequately ventilated so the indoor air stagnates, creating persistent odors and/or accumulated pollutants, such as stale tobacco smoke and fumes from carpet adhesives, copying machines, etc. The occupants of such buildings experience various symptoms, including respiratory distress, headaches, nausea, sleeplessness, and inability to concentrate, some of which may be causally related to the indoor environment and others perhaps attributable to the power of suggestion.

sickle cell trait Hemoglobin S, an abnormal variant inherited as a recessive genetic characteristic, causes distortion of the shape of red blood corpuscles, leading to the serious, potentially fatal condition of sickle cell anemia. This is a hemolytic anemia caused by destruction of abnormally shaped erythrocytes. The heterozygous condition is the sickle cell trait. This trait confers a survival advantage in regions where malaria has been prevalent because affected blood corpuscles are resistant to the malaria parasite. This explains the high prevalence of the sickle cell trait among populations from the eastern Mediterranean (Cyprus, Lebanon) and Sub-Saharan Africa.

sickness impact profile A questionnaire-based survey instrument that assesses the physical and psychological consequences of chronic disease, especially respiratory disease. The questions are in two domains (physical and psychosocial) and 12 categories (sleep and rest, eating, work, home management, recreation and pastimes, ambulation, mobility, body care and movement, social interaction, alertness behavior, emotional behavior, and communication).

sick role A term used by medical sociologists to describe the behavior pattern of persons who have become ill, especially when they are confined to a hospital bed. It is characterized by loss of autonomy, dependency, and variable sets of emotions, e.g., anger, passivity, tearfulness.

SIDA 1. Syndrome d'immunodéficience aquise (French) and síndrome de imunodeficiência adquirida (Spanish) for ACQUIRED IMMUNODEFICIENCY SYNDROME (AIDS). 2. Acronym of the Swedish International Development Agency.

side effect A consequence, other than that intended, of a therapeutic or preventive intervention. This may be an adverse effect or, less commonly, a beneficial one.

sidestream smoke Smoke from combusted or smoldering cigarette tobacco that has not been filtered through a smoker's respiratory tract and therefore contains higher concentrations of toxic products, including carcinogens and irritant aldehydes, than does exhaled tobacco smoke.

SIDS Acronym for SUDDEN INFANT DEATH SYNDROME.

sievert (Sv) The Système International (SI) unit of radiation dose, named for the Swedish physicist Rolf Sievert (1896–1966). It is the unit of radiation dose equivalent, replacing the rem (1 Sv equals 100 rem). Some types of radiation are more harmful than others for the same absorbed dose: an absorbed dose of alpha radiation causes 20 times as much biological damage as the same dose of beta radiation. Humans can absorb as much as 0.25 Sv without immediate ill effects; 1 Sv may produce radiation sickness; and more than 8 Sv is fatal.

signal-to-noise ratio The ratio of desired data or information to all extraneous and unwanted information with which it can be confused.

significance Something that is meaningful. See STATISTICAL SIGNIFICANCE, which should be clearly distinguished from clinical significance, public health significance, and social, emotional, and political significance, which do not abide by the laws of probability but rely on judgment, anecdotes, emotions, etc., that, depending on the context, may be as important, or more so, than associations unlikely to occur by chance.

sign language See AMERICAN SIGN LANGUAGE (ASL).

silage A crop that is harvested and used for animal fodder. When stored in a silo, decomposition can lead to production of METHANE. Mold, fungus, and disease-carrying vermin may also be associated with silo storage. See also FARMER'S LUNG.

silica, silicon (Si) A nonmetallic element, second-most abundant in the world, occurring in rocks, clay, soil, and sand and used to make glass; supposedly rather inert but biologically active when inhaled as fine dust. Inhaled silica dust causes silicosis, progressive disabling pulmonary fibrosis.

silicosis The form of pneumoconiosis caused by inhalation of silica dust, a disease of miners who work underground in hard rock containing a high silica content, and various other occupational groups. Silicosis causes progressive fibrotic pneumoconiosis that continues after exposure ceases and ultimately causes death from right-sided heart failure (cor pulmonale). Coal miners sometimes get silicoanthracosis, and the common combination with tuberculosis is called silicotuberculosis.

silo-filler's disease An inflammatory bronchiolitis and pneumonitis with pneumonia and pulmonary edema in severe cases, due to inhaled fumes of nitrogen oxides that are produced by fermenting silage; an occupational disease of farmers and other exposed agricultural workers. See also FARMER'S LUNG.

simulation An artificial replication of a natural phenomenon, conceptualized and usually constructed to study the operation and interaction of parts of the phenomenon. It may be an abstract simulation, e.g., a mathematical model, or a physical simulation.

single-parent family A parent-child family consisting of one parent and child(ren). The most common is a mother-led family, originating either because the mother was never a partner of the father of the child(ren) or because of separation, divorce, desertion, or death of the male head of the household. Children of single-parent families are vulnerable to social, economic, and emotional problems that can often be demonstrated to be associated with the family structure and function. However, children may be less disturbed in a single-parent family than in a dysfunctional family with two parents.

sink The collection place for waste water in kitchens, bathrooms, etc. A CARBON SINK collects and chemically or biologically transforms atmospheric carbon dioxide.

sin tax A sales tax on nonessential, "health-harming" consumer goods, e.g., tobacco, alcohol, candy, or luxury goods, such as fur coats and jewels, that some people regard as "sinful" to own. The popular belief is that taxes raised by the sale of such products are earmarked for health, education, and needed social services. In reality, this rarely happens.

sintering Fusion of particles of material at temperatures below their melting point in order to produce a porous product. The process can generate fumes that are often toxic.

situation analysis Assembly of all pertinent information about a situation as a preliminary to developing strategies and tactics to deal with it. Health situation analysis consists of gathering all the available vital and health statistics, including epidemiological data and a census of the current and projected health facilities and human resources, as a preliminary to development of strategic and tactical plans to deal effectively and efficiently with the situation.

skew distribution An asymmetrical unimodal distribution in which values tail off more slowly in one direction than the other. Often it is a log-normal distribution. A positive skew distribution has a longer tail of high values than of low ones; a negative skew distribution has a longer tail of low values. Mean, median, and mode do not coincide as they do with a normal distribution.

skill development The provision of education and training to facilitate proficiency at expected tasks or new tasks that previously could not be performed. This is an important part of capacity building and of rehabilitation in which people who have been incapacitated by injury or illness are equipped with new skills to enable them to work. An example is computer keyboard skills to enable disabled manual workers to obtain office employment.

skill set The term used by behavioral and social scientists to describe the activities that people are able to perform at a satisfactory level, e.g., reading, calculating costs for housekeeping, cooking.

skin cancer The most common variety of cancer, occurring in three main forms: basal cell cancer (rodent ulcer); squamous cell cancer; and malignant melanoma. The last of these is most dangerous, often invasive and metastasizing to distant organs.

skin piercing Pierced ear-lobes for earrings are very common among women and increasingly among men in high-income countries. Other variations of body piercing are a fashion or status symbol in some preliterate cultures, and a fad principally among adolescents and young adults in some sectors of society in rich industrial nations; these individuals have their ears, noses, eyebrows, tongues, nipples, and genitalia pierced and metal or plastic decorations inserted. Tattoos may be another feature of this custom, which may be most common among people outside the mainstream of society, who may have other behaviors, e.g., RECREATIONAL DRUG use, that put them at risk of adverse health outcomes.

skin test A diagnostic test in which a small drop of antigen is placed on a scarified skin surface or injected intradermally to provoke a reaction. The MANTOUX TEST is an example; others are the reagents used by allergists to determine which allergens cause asthma, hay fever, etc.

sleep apnea A potentially serious condition in which respiration becomes sluggish or ceases altogether for periods as long as 30 seconds, often repeatedly many times each night, during deep sleep. It is usually caused by obstruction of the airway as muscles relax during sleep. The danger arises because of the risk that cerebral ischemia can damage higher cortical functions, leading to lasting symptoms such as memory loss, or, in more severe cases, can interfere with essential brainstem activity.

sleep deprivation syndrome A cluster of psychological and neurological symptoms and signs that occur in prolonged periods without sleep, including disorders of perception and mood, sluggish reflexes, errors of judgment, or loss of manual dexterity, making work with machinery, etc., hazardous.

sleep disorders This term covers several conditions, including insomnia, narcolepsy, sleep apnea, nocturnal cramps, and restless legs syndrome. INSOMNIA is commonly caused by anxiety, depression, or physical conditions, such as urinary frequency. SLEEP APNEA has several causes, including flabby muscles in the upper airway (floppy uvula) and defective brainstem regulation of respiratory rhythm. Narcolepsy is an uncommon condition in which an overwhelming desire to sleep occurs during what are otherwise normal waking hours.

slim disease The name for AIDS in Uganda and adjacent nations in Africa, signifying the wasting, or cachexia, that is a common feature of AIDS, often complicated by coexistent tuberculosis.

slipped disk Syn: prolapsed intervertebral disk. An orthopedic condition, usually the result of a sudden weight-bearing stress on the vertebral column under ergonomically unfavorable conditions that exposes the soft elastic tissue between the vertebrae to pressure, causing herniation. This usually presses on nerve roots and causes severe pain, commonly sciatica.

slippery elm The mucilaginous interior surface of elm tree bark contains astringent alkaloids and is a traditional herbal remedy for various complaints, including gastrointestinal irritation, menstrual irregularities, and renal dysfunction. It has been used, although without proven efficacy, as an abortifacient.

slow virus diseases A miscellaneous group of progressive neurological diseases that have been attributed to infection with hypothesized slowly acting viruses with a long incubation period. Some, notably KURU and CREUTZFELDT-JAKOB DISEASE, have been demonstrated to be caused by a PRION, but the hypothesis of a slow-acting, long-incubation-period virus remains viable for others, including multiple sclerosis.

sludge Accumulated solid or semisolid waste matter deposited as a layer below supernatant liquid. Sewage sludge is aerobically and anaerobically digested, free of pathogens and offensive smells, and can be safely used as organic fertilizer. Industrial sludge is the solid or semisolid waste matter from industrial processes and often contains toxic material.

slum housing The main characteristics of all forms of slum housing, whether dilapidated former mansions, SHANTYTOWNS, tenements, or multistory apartment buildings, are overcrowding and poor infrastructure services. Many have inadequate sanitary and health care services, and many who live in slum housing have multiple social and medical problems.

slurry A viscous liquid suspension of manure used for fertilizing fields. The same word is used to describe liquid suspensions of solid waste in industrial waste sites and for liquid suspensions in many industrial processes.

smallpox Syn: variola (major and minor). A highly contagious virus disease that occurred in devastating epidemics with mortality rates as great as 30% to 40% until smallpox (cowpox) vaccine was successfully tested in 1796–98 by EDWARD JENNER (1749–1823). Smallpox declined in ferocity in the late 19th century, but epidemics continued until

the 1960s, when the WHO launched a global smallpox eradication campaign. The last case outside a laboratory occurred in Somalia in 1979, and the disease was declared eradicated by the World Health Assembly in 1980, but the virus has been maintained in secure laboratories in several countries and is regarded by several national leaders as a potential weapon of biological warfare or BIOTERRORISM. See also VARIOLATION.

smog An atmospheric mixture of smoke and fog. The "smoke" often consists of concentrations of air pollutants from combusted automobile exhaust fumes and industrial processes, and can be harmful to the very young, the elderly, and people with chronic cardiovascular and respiratory disease. Severe smog episodes frequently occur during heat waves and sometimes in cooler weather in urban areas, causing exacerbation of chronic cardiovascular and respiratory diseases and an upward surge in death rates among the most vulnerable. Many urban regions have "smog alert" messages on radio and television when conditions favor occurrence of severe episodes of smog, advising vulnerable people to remain indoors. Smog alerts are an indicator of inadequate control and prevention of emissions. A better approach is to reduce carbon emissions. See AIR QUALITY INDEX, LONDON SMOG, and LOS ANGELES SMOG.

smoke Suspended atmospheric particulate matter due to combustion of carbon-based fuels. The composition varies widely. It often includes toxic aerosols and solid particulate matter, e.g., toxic polyaromatic hydrocarbons (PAHs). High concentrations of inhaled smoke can be fatal.

smoke abatement Policies, practices, procedures, and methods aimed at reducing, preferably eliminating, atmospheric pollution with smoke from combusted carbon fuels. The sources of smoke may be industrial furnaces and generators, or domestic cooking and heating fires, or both. The largest global source of smoke is biomass fuel combustion in domestic stoves. Smoke abatement measures include the use of smokeless fuel (this is not necessarily nonpolluting) and establishment of smokeless zones as in some European cities since the mid 20th century.

smokeless tobacco Tobacco in a form that enables the user to satisfy nicotine addiction without combusting the dried leaves. Two common forms are chewing tobacco and snuff, which is fine-powdered tobacco leaves retained for long periods in the mouth in the buccogingival pouch or inhaled. Chewing tobacco causes ulceration and ultimately cancer of the tongue or gums, and snuff causes perforation of the nasal septum and cancer of the nasal mucosa or paranasal sinuses.

smoking Unqualified, this word refers to TOBACCO smoking, which became popular and socially acceptable among European and American men in the 18th and 19th centuries. During and after World War I, cigarette smoking, the most dangerous form, increased rapidly among men, and it gained social acceptability among women in the 1930s and 1940s. In the mid-20th century, it was a widespread social custom when introduced to strangers to offer a cigarette. The addictive properties of NICOTINE had been empirically understood long before then and were confirmed by many pharmacological studies in the final third of the 20th century. The prevalence of smoking began to decline among men in the United Kingdom and the United States after the mid-20th century but increased sharply among girls and women. In the late 20th and early 21st centuries, smoking became increasingly prevalent in low- and middle-income countries, with female rates lagging behind those of men. Pandemic respiratory and other cancers and increasing coronary heart disease and stroke follow cigarette smoking trends, with a lag time of about 3 decades. Smoking control measures have often been ineffectual unless reinforced by consistent strong government support, e.g., with strict enforcement of policies that prohibit smoking in many public places. Tobacco companies and their advertisers wield enormous economic and political leverage and have successfully thwarted most efforts to reduce the appeal of smoking to new child addicts. Smoking therefore remains among the most pervasive and intractable public health problems in the world. The WHO FRAMEWORK CONVENTION ON TOBACCO CONTROL (FCTC), approved by the World Health Assembly in 2003 and ratified by 57 nations as of 2005, came into effect in February 2005. The FCTC outlines strategies and tactics to deal with the problem. Time will tell how effective this will be.

smoking cessation program An organized activity sponsored by national or local public health departments and/or voluntary agencies such as FOUNDATIONS dedicated to prevention and control of cancer and heart disease. Features of successful smoking cessation programs include social and moral support, nicotine patches or lozenges, and the creation of nonsmoking environments.

Snow, John (1813–1858) A London physician, a founding figure of modern epidemiology, and a pioneer anesthetist. Snow's main contributions to epidemiology were his demonstrations of the importance of logical reasoning, the use of spot maps to display the progress of epidemics of CHOLERA, and the application of rigorous numerical methods in which comparisons were based on proportions or rates rather than merely on general impressions and anecdotes.

social anthropology See ANTHROPOLOGY.

social assistance See WELFARE.

social barriers Impediments such as educational, occupational, and cultural differences in manner of dressing, speaking, and eating food that cause one group of people to avoid or minimize social intercourse with another. The process works in both directions and in many ways; e.g., people in poverty may be ashamed to be seen in a doctor's waiting room because their clothes are shabby.

social capital The processes and conditions among people and organizations that lead to their accomplishing a goal of mutual social benefit, usually characterized by interrelated constructs of trust, cooperation, civic engagement, and reciprocity, reinforced by networking.

social change 1. The process of altered status, values, behavior, and mode of speech and dress that accompany social mobility. 2. The alteration of a society as its level of wealth and other resources changes. This is normally a slow process from one generation to the next, documented by social historians. It may be accelerated by extraneous events, for example the great increase in female participation in the wage-earning workforce in World War II that was accompanied by other rapid changes in nutritional status and in sexual and other health-related behavior.

social class A stratum of society comprising people of similar incomes and occupational groups and sometimes similar interests, values, political loyalties, and ways of speaking. This is an important sociological concept. Lay thinking often arranges people into three groups: upper, middle, and lower classes. Most people identify themselves as middle class, and they may use pejorative expressions such as "elite" to describe the upper class and look down on those they regard as lower class, formerly called "the great unwashed" and now known by several epithets. Another way to classify people is to sort them into clerical or manual, "white-collar" or "blue-collar" workers. Social class differences are often associated with cultural and behavioral differences, as well as with more obvious differences in income and living conditions. See also INEQUALITIES IN HEALTH, REGISTRAR GENERAL'S OCCUPATIONAL CLASSIFICATION, and SOCIOECONOMIC CLASSIFICATIONS.

social classification A system for arranging the people in a national population into groups that are mutually exclusive and internally consistent, with meaningful predictive properties. A system used for many years in Britain was the REGISTRAR GENERAL'S OCCUPATIONAL CLASSIFICATION of the British people into five social classes. In the United States, a

SOCIOECONOMIC CLASSIFICATION based on a combination of income and occupational group is often used.

social contract A term dating to the English philosopher Thomas Hobbes (1588–1679) and made explicit by Jean-Jacques Rousseau (1712–1778) that describes the desirable and usually mutually accepted forms of interaction among individuals and groups in their social environment. Modern political philosophers give the term a particular meaning: an unwritten agreement regarding rights and responsibilities between a state and its citizens.

social Darwinism A 19th century political and economic philosophy developed by the British philosopher Herbert Spencer (1820–1903) that projected the concept of "survival of the fittest" onto the social fabric of early industrial civilization, based on the notion that those who deserved to succeed by reason of their superior intelligence, cunning, or ruthlessness would do so, whereas the "weaker" ones would not and would be eliminated in subsequent generations. The weaker ones were usually the sickly ones, for whom there was no place in this social order. Public outrage at the consequences of this predatory view led it to be displaced by concepts of SOCIAL JUSTICE. It has returned in modified form in the modern neoconservative political movement.

social distance See SOCIAL BARRIERS.

social epidemiology The epidemiological study of the social determinants and social distribution of disease and states of health. It is the interface of epidemiology with sociology, political science, economics, and social and cultural anthropology. It includes studies of personal and population health in the context of behavior, social networks, and determinants such as ethnicity, socioeconomic status, and housing conditions. It may use a LIFE COURSE approach that attempts to place current states of health in the context of formative social, economic, and cultural determinants. In intervention studies, it seeks to modify adverse factors and ameliorate determinants that can enhance good health.

social evolution The process of change in customs, values, or behavior in a society that may go on slowly from one generation to another or more abruptly when there is a radical disruption, such as may be caused by war or revolution. An example with major implications for health was the transformation of society brought about by the internal combustion engine and the rise in road and air transport, and the decline of home entertainment by performing family members and its replacement by gramophone records, then by radio and television, which can have great utility as an

educational tool but also encourages indolence and its adverse health consequences.

social history 1. Inquiry into the social circumstances of individuals and families in order better to meet their health care needs. 2. The historical study of social conditions, changing values, etc.

social indicators Criteria, often UNOBTRUSIVE MEASURES based on census data, that reveal aspects of society, e.g., literacy levels, proportions of elderly people living alone, occupancy in relation to number of bedrooms (an indicator of crowding), and ownership of cars, televisions, and computers.

social insurance See SOCIAL SECURITY.

social isolation A condition in which an individual lacks connections to family, friends, or others and lacks access to a SOCIAL SUPPORT SYSTEM. Socially isolated people are more vulnerable than others to many conditions, including psychosocial problems and complications when they experience conditions that render them housebound.

socialization In sociology, the process of behavioral and value change that people undergo on joining a cohesive group, such as a class of medical students, a firm of lawyers or stockbrokers, an elite military regiment, or any other group that has its own dynamics. Not to be confused with the political process of socializing, which means using taxes to pay for a public service, such as medical and hospital care.

social justice The concept and implementation of EQUITY. One philosophical justification for advances in public health is recognition that many disparities in health are caused by deprivation and that alleviation of these disparities requires correction of deprivation. The adverse impact on health was a powerful incentive to eliminate child labor, slavery, and racial segregation, to elevate the status of women in society, and in all other ways to aspire to a just and equitable society.

social marketing The methods based on commercial marketing techniques, used in health-promotion programs to raise awareness of actions that may be adopted by individuals and groups to enhance their health.

social medicine A term that came into vogue in the United Kingdom with the appointment of a distinguished clinician not identified with public health, John Ryle (1889–1950), as the first professor of social medicine at Oxford University in 1938. Ryle's concept of social medicine was of medical practice that treated the sick by ameliorating adverse social conditions, such as poverty and unemployment, that contributed to or caused their illnesses. Ryle combined this approach with scientific study of the relationship of disease to social conditions and stimulated the postwar rise of epidemiologically based public health science that was called "social medicine" in most British universities until the term became confused with socialized medicine and acquired negative associations. See also COMMUNITY MEDICINE.

social mobility Movement of individuals between different levels of the social hierarchy. Upward social mobility typically means movement from unskilled working class ("blue-collar") origins to higher paying and higher status "white-collar" professional ("intellectual") roles in society. The main lever that permits upward mobility is access to higher education, regardless of family income. Downward mobility often occurs because of physical or intellectual impairment, or economic and social disruption with displacement from origins, as by violent armed conflict, so biologists from Baghdad drive buses in Birmingham and barristers from Bosnia flip burgers in Boston. Health status generally improves with upward mobility and deteriorates with downward mobility, but in the latter case deterioration of health status, especially mental health, may accelerate downward mobility.

social network The communication links among individuals that function via family connections, neighborhood, workplace, recreations, and today the Internet. Epidemiological studies show a consistent positive correlation between strong social networks and favorable health status, although the relationship is not necessarily causal.

social pathology Structural and functional malfunction of society associated with pervasive problems that often have adverse consequences for health. It is often difficult to discern causal linkages, but an example is the associations among unemployment, alcohol and substance abuse, family violence, broken families, vandalism, street crime, and premature death that are a common feature of inner city slum housing.

social problems A range of adverse conditions in society, sometimes called "social pathology," that have obvious adverse effects on personal and population health, e.g., family breakdown, unemployment, overcrowding, and slum housing. There is often a vicious circle in which the social problems or conditions aggravate health problems, such as alcohol or substance abuse, that in turn make the victims even less employable.

social psychiatry a branch of psychiatry that emphasizes the importance of social groups and families and bases its therapeutic methods on these groups. It is both an approach to diagnosis and a treatment method based on the concept of the THERAPEUTIC COMMUNITY.

social safety net A combination of tax-supported, voluntary, and charitable community agencies that provide services for many kinds of disadvantaged people in most liberal democratic nations, as well as in socialist nations such as Cuba. The disadvantaged people include single-parent, mostly mother-led families who are dependent on WELFARE for financial support, unemployed and unemployable people, elderly and shut-in people, people with chronic impairments, and those with disabilities or handicaps.

social science search engines Several Internet search engines are available to assist in locating abstracts and other information about the social sciences. These include a UK-based search engine, http://www.sosig.ac.uk/harvester.html, and data bases on demography, sociology, gerontology, economics, etc.. See http://www.searchengineguide.com/pages/Social_Science/.

Social Security A national system of public insurance, into which income-earning citizens pay a regular contribution to generate a collective capital fund that in theory provides the basis for retirement and disability pensions. Social insurance systems exist in most democratic nations, and in many they are insulated from access by governments who might seek to use this source of funds as an alternative to raising taxes to pay for current expenses. Not all are fiscally sound, because of inadequate contributions or failure to allow for AGING OF THE POPULATION as members of the baby boom generation retire. Social Security is an established feature in affluent nations. Low- and middle-income nations mainly rely on family and informal support systems.

Social Security Act US federal legislation enacted in 1935 with many subsequent amendments. It originally provided ENTITLEMENTS to meet the economic needs of elderly and retired people, the disabled, and the needy. It incorporates a compulsory insurance program; unemployment insurance; aid for families with dependent children or blind and disabled persons, etc. The provisions are set out in about 20 numbered TITLES of the Social Security Act. Most other industrial nations have similar legislation of varying effectiveness and comprehensiveness.

social services A range of community services provided by agencies that usually function at local government level, often combining publicly administered and funded agencies and a range of private and voluntary services that include social work, usually provided by professionally trained social workers, with special services for those with special needs, such as day care, Meals on Wheels, free hot meals for destitute street people, distress centers, drop-in centers, etc.

social stratification Even the most egalitarian societies have some hierarchical structure, and in all democracies there are distinctions on the basis of education, income, occupation, cultural differences, and social mores related to prior schooling and membership in faith-based and many other institutions of society. Inevitably, some of these are perceived as having higher social standing than others; thus "social stratification" is a useful term to describe them. Health status often correlates with social standing in most social strata.

social support systems Apart from official SOCIAL SAFETY NETS that exist in most Organization for Economic Cooperation and Development (OECD) nations, family, friends, and neighborhood networks provide an informal social support system for most people in urban societies. Informal social support systems have long been perceived as more supportive in rural communities than in urban ones, but reality does not always accord with this. See also SOCIAL NETWORKS.

social work The professional activity carried out by trained social workers to help individuals, groups, and communities to enhance or restore their capacity to achieve full social functioning and create societal conditions favorable to this goal. Social work practice is usually case based, and seeks to restore capacity when it is impaired, working with clients to achieve this end. The qualifying degree for social workers is Master of Social Work (MSW).

sociobiology A concept expounded in *Sociobiology: The New Synthesis* (1975) by the American entomologist and ecologist Edward O. Wilson (b. 1929). Wilson defines sociobiology as the systematic study of the biological basis for social behavior. He asserts that altruism and other desirable behaviors confer evolutionary benefit by enhancing reproductive fitness. Geneticists and evolutionary biologists criticize this concept, but it is intuitively appealing. It is a difficult set of beliefs to verify or refute.

socioeconomic classifications Social planners, epidemiologists, vital statisticians, and others have wrestled with the problem of classifying people according to their place in society. An early method was the United Kingdom's REGISTRAR GENERAL'S OCCUPATIONAL CLASSIFICATION, which requires an answer to a single question about occupation.

This has the virtue of simplicity but has several limitations; for instance, income and living conditions do not necessarily relate closely to it. The scale invented by the American sociologist A. B. Hollingshead requires several questions about income, educational level attained, occupation, and housing conditions (owned or rented home). A similar scale created by the Australian social scientist Alexander Congalton relates residential address to the municipal tax rate of the property as an UNOBTRUSIVE MEASURE of personal wealth. The aim of all such classifications is to throw light on other variables, such as health-related behavior. It may be best to develop specific questions regarding income, occupation, housing conditions, expenditure on amenities, etc., rather than to use existing survey instruments, if that is the aim of the classification.

socioeconomic status (SES) A descriptive term for the position of persons in society, based on a combination of occupational, economic, and educational criteria, usually expressed in ordered categories, that is, on an ordinal scale. Many classification systems have been proposed, from a simple division according to occupation, which usually relates closely to income and educational level, to more complex systems based on specific details of educational level, income, occupation, and sometimes other criteria, such as whether the usual place of dwelling is owned or rented and the ratable value of the dwelling. Other factors, including ethnicity, literacy, and cultural characteristics, influence socioeconomic status, which is an important determinant of health.

sociogram A diagrammatic representation of the lines of communication among groups of people, showing the frequency of communications and the directions in which they flow.

sociology The scholarly study of society, an ancient pursuit dating at least to classical Greece, if not earlier, that was systematized with linkages to economics, politics, history, demography, and vital statistics by 19th century scholars, including the French social scientist Émile Durkheim (1858–1917), the German sociologist Max Weber (1864–1920), the German political philosopher Karl Marx (1818–1883), and a host of 20th century successors. Modern sociology is concerned with the analysis of social problems and with explanation of social phenomena and trends, and has a broad interface with public health, through social work, medical sociology, community surveys and social research, and social epidemiology, and in diverse other ways.

soil conservation Measures designed to minimize soil erosion by the action of water or wind, e.g., contour plowing to minimize runoff of rainwater, planting soil-binding plants to avoid soil loss due to wind erosion, etc.

soil contamination A common form of pollution with many causes, including leakage from oil or other service station wastes and leaching from landfill sites, industrial waste sites, etc. It is dangerous when contaminants, e.g., dioxins, PCBs, and toxic metals such as lead, mercury, or arsenic, are absorbed and metabolized by food crops and enter the food chains of animals or humans.

sojourn time Syn: detectable preclinical period. The interval between the detectability of a condition on screening and the stage when the condition presents clinically, i.e., the interval during which the condition can potentially be detected or diagnosed. Life-threatening diseases such as breast cancer often can be detected by clinical examination during the sojourn time.

solar radiation Light and energy from the sun that gives life to the earth includes all wavelengths, from extremely short ionizing through the visible light spectrum to infrared and longer wavelength radiation. Although solar radiation confers life and health, excess of some of the shorter wavelength ionizing radiation is harmful, increasing cancer and cataract risks.

solid waste Refuse of domestic, agricultural, commercial, and industrial origin, including semisolid sludge, discarded paper and containers, waste products of industrial processes, street sweepings, a mixture of materials only some of which are organic and can decompose and only a little of which can be recycled and reused. Disposal of solid waste presents many challenges. See also WASTE DISPOSAL.

sonography A method that uses sound waves to assess the presence of solid substances in a fluid medium. It is used to detect depth in the sea, the presence of schools of fish, and mines and enemy submarines during warfare, and in obstetrics, by means of ultrasonography, to delineate the dimensions of the fetus.

soundex code An alphabetical sequence of letters that is used to create a phonetic representation of personal and family names in RECORD LINKAGE systems.

soup kitchen A service established during times of hardship, notably in the Depression of the 1930s, by agencies such as the SALVATION ARMY to provide a hot meal for destitute people; such services are now widespread throughout the industrial world, serving mainly the needs of homeless people.

sour gas A general term for acidic natural gases, natural or petroleum gas containing hydrogen sulfide, sulfur dioxide, or mercaptans. A concentration of 1 part per million is perceptible and 3 parts per million is toxic. Two sour gases associated with oil and gas drilling and production are hydrogen sulfide and carbon dioxide. Sulfur and nitrogen oxides, generated by oxidation of sulfur- or nitrogen-bearing materials, are also acidic but do not occur in the anaerobic conditions of the subsurface.

Southern blot An electrophoretic method of testing for nucleic and acid-base composition of antibodies, invented by the British biologist E. M. Southern. A test commonly used in molecular biology and genetics to check for a match between DNA molecules. DNA fragments are separated by electrophoresis, transferred or "blotted" to membrane filters, and hybridized with radiolabeled probes to detect specific base sequences with the probes.

spa A place with access to natural hot springs used for therapeutic and/or recreational purposes. Hot springs are rich in dissolved chemicals, such as magnesium sulfate. Spas have been used for many centuries in Europe for recreation and to treat conditions such as rheumatism. The word also describes small manufactured heated pools, which sometimes have thermal or biological hazards, such as providing a nidus for propagation of LEGIONNAIRES DISEASE.

special education The term used to describe the system and curriculum designed to meet the needs of children with intellectual impairments and sometimes those with physical disabilities such as cerebral palsy that make regular classroom teaching and learning difficult or impossible.

special needs clinic A clinic, usually in a children's hospital or service, to treat conditions such as intellectual impairment, Down syndrome, etc.

specialty boards See AMERICAN BOARDS.

species A group of organisms that resemble one another closely in appearance and genetic makeup. Members of a species can breed with others of the same species but generally not with other, even closely related, species. In taxonomy, a species is the division below a genus.

specificity Syn: true negative rate. The ability of a diagnostic or screening test to identify correctly persons who do not have the disease for which the test is done.

spectrophotometry A method of examining the atomic and molecular structure of a substance by dissolving it in water or other suitable solvent, illuminating it with a powerful light source, and studying the spectrum that it produces.

spectroscopy An analytic examination of the electromagnetic spectrum produced when radiant energy is emitted or absorbed by a substance. An optical spectroscope is a prism that separates visible light into separate wavelengths. Other wavelengths of electromagnetic radiation can be separated into component parts by suitable equipment, in order to identify molecules, elements, and compounds of which substances are made. Thus, spectroscopy is a method to identify the composition of a substance.

speech disorder A condition that may be inborn or acquired, sometimes with clearly defined pathology, such as brain damage, sometimes apparently of psychological origin, including stuttering, dyslexia, aphasia. Some speech disorders respond well to speech therapy.

speed The street name for amphetamine, dextroamphetamine, and related substances used as illicit addictive drugs. Overdoses can precipitate cardiovascular collapse, and long-term use can cause psychosis, such as paranoid delusions.

spermatozoan (Plural: spermatozoa) The male gamete, the active ingredient of semen, discharged in the hundreds of millions in an ejaculate. Only one reaches and fertilizes the ovum—rarely, two, in the case of dizygotic twins. Spermatozoa survive for as long as 72 hours in the vagina and uterus but are fragile, easily damaged by disease and drugs, and inactivated by spermicide contraceptives.

spina bifida A NEURAL TUBE DEFECT in which the lower end of the vertebral column fails to close, leaving the lower end of the spinal cord and cauda equina exposed and the nerve fibers incompletely developed. It is a serious congenital malformation often associated with loss of bladder and bowel control with frequent recurrent bladder infections requiring aggressive control with antibiotics. Even the milder form called spina bifida occulta, in which there is little or no outwardly visible anatomical defect, can be associated with severe neurological damage. This birth defect is associated with prenatal maternal FOLIC ACID deficiency. Incidence is reduced by folic acid supplements before and during early pregnancy.

spinal manipulation Originally the domain of Turkish masseurs and those practicing CHIROPRACTIC, spinal manipulation is applied by physiatrists and physiotherapists among others, using vigorous flexion, extension, massage, etc., to treat backache.

spirochete A group of bacteria characterized by spiral shape and motility. The best known member of the group is *Treponema pallidum*, the causative organism of SYPHILIS.

spongiform encephalopathy See TRANSMISSIBLE SPONGIFORM ENCEPHALOPATHY.

sporadic Descriptive of a disease that occurs haphazardly from time to time with no discernible pattern, rather than in any recognizable epidemic or endemic pattern.

spore The survival mode of a small, often single-cell organism, such as a bacterium or protozoan, usually a shell or case that provides some protection for the organism from harsh environmental conditions, such as excessive dryness or cold.

sporozoite See MALARIA LIFE CYCLE.

sports medicine The branch of medical practice dealing with enhancing fitness to engage in sports and the prevention and treatment of injuries related to athletics and sporting activities. Nutrition is a core discipline. There is considerable emphasis on treatment of injuries to joints, ligaments, muscle strains, etc. There is also much emphasis on improving muscle strength and endurance, some of which involves the use of drugs that increase muscle mass and strengthen muscles but also have harmful cardiovascular and metabolic effects and have been banned by the International Olympic Committee and other sporting associations. An important aspect of sports medicine is prevention and detection of the use of performance-enhancing substances. Another development is in sports psychology, which aims to create the will to win.

sporulation The process of forming spores.

spot map A method of displaying the geographical distribution of a disease, sometimes helpful in epidemic investigation, in which cases of a disease of interest are plotted on a map. From the distribution, it may be possible to make inferences about the origin of a point-source epidemic and its mode of spread and thus initiate suitable control measures.

sprue Syn: malabsorption syndrome. A condition in which ingested fats are imperfectly absorbed and digested, causing fatty diarrhea (steatorrhea) and reduced intake of fat-soluble vitamins. It is most common in the tropics. Celiac disease, caused by an inborn metabolic disorder, is a similar disorder in its clinical manifestations.

spurious correlation Syn: nonsense correlation. A relation between two variables that is statistically significant but lacks biological, social, or other plausibility. If statistical significance is accepted at the level of 5% (i.e., $p < 0.05$), one in 20 correlations will be "statistically significant" by the operation of chance alone, regardless of any other meaning they may or may not have.

squatter settlement An informal place of shelter for displaced or homeless people, often using makeshift materials such as discarded packing cases, cardboard boxes, etc., lacking any sanitary facilities or other essential infrastructure. The term implies that a squatter settlement is temporary, but it often evolves into or merges with an existing shantytown or slum.

stack effect The physics of gases determines that the hot gaseous emissions from factory, smelter, and furnace chimney stacks will rise into the atmosphere and be blown by the wind as a PLUME of emissions, including gases, airborne particles, and trace amounts of many chemical compounds, including toxic metals such as lead, mercury, and arsenic. These descend to the earth's surface as FALLOUT, which is a major contributing factor to environmental pollution.

stack effluent The gases, fumes, and suspended particulates emitted from a factory or furnace smokestack. It has been customary since the beginning of the industrial revolution to use this method to disperse emissions, in the belief that atmospheric dilution would somehow eliminate the toxic ingredients. Of course, nothing of the sort happens. Instead, all the toxic substances in the effluent—trace amounts of lead, mercury, arsenic, carcinogenic hydrocarbons, many other toxic substances, etc.—are dispersed as fallout over a wide area in the PLUME.

staging of disease A formal procedure in the management of cancer using a combination of clinical, radiological, imaging, and pathological evidence to categorize cancer cases, e.g., breast cancer, into stages indicating how advanced the disease process is, its appropriate treatment, and its prognosis. Staging of cancer is based on the TNM (tumor, nodes, metastases) classification, i.e., the nature and configuration of the tumor at the primary site, the presence and extent of affected regional lymph nodes, and the extent if any to which metastases have proliferated. A clinically more useful method for some cancers is a numerical staging system. Stage I is suitable for localized resection; stage II requires regional resection; stage III needs radiotherapy and/or chemotherapy; and stage IV is terminal or preterminal cancer for which only palliative care is possible. Several other staging systems have been developed for cancer, for conditions such as AIDS, and less consistently for

some other prolonged diseases associated with progressive deterioration.

stakeholder A person, group, or entity, such as a commercial corporation, that has a financial or other interest in a policy or program and seeks or merits a voice in decision making.

standard An established and accepted basis for comparison, a technical specification, results or findings from a recognized study. See also CRITERION and NORM.

standard deviation The most widely used measure of spread or dispersion from the central value of a frequency distribution. It is the positive square root of the variance from the mean or central value of the individual measurements in the distribution.

standard error The standard deviation of an estimate. The term often refers to the standard deviation of the observed mean, represented by the symbol σ and calculated from a sample and the true population mean.

standardization This term describes several alternative methods to adjust sets of data in ways that reduce the distorting effect of variables, such as differences in the age structure, that might otherwise confound comparisons of two or more populations being made for other purposes. Direct standardization uses weighted averages of specific rates in the study population based on distributions in a specified STANDARD POPULATION and comparing these with the rates that would be expected in the standard population. Indirect standardization is used when the specific rates in the study population are unknown or unstable. It requires projection of averaged specific rates in the standard population onto the study population, weighting these with distributions in the study population, then calculating the standardized incidence ratio or STANDARDIZED MORTALITY RATIO (SMR).

standardized incidence ratio The ratio of the incident number of cases of a condition in the study population to the number that would be expected if the study population had the same incidence rate as a standard population. This is an infrequently used parameter.

standardized mortality ratio (SMR) The ratio of the number of deaths in a study population to the number that would be expected if this population had the same distribution as a standard population. The SMR is usually expressed as a percentage.

standard metropolitan statistical area (SMSA) An entity defined by the US Census

Bureau as an urban metropolis and its immediate environs with defined jurisdictional boundaries.

standard occupational classification (SOC) The categorization of occupations used in the United States and, with modifications, in several other countries, including Canada. The SOC lists 23 broad categories, 96 minor groups, 449 broad occupational groupings, and 822 specific occupational types. It is used to collect and analyze data on types of work by the US Department of Labor and other government agencies. See http://www.bls.gov/soc/home.htm for details.

standard operating procedure The specified routine or "textbook" way of proceeding with a process, such as laboratory testing or manufacturing ingredients. It follows a formal protocol. In practice, it has often evolved from empirical experience rather than from textbooks and is refined by measures such as process analysis, monitoring, and evaluation.

standard population A population used for STANDARDIZATION. Any population can be used for this purpose provided its age and sex structure are precisely known. Examples include Sweden in 1940, the US census population of 1990, etc.

standard setting Establishment by one or more of several methods of a set of criteria, e.g., for occupational exposure levels to workplace pollutants. The methods commonly require consensus development based on input from empirical observations, animal models, epidemiological studies, other toxicological findings, ergonomics, etc.

standing orders A formal protocol specifying how to proceed in any commonly occurring set of circumstances, sometimes set out in bylaws or other written guidelines of an organization, such as a public health department. Standing orders do not have the legal force of regulations but are intended to replace or augment ad hoc decision making in an organization.

staphylococcal enterotoxin The ENTEROTOXIN produced when staphylococci, often introduced by food handlers, reproduce in prepared food such as dishes containing cream, salad dressing, custard, eggs, barbecued chicken, etc., stored at room temperature for more than an hour or so. This toxin is tasteless, odorless, and heat stable. It often causes explosive bouts of vomiting followed by diarrhea and sometimes extreme prostration, with an incubation time of a few hours after eating the contaminated food.

staphylococcal infections The staphylococcus is ubiquitous. *Staphylococcus aureus* resides on the skin, in pores of the skin, in the nose, around the rectum, etc. When it finds a hospitable niche, such as a hair follicle, it can grow and form an inflamed lesion—a pimple, boil, or carbuncle. More invasive infections are impetigo, cellulitis, occasionally septicemia, pneumonia, osteomyelitis, endocarditis, often caused by antibiotic-resistant strains.

starvation The condition that occurs with prolonged deprivation of food, i.e., essential nutriment. This occurs under several circumstances, including warfare when food production, distribution, and supply are disrupted; severe prolonged drought or other natural disaster that prevents production or ripening of food crops, often compounded by inadequate distribution systems; or enforced restriction of food intake, as in concentration camps. It occurs to individuals as a consequence of some diseases, including severe intestinal parasitic infections, certain cancers, sprue, etc. Survival in extreme starvation is possible for as long as several weeks, depending on prior nutritional status and physical fitness. Often there are differential rates at which deprivation of essential nutriment causes clinical symptoms and signs. Kwashiorkor is primarily due to protein deficiency; marasmus is generalized calorie deficiency. Vitamin deficiency may occur first, e.g., thiamine deficiency causing beriberi. See also FAMINE, MALNUTRITION, and MARASMUS.

state, or provincial (public), health department The public health department responsible for providing public health services for all the people of a specified regional jurisdiction. In most nations that have this arrangement of public health services, the ESSENTIAL PUBLIC HEALTH SERVICES provided include communicable disease surveillance and control, environmental health services (some are provided at the national and some at the local level), specific health care for vulnerable groups, health promotion and education, chronic disease prevention, health services administration, management, and evaluation.

statins A family of compounds that have the effect of reducing serum cholesterol levels. They reduce LDL cholesterol more than other types of drugs by inhibiting an enzyme that controls the rate of cholesterol production in the body and increasing the liver's ability to remove the LDL cholesterol in the blood. They have become the most widely prescribed medication in North America in the early 21st century because of their presumed beneficial effect on reducing the risk of coronary heart disease. They have some undesirable side effects, including arthritis-like joint and muscle pain and mood disorders. See http://nhlbisupport.com/chd1/meds1.htm for details. Clinical trials have demonstrated their efficacy, but skeptics question the rationale for drug-induced cholesterol reduction rather than diet and exercise to achieve the same end result.

statistical significance A characteristic of a phenomenon or an observation that is unlikely to have occurred by chance. The definition of "unlikely" is variable. In the physical sciences, engineering, etc., an event that is unlikely to occur by chance more often than about once in a million times might be required for an assertion that it is statistically significant. In the biological and medical sciences and in clinical epidemiology, it is a matter of judgment, but events that would be unlikely to occur by chance more than once in 20 times, i.e., with a probability $p < 0.05$, are often accepted as statistically significant. A more rigorous test requires a probability of less than 1 in 100 ($p < 0.01$). See also RANDOM and RISK.

statistics The science, art, and technique of collecting, summarizing, analyzing, and interpreting numerical information that is subject to chance or systematic variations. The word originated as the noun to describe numerical information about the state or nation. It describes any observable phenomenon that demonstrates variability. VITAL STATISTICS deals with the statistics of vital events, i.e., events concerned with the facts of life, such as birth, marriage, death, divorce, separation, etc. Biological statistics, or BIOSTATISTICS, is concerned with the statistical analysis of biological events, including those related to human health and disease.

stem cell An undifferentiated parenchymal cell that develops into a particular kind of specialized cell, e.g., blood-forming, renal tubules, and can sometimes be used in tissue transplants. Fetal embryonic stem cells are preferred for some research and clinical applications, but there are both practical and ethical problems in recovering these, and in some countries access to them is denied.

stereotype Ideas that are preconceived, often prejudicial, about certain kinds of individual or patterns of behavior.

sterile 1. Incapable of sustaining life, especially pathogenic microorganisms. 2. Incapable of fertilizing or being fertilized, i.e., incapable of conceiving.

sterilization 1. The process of rendering free from pathogens and other organisms capable of breeding or reproducing. In medical care, cleaning and purifying with ANTISEPTICS (i.e., rendering sterile) the skin surface and the surgical instruments to be used on it, so that infectious agents will not be introduced during a surgical operation. 2. A surgical or medical procedure that renders a person incapable of fertilization, i.e., producing a zygote that can implant and develop into a fetus.

Male sterilization is usually performed by VASECTOMY, i.e., ligation and excision of a short portion of the vas deferens, so spermatozoa cannot pass from the testes to form the active ingredient in semen. In females, the usual procedure is ligation and excision of the fallopian tubes. Medical sterilization follows the use of certain drugs or exposure to certain environmental toxins, or exposure to large doses of ionizing radiation.

steroids A group of organic compounds comprising four conjoined benzene rings with other elements and moieties attached at various positions, mostly manufactured in the liver, found in bile, and including several that are essential hormones, i.e., adrenal and sex hormones. The word means any organic compound in this class but most commonly applies to synthetic anabolic steroids, which have been much used by bodybuilders and competitive athletes to improve their performance. Their use is prohibited in most sports, including the Olympic Games, because those who use them have an unfair advantage and because of the associated health risks. See also ANABOLIC STEROIDS.

sterols A subgroup of alcohol compounds of steroids, the most important of which are the lipoproteins and cholesterol, implicated in ATHEROSCLEROSIS.

stigma The word comes from ancient Greek, in which it meant a mark of disgrace or shame, or the brand of a slave made with a red hot iron. In modern usage, it means a shameful or disgraceful sign or condition. Some diseases or conditions carry a social or cultural stigma, notably syphilis and other sexually transmitted diseases, HIV/AIDS, alcoholism, formerly tuberculosis (because of its frequent association with vagrancy, alcoholism, and crime), and mental disorders that cause people to act oddly. HIV/AIDS carries a stigma because many people disapprove of behaviors, such as homosexual intercourse and intravenous drug use, that lead to high risk of the condition. It is important for health workers to spurn such prejudices and their corollary, victim-blaming.

stillbirth Syn: fetal death. Death of a fetus before complete expulsion or extraction from the uterus of a product of conception, regardless of the duration of pregnancy.

sting The lesion inflicted by a biting or stinging insect (spider, scorpion, wasp, bee, flea, etc.) or animal (e.g., a snake). Such an injury is sometimes toxic, anaphylactic, or poisonous. In parts of the world where the principal fuel for cooking and heating is biomass, e.g., agricultural waste, bites and stings from poisonous insects and animals are a significant public health problem for those who gather fuel, who are mainly women and girls. In south and southeast Asia, Africa, and parts of South America, this is an important occupational health risk.

stochastic process Syn: statistical process. A process that is determined by chance; a random function. The function may be defined by time intervals, when it is called a time series, or by space (length, breadth, depth), which is called a random field. Examples include medical data, such as individual electrocardiograms, blood pressure, or temperature, and the fluctuations in incidence of new cases of many communicable and noncommunicable diseases.

Stopes, Marie (1880–1958) British botanist, feminist, and activist who wrote extensively on marriage, family life, and especially family planning or birth control. In 1921, she founded in London the first clinic for women where educational material and contraceptive supplies were available. Although opposed initially, her ideas and methods took root in the tolerant political climate after World War I. Her books, *Married Love* and *Wise Parenthood*, both published in 1918, and many other writings, sold widely.

strategic planning In the health sector, as in all others, planning may be ad hoc or carefully considered and long range, taking note of predictable health-related contingencies, such as seasonal variations in disease patterns, changing demographics, etc. Planning that takes all such factors into account can legitimately be described as strategic. Ideally, it begins with a vision of what the ultimate aims are, includes a mission statement, and spells out steps and stages of the plan, methods and procedures, financial estimates, proposed evaluation methods, etc.

strategy 1. A formally planned set of actions to deal with a problem, with the implication that it is a long-range plan rather than a short-term, ad hoc solution. Tactics are the details of a strategic plan. 2. In GAME THEORY, a strategy is a mathematical function. 3. Research strategy is emphasized in many graduate programs, and tends to a adopt a stereotype pattern with a formal series of steps that, if interpreted literally, can stifle originality and creativity.

stratification The process of separating members of a population into groups according to predetermined criteria, such as age, sex, occupation, i.e., compiling a stratified sample. This is commonly done in observational studies as a way to reduce the effect of confounding variables. For example, when investigating environmental cancer risks due to domestic radon gas exposure, it is desirable to stratify the study and control groups by smoking status and occupational groups because these are known cancer risk factors that could confound the results.

stratosphere The atmospheric layer extending from about 11 to about 20 km above the earth's surface, where low pressure means rarefied air. At its upper extremity is the ionosphere, where the action of solar radiation on oxygen produces ozone, which provides some protection from the harmful effect of short wavelength solar ultraviolet radiation.

street gang Typically a group of young people, preteens, teenagers, young adults, with a loose-knit, rather than closely cohesive, social structure. Members provide mutual support and engage collectively in behavior that may be benign or malicious, involving petty or major crime. Young people who become members of street gangs may be initiated in health-harming habits, including tobacco, alcohol, and substance abuse and sexual promiscuity. Intervention by social workers, school teachers, and local public health departments may direct a gang's energies toward more socially desirable ends, such as helping to care for isolated elderly housebound people.

street person A person who either lives on city streets, i.e., a homeless person, or spends virtually all waking hours on city streets but perhaps has a dwelling in which to sleep. Street people in low-income countries include street children, abandoned children who survive by petty crime and prostitution. Everywhere they include people with various forms of mental illness, substance abuse, and chronic alcoholism, and unemployed, homeless people who forage for sustenance in garbage bins, etc. Street people, especially street children, have a host of health problems, including deficiency diseases, diseases associated with exposure to the elements, violence, tuberculosis, HIV/AIDS, etc. See also STREET GANG.

streptococcal infection Streptococci cause several diseases. Group A hemolytic streptococcal infections include acute pharyngitis, impetigo, erysipelas, scarlet fever, rheumatic fever, acute nephritis, and puerperal fever, the last of which, called childbed fever at the time, was a common cause of death in the immediate postnatal period in the days before antisepsis. This still occurs in some rural regions of low-income countries where child-birth antisepsis is inadequate. All these diseases are preventable by attention to asepsis, and most respond to antibiotics.

streptomycin The first broad-spectrum antibiotic to be effective against tuberculosis, discovered by the Russian-born American microbiologist Selman

Waksman (1888–1973). It works by inhibiting protein synthesis in bacteria.

stress An environmental, social, behavioral factor or combination of factors capable of inducing responses that are helpful in fight-or-flight survival situations, desirable in moderation to provide incentives but under some conditions may be harmful to physical, mental, and/or emotional health by destabilizing the neural, psychological, and/or endocrine equilibrium of the body. When the human body is exposed to stress, psychological, neurological, metabolic, and hormonal reactions are induced. Prolonged or repeated exposure to stress causes lasting changes known as the GENERAL ADAPTATION SYNDROME.

stress diseases A miscellaneous group of disorders with onset and recrudescence frequently associated with emotional or work-related stress. These conditions include hypertension, peptic ulcer, atopic dermatitis, migraine headaches, menstrual irregularities, and others. In almost all such conditions, other etiological factors can be identified; e.g., peptic ulcer is associated with *HELICOBACTER PYLORI* infection. Stress per se is not a sufficient cause of these conditions.

stress management A broad variety of environmental, personal, and interpersonal interventions that can be deployed by professional health workers and others to identify the sources of and reduce stress levels, and to enhance the body's efficiency in coping with stress. Meditation, yoga, and psychotherapy may also be beneficial approaches to stress management.

stroke A hemorrhage or thrombosis in a blood vessel in the brain, one of the most common causes of death in old people, formerly more common than now among the middle-aged, in whom it presented as a complication of undetected and untreated high blood pressure.

strongyloidiasis A tropical and temperate-zone infection with filarial helminths (*Strongyloides stercoralis* and *S. fuelleborni*) that enter the human body by penetrating the skin, migrating through the lungs, where they cause bronchitis, and residing in the duodenum and small intestine. It is often symptomless but can be debilitating, especially in immunocompromised persons, such as those with AIDS.

strontium (Sr) A metallic element, one of the "rare earths" that burns with a bright red flame, so is used in flares and fireworks. As radioactive strontium, it occurs in trace amounts in the fallout from nuclear explosions, is absorbed into food chains, and is concentrated in cows' milk,

which after the nuclear weapons tests in the 1950s and 1960s contained significant amounts of Sr_{90}. This was absorbed and deposited in the bones and teeth of milk-drinking children in fallout zones.

structural adjustment A policy of the International Monetary Fund (IMF) and the World Bank that has been implemented since the 1980s. Its aim is to ensure that nations receiving loans from the IMF and the World Bank run their economies in a manner that will generate foreign exchange to repay the loan. This requires them to focus on income-generating luxury foods, flowers, etc., for export rather than on food for themselves; privatize many essential public services; charge user fees for health care and education; and, in short, create a capitalist economy. It is a harsh monetary policy, based on economic and social theories that are meaningless in most subsistence economies, and it ignores culture and traditions. Its consequences include export of capital and skilled workers from poor countries, increasing impoverishment, and widening of the gaps between rich and poor. Its adverse effects on health are now widely recognized.

structured abstract A systematic way to organize the summary of a research study when it is published in scientific journals. The aim is to present information in a logical order, such as aims or objectives, design, methods and procedures, outcome measures, setting and study subjects, results, and conclusions. Many peer-reviewed medical and scientific journals require authors to submit articles in this form.

student health services This term is usually applied to health services at the tertiary education level, i.e., for adolescents and young adults, where the health problems include many associated with the stresses and strains of emotional development and the increasing intellectual challenges of higher education. Thus, there is more emphasis on mental health than in health services provided for younger school children. See also SCHOOL HEALTH SERVICES.

Student's *t* test A statistical test for the degree of similarity or difference between two or more distributions, invented by the British mathematician W. S. Gossett, who published under the pseudonym "Student" because of the conditions of his employment.

study design See RESEARCH DESIGN.

styrene Syn: polystyrene, vinylbenzene. A widely used chemical from which plastic products, fiberglass, etc., are manufactured. It is a neurotoxin, mutagenic, and possibly carcinogenic to workers engaged in the manufacture of polystyrene products.

subculture 1. In sociology, a section of society that has behaviors and values that are identifiably distinct and different from those of the general population. Examples include certain occupational groups, including lawyers, physicians, members of some societies and clubs, and motorcycle gangs. 2. A bacterial culture made from a previously cultured organism, usually one that is a mixture of several organisms, which can be separated in subcultures favoring one over the others.

sublimation 1. Transformation from a solid to a gaseous state without passing through a liquid phase. 2. In psychology, the psychoanalytic theory whereby perceived "unhealthy" desires and urges are redirected into other consciously controlled activities, e.g., artistic creations.

subliminal stimulus A sensory stimulus that does not quite impinge on consciousness. For instance, cinematic moving pictures in which one image is replaced by a printed message are viewed without conscious perception of the message, although neuropsychological tests reveal that the image is nonetheless retained in memory.

subsistence economy An economy that provides the bare minimum requirements for survival. It functions mainly in the absence of cash, and people sustain themselves by drawing upon limited resources in their immediate environment that may be inadequate or barely adequate for survival.

subspecialist Syn: superspecialist. A specialist in medicine or surgery whose field of expertise is confined within a narrow range, such as microsurgical repair of severed nerves or the use of flexible fiberscopes for endoscopic examination of the bronchial tree or the esophagus and stomach. The prefixes "sub" and "super" are often interchangeable, but superspecialists are sometimes regarded as exceptionally proficient at specific technical procedures, whereas subspecialists are those who have confined their work within a very narrow range but may not necessarily possess exceptional ability or skills. A problem arises when medical care is fragmented among narrowly specialized fields if patients and their families cannot identify who is ultimately responsible and accountable in the event of mishaps in care.

substance abuse Nontherapeutic use of any licit or illicit material or chemical compound with the intention of altering the state of consciousness or emotions, especially if done repeatedly or habitually. The substances include prescription drugs, illegal drugs such as heroin and cocaine, alcohol, and fumes from solvents, glue, gasoline. A few substances that alter states of consciousness are culture-specific. Their use or abuse depends on availability, cost, and custom. Examples include coca leaves, betel nut, marijuana, peyote, and crystal meth.

Substance Abuse and Mental Health Services Administration (SAMHSA) The division of the US Department of Health and Human Services responsible for action aimed at prevention and control of substance abuse. The range of services and activities of SAMHSA extends from primary prevention through medical care in such settings as detoxification centers to law enforcement. See http://www.samhsa.gov/index.aspx for details.

sudden infant death syndrome (SIDS) Syn: cot death, crib death. A condition, or group of conditions, that leads to sudden, unexpected death in infancy between a few weeks and about 9 months of age. The possible causes include cardiac-respiratory crises, possibly associated with exposure to tobacco smoke, overwhelming infection, and electrolyte imbalance. There is a strong association with high concentration of environmental tobacco smoke in the place where the infant sleeps. Another association may be with sleeping posture, and placing infants to sleep in the prone position seems to help reduce the risk of SIDS. Many SIDS deaths are never adequately explained.

suffocation Obstruction of the airway and oxygen lack, e.g., by strangulation, or by a gas such as carbon dioxide that displaces oxygen. It is a mode of immediate cause of death.

suicide The act of taking one's own life. This may be done in ways that leave no room for doubt about intent, e.g., shooting oneself in the brain, hanging, leaping from a great height, or inhaling poisonous gas fumes, or tentatively, as attempted suicide, by an act that unless interdicted or interrupted would result in self-destruction, e.g., deliberately taking an overdose of sleeping pills. Violent suicidal death is sometimes concealed, as in some single-vehicle, high-speed crashes. A suicidal gesture is an act that the perpetrator believes others will interpret as an attempt to commit suicide and may be a way for an emotionally disturbed or distraught person to send a distress signal that could prompt others to provide needed help.

suicide prevention Suicide is frequent enough in some populations, for example marginalized young people in indigenous communities in affluent nations, that programs aimed at preventing it have high priority. Methods and procedures such as psychotherapy, provision of emotional and social support, use of mood-modifying drugs to relieve severe depression, and miscellaneous other measures, e.g., awareness-raising educational programs, can be deployed. Probably the most effective strategy is to identify and intervene with high-risk groups and provide improved training and career opportunities to motivate school children and youth in high-risk populations, such as young people in indigenous communities.

sulfanilamide The generic name for a synthetic pharmaceutical preparation that was the first effective drug against bacterial infection with pneumococci, gonococci, etc. It was developed in 1938 in Germany and Britain by the German scientist Gerhard Domagk (1895–1964). He received the 1939 Nobel Prize in Physiology or Medicine for his discovery. Many bacteria, unfortunately, soon became resistant.

sulfites Salts of sulfurous acid, some of which are produced by ACID PRECIPITATION and contribute to the environmental damage this causes, as well as to the pulmonary damage caused by inhaling air laden with sulfur-containing industrial emission products.

sulfur (S) A yellow nonmetallic element naturally occurring in elemental form in volcanic eruptions and in many compounds in which it replaces oxygen in chemical bonds.

sulfur dioxide (SO$_2$) A pungent, choking, poisonous gas that is an ingredient of combusted carbon fuels, in which sulfur compounds occur as trace contaminants. In contact with rain or moisture in the atmosphere, it forms sulfuric and sulfurous acid, as in ACID PRECIPITATION. This causes serious respiratory irritation and inflammation, leading to chronic bronchitis and emphysema in urban regions with high levels of atmospheric pollution.

sullage Syn: gray water. Dishwater, bath water, etc., i.e., water that has been used for washing dishes, clothes, or the body and therefore is unfit for drinking but can be used for irrigation or watering garden vegetables and flowers.

sunburn Erythematous inflammation of skin exposed for too long to sunlight, most noticeable in fair-complexioned people. How long is "too long" is inversely related to cutaneous protective melanin pigment and to the intensity of solar radiation. Solar radiation that enters the atmosphere obliquely, i.e., at high latitudes, has had a high proportion of short-wave ultraviolet radiation filtered out by the atmosphere before it reaches the earth's surface and is therefore less harmful than tropical sunlight to very fair-skinned people, for whom acute sunburn is a hazard of tropical vacations.

sunlight Syn: actinic radiation. Sunlight is life giving, required for germination of most forms of plants, and directly or indirectly necessary or beneficial for most other living things. As well as visible light, sunlight comprises ultraviolet and infrared radiation.

sunscreen Cream or lotion containing ingredients that scatter solar radiation and thus block access to the skin surface by harmful levels of ultraviolet radiation, thereby reducing the risk of sunburn and skin cancer. Most contain compounds of oxybenzone and/or para-aminobenzoic acid and come in varying strengths, some of which permit enough radiation to penetrate for tanning to occur.

Superfund The US Resource Conservation and Recovery Act of 1976 allocated financial funds to cleaning up designated toxic waste sites and other hazardous environments, rehabilitating BROWNFIELDS, etc., and was reinforced by further legislation in 1980. More information is available at http://www.epa.gov/superfund/.

support group A usually informal group of friends, colleagues, etc., who provide emotional and social support at times of trouble. Epidemiological evidence suggests that the availability of a support group reduces the risk of adverse health outcomes from common serious diseases.

support system See SOCIAL SUPPORT SYSTEMS.

suppression of information The situation in which important and relevant facts and conclusions that are in the public interest to be disclosed are concealed or withheld from the public domain. Important scientific advances are normally communicated as soon as possible to the scientific community, but there are exceptions, as during World War II, when medical discoveries, such as effective ways to treat wound infections and malaria, were military secrets. As of the late 20th century, pharmaceutical manufacturers and the scientists who work for them are sometimes secretive about the compounds they are studying, and government biomedical scientists also may be obliged to suppress their results, usually in the interest of national security.

suprarenal gland disorders The suprarenal or adrenal glands are paired endocrine organs located just above the kidneys. They function interactively with the pituitary and hypothalamus and are essential to effective control of blood pressure, body chemistry, metabolism, and immune responses. Disorders include Addison's disease, a generalized chronic wasting and debilitating condition often accompanied by skin pigmentation, formerly sometimes a complication of advanced tuberculosis.

surface water Water that collects on ground surface after rain, seepage from a spring, etc. In many environments, it is a breeding ground for insect vectors, such as mosquitoes. Surface water is generally contaminated, e.g., by feces, but is nevertheless often the source of drinking water in low-income countries.

surfactant A substance that reduces the surface tension of a liquid. Examples include naturally occurring substances in bronchial secretions that prevent accumulation of gelatinous sputum, and domestic and industrial detergents.

Surgeon General In the United States, the chief medical official in the US Public Health Service; the same designation applies to the chief medical officer in the armed services of the United States and several other nations that adopt the same nomenclature for medical military ranks. See http://www.surgeongeneral/gov/.

surgery 1. The branch of medical practice that uses operative procedures, rather than medication, to treat disease. 2. In Britain, the name for a doctor's office or consulting rooms.

surrogate A person appointed to act in place of another. In the health sector, the word usually applies to a surrogate parent and specifically to a woman who "leases" her womb to a couple or another woman who is unable to carry a pregnancy, e.g., because of prior hysterectomy or disease of the uterus or adnexum. There are troubling ethical and moral issues involved. In some nations, surrogacy is legally permissible, provided it is not done for financial gain; in others, it is banned.

surveillance Systematic, ongoing collection, collation, and analysis of health-related information that is communicated in a timely manner to all who need to know which health problems require action in their community. Surveillance is a central feature of epidemiological practice, where it is used to control disease. Information that is used for surveillance comes from many sources, including reported cases of communicable diseases, hospital admissions, laboratory reports, cancer registries, population surveys, reports of sickness absence from school or work (in which a sudden sharp rise in numbers may signal the onset of an epidemic), and reported causes of death, in which again a sudden rise in numbers, for instance of deaths from pneumonia, may signal the onset of epidemic influenza.

survey An investigation in which information is collected systematically but often without a formal research design to test a hypothesis. Surveys commonly consist of questionnaires or interviews, less commonly of physical examinations or measurements or targeted laboratory tests. The information is often complex and is collected by means of a SURVEY INSTRUMENT, such as a set of carefully composed questions that have been tested for validity and consistency, as in the Health and Nutrition Examination Surveys of the US National Center for Health Statistics.

survey instrument A term used mainly in the social and behavioral sciences to describe the protocols such as questionnaires, interview schedules, or other sets of questions used in social research.

survival analysis The analysis of information gathered by followup of a group of individuals who have received some sort of intervention, usually with the aim of evaluating the efficacy of a therapeutic regimen.

survival curve A graphical display of the number or proportion of an exposed population that remain alive at specified intervals after an exposure to a risk or an event of interest. Survival curves are often used to display the survival rates at specified intervals after diagnosis and/or treatment for many conditions, such as various kinds of cancer.

survival of the fittest A phrase often loosely used to mean survival of the physically fittest in hostile or environmentally challenging conditions. The way the concept was described by the English scientist Charles Darwin (1809–1882) in his works on evolution (using the term "natural selection"), it means reproductive or genetic fitness, i.e., survival into future generations of characteristics recognized since Darwin's time as genetic, and in this sense it is an essential feature of EVOLUTION.

survival rate A numerical statement of the portion of the population remaining alive at a specified time after a life-threatening exposure or event. It may be a true rate, but often it is a number rather than a true rate, because the population at risk, the time and duration of exposure, and/or other necessary parameters to calculate a true rate cannot be accurately ascertained.

survival value Qualities that confer an advantage on individuals or species by enabling them to survive adverse environmental circumstances and subsequently reproduce. Examples include spore formation by certain microorganisms, camouflage coloration of moths and birds, etc.

susceptibility Vulnerability, often specific to particular threats, e.g., from pathogens.

suspended particulate matter Substances smaller than about 20 microns that remain in the atmosphere for extended periods because their small mass is not immediately influenced by the force of gravity. Particulate matter smaller than 10 microns can be inhaled, and particles smaller than 2.5 microns can be inhaled and penetrate to the alveoli.

sustainable development This term describes the process of modification of the environment that remains ecologically in balance, so sufficient resources such as crops can be harvested or extracted without degrading the environment or irreversibly damaging the ecosystem. By definition, extraction of nonrenewable resources, such as oil, natural gas, and minerals, cannot be sustainable because the supply of these resources must eventually be exhausted. In sustainable development, the supporting ecosystem remains intact and can continue indefinitely.

sweating sickness A disease that occurred in several large epidemics and many small outbreaks in medieval Europe, with a clinical picture described in meticulous detail by several competent clinical observers; it was characterized by fever, respiratory distress, and profuse sweating. No disease resembling this has been seen for several hundred years, so sweating sickness appears to have been an evanescent phenomenon.

sweatshop A workplace sometimes identified with the UNDERGROUND ECONOMY employing people who may not be able to work legitimately, e.g., because they are illegal immigrants, often in unhealthy, dangerous conditions where occupational injury is prevalent.

swimmer's itch Syn: cercarial dermatitis. A subcutaneous eruption caused by penetration of cercarial larvae that may or may not be able to develop in a human host. Often the condition is caused by larvae of cercariae that are rejected by the human host and die in situ. Information is available at http://www.cdc.gov/ncidod/dpd/parasites/schistosomiasis/factsht_cardmermatitis.htm.

swine influenza A strain of influenza A that was traced to its origin in swine in 1976, and caused a small localized outbreak of virulent influenza that killed at least one serviceman in a military camp in the United States. All indications were that this could be the beginning of a very large epidemic, but for whatever reason this did not materialize. The Centers for Disease Control and Prevention was able to rapidly prepare and distribute large quantities of a specific vaccine, and this was given to some 20 million people. About 80 of them subsequently contracted Guillain-Barré syndrome with paraplegia. This was wrongly attributed to the vaccine until it was realized that the number of cases during the period in question was no greater than would be expected by chance. But by the time this was realized the harm had been done, and many people still believe that influenza vaccine carries significant risk of this complication.

symbiosis A relationship between two or sometimes several dissimilar species of organism in which they live together in the same ecosystem in a mutually beneficial relationship. If only one species benefits, the relationship is described as commensal, and if one benefits at the cost of harm to the other, the relationship is described as PARASITISM.

sympathetic nervous system Part of the autonomic nervous system, including nerve ganglia alongside the spinal cord and the vagus nerve. The sympathetic nervous system controls essential and mainly automatic functions such as heart rate and respiration. It is the part of the nervous system that responds to fear, prepares the body for "fight or flight" in emergencies, and slows or shuts down nonessential functions. Its action increases heart rate, blood pressure, and cardiac output; diverts blood flow from the skin and intestines to skeletal muscle; dilates the pupils and bronchioles; contracts sphincters; and mobilizes fat and glycogen.

syndrome A set of symptoms and/or clinical signs that usually occur together and are inferred to be caused by the same disease or underlying condition, or a condition characterized by a set of associated symptoms and/or signs. A great many syndromes are known, and many are identified by specific names, often by an eponym commemorating the person(s) who first described them. Since some syndromes can have more than one cause, it is important always to diagnose this and treat it appropriately, rather than use symptomatic treatment only.

syndromic approach to treatment A method of treatment based on the assumption that all or the majority of patients presenting with a certain cluster of symptoms and signs have the same condition, and that therefore all can be treated in the same way. It is a justifiable "shortcut" when a dangerous epidemic occurs, especially if resources are limited. The method has been used in India to treat large numbers of village women with vaginal discharges on the assumption that their condition is due to bacterial infection, but when samples of these women have been investigated bacteriologically most show no evidence of bacterial infection.

syndromic surveillance Surveillance based on enumeration of clusters of symptoms rather than on diagnosed cases of the disease under surveillance.

synergism The collective action of two or more factors that is greater than the sum of their actions would be separately, the synergistic effect.

syphilis Until the appearance of HIV/AIDS, this was the most serious and deadly of the sexually transmitted diseases. It seems to have appeared for the first time in Europe in the late 14th or early 15th century, probably imported from the Americas in the early days of European colonization, or perhaps a newly emerged pathogen. It occurred in florid epidemic form and was rapidly recognized to be spread by promiscuous sexual intercourse. It was given names descriptive of its appearance and supposed place of origin, such as "the pox," "the French disease," "the Spanish disease," "le mal anglais," etc. It was the first and worst VENEREAL DISEASE. After its initial appearance in Europe, it slowly changed its character from a fulminating, acute, and often rapidly fatal disease to a more chronic form with a primary chancre on the genitals or mouth at the site of infection, soon followed by a macular skin rash, a latent period, then tertiary syphilis affecting the central nervous system, the cardiovascular system, and sometimes other organs. The causative organism, the spirochete *Treponema pallidum*, is a delicate obligate parasite that responds to several antibiotics. For several decades after the 1950s, syphilis was well controlled and became uncommon, but it has entered a period of resurgence, mainly among persons with compromised immune systems because of HIV/AIDS infection.

syringe jaundice An obsolete name for HEPATITIS B that recognized a correlation between the disease and prior use of a hypodermic or intravenous infusion with a contaminated needle.

systematic error A consistent bias due to faulty instruments that yield incorrect readings or results, e.g., because of calibration, wrong dilution of reagents, etc.

systematic review A method of analysis based on pooled data from as many sources as possible,

preferably, but not necessarily, using exactly comparable research studies. In this respect, a systematic review may not be quite the same as a META-ANALYSIS, which relies on comparable studies. The aim is to make maximum use of the best available evidence from all available sources in EVIDENCE-BASED DECISION MAKING. See also COCHRANE COLLABORATION.

systematized nomenclature of human and veterinary medicine (SNOMED) A methodical taxonomical system for naming diseases and procedures developed by the American College of Pathologists. It is somewhat cumbersome and has not caught the imagination of most of the health professionals for whom it was designed. See http://www.snomed.org/snomedct/.

Système International (SI) d'Unités (in English, International System of Units, abbreviated to SI units) A set of measurements of physical variables based on a more rational examination of the properties of length, mass, time, radiation, etc., than the traditional measurements and nomenclature. SI units have been widely adopted in the physical sciences, meteorology, etc., especially in many European nations, but traditionalists in the English-speaking world have been rather reluctant to adopt SI units

systems analysis The scientific evaluation of data from component parts of a functioning system, such as a public health service or its components, e.g., immunization programs. The analysis examines and evaluates distinct elements of the system, such as input, output, and feedback loops.

systems theory The branch of scholarly inquiry that examines phenomena to discern whether and how they are related and seeks to define the underlying natural laws or systems that govern their activities. Systems theory has been used in studies of human behavior and interactions, that by analogy with physiological systems are considered to abide by more or less predictable laws. The methods of so doing are called SYSTEMS ANALYSIS.

T

taboo From a Polynesian word meaning a sacred prohibition, taboo has passed into international usage to describe behavior, places, people, and social roles that are unacceptable. Some taboos are wide-spread among human societies, although they are not universal. Examples include incest, killing one's own children, killing others. Inhibitions on these behaviors are personal, familial, and societal, and sanctions against violation are reinforced by laws almost everywhere. Taboos have health implications, which, depending on circumstances, may be beneficial or detrimental, such as when they inhibit sexual relationships or specific food items.

TAB vaccine The killed bacterial vaccine that provides immune protection against typhoid and paratyphoid A and B infection. The vaccine can induce severe localized and sometimes systemic reactions with fever and malaise, so it is not desirable as a routine procedure, but vaccination against typhoid is recommended for travelers going to endemic regions.

taeniasis Infection with the pork tapeworm, *Taenia solium*, or the beef tapeworm, *T. saginata*. These enter human hosts as cysts in raw or undercooked pork or beef, respectively, and mature in the intestinal tract, where they develop into mature adult TAPEWORMS. The eggs are consumed by the animal host (pigs or cattle, respectively), penetrate the intestinal wall, and are carried in the bloodstream to muscle tissues, where they form cysts, visible to the naked eye as "measly" pork or beef. Self-infection is possible with some species, as the condition known as CYSTICERCOSIS.

tailings The worked out residue left over after active mineral content has been extracted from the coal or mineral ore collected at a mine. In the case of coal mines, these are usually called slag heaps. The tailings from mineral ore vary considerably in usefulness and actual or potential health hazard. Some mine tailings make useful building material, e.g., as part of the solid ingredient in cement. Radium and uranium mine tailings emit radon gas for many years and are hazardous to health if used as building material. Some mine tailings contain lead, arsenic, and other toxic minerals in significant trace amounts.

talc Amorphous hydrated magnesium silicate, used as a dusting powder, e.g., to lubricate the insides of surgical gloves. Occupational exposure, for example, in mining and refining, can cause PNEUMOCONIOSIS unless workers are protected from the risk of inhaling silica dust by wearing respirators. Talc may also be contaminated, for instance, by trace amounts of arsenic.

tamoxifen Synthetic nonsteroid estrogen antagonist that acts specifically as a therapeutic agent in the treatment and prevention of breast cancer. It retards or reduces the proliferation of some varieties of breast cancer but not others. Beneficial side effects include reduced osteoporosis and a cholesterol-lowering effect, but it may also induce corneal opacities, venous thrombosis, and depression. Large-scale clinical trials have demonstrated that efficacy outweighs adverse side effects. See http://www.fda.gov/cder/news/tamoxifen/default.htm for details.

tanning 1. Processing of animal hides to produce leather, a craft dating to prehistoric times. After cleansing, hides are treated (cured) using bark or other vegetable matter containing tannin, thus the name. Modern methods employ ammonia, chromium salts, and other toxic chemicals that expose workers to various hazards. 2. Increased melanin pigment in the skin that imparts a brown color. Exposure of the dermis of fair-skinned people to solar or ultraviolet radiation causes varying degrees of erythema (SUNBURN), and the melanocytes produce melanin that tans the skin, which many people with fair complexions consider attractive. If enough sunlight is not available, tanning salons have become a popular alternative. Ultraviolet radiation from sunlight or tanning salons increases the risk of skin cancer and malignant MELANOMA.

tapeworms Segmented helminth intestinal parasites that fasten on the epithelial wall of the intestine where the 1- to 5-mm head is dwarfed by multiple segments that may extend to many meters in length. Each segment is a self-contained unit that produces eggs in prodigious numbers and is eventually shed in feces, where eggs can be consumed by the animal host. See TAENIASIS. The principal varieties are the pork tapeworm, *Taenia solium*, and the beef tapeworm, *T saginata*, and *Echinococcus* species.

tap water The water that emerges from taps in homes, public buildings, etc., and standpipes in low-income countries, where a single standpipe may service many families. Tap water usually comes from a reservoir. It may or may not have been partly purified by filtration and disinfected by chlorination, but it may still contain toxic or other chemicals and some pathogens, e.g., Giardia, cryptosporidium, and sometimes more dangerous pathogens such as *Salmonella typhi*. When there is doubt, water should be further tested and treated by boiling before it is used for drinking, cleaning vegetables, or cooking.

tar A gelatinous black substance occurring naturally as deposits of decomposed carboniferous plants or as a by-product of coal, used to seal roads and roofs. Because it contains benzapyrene, which is a carcinogen, tar workers are at increased risk of skin cancer from exposure. See also COAL TAR.

Tarasoff v. Regents of the University of California A landmark legal judgment in 1969 that established the principle according to which it can be legally, as well as ethically, justifiable to violate an explicit or implicit promise of confidentiality. In *Tarasoff*, the court held that there is a legal and moral duty for a medical attendant to violate an oath of secrecy if doing so can save the life of an innocent person. The precedent has been accepted and adopted in many jurisdictions throughout the world and applies in public health practice. There are many discussions in legal and ethical publications. See http://www.publichealthlaw.net/Reader/docs/Tarasoff.pdf.

target Syn: objectively verifiable indicator. In the language of health planning, an explicitly stated outcome of a program, to be achieved by a specified date and stated in quantitative terms, e.g., vaccination of all infants against vaccine-preventable diseases or reduction of teenage smoking rate by specified amounts at specified dates. The quantitative element distinguishes targets from OBJECTIVES, which are more general statements of the aims of a program. Targets have three elements: quantity, quality, and time.

target organ The organ singled out by a pathogen and by specific intervention agents used to prevent or treat the disease caused by this pathogen. Lungs, gastrointestinal tract, kidneys, and liver are common target organs.

target population A specified subset of the population for whom a health-related intervention is specifically intended, e.g., infants, for whom immunization programs are designed and intended.

task force A committee established to address a particular problem or issue. When this problem has been dealt with in a satisfactory manner, the task force is disbanded ("self-destructs").

tattoo Colored pigment implanted in or injected into the dermis, usually for decorative purposes, occasionally an accidental consequence of an explosion that injects pigmented fragments. Tattoos have been part of many human cultures for at least several millennia. Among the New Zealand Maori and other Polynesian cultures, tattoos are traditional symbols of standing in the community. Among sailors, members of the armed forces of many nations, and a small proportion of others, mostly young adults, tattoos are a status symbol. The process carries a risk of introducing serious pathogens, including HIV and hepatitis, but other aspects of lifestyle that may be prevalent in the same people probably carry a higher risk of infection.

taxon A term for a member or entity in a classification group, such as a genus, species, or family of organisms in a taxonomy (plural: taxa).

taxonomy A systematic classification of entities into related groups. A DISEASE TAXONOMY is an orderly classification of diseases into groups on the basis of their underlying causal agents, such as infectious pathogens or trauma, or their anatomical or functional relationships, such as diseases affecting the cardiovascular system or mental, emotional, and personality disorders. The Linnaean taxonomy is arranged hierarchically, into kingdom, phylum, class, order, family, genus, species, and individuals.

Tay-Sachs disease A lethal hereditary disease due to deficiency of an enzyme, hexosaminidase. This leads to accumulation of metabolic end products and causes paralysis, mental retardation, blindness, and death in early childhood. The defect occurs on chromosome 15 in about 2% of Ashkenazi Jews. Genetic counseling among higher-risk subgroups of this population has helped to reduce the incidence of Tay-Sachs disease. The disease is named for the British physician Warren Tay (1843–1927) and the American neurologist Bernard Sachs (1858–1944).

T cells Also called T-helper lymphocytes, these lymphocytes manufacture antibodies to enhance cell-mediated immunity to many viral and bacterial diseases. HIV infection destroys T cells, thus leading to progressive decline of T-lymphocyte production. Therefore, T-lymphocyte cell count, and especially the T4 cell count, is an indicator of the progress of HIV/AIDS.

t-**distribution** A mathematical model that defines the relationship between two or more sets of data, used to determine whether they are significantly different. The *t*-distribution is the quotient of sets of independent random variables, in which the numerator is a standardized normal variate and the denominator is the square root of a quotient of a chi square distributed variate and its number of degrees of freedom.

technical efficiency The aspect of EFFICIENCY that is determined by the quality of equipment used in a process or procedure and the competence of the person using the equipment.

technology assessment The evaluation of innovative technologies in the health sector includes epidemiological studies, e.g., clinical trials, outcome studies, economic evaluation, and cost-benefit, cost-effectiveness, and quality-improvement studies. These have been applied to many modern medical technologies, such as diagnostic imaging and cardiac and laparoscopic surgery.

technology transfer The term used by UN agencies and nongovernmental organizations to describe the process of importing ideas, techniques, and equipment, usually from rich industrial nations to low-income developing countries as part of the process of moving them toward the standards of wealthier countries. This is part of the process of closing the INGENUITY GAP. The term also refers to the process of developing practical applications of new scientific discoveries. Technology transfer also occurs between middle- and low-income countries, where it is described as south-south cooperation.

tectonic plates The theory of plate tectonics—that the earth's lithosphere is composed of large semirigid plates that float on the underlying molten core—explains natural phenomena, including earthquakes and tsunamis caused by movement of one plate on another; volcanoes, which occur at sites where the molten core escapes between plates; and the distribution of plant and animal species that relates to the position of large continental land masses in earlier geological eras.

teenager Literally in the age range of 13 to 19 years inclusive, but in popular speech the age range is less precisely defined and is often understood to mean an adolescent between puberty and adult, that is, someone who has not yet attained full maturity.

teleconference A meeting conducted by telephone with geographically dispersed participants all connected to the same telephone number. A videoconference augments speech with television images of those taking part, and a net meeting uses Internet connections among all participants in real time. These methods are increasingly used, for instance, in nationwide discussions by public health officials to set and implement public health policies, including many related to urgent problems, such as dangerous disease outbreaks and disaster management. Teleconferences are widely used also in continuing education programs.

telemedicine The use of electronic methods, especially television and the Internet, in distance education and disease management, including training in technical and manipulative procedures, sometimes to conduct surgical or obstetric procedures in remote locations with guidance from experts located in a major medical center. Telemedicine has been applied in control of epidemics by WHO experts and others in remote places such as parts of Sub-Saharan Africa and in disaster management.

temperance movement An international collectivity that aims to reduce alcohol consumption substantially or, preferably, eliminate it altogether. The movement originated in nonconformist Protestant churches to counteract the social disruption associated with drunkenness in the United States and Europe in the late 19th century, and reached its zenith

in the US experiment with Prohibition. That experiment failed, but the movement survives, bolstered by organizations such as Al-Anon (family members and victims of ALCOHOLISM). The movement proclaims the health benefits of abstinence from alcohol and thus aspires to achieve societal benefit.

temporal relationship An essential feature in interpretation of events is their relationship to one another in time. In all causal relationships, the cause must precede the effect.

tendinitis Syn: tenosynovitis. An inflammatory lesion affecting tendons and/or the synovial joints that the tendons activate, usually related to repeated stresses. One form of it that is usually occupational and related to unsatisfactory ergonomic circumstances is REPETITIVE STRAIN INJURY (RSI).

tenement A multiunit, high-density, low-rental apartment building or rooming house, usually on several or many floors, often dilapidated, sometimes occupied by problem families. Tenements may be overcrowded, favoring transmission of communicable diseases, may be fire hazards, and are often the site of conflict situations and violent behavior among occupants.

teratogen An agent that acts on the early developing embryo to induce departures from normal growth and development, causing fetal malformation.

terminal care Medical and supportive social and psychological care at the end of life. It differs from palliative care in that the emphasis is primarily on ensuring comfort in the transition from life to death.

terrorism Violent attacks against citizens, governments, and their infrastructure, conducted by aggrieved groups, factions, or individuals, intent on killing and injuring noncombatant people and disrupting services, causing intimidation and fear, aiming to draw attention to the cause that the terrorist individual or group seeks to promote. The definition of terrorism is to some extent subjective. One person's terrorist may be another's freedom fighter, seeking to hit back at a repressive regime. Terrorist attacks may have public health dimensions because they may damage essential infrastructure or because terrorists seek to harm population health or disrupt food production. Spain, Pakistan, parts of Africa, Sri Lanka, Israel, Iraq, Colombia, and other countries are chronically afflicted with terrorist attacks. The United States had a dramatic episode in 2001, when terrorists hijacked passenger aircraft and flew them into the twin towers of the World Trade Center in New York and the Pentagon in Washington, DC. This transformed American policies and public attitudes toward security, which became a higher priority than personal liberty for some. In 2005, major terrorist attacks occurred in Britain and Indonesia. Experience has demonstrated that identifying and eliminating or alleviating the motives for terrorism are more effective countermeasures than aggressive crime control tactics. Terrorists come from many ethnic and religious backgrounds and tend to be young, well educated, and rarely religious fanatics but are convinced that their cause is just. See also BIOTERRORISM.

tertian fever Fever that recurs every third day, i.e., with bouts of fever at 48-hour intervals, that characteristically occurs with *Plasmodium vivax* malaria.

tertiary care Specialized highly technical diagnostic and therapeutic services that are usually available only in large hospitals or major medical centers. Often the most advanced tertiary care services are located in teaching hospitals associated with medical schools and universities.

test case In medical law, such as in tort liability where an occupational or environmental exposure causes harm, this is an action that if successfully argued can become the basis for claims in other cases or a class action suit.

testicular toxins These are chemicals that impair spermatogenesis. They include lead compounds and organic pesticides, notably dibromochloropropane (DBCP).

testosterone The male sex hormone, produced primarily by the testes, also in both sexes by the adrenal cortex, and in small quantities by ovaries. Testosterone stimulates development of male sex organs and secondary sexual characteristics and may contribute to aggressive behavior.

test-retest reliability A method of calibrating equipment, verifying the validity of findings, and assessing the dimensions of instrumental error conducted by repeating the same test several or many times under conditions as nearly identical as feasible. See REPRODUCIBILITY.

tetanus A generalized disease due to the toxin produced by the anaerobic organism *Clostridium tetani*, which usually invades the body in a laceration or compound fracture that was inadequately cleaned and in which dead, i.e., anaerobic, tissue is present. Another entry route is contamination of the umbilical cord of a newborn infant, leading to neonatal tetanus. Tetanus may follow treatment or preventive procedures, such as circumcision or injections undertaken under poor hygienic conditions. The tetanus toxin causes muscle spasms and rigidity of voluntary and respiratory muscles that is fatal unless treated. The natural habitat of *C. tetani*

is the soil. The spores enter the body when the skin is lacerated and flourish, especially when there is necrotic tissue. Until the development of tetanus antitoxin, tetanus caused innumerable deaths from battle wounds, as in the American Civil War.

tetanus neonatorum Syn: neonatal tetanus. Tetanus that occurs in newborns, typically 10 to 14 days after delivery. In some cultures in which the umbilical cord was crushed, as by being ground between two stones, or where the cut end was not cleansed and disinfected, neonatal tetanus was a frequent and tragic cause of neonatal mortality. Education, eradication of unhygienic customs, and tetanus toxoid prophylaxis for pregnant women to protect their infants have greatly reduced the risk, but it still causes as many as 200,000 deaths annually in low-income countries.

tetany Abnormal excitation of voluntary muscles that causes them to contract spasmodically. The physiological reason is calcium ion deficiency or loss, which occasionally happens with the sudden onset of electrolyte imbalance caused by severe diarrhea and vomiting, or it can be due to deficiency disease of the parathyroid glands, or even transiently to hyperventilation and serum carbon dioxide depletion that disrupts normal electrolyte balance.

tetrachlorethylene A chlorinated organic solvent used in dry cleaning and for many industrial purposes. It sometimes contaminates aquifers that are a source of drinking water, e.g., when industrial waste or dry cleaning effluent is released indiscriminately into the environment. It is a neurotoxin, a hepatotoxin, and a reproductive toxin.

tetrachlorodibenzodioxin See DIOXIN.

tetracyclines Broad-spectrum antibiotics effective against a wide range of common pathogenic bacteria, synthetically manufactured to resemble naturally occurring compounds produced by certain fungi and molds. Unfortunately, many bacteria have developed resistance, aggravated by widespread use of this family of antibiotics in animal husbandry as growth promoters.

tetrahydrocannabinol (THC) The active alkaloid ingredient in MARIJUANA.

T4 lymphocyte The white blood cells responsible for producing antibodies, i.e., for developing and strengthening cellular immunity. Decline in the T4 lymphocyte cell count when they are attacked and destroyed by HIV infection is a prognostic indicator of the progress of HIV/AIDS.

thalassemia A group of inheritable diseases of hemoglobin synthesis in which abnormal hemoglobin molecules cause red blood corpuscles to be malformed and thus destroyed in the spleen, producing hemolytic anemia that may be mild or severe, even lethal, depending on the underlying specific genetic defect. People with thalassemia are resistant to infection with malaria parasites, which accounts for the geographical and ethnic distribution of the disease in regions of high malaria endemicity from which people with thalassemia originally came. Many victims require repeated blood transfusions to overcome severe hemolytic anemia. See http://www.marchofdimes.com/professionals/681_1229.asp for a useful fact sheet on the condition and its management.

thalidomide A synthetic drug widely used as a mild hypnotic and sedative in the 1950s and early 1960s until its devastating teratogenic effects on early fetal development were identified. It causes reduction defect of the limbs, and its manufacture and use ceased. It has since been found to be an effective therapy in some otherwise intractable malignant neoplasms. In 1998, the US Food and Drug Administration approved thalidomide for use in treating leprosy symptoms and initiated studies of its efficacy in AIDS, lupus, macular degeneration, and some cancers. Information is available at http://www.fda.gov/cder/news/thalinfo/default.htm.

theories of illness See ILLNESS THEORIES.

theory A belief system based on observation and supposition; compare AXIOM, canon, and HYPOTHESIS. Many scientific theories are based on observation or INFERENCE, some on experiments, including THOUGHT EXPERIMENTS. All commonly applied theories in the natural and public health sciences are subjected to frequent tests of their validity and are vulnerable to refutation. For example, the MIASMA THEORY of disease causation was refuted, whereas the GERM THEORY prevailed. The theory of evolution is denied by some people but is confirmed by DNA studies and empirical observations of how resistance develops to antibiotics and insecticides.

therapeutic community An approach to community-based management of psychiatric and related disorders, including emotionally disturbed adolescence, substance abuse, and mental retardation. In Scotland, the therapeutic community was pioneered by a psychiatrist, Maxwell Jones (1907–1990), who dismantled a long-stay custodial mental hospital and integrated patients into local towns in miscellaneous occupations. Many similar therapeutic communities have been established elsewhere in the United Kingdom and Europe and subsequently in the United States and Canada. The same term describes establishments such as Boys

Towns, for emotionally disturbed and delinquent youths, and facilities for rehabilitation of substance abusers; evaluations often reveal lower rates of recidivism of disturbed youths than in reform schools, but therapeutic communities have been less successful in treating and rehabilitating substance abusers. Sheltered workshops for mentally retarded young people and adults may be another form of therapeutic community. There is a tradition of caring for the mentally ill in some European villages dating from medieval times.

thermography The use of infrared photography to identify "hot spots," tissues that generate above-average and below-average amounts of infrared radiation, such as certain kinds of neoplasms of the breast. Thermography was advocated as an alternative to x-ray mammography because it does not expose the radiosensitive breast tissue to ionized radiation, but evaluation demonstrated unsatisfactory sensitivity, so it fell out of favor.

thiamin Syn: vitamin B_1. A water-soluble member of the vitamin B group. Thiamin plays an essential role in cell metabolism of carbohydrates and is required to convert carbohydrates to energy. Deficiency occurs when diets are lacking in whole grains, meat, yeast, potatoes, and peas, and severe deficiency causes the disease known as BERIBERI.

third age A popular euphemism in Commonwealth nations for the period of life that follows retirement, associated especially with new vocational choices, and entering or re-entering courses of study or educational programs at the community college or university level.

third party 1. A term used in the insurance industry to designate the insurance carrier, i.e., the organization or agency that pays for services rendered by health professionals for sick or injured persons. 2. The name for mandatory liability insurance required by licensed automobile drivers.

third world A term that originated in French (*tiers monde*) in the 1950s to distinguish the low-income, nonaligned nations of Africa, Latin America, and south Asia from those aligned either with the Western democracies or with the Soviet bloc and communist China. The collapse of the Soviet Union and the end of the Cold War made this term obsolete.

thorium (Th) Radioactive metallic element with several isotopes, one with a half-life of 1.39×10^{10} years. Thorium as Th_{232} is used in NUCLEAR REACTORS to "breed" fissile uranium 233.

thought experiment A method of investigation used mainly in physics and astronomy, famously by the German-Swiss-American theoretical physicist

Albert Einstein (1879–1955) to prove his theories of relativity. Thought experiments have been used in theoretical epidemiology, for example, by the British malariologist RONALD ROSS (1857–1932) in mathematical models of malaria epidemics.

Three by five (3×5) initiative The WHO global TARGET to provide three million people living with HIV/AIDS in low- and middle-income countries with life-prolonging antiretroviral treatment (ART) by the end of 2005. It is a step toward the GOAL of making universal access of HIV/AIDS prevention and treatment accessible for all who need them as a human right. Details are available at http://www.who.int/3by5/en/.

Three Mile Island A nuclear power plant near Harrisburg, Pennsylvania, where a nuclear accident in 1979 came close to causing a meltdown that could have had catastrophic consequences. The original problem was mechanical failure in the cooling system that led to overheating of the nuclear fuel. No one was injured or killed, but if the situation had progressed to cause nuclear fallout, a heavily populated region would have had to be evacuated and might have been rendered uninhabitable for decades or longer. Publicity surrounding this event deterred political decision makers in the United States from further investment in nuclear power plants.

threshold In communicable disease epidemics, the perceived incidence level at which action such as a public immunization program is taken to control the epidemic.

threshold dose The amount of a drug or other substance that induces a physiological or clinical reaction. At lower levels there is no perceptible reaction.

threshold limit value (TLV) The criteria for exposure levels to toxics set by the American Conference of Government Industrial Hygienists that superseded the older MAXIMUM ALLOWABLE CONCENTRATIONS (MACs), and have to a large extent been replaced by PERMISSIBLE EXPOSURE LIMITS (PELs).

thrifty phenotype hypothesis See BARKER HYPOTHESIS.

thrush A *Candida albicans* fungus infection of the mouth or vagina that causes white plaques and a painful inflammatory zone around each lesion. It is common in bottle-fed infants, debilitated elderly people, and anyone with a compromised immune system, as in HIV/AIDS. Infant thrush usually resolves without specific treatment. Antifungal mouthwash or lozenges relieve adults, but if the condition is a complication of HIV infection it tends to be indolent and to resist treatment.

thymine A heterocyclic pyrimidine compound, one of the four essential amino acids that comprise RNA, together with adenine, cytosine, and guanine.

thyroid The endocrine gland located in the neck embracing the larynx. It secretes thyroxine, the hormone that controls metabolism by increasing protein synthesis, raising the basal metabolic rate, and increasing heat production. The activity of the thyroid is controlled by thyroid-stimulating hormone, which is produced by the anterior lobe of the pituitary gland, and this in turn is at least partly influenced by neural impulses, including those associated with emotions. The thyroid gland and its function are sensitive to dietary iodine intake because iodine is required to synthesize thyroxine. IODINE DEFICIENCY leads to hypothyroidism and goiter.

thyroid cancer A highly malignant neoplasm that has a high incidence in populations exposed to radioactive iodine, e.g., populations in the fallout plume zone after the CHERNOBYL nuclear reactor disaster and, earlier, Hiroshima and Nagasaki atomic bomb survivors.

thyroid gland disorders Two common categories are cretinism and adult hypothyroidism, generally associated with IODINE DEFICIENCY, and thyrotoxicosis or hyperthyroidism, which may be secondary to pituitary or suprarenal gland dysfunction or a primary disease of the thyroid, which is an autoimmune disease characterized by abnormally high metabolic rate, fast pulse, often exophthalmos, menstrual irregularity or cessation, excitability, hyperactivity, and weight loss. This is a life-threatening disease formerly treated by surgical removal of much of the thyroid gland, now usually by medication, including sometimes radioactive iodine.

tick-borne diseases A miscellaneous group of communicable diseases that may be caused by viruses (encephalitis, hemorrhagic fever), rickettsia (typhus, Rocky Mountain spotted fever, Q fever), bacteria (Lyme disease, relapsing fever), and protozoa (babesiosis). Most tick-borne diseases are zoonoses, and they are transmitted to humans by ticks that primarily infest the animal host. Control measures vary. Some respond to elimination of ticks from animal hosts; others require ecological approaches to deal with the ticks' habitat. For further information, see http://www.cdc.gov/ncidod/diseases/list_tickborne.htm.

tick paralysis Certain varieties of hematophagous ticks remain attached to their mammalian host (animal or human) for prolonged periods, during which they become engorged with blood while they inject a neurotoxin that causes paralysis of peripheral muscles. The neurotoxin is powerful enough to kill domestic animals and children if the tick is undetected.

time-place cluster See CLUSTER.

Times Beach A small city in Missouri that was evacuated by order of the Environmental Protection Agency in 1983 after dangerous concentrations of dioxins were found in the soil, which, in order to reduce dust, had been sprayed with oil containing dioxins. This was one of several environmental and ecological disasters in the late 1970s and early 1980s that galvanized public opinion in the United States, leading to more stringent regulation of environmental hazards.

time series Any sequential measurements continued over a period that aim to reveal changing trends over time.

time-weighted average A unit of measurement used in industrial toxicology, signifying the environmental concentration of a toxic substance to which workers are exposed during a working day of designated duration, usually 8 hours.

tinea A group of fungus infections of the skin. Tinea pedis, or ATHLETE'S FOOT, is the most common; tinea capitis, or ringworm, occurs mainly on the scalp, occasionally elsewhere on the body or in the groin. Another variety of tinea causes chronic paronychia, infection of the bed of the fingernails.

tinnitus The sensation of a high-pitched noise in the ears, a common complaint associated with hearing loss among workers and others, e.g., music patrons exposed to loud noise.

tissue committee The name for the quality control and accountability committee that is required by American Hospital Association rules in all approved hospitals where surgical procedures are conducted. The preoperative and postoperative diagnoses and the number of nondiseased organs and tissues surgically removed as a proportion of all surgical procedures are indicators of the diagnostic acumen of individual surgeons. Similar committees exist for the same purpose in other upper-income nations with quality assurance rules and well-organized hospital services.

tissue culture Maintenance of living animal tissue in vitro, i.e., outside the body; a method of culture used to study physiological and pathological processes and to cultivate pathogenic organisms, especially viruses. Under some circumstances, live cells can be maintained and continue to divide indefinitely. Some vaccines can be prepared from tissue cultures.

Title III services 1. A range of medical and social services for Americans 60 years of age and older that are financially supported by the Older Americans Act. The services covered include meals, legal assistance, transport, homemaker services, health promotion and disease prevention, and medical care. 2. Provision of comprehensive primary care services to people living with HIV/AIDS under the Ryan White Act is also designated Title III; see http://hab.hrsa.gov/programs/factsheets/titleiii.htm.

Title IV This section of the US Social Security Act provides foster care for dependent children.

Title IX This section of the US Education Amendment Act of 1972 prohibits most forms of sex discrimination in education. One of its main consequences has been increases in funds for sports scholarships. Its effects on scholastic opportunities have been mixed.

Title VII This section of the US Civil Rights Act guarantees equal employment opportunities.

Title XIX This is the 1965 amendment to the US Social Security Act that established the federal Medicaid program, providing health care to indigent and medically indigent persons.

titration A method of analysis used mainly in chemistry and immunology. In chemistry, it consists of slowly mixing a reagent into a solution until an identifiable end point, such as a color change, occurs. The concentration or quantity of the reagent at this end point is the basis for calculating quantitative and/or qualitative characteristics of the solution under investigation. In immunology, similar methods are used to calculate antibody titer in serum.

TNM classification A classification system for defining the stages of malignant neoplasms that takes into account T, the tumor size; N, the presence or absence of cancerous regional lymph glands or nodes; and M, the presence and extent of metastases.

tobacco The broad-leaf plant that contains NICOTINE. The dried, cured leaves can be rolled into cigars or used to make pipe tobacco, cigarettes, snuff, or chewing tobacco. Because of its addictive ingredient, nicotine, tobacco is a lucrative cash crop and has been the basis for an expanding industry for several hundred years.

tobacco addiction A worldwide and extremely common addiction, often beginning in childhood. Skillful and often devious marketing strategies secure a steady supply of new child addicts to tobacco, even in jurisdictions where advertising is banned or tightly controlled; the subliminal or covert appeal is to the notion that smoking is a token of maturity and rebellion against oppressive adult parental authorities. Females seem to be more susceptible to addiction than males and usually have greater difficulty in weaning off the addiction should they attempt to quit smoking. Tobacco addiction causes many cancers and chronic disabling respiratory diseases.

tobacco control The multiple harmful effects of ingredients in tobacco smoke and of nicotine itself were not thoroughly investigated until the second half of the 20th century, by which time the transnational tobacco industry had become so rich, powerful, and politically influential that it has been able to fend off many lawsuits and tort claims brought against it, and to impede the passage of laws and regulations aimed at reducing the harm done by tobacco addiction. Tobacco control involves five steps: 1. Recognition that tobacco is a public health problem; 2. Understanding what causes the problem, i.e., subtle social, cultural, and emotional pressures, plus pharmacological addiction; 3. Capability to deal with the causes; 4. The belief (sense of values) that the problem is important and worth solving; and 5. Political will. (These five steps are required to solve all public health problems.) In 2003, the World Health Assembly reached agreement among member states of the WHO to approve the FRAMEWORK CONVENTION ON TOBACCO CONTROL (FCTC), which embodies part of all these five steps. The final step, however, may be difficult to implement.

tobacco industry A huge, lucrative, transnational industry with annual gross revenues greater than those of many nation states. The wealth of the tobacco industry derives from the addictive property of NICOTINE, and the wealth confers political influence. Most national governments extract substantial tax revenues from the tobacco industry, so they have had little or no interest in restricting sales. This began to change in some industrial nations toward the end of the 20th century, when the harmful properties of tobacco smoking became widely known. The tobacco industry reacted with aggressive marketing strategies that targeted women, children, and people in developing countries. Tobacco companies also diversified, buying corporations in other sectors of the economy. Member states of the United Nations ratified the FRAMEWORK CONVENTION ON TOBACCO CONTROL (FCTC) at the World Health Assembly in 2003.

tocopherol See VITAMIN E.

toddler A descriptive term loosely age-related, describing a small child who is in the process of learning to walk, i.e., in the age range of about 9 to 18 months. The popular media often describe children aged 1 to 2 years as toddlers, and some pediatricians set a lower age range. It is a variable and vague period of early childhood, and because of the variability the term is preferably avoided.

tolerable daily limit The estimated amount of a substance to which workers and others can be exposed on a day-to-day basis without experiencing any harmful effects. This is a loose standard with no legally binding force.

tolerance 1. In instrumentation, the limit of allowable error. 2. In immunology, ability to accept antigenic stimuli without adverse reaction. 3. In pharmacology and therapeutics, the increasing dose of a drug required with repeated use to induce the same effect. 4. In sociology, the ability to remain equable and comfortable with individuals and groups whose beliefs and behavior are alien or different in ways that can provoke hostile reactions.

toluene Methyl benzene, a colorless, volatile, liquid solvent with many important industrial uses. It is a mucous membrane irritant and a neurotoxin. Its fumes are intoxicating and narcotic, so it is among substances used illicitly by solvent-sniffers.

tomography A collective name for several diagnostic imaging methods and procedures with which it is possible to construct a three-dimensional image of internal organs. It may use either ultrasound or radiation. The technique consists of rotating a radiation detector around the patient so the image gives three-dimensional information. In plain film tomography, the source of x-rays and the photographic film move around the patient to produce an image of structures at a particular depth within the body, bringing them into sharp focus, leaving structures above and below them out of focus. Computerized tomography produces an image of a slice through the body at a particular level. Tomography exposes patients and technicians who operate the equipment to ionizing radiation, but modern radiation protective measures ensure that the risks are minimized, and the benefits of diagnostic accuracy are considerable.

tonne The SI unit of mass. One tonne equals 1,000 kilograms.

topsoil The uppermost biologically active layer of the lithosphere, comprising earth with a high content of organic matter. Most important to agriculture, some of this is relevant to health, e.g., because of the presence of antibiotic-producing fungi, pathogens, cysts, and eggs of parasites.

tornado An extremely violent and powerful wind storm in which a rotating column of air forms between a low cumulonimbus cloud and the land below, generating wind speeds of 300 km/hour or more with powerful updrafts. It characteristically occurs in the South and Midwest of the United States. The destructive high winds can do great damage, usually over a narrow path.

tort An injury or wrong; or the breach of a duty imposed by law that leads to injury or wrong. A toxic tort is a breach of the law relating to occupational or environmental exposure to toxins. Tort lawsuits often arise in occupational and environmental health problems and not infrequently as a consequence of mishaps in health care, including some in public health services.

torture Deliberate, systematic infliction of physical and/or psychological stimuli causing pain, prolonged sleep deprivation, or profound emotional distress, with the intention of extracting information, forcing a confession, or transforming a political viewpoint, or just to humiliate and degrade the victim who differs from the torturer(s) in a meaningful way, such as in race, religion, or political beliefs. Torture has been a feature of human societies throughout history, and despite United Nations resolutions and declarations it continues to be widely used. In some countries, it has been and still is practiced at a communal level, as part of a process of ETHNIC CLEANSING, with the aim of driving an unwanted minority away from their homes and habitat. At this level, it becomes a public health problem. Its consequences usually include permanent physical and psychological damage to the victims

total fertility rate The average number of children a woman would bear if all women live to the end of their childbearing years and have children according to a given set of age-specific fertility rates. It is the sum of age-specific fertility rates multiplied by the number of years in each age interval, typically 5.

total suspended particulate matter (TSP) All the solid and aerosol substances that are small enough and light enough to remain suspended in still air, including dust, fumes, smoke, droplets, particles of inorganic and organic compounds, plant spores, pollen, etc.

Townsend score An index of the social and economic deprivation of a locality, such as an administratively defined region in a city. It is based on the composite score for four proportions: unemployed residents older than 16 years, as a percentage of all economically active residents aged older than 16 years; proportion of households in the area with 1 person per room and over; proportion of households with no car; and proportion of households not owning their own home. It is used in the census and in population surveys in the United Kingdom. It was developed by the British sociologist Peter Townsend (b. 1929). The Townsend score is considered the best indicator of material deprivation currently available.

toxicant A toxic substance introduced into the environment, such as a pesticide. A substance that causes poisoning typically of a pest or unwanted species but that may harm other species, including humans.

toxicity testing A procedure for assessing the safety of chemicals, especially newly developed chemical compounds, that should be mandatory for all, but because there are so many new chemical compounds, those that are chemically closely related to existing compounds known to be safe are often allowed into commercial production and use without formal toxicity tests. The aim is to ensure there are no significant toxic hazards, and ideally that there are no risks of carcinogenesis, teratogenesis, or mutagenesis. In real terms, however, evidence of these possible hazards may come only after the fact, as has happened, e.g., with THALIDOMIDE.

toxic oil syndrome An apparently unique foodborne epidemic that occurred in Spain in 1981 and was traced to a contaminated batch of cooking oil. The nature of the contamination was never precisely identified, but it may have been an aniline derivative that was inadvertently used to adulterate olive oil that had been diluted with rapeseed oil. The symptoms were respiratory, gastrointestinal, renal, and neurological. Several hundred people ultimately died of the 20,000 originally affected.

toxicology The study of the toxic effects of chemicals, such as environmental contaminants, drugs, and atmospheric or water pollutants. This is an important specialty in environmental health.

toxic shock syndrome An acute, life-threatening, reaction to staphylococcal enterotoxin (more than 50% case fatality rate) caused by enterotoxin absorbed from vaginal tampons. There was an epidemic of this condition after the commercial release of superabsorbent vaginal tampons that could be retained for many hours; unfortunately, they were a favorable culture medium for staphylococci and other potential pathogens.

toxic tort A legal claim for damages due to injury or other harm resulting from exposure to environmental toxin(s) or adverse toxic effects of a pharmaceutical preparation.

toxic waste Industrial, commercial, domestic, and hospital solid or liquid waste that is itself toxic or contains toxic substances. There is such a wide variety that simple classification is impossible. It consists of or includes heavy metal compounds, e.g., lead or mercury, other metallic compounds; arsenicals; petrochemicals and their by-products, including carcinogens; corrosive substances; and many other varieties of poisonous substances.

toxic waste disposal A complex challenge because many varieties of toxins are produced as industrial by-products. They include volatile and nonvolatile liquids; organic and other dusts; solids; corrosives; metabolic, neurological, hepatic, renal, gonadal, and other organ-specific poisons; and mixtures of several varieties. Disposal methods include recycling and recovery of useful ingredients; incineration; storage in ponds, landfill sites, disused mine shafts, etc.; dumping at sea; exporting to low-income countries; and illegal dumping. Some methods merely postpone the problem for future generations to deal with, as with radioactive waste disposal. Toxic waste disposal is one of the great unsolved problems of industrial civilization. See also BROWNFIELDS.

toxin A poisonous substance, biological or metabolic product, or medicinal compound of biological origin. It may be an antigenic poison or venom of plant or animal origin or produced by or derived from microorganisms. Toxins may cause disease, even when present at low concentration in the body.

TOXLINE This is a searchable data base of publications on toxicology maintained by the US National Library of Medicine. This and TOXNET, a searchable data base of information about toxic substances, are accessible through the National Library of Medicine Web site, i.e., http://*www.nih .nlm.gov/toxline* and http://*www.nih.nlm.gov/ toxnet*. These Web sites can provide answers to many inquiries that local public health staff receive from worried citizens.

toxocariasis Syn: visceral larva migrans. An infection of tissues and organs by the larval stage of *Toxocara canis*, a parasitic helminth of dogs, usually affecting children who ingest the eggs.

toxoid A bacterial or other toxin that has been treated with formaldehyde to reduce its toxicity without reducing its antigenic property. Diphtheria vaccine and tetanus vaccine are prepared from toxoids.

toxoplasmosis A systemic zoonotic infection of mammals and birds caused by the protozoan *Toxoplasma gondii*, transmitted to humans in cat feces or poorly cooked meat. It may be latent or asymptomatic, but it usually causes a mild influenza-like illness with lymphadenopathy that can be serious in immunocompromised persons. Infection during pregnancy can cause congenital toxoplasmosis, and although most infants are unaffected or have very mild disease, stillbirth, severe malformations of the skull and eyes, or active infection in the liver can occur. Infection can be detected by serology, and pregnant women can be treated with antibiotics such as spiramycin. See http://www.cdc .gov/ncidod/dpd/parasites/toxoplasmosis/factsht_ toxoplasmosis.htm.

trace elements Elements or their compounds that are present in trace amounts, i.e., amounts that are usually measured in parts per million or parts per billion. Several have an essential biological effect. An example is sodium fluoride, which is present in trace amounts in some natural sources of drinking water, and provides essential strengthening to dental enamel.

tracer A slang or jargon term for a substance or phenomenon that indicates what is happening and how a process works. A "tracer condition" is one that is easily diagnosed and that indicates by its prevalence a significant way in which the health care system is performing. For instance, a high prevalence of uncorrected refractive error indicates inadequate optometry or ophthalmic services. A tracer substance may be used in many ways, for instance, fluorescein dye is used as a tracer to detect possible seepage from sewer pipes to water-supply pipes.

trachoma An acute or insidious chronic conjunctival infection caused by *Chlamydia trachomatis* that if untreated causes severe ocular damage, often blindness. It is transmitted by flies or infected mucus secretions from the eyes or nose of infected children by direct contact. It is endemic in arid parts of the world, especially among children for whom hygiene is poor. For more information, see http://www.who.int/water_sanitation_health/ diseases/trachoma/en/.

trade secret Copyright and patent laws permit keeping secret the details about many industrial processes, ingredients, and composition of industrial products, often even when occupationally related disease occurs as a result of exposure to toxic substances used in these processes. This can lead to an adversarial relationship between regulators and industrialists, requiring resolution in a court of law or by enacting specific legislation.

trade union An organized group of workers in a particular occupation or group of occupations that uses its collective power to negotiate with employers for improved working conditions. Reduction or preferably elimination of occupational health hazards has always had a high priority on the agenda of most trade unions.

tradition One of the fundamental features of a culture that is part of the collective memory or unwritten history of a definable community, social group, or nation; it often has implications for human health. For example, several traditions and customs associated with childbirth can be harmful or dangerous to infant or mother or both, including traditional methods of severing the umbilical cord (crushing between stones); swaddling (tightly constricting the infant in sheets); and, in Western industrial nations, confining women in bed for prolonged periods after childbirth, risking thromboembolic and other complications.

traditional birth attendant (TBA) Usually, a rural village woman in a low-income country, trained by apprenticeship or self-taught by experience and observation, seldom acquainted with basic principles of hygiene and sanitation, and often associated with high maternal and neonatal morbidity and mortality rates. In countries where this system prevails, the WHO has encouraged the provision of simple training and education for traditional birth attendants, but the effectiveness of this training is a matter of controversy. Formal comprehensive training of TBAs is a preferable approach.

traditional medicine Systems of medical practice, such as the use of local herbal remedies, that have survived for many centuries. Many originated in preliterate societies in which knowledge about effective ways to treat and sometimes to prevent disease were transmitted by word of mouth from older to selected younger members of the cultural group. Two widely used forms are AYURVEDIC MEDICINE and Chinese traditional medicine, including acupuncture. Both of these are organized professionally and have acquired some modern features. Traditional medicine systems are a mixture of common sense, remedies empirically demonstrated to work, and other approaches to healing that may in some respects be very effective, but in others no more effective than BLACK MAGIC or WITCHCRAFT.

traffic crash Syn: motor vehicle accident (MVA). The term preferred by some purists who dislike using the word "accident," which implies an unavoidable and unpredictable event, whereas epidemiological and other evidence shows that many traffic crashes are predictable, caused by factors that can be classified in terms of the epidemiological triad of host, agent, and environment. Host factors include risk taking; excessive speed; and impairment of judgment by alcohol, drugs, or disease. Agent factors include faulty vehicles with defective brakes or steering or other malfunction. Environmental factors include unsafe road conditions, poor grading, insufficient visibility, and the like.

tranquilizers Pharmaceuticals that act as sedatives and mood modifiers that can be used to treat a range of psychological problems, including common neuroses, behavior disturbances, insomnia, and phobia. These are mainly chronic and not life-threatening conditions. Benzodiazepines are a popular variety. One problem is that many psychological disorders treated with tranquilizers are chronic, even lifelong, and some tranquilizers have long-term adverse effects.

transborder pollution The situation that arises when polluting atmospheric emissions or toxic effluent discharged into waterways cross the border between nations or jurisdictional regions. The problem this presents depends on the existence and efficacy of political agreements on the two sides of the border. It was sometimes extremely difficult to deal with when former Soviet bloc nations were responsible for causing the pollution, and remains difficult among some jurisdictions in Europe, Asia, and the Americas.

transcendental meditation A system of meditation popularized in the 1950s by an Indian mystic, Maharishi Yogi, that consists of deep breathing, attempting to rid the mind of conscious thoughts, and repetition of a mantra for 10- to 20-minute sessions. It is claimed to enhance mental and physical well-being and may help to lower blood pressure in some cases of moderate to severe hypertension.

transcription The process of copying DNA strands to RNA that occurs in cell division. This occurs by polymerization of ribonucleotides into a strand of RNA in a sequence complementary to that of a single strand of DNA. By this means, the genetic information is matched. The process is mediated by a DNA-dependent RNA polymerase.

transdisciplinarity A logical philosophical method of studying complex problems that rejects the reductionist approach of conventional scientific method in favor of integrating ideas from diverse scholarly fields in order to deal with the inherent complexity of some urgent problems of the present human situation. The aim is to evolve a conceptual framework that embraces and seeks to mobilize ideas from every pertinent scientific and scholarly discipline: physical, biological, social, and behavioral sciences; economics; politics; and the humanities. Many problems in public health benefit from the transdisciplinary approach. Examples include urban housing; social integration and health promotion in ethnically diverse communities; regional and urban transport; pollution control; global ecosystem change; and the causes and control of chronic, low-intensity violent armed ethnic conflicts.

trans fats, trans fatty acids The collective name for a group of synthetic fats produced by hydrogenating vegetable oils. So-called FAST FOOD and JUNK FOOD may have high concentrations of trans fats. Modern technologies have succeeded in greatly lowering the concentration of trans fatty acids used in the manufacture of margarine. Trans fats are particularly prone to aggravate arterial degenerative changes. Useful information including trans fat content of common foods is available at http://www.fda.gov/fdac/features/2003/503_fats.html.

transference The psychoanalytic concept of transfer of bonds of affection or hostility from a parent to a therapist with whom an emotionally disturbed individual has a long-term therapeutic relationship. This phenomenon in psychotherapy can also occur in social work.

transfusion Intravenous infusion of fluid, electrolytes, and usually blood corpuscles into a recipient who needs some or all of these ingredients because injury, shock, or illness have caused a deficiency. The word "transfusion" unqualified usually refers to a blood transfusion. Other kinds include emergency on-site transfusion of fluid and electrolytes at the scene of serious accidents, in battlefield conditions, etc. Blood must be correctly matched and typed to minimize, and preferably avoid, the risk of transfusion reactions. Transfusion of mismatched blood can be fatal or induce extremely serious hemolysis, e.g., with damage to the renal system.

transgenerational effects The effect on the next generation—or possibly several subsequent generations—of pharmaceutical or illicit drugs, ionizing radiation, or environmental exposure to toxic substances. This may be expressed in several ways, for instance, as chromosomal abnormalities and premature sexual maturation in children born to mothers exposed to diagnostic doses of ionized radiation in early pregnancy, or malformations of the genital tract in the offspring of women who took diethylstilboestrol in early pregnancy. It is too soon to know how many subsequent generations may be affected.

transgenic organism An organism, such as a mouse, that has a genome that incorporates and expresses genes from another species, created by genetic engineering. This is done by inserting the foreign gene into the fertilized egg or early embryo of the host. Transgenic organisms have important potential medical application, although ethical implications of this technology are quite troubling for many people. They also have considerable commercial potential.

transient ischemic attack An acute episode of neurological disruption, such as hemiplegia, presumably caused by disruption of blood supply to part of the brain, that lasts less than 24 hours. Symptoms lasting longer than 24 hours meet the clinical definition of a stroke.

transition states Nations in transition from totalitarian rule, mainly under the aegis of the former USSR, to liberal democracy. Many such nations have had unfavorable mortality trends since the late 1980s: the trends for premature mortality among males have been among the least favorable in the world. In Russia in the late 1990s, there were 2.5 million excess male deaths compared with the already elevated rates of 1991. Cardiovascular disease and violence were the largest contributors to excess mortality. There was a widespread failure to develop effective control programs for chronic diseases and for injury and violence, often associated with excessive alcohol use.

translocation An intranuclear biological process whereby part or all of a chromosome with its genes detaches from its position and attaches to another chromosome or to a different position on the same chromosome. Either form of translocation can result in a mutation of the phenotype.

transmissible spongiform encephalopathy A class of relentlessly progressive degenerative neurological diseases, including kuru, classical and variant CREUTZFELDT-JAKOB DISEASE of humans, scrapie in sheep, and BOVINE SPONGIFORM ENCEPHALOPATHY (mad cow disease) in cattle. All are transmitted by PRIONS, or infectious proteinaceous particles, formerly thought to be slow viruses. The pathogenesis of these conditions is obscure, but a possible course of events is that ingested pathogenic prions activate pathological changes in host neurological tissue. It remains uncertain whether prions should be considered to be living organisms or, more likely, nonliving protein that is capable of replication in the body under appropriate circumstances. Information is available at http://www.ninds.nih.gov/disorders/tse/tse.htm.

transmission of infection Infectious agents can be transmitted to susceptible hosts in any of several ways: Direct transmission occurs person to person by intimate contact, such as with sexually transmitted diseases or by DROPLET spread or by way of FOMITES. Indirect transmission by means of a

COMMON VEHICLE, such as water-borne, food-borne, or air-borne spread, or via contaminated blood or blood products, can lead to infection of many people remote from the original source; VECTOR-borne infection is most usually by way of insect vectors. Other routes include infection transmitted to susceptible human hosts from an animal that may or may not have overt evidence of a zoonosis, and direct transmission from an environmental source, such as tetanus spores, which enter directly from the soil or other nonliving source.

transpiration That part of the hydrological cycle in which water passes from vegetation to the atmosphere by metabolic action of sunlight on the green leaves of plants in which carbon dioxide is absorbed and oxygen and water vapor are released.

trauma service Syn: accident and emergency service, casualty service. A specialized emergency medical service (EMS) equipped with specialized ambulances and paramedical personnel trained in all aspects of emergency care, including provision for on-site intravenous infusions, etc.

traveler's diarrhea Syn: Montezuma's revenge, turista, gippy tummy, Delhi belly, etc. A general term for any of several forms of malaise with loose stools that commonly afflict persons during their travels, usually caused by enterotoxigenic *Escherichia coli*, sometimes by NOROVIRUS or more serious pathogenic organisms, such as shigella dysentery, sometimes merely by unfamiliar diets.

travel medicine Syn: EMPORIATRICS. The branch of medical practice concerned with prevention, diagnosis, and treatment of diseases associated with travel. This includes protecting people from diseases that occur in their region of destination that are not encountered in their home country and identifying and treating diseases imported by returning travelers.

treadmill exercise test A method of assessing cardiovascular fitness and vital capacity by measuring and recording heart rate, blood pressure, electrocardiographic changes, etc., during periods of standardized exercise on a treadmill.

tremor Involuntary muscle movement, affecting in particular the small muscles of the hands and sometimes other parts of the body, e.g., facial muscles, occurring as a consequence of disruption of neuromuscular coordination, neurological disease, etc.

trench fever Syn: quintana fever. An obsolete term for a disease that is now rare, resembling typhoid, caused by *Bartonella quintana* with the body louse as vector. Cases have been reported among persons with AIDS and among destitute urban homeless people.

trench foot See IMMERSION SYNDROME.

trend A series of measurements in which variables show a pattern of increasing or decreasing magnitude over time; when they are plotted on a graph, a trend line is perceptible.

triage A process originally developed during wartime conditions for rapid sorting of injured and ill patients into groups comprising those for whom immediate emergency treatment offers only slim or no hope of survival, who are given symptomatic treatment only; others for whom immediate critical care services offer a reasonable chance of survival; and those who can wait a while for treatment because their condition is less serious. The primary aim of triage is to identify persons in the middle group who can be expected to survive if given immediate care.

tributyl compounds These compounds, e.g., tributyl tin, are used as marine antifouling agents. They are toxic and irritant in undiluted form and pollute the marine environment.

trichinosis Syn: trichinellosis. Infection with the parasitic roundworm *Trichinella spiralis*, which usually passes the adult stage of its life cycle in rats or swine. Humans are infected by eating undercooked or raw meat containing encysted larvae, which migrate to many tissues and organs, including the brain, heart, etc., and can cause serious disease. A fact sheet is available at http://www.cdc.gov/ncidod/dpd/parasites/trichinosis/factsht_trichinosis.htm.

trichloroethylene A volatile organic solvent and a central nervous system depressant that induces loss of consciousness when inhaled.

trichomoniasis A protozoan infection of the female genital tract that causes offensive vaginal discharge and (rarely) urethral discharge in infected men. It is a common disease that is usually sexually transmitted, but it may be introduced into the vagina by poor personal hygiene and exposure to vaginal discharge of another woman, for instance, from moisture on a lavatory seat.

trichuriasis Intestinal infection with the whipworm parasite, *Trichuris trichiura*.

triglycerides Syn: triglycerols. A neutral compound of three fatty acids, commonly stearic, oleic, and palmitic acids, an energy store of adipose (fat) cells in animal and human bodies, which metabolize to glycogen and glucose for release as energy. Triglycerides are a major component of most Western diets, and high dietary intake is responsible for much obesity, non-insulin-dependent diabetes, and coronary heart disease. A useful fact sheet produced by the American Heart Association is available at http://www.americanheart.org/presenter.jhtml?identifier=4778.

trihalomethanes A class of organic chemical compounds that include chloroform and several chlorine plus bromine compounds, most of which have cumulative toxic properties if ingested in small quantities over prolonged periods. Some are metabolic breakdown products of organic matter in drinking water that has been chlorinated to kill pathogens. Long-term ingestion of chlorinated drinking water with high trihalomethane concentration is a suspected cancer risk.

trinitrotoluene (TNT) An explosive compound of toluene discovered by the Swedish chemist Alfred Nobel (1833–1896) and used in dynamite and other explosives. Because it is a powerful vasodilator, it is used to relieve angina pectoris. Workers exposed over long periods have a high prevalence of chronic cardiovascular disease and hypertension.

triple-blind study A DOUBLE-BLIND STUDY in which, as well as withholding information from study subjects and investigators, the statistician performing statistical analysis of the results is not informed about which subjects were in the control group, or the expected results of the analysis.

trisomy The presence of an additional chromosome, as well as the normal two, in all somatic cells that is believed always to be associated with congenital abnormalities. Several chromosome disorders are due to trisomy, including DOWN SYNDROME and Klinefelter's syndrome. Trisomy 21 is the chromosome abnormality of Down syndrome.

tropism Movement of part or all of an organism in response to a stimulus, such as exposure to sunlight (phototropism). Movement of spermatozoa up the vagina and through the cervix is a response to the stimulus of a chemical tropism.

troposphere The layer of the atmosphere between the earth's surface and the STRATOSPHERE.

trypanosomiasis A disease caused by parasitic protozoa of the genus *Trypanosoma*. The two most important such diseases are CHAGAS DISEASE (South American trypanosomiasis) and African trypanosomiasis, or sleeping sickness. This is transmitted by the TSETSE FLY, and is confined to ecosystems in equatorial central and east Africa, where these flies flourish. It affects domestic and wild animals and humans, in whom it causes a progressively debilitating disease that terminates in coma and death

unless treated. For further information, see http://www.who.int/tdr/diseases/tryp/default.htm.

tryptophan One of the essential amino acids. It is the precursor of the neurotransmitter serotonin and of niacin. Average dietary intakes of tryptophan in dairy products, legumes, and other protein-rich foods are more than adequate to meet niacin requirements, without the need for additional niacin in the diet.

TSE See TRANSMISSIBLE SPONGIFORM ENCEPHALOPATHY.

tsetse fly Any of six varieties of *Glossina*, a blood-feeding blackfly indigenous to parts of tropical central Africa. This is the vector for African trypanosomiasis, commonly called sleeping sickness and also a major cattle disease.

tsunami A pressure or shock wave that travels at up to 400 km/hour in the ocean, caused by an undersea earthquake, subsidence, coastal landslide, or volcanic activity, producing a wave or series of waves as great as 10 meters high. Tsunamis cause sudden change, often a precipitous drop followed by an increase, wrongly called a tidal wave, in sea level along a shelving coast. This inundates land near the coast and, in heavily populated areas, there may be great loss of life. On December 26, 2004, shifting TECTONIC PLATES near Sumatra caused an undersea earthquake with a magnitude of 9.5 on the RICHTER SCALE that generated a tsunami responsible for about 300,000 deaths, the largest natural disaster of modern times.

t **test** See STUDENT'S *T* TEST.

tubal ligation A method of sterilization of women to prevent pregnancies, consisting of excision of a segment of the fallopian tubes and ligating the cut ends in order to prevent the passage of ova to the uterus.

tuberculin test A skin test for the presence of antibodies to tuberculosis. See MANTOUX TEST.

tuberculosis Syn: TB. A ubiquitous bacterial disease since prehistorical times, caused by *Mycobacterium tuberculosis*. An estimated one-third of the world's population is infected with TB, but only a small proportion have active disease, most commonly of the lungs although other organs may be affected. Many who have good nutrition and immune defenses readily overcome their primary infection. Those who develop progressive pulmonary tuberculosis are predominantly at the lowest income level, often undernourished and living in crowded conditions that encourage spread. Increasingly, those with progressive disease are persons with compromised immune systems because of HIV disease. The TUBERCULIN test for the presence of infection is unreliable when the immune system is compromised. Tuberculosis is a major global public health problem. The spread of severe poverty in low- and middle-income countries and of homelessness and destitution in affluent nations, as well as proliferation of resistant organisms, has led to the re-emergence of tuberculosis as a serious problem for world health. For more information, see http://www.cdc.gov/nchstp/tb/faqs/qa.htm and http://www.who.int/tb/en/.

tularemia A zoonosis caused by *Francisella tularensis* that occurs in rabbits and similar animals in western North America and is transmitted by ticks to humans. It causes a disease that, in its severe form, somewhat resembles plague.

twin studies Research by geneticists, epidemiologists, behavioral scientists, and child development specialists that focuses on twins, especially identical twins, seeking to examine similarities and differences attributable to genetic and environmental factors. For instance, identical twins may be mirror images of each other, or collateral "carbon copies," both right-handed with fingerprint whorls, hair parting, etc., running in the same direction, and personality tests may reveal similar or opposite tendencies. A popular field of study has been of identical twins reared apart, seeking evidence of the impact of environmental, social, and behavioral differences on mental health. Many intriguing results have emerged, for example, about unexplainable concordance of emotions and responses to stress and other stimuli that seems to persist throughout life.

2,4,5-T 2,4,5-Trichlorophenoxyacetic acid, a chlorophenoxy broad-leaf herbicide used to kill weed trees in commercial softwood pine forests and as a domestic weed killer. It is a suspected carcinogen and teratogen and a risk factor for lymphoma. It was one of the active ingredients of the herbicide AGENT ORANGE (the other was 2,4-D). It is banned in the European Union.

two-tail test A statistical test, e.g., chi square test, that examines both ends of a frequency distribution.

2,3,7,8-TCDD 2,3,7,8-Tetrachlorodibenzodioxin, a member of the family of DIOXIN compounds that was a contaminant in a broad-leaf herbicide used to kill weed trees, and as AGENT ORANGE, used in massive quantities by the US forces in Vietnam in the late 1960s and early 1970s. It is a carcinogen, a mutagen, and a teratogen. Its manufacture and use ceased in the late 1970s, but the delayed after effects, notably malignant disease, continued to occur for several decades.

two-tier system A health care system in which publicly funded and privately financed services exist side by side (or one above the other, implicitly the private system superior to the public one).

type I error Syn: alpha error. The error of wrongly rejecting a true null hypothesis, i.e., declaring that there is a significant difference when in reality there is not.

type II error Syn: beta error. The error of not rejecting the null hypothesis, i.e., declaring that a difference does not exist between sets of data when in fact a difference does exist.

type A behavior, type B behavior In 1959 two American cardiologists, Meyer Friedman (1910–2001) and Ray H. Rosenman (b. 1920) described personality profiles they designated type A and type B, associated, respectively, with high and low risk of coronary heart disease. The type A personality profile is characterized by ambition, competitive drive, impatience, aggressive tendencies, and argumentative conversational style. The person with type B personality is more patient and reflective, listens carefully, and decides without hurrying. Much work has been done on the relationship of these personality types to cardiovascular and other diseases, risk of accidents, and other correlates. Although the findings are somewhat inconsistent, there does appear to be a weak association of personality to the risk of getting or dying of certain diseases, including coronary heart disease.

typhoid Syn: enteric fever. A serious systemic disease usually transmitted by the fecal-oral route or by water or food contaminated with the causative pathogen *Salmonella typhi* or one of its relatives. It was formerly common, but sanitation and safe drinking water supplies have virtually eliminated it in modern urban settings, although occasional imported cases and small epidemics still occur. The symptoms include fever to 39°C to 40°C, slow pulse rate, loss of appetite, diarrhea, stomach pains, and a distinctive rash. Diagnosis is made by blood or stool culture and the WIDAL TEST for salmonella antibodies. Typhoid formerly had a case fatality rate of 10% to 20% but responds well to antibiotics, such as ampicillin and ciprofloxacin. An asymptomatic carrier state follows recovery in about 5% of cases. Vaccines for typhoid and paratyphoid are recommended for travelers to regions where the disease is common. For more information, see http://www.cdc.gov/ncidod/dbmd/diseaseinfo/typhoidfever_g.htm.

Typhoid Mary The original Typhoid Mary was Mary Mallon (c. 1870–1938), an itinerant Irish immigrant cook who infected at least 22 people with typhoid in New York in 1900 to 1907, was identified as a typhoid carrier, and incarcerated in a quarantine hospital. After she was released, she obtained work as a cook in a maternity hospital, where she infected an additional 25 people, 2 of whom died. She was seized again and spent the rest of her life imprisoned in quarantine. Her plight as an unwitting and, in her eyes, innocent agent of a deadly disease has inspired several poems and novels. The term "Typhoid Mary" is occasionally used to describe anyone who unwittingly transmits infection to others.

typhus fever Syn: epidemic louse-borne typhus. A serious epidemic disease caused by *Rickettsia prowazekii*, transmitted by the body louse. It has a high mortality rate if untreated. Typically, it is associated with dirty, verminous clothing and overcrowding, as in campaigning armies, prisons, and concentration camps, such as in World War II. In 1944, an impending serious epidemic in Naples was controlled by treating the entire population with DDT powder to kill body lice.

U

UHT Acronym for ultra-high temperature, a method to pasteurize milk and dairy products, often used for the small containers of milk and coffee creamer in restaurants and hotel rooms.

UICC Union Internationale Contre le Cancer, French for International Union Against Cancer, an international private voluntary organization with headquarters in Paris, that raises funds and sponsors research and treatment of cancer.

UK Public Health Association The British organization for public health professionals. It is a professional association that holds scientific meetings, publishes a journal and newsletter for its members, advises the British government, is an advocacy group, and liaises with the EUROPEAN PUBLIC HEALTH ASSOCIATION. See http://www.ukpha .org.uk/ for details.

ultrasonography A method of imaging that depends on differential reflection of ULTRASOUND waves by tissues and organs of varying density. It is used mainly in obstetrics to detect fetal abnormalities and to outline the configuration of the early developing fetus. Enough detail can be discerned by 12 weeks' gestation to determine the sex of the fetus and to detect gross structural anomalies. It can also detect and delineate renal calculi, gallstones, and some abdominal cysts and tumors.

ultraviolet radiation Electromagnetic radiation with a wavelength just too short to be visible. Solar ultraviolet radiation has three defined wavelengths designated UVA, UVB, and UVC. The UVC wavelength, of 200 to 290 nm, is the most biologically active, but it is blocked by stratospheric ozone, and little or none of this wavelength reaches the earth's surface; UV-B, with a wavelength of 290 to 320 nm, penetrates to the earth's surface in amounts inversely proportional to the concentration of atmos-

pheric ozone, which is formed by the action of UV radiation on oxygen; and UVA, with a wavelength of 320 to 400 nm, penetrates the stratospheric ozone layer and reaches the earth's surface, where its main effect on humans is to cause erythema and tanning of fair-skinned people. UV radiation can be lethal for microorganisms, protozoa, etc. Excessive or repeated exposure to UV radiation impairs immune responses, increases the risk of cataract development, and induces malignant changes in the skin, i.e., squamous and basal cell carcinoma and malignant melanoma. Useful information about measuring and monitoring UV radiation flux in the United States is available at http://www.arl.noaa .gov/research/programs/uv.html. Global information is available at http://www.srrb.noaa.gov/UV/ http:// www.unep.org.

umbilical cord The blood vessels—a vein and two arteries—enclosed in a mucous-epithelial sheath, responsible for carrying oxygen and nourishment from mother to fetus and carbon dioxide and metabolic waste products from the fetus back to the mother via the PLACENTA. It is severed after birth, and the stump shrivels, leaving a scar, the navel. Poor hygiene in cutting the umbilical cord can allow anaerobic tetanus spores to gain entry to the ischemic stump of the cord, causing neonatal tetanus, a common cause of early neonatal death in low-income countries.

UNAIDS See JOINT UNITED NATIONS PROGRAMME ON HIV/AIDS.

UNCED United Nations Conference on Environment and Development, a landmark conference in Rio de Janeiro, Brazil, in 1992, at which the RIO DECLARATION on sustainable development was approved. This led to the KYOTO PROTOCOL on reduction of carbon emissions.s Information is available at http://www.ciesin.org/TG/PI/TREATY/ unced.html.

uncertainty A reality in public health planning and practice is unreliable information, leading to estimates based on flawed and invalid assumptions, and only partially predictable or unpredictable future trends. An approach being used by the WHO and other agencies is to make the best possible estimates and quantify the level of uncertainty using analytic methods similar to Bayesian statistics.

uncertainty analysis A form of analysis that recognizes and attempts to quantify the effects of several kinds of error and uncertainty that might affect the applicability of study findings to a specific public health problem in a specified population and setting. These could include random and systematic errors in studies used to predict effects, and uncertainty about exposure levels in the population of interest. Software programs that sample from and propagate uncertainty distributions increase the feasibility of uncertainty analysis.

UNCSD The United Nations Conference on Sustainable Development, renamed before it took place in 2002 in Johannesburg as the WORLD SUMMIT ON SUSTAINABLE DEVELOPMENT (WSSD).

underachiever A term for a person, often in the middle level of the educational system, who according to intelligence tests or other indicators should be capable of doing better than the examination results actually show. Similar criteria are used to label underachievers at later stages of life. The situation is sometimes explained by physical, emotional, or mental disorder and/or by social or cultural circumstances. It merits investigation and intervention when there is a significant level of underachievement.

underclass Persons at the lowest level of the socioeconomic pyramid in industrial nations, comprising the unemployed, working poor, and persons in low-paid, temporary, and part-time work, often only marginally connected to the mainstream of society, lacking power and influence, and sometimes experiencing intractable mental and physical health problems. This is a common situation among high proportions of indigenous people who remain at a perpetual social and economic disadvantage in some countries. The underclass may also include high proportions of illegal immigrants and "guest workers," who have had no prior health screening and may harbor communicable diseases, including tuberculosis and intestinal parasites.

under 5 mortality rate The estimated probability of dying between birth and the fifth birthday, in life table notation, $_5q_0$. It is usually expressed as the ratio of deaths in those younger than 5 years to 1,000 live births and is regarded as one of the most useful and sensitive indicators of child health in low- and middle-income countries, where it may not be practicable to calculate infant mortality rates for the whole population. Instead, the under 5 mortality rate is estimated from responses of women in reproductive ages to questions in a DEMOGRAPHIC AND HEALTH SURVEY about the number of children they have borne and the number still alive. The rate can be directly estimated if detailed birth histories are available or indirectly estimated if only summary information is available.

underground economy An entirely unregulated economic system in which goods and services are exchanged by bartering and/or by cash transactions without any formal paper record. See also GRAY MARKET.

underlying cause of death The disease, injury, or pathological condition that initiates the chain of events leading to death. The attending physician or other individual responsible for writing the death certificate attributes the death ultimately to this condition, and this is used in the compiled statistical tables of causes of death.

undernutrition Insufficient intake of calories, which most often occurs during periods of food shortage less severe than FAMINE and not severe enough to cause MALNUTRITION. It can also occur with fad diets, e.g., those sometimes adopted by persons seeking to lose weight.

underprivileged Descriptive of the state of being deprived of opportunities to advance in life and work, often because of poverty, ignorance, and lack of employment opportunities.

underreporting Incomplete provision of information about conditions for which data are required, especially in the interests of the public health. This is the bane of health information systems and of a comprehensive record of the status of many aspects of life. Underreporting of diseases, especially sexually transmitted diseases and to a lesser extent other communicable diseases, can occur for many reasons, for instance because the affected individuals never come into contact with anyone from the health care system or because health professionals do not identify the condition or fail to report the case to the public health information system. The consequence is distorted health statistics, and consequently inadequate planning and actions.

underserved community Guidelines and numerous studies provide information about the per capita requirements for all the principal components of a health care system. Another way that health planners operate is simply to calculate the per capita numbers of health professionals for the entire jurisdiction they administer and examine departures from the "average" that indicate (in theory) whether a community is underserved. Typically, rural regions and communities that are occupied predominantly by people in the lowest socioeconomic classes are underserved.

underworld The part of the economy that derives income from criminal activities, some of which have important implications for health, notably drug trafficking, prostitution, and people smuggling. Because of the health consequences of some criminal activity, it may be useful for public health officials to be able to communicate with the underworld, but there would be political objections and it would be difficult to do and to maintain a line of communication and mutual trust.

undocumented person A person, an "alien" in US usage, who enters and remains in a country without passing formally through the official procedures carried out by immigration and/or border control officials who maintain official records of immigrants, temporary visitors, guest workers, etc. Such people are often employed illegally or in the underground economy and, among other things, usually lack official access to health care and educational services for their children.

UNDP See UNITED NATIONS DEVELOPMENT PROGRAMME.

undulant fever See BRUCELLOSIS.

unemployment The situation that exists when people seeking gainful employment are unable to obtain it. This is often expressed as an unemployment rate, the number of persons seeking work divided by the total number in the workforce, working and nonworking. Unemployment is associated with a range of social and health problems, especially when it is a chronic or semipermanent condition.

unemployment insurance In the United States and several other countries, this is an official program partially or fully funded by taxation or compulsory levy from employers and/or salaried workers (e.g., as a payroll tax). Eligible workers who lose their jobs receive a weekly stipend sufficient for subsistence for a specified period.

unemployment rate A statistical indicator of the state of the nation's industrial economy. It is the proportion of the population eligible for and seeking work who are unemployed. Published statistics often dissect the total unemployment rate into age-specific rates and sometimes into other

categories, such as occupational, regional, and ethnic groups. It can underrepresent reality when there are large numbers of unemployed who have given up searching for work.

UNEP See UNITED NATIONS ENVIRONMENTAL PROGRAMME.

UNESCO See UNITED NATIONS EDUCATIONAL, SCIENTIFIC AND CULTURAL ORGANIZATION.

UNFPA See UNITED NATIONS POPULATION FUND, formerly called the United Nations Fund for Population Activities, thus the initials, which have remained unchanged..

UNHCR See UNITED NATIONS HIGH COMMISSIONER FOR REFUGEES.

unhealthy diets Sometimes a matter of opinion rather than fact, these are diets that parents and others disapprove of for children. Pediatricians, nutritionists, and authors of magazine articles often object, but such diets are widely promoted in TV and other advertising. They cover a wide range but have some common features, including carbonated soft drinks with a high sugar content; fatty foods, especially foods with a high content of TRANS FATS; and diets that contain little or no fresh fruit and vegetables. This is a vague term best avoided.

UNICEF See UNITED NATIONS CHILDREN'S FUND.

uniform data set The range of items of information recommended by the US National Center for Health Statistics that are required for detailed, valid, reproducible statistical analysis of health status. It includes demographic, socioeconomic, and clinical data. Many organizations and agencies in the health field have developed and advocate use of their own uniform data set. Unfortunately, there are so many variations that the use of the word "uniform" is a misnomer. Much depends on the purpose for which uniformity is required.

uniformed services See ARMED SERVICES.

unintended consequences A useful phrase that usually describes unfortunate or undesirable consequences of policies and practices that had good, indeed, the best intentions. Conversely, it may describe unexpected favorable outcomes not considered at the planning stages of a program. An example of disastrous unintended consequences was the occurrence of arsenic poisoning in Bangladesh after water pumps were installed to overcome the hazard of bacterial waterborne disease in contaminated surface water; unfortunately, the subsurface soil strata over a wide region contained a high content of arsenic salts. An example of good unintended consequences is strengthening of parent-teacher relations as a result of a school safety program.

unions Syn: labor unions. See TRADE UNION.

unique identifiers Items of personal identifying information used in RECORD LINKAGE that reduce to a minimum the likelihood of confusing two or more individuals, e.g., because they have the same or closely similar names.

unique identifying code A systematic method of assigning numerical codes to individuals for such purposes as identity cards, income tax records, or driver's licenses. Nations such as Sweden that use a unique identifying code generally base it on a sequence of digits for birth date, birth place (with postal code or administrative jurisdiction code), sex, first and last birth names of the mother or father, and additional digits or alphabet letters to ensure separate identification of individuals from twin or multiple births. Unique identifying numbers or a system for uniquely identifying individuals are a prerequisite for RECORD LINKAGE.

United Kingdom Public Health Association See UK PUBLIC HEALTH ASSOCIATION.

United Nations The initiative in global governance inaugurated in 1945 that evolved from the coalition of nations opposed to the regimes of Nazi Germany, Italy, and Japan in World War II. It consists of the General Assembly, where all member nations are represented and discuss issues of common concern, and the Security Council, with five permanent members: China, France, Russia, the United Kingdom, and the United States, each with veto power over resolutions, and a rotating membership of 10 other nations voted in at periodic elections. The UN has achieved a great deal, but its initiatives are often frustrated. Attempts to reform the United Nations and the Security Council have not yielded meaningful change as of 2005. For details of the United Nations Charter, activities, agencies, etc., see http://www.un.org.

United Nations agencies and programs The United Nations (UN) is responsible for administering a large number of multilateral agencies, many of which are identified and best known by acronyms. Several UN agencies have direct or indirect responsibility for aspects of human health, notably the WORLD HEALTH ORGANIZATION, UNITED NATIONS CHILDREN'S FUND, FOOD AND AGRICULTURE ORGANIZATION, UNITED NATIONS ENVIRONMENTAL PROGRAMME, UNITED NATIONS HIGH COMMISSIONER FOR REFUGEES, WORLD FOOD PROGRAMME, JOINT UNITED NATIONS PROGRAMME ON HIV/AIDS, and UNITED NATIONS POPULATION FUND.

United Nations agreements on human rights The United Nations has convened and/or sponsored a series of conferences and conventions on aspects of human rights, including the UNIVERSAL DECLARATION OF HUMAN RIGHTS, covenants on civil and political rights, conventions against torture and genocide, the conventions on the rights of women and the rights of the child; the UN has also reaffirmed and revised the original GENEVA CONVENTIONS. The United Nations Charter itself also addresses human rights. All the UN agreements, conventions, covenants, and related documents are accessible at http://www.hrweb.org/legal/undocs.html.

United Nations Children's Fund The acronym UNICEF originally stood for United Nations International Children's Emergency Fund. Although the name was shortened to the United Nations Children's Fund in 1953, the acronym survived because it was so widely recognized it had become a noun. In 1965, UNICEF was awarded the Nobel Peace Prize for its work on child advocacy. In the 1970s, UNICEF assumed a global leadership role in dealing with health problems affecting children. In 1990, it sponsored the WORLD SUMMIT ON CHILDREN. This drafted the DECLARATION OF THE RIGHTS OF THE CHILD, affirming the right of all children to health, education, and freedom from oppression and slavery. This declaration has been ratified by all the world's nations except the United States and Somalia. Details of UNICEF's activities are at http://www.unicef.org.

United Nations Convention on the Rights of the Child See WORLD SUMMIT ON CHILDREN.

United Nations Development Programme (UNDP) The aim of this UN agency is to advance the process of social, economic, and health improvement in low-income nations. It offers technical advice and assistance and unconditional low-interest loans, so at times it is at cross purposes with the INTERNATIONAL MONETARY FUND and the WORLD BANK. (Although IMF and World Bank loans are also at low interest, they have more conditions and restrictions than those of the UNDP.) The UNDP annually reviews and ranks development levels using the UN's HUMAN DEVELOPMENT INDEX, thus tracking and monitoring progress or deterioration. See http://www.undp.org for details,

United Nations Educational, Scientific and Cultural Organization (UNESCO) This UN agency, based in Paris, has programs in many fields, including literacy, knowledge and technology transfer, preservation of the world's natural and cultural heritage, enhancing scientific expertise, and the interfaces among the sciences and education, culture, and technology. For details, see http://www.unesco.org.

United Nations Environmental Programme (UNEP) This UN agency has its headquarters in Nairobi, Kenya. It is concerned with monitoring and surveillance of environmental conditions (air, water, land, forests, wilderness regions, ecosystems, wildlife, etc.) worldwide. Details are available at http://www.unep.org and http://www.unep.ch.

United Nations High Commissioner for Human Rights The office within the United Nations family of agencies that is concerned specifically with upholding human rights, monitoring reported violations, and initiating action to ensure that human rights are restored and maintained. For details, see http://www.ohchr.org/english/.

United Nations High Commissioner for Refugees (UNHCR) This UN agency has the task of caring for and arranging resettlement of refugees and internally displaced people who have lost their usual home and habitat as a result of natural or manmade disasters, mainly the latter, people displaced by violent armed conflict. At any given time there are usually 18 to 20 million such people, some of whom have become permanent refugees. See http://www.ohchr.org/english/.

United Nations Office on Drugs and Crime (UNODC) The Vienna-based UN body entrusted with the responsibility for coordinating and providing leadership for UN drug-control activities, and one of the sponsors of UNAIDS. For details, see http://www.unodc.org.

United Nations Population Fund Formerly known as the United Nations Fund for Population Activities (UNFPA), this agency supports and sponsors research and service in the field of human reproduction, with emphasis primarily on problems related to reproductive health of women in developing countries. See http://www.unfpa.org/ for details.

United Nations Special Programme on AIDS See JOINT UNITED NATIONS PROGRAMME ON HIV/AIDS.

United States Department of Agriculture (USDA) This agency has responsibility for important aspects of animal health, including safety of meat for human consumption. For details, see http://www.usda.gov.

United States Pharmacopeia (USP) A publication established in 1820 that contains legally recognized standards of identity, strength, quality, purity, packaging, and labeling for drug substances, dosage forms, and other therapeutic products, including nutritional products and dietary supplements. Since 1975, it has included the British National Formulary, with information on excipients. It is frequently revised and updated, most recently in 2005. For details, see http://www.usp.org/USPNF. For the British equivalent, see BRITISH NATIONAL FORMULARY.

United States Public Health Service (USPHS) This large federal agency has several important agencies or divisions: Centers for Disease Control and Prevention; National Institutes of Health; Food and Drug Administration; Agency for Toxic Substances and Disease Registry; Indian Health Service; Agency for Healthcare Research and Quality; Substance Abuse and Mental Health Services; Health Resources and Services Administration. See http://www.usphs.gov for current organization and details of activities of agencies and divisions.

universal coverage 1. Applied to medical and hospital insurance, this means that the insurance policy covers all contingencies without significant exclusions. 2. The term can also mean social, medical, and hospital coverage for everyone in a political jurisdiction, as in Sweden and the United Kingdom.

Universal Declaration of Human Rights This declaration arose from discussions at the newly formed United Nations in 1948. It was drafted by a Canadian diplomat, John Peters Humphrey (1905–1995) with the encouragement of Eleanor Roosevelt (1884–1962), widow of the US President Franklin D. Roosevelt, and endorsed by almost all member states of the UN. It declares that all humans are born free and equal in dignity and rights; all have freedom of thought, expression, opinion, the right to own property, and freedom of movement and residence within their state or nation; it proclaims equality before the law, the right to nationality and citizenship, the right to marry and have a family and to participate in the cultural life of the country. The right to health is embodied within the Declaration. It prohibits slavery, arbitrary arrest, detention, and exile, and affirms that all people in all nations that sign the Declaration have a duty to uphold all the rights specified in the Declaration. See http://www.un.org/Overview/rights.html.

universal donor In theory, a donor of blood group O, Rh negative, whose blood can be transfused to any recipient, but in practice there is really no such donor: blood for transfusion must always be precisely matched.

universal precautions Procedures followed by health workers with all patients when there is a risk that any of their patients could infect them, or indirectly through them infect others with dangerous contagious diseases such as EBOLA FEVER, SEVERE ACUTE RESPIRATORY SYNDROME (SARS), or MARBURG disease. Universal precautions include use of gown, gloves, mask, face shield or goggles, and immediate access to hand-washing facilities. All clothing, dressings, etc., that have been in contact with patients are discarded and sterilized immediately after use. Where possible, all potentially or suspected contagious patients are segregated.

universal product code The identifying number and/or bar code that can be found on almost all retail products, with sequences of numbers that identify the manufacturer and the product and give other details, such as the nature and composition of the product. In the health sector, the product number identifies details such as pharmacological action of drugs.

universal recipient A person of blood group AB Rh positive, who in theory can receive blood of any ABO group without adverse transfusion reaction; in practice blood for transfusion must always be precisely matched.

universe In epidemiological and social science research the population pool from which a SAMPLE is selected.

unleaded gasoline Hydrocarbon gasoline that either has no additives or uses antiknock additives other than lead. It is less environmentally harmful than leaded gasoline, which can be a serious contributor to the risk of lead poisoning in exposed populations.

unobtrusive measures A miscellaneous group of observational methods to assess behavior without asking direct questions and without influencing the behavior of the population that is being observed. For example, cigarette-smoking behavior can be inferred from sales statistics and from visual evidence, such as discarded cigarette butts.

UNODC See UNITED NATIONS OFFICE ON DRUGS AND CRIME.

unprofessional conduct A general term for behavior by a health professional, usually a physician or nurse, that falls in the category of negligence, incompetence, or misconduct or is unacceptable for other reasons, such as violent outbursts of bad temper. The use of this term leaves open the nature of the behavior, other than indicating that it is unacceptable and usually requires disciplinary or corrective action.

unproven remedies A large class of interventions, including some traditional healing methods and medications, some modern medications, technical equipment and devices, certain types of massages and manipulations, and unconventional psychotherapeutic approaches, that are resorted to by patients or their close kin in search of a cure

for conditions that are often incurable, such as advanced cancer or progressive degenerative neurological disorders. Some are quackery, fraud, and deliberate deception for gain, and many are futile, albeit well-meaning, attempts to achieve cure or remission. Some provide comfort by signaling that something, rather than nothing, is being done to help in a desperate situation, and some have a placebo effect, but usually sick people are better off without such supposed remedies. Traditional healing methods are in some respects in a separate category because, although their efficacy is usually unproven, at least they have stood the test of time in not causing too many deaths or obvious adverse consequences.

unsaturated fatty acids A group of fatty compounds with double- or triple-bonded carbon atoms, that are metabolized and stored in the body and contribute to the formation of atheromatous plaques. They have one (monounsaturated) or more (polyunsaturated) double bonds between carbon atoms. Each double bond takes the place of one hydrogen atom. The double bond imposes a kink in the molecule, making unsaturated fatty acids less easy to pack together. Consequently, unsaturated fats are usually liquid (oil) at room temperature. Diets rich in polyunsaturated fats are generally considered somewhat less likely than other high-lipid diets to be associated with development of obesity and coronary heart disease.

untouchables Among Hindus in India, the people of the lowest CASTE, who are identified and regarded by other Hindus as persons with whom they can have no social contact and only the minimal contact necessary to demand of them menial tasks or services that no one else is willing to perform. Health experience and access to health care are poor compared with those of members of other castes. The caste system is breaking down in modern India under pressure from political and economic change and tends not to be as powerful in the Hindu diaspora as in the Indian Subcontinent, but "untouchability" remains a social disability, despite the fact that some members of this caste have achieved international scientific prominence or high political office.

upper-body obesity Syn: abdominal obesity, android obesity. Obesity characterized by increased waist circumference and ratio of waist to hips, and increased skinfold thickness of hips. This form of obesity often signifies excess intraabdominal fat and is associated with hypertension and an increased risk of non-insulin-dependent diabetes, coronary heart disease, and stroke. It may also be associated with antiretroviral treatment for AIDS. These outcomes are only weakly and inconsistently associated with obesity that is more evenly and peripherally distributed.

upper respiratory tract infection (URTI or URI) An inflammatory and usually infectious condition of the upper respiratory tract, that is, of the throat, nose, nasal sinuses, tonsils, and pharynx. Usually this is a COMMON COLD, but similar symptoms occur in the prodromal stages of measles, influenza, and other serious conditions. URIs are a massive public health problem, causing more loss of time from work than any other condition. Technically, the term applies to any infection or inflammatory condition of the upper respiratory tract.

uppers A street name for Benzedrine and similar illicit drugs taken to elevate mood and induce wakefulness and a state of excitement. The converse, "downers," for hypnotic or sedative drugs, has never gained currency.

upstream determinant A determinant of disease that has an indirect but obvious effect on risk factor(s) for disease. For example, poverty is an upstream determinant of childhood malnutrition; affluence is an upstream determinant of coronary heart disease because it tends to be associated with risk factors such as diets rich in lipids, but it may also be an upstream determinant of reduced risk if it is associated with knowledge of risk and protective factors and the capacity to maximize benefit from these. See PROXIMAL and DISTAL RISK FACTOR.

upstream intervention The concept of anticipating adverse effects of situations and events that, if unchecked, could lead to potentially harmful health consequences, in order that relevant early intervention can be initiated to break the causal chain. For example, education of adolescent school children about traffic rules and road safety can be an effective upstream intervention to reduce the risk of traffic injury. See also PROXIMAL RISK FACTOR.

upward mobility The sociological process of a person achieving a higher socioeconomic status than earlier in life. This happens when a child of working class parents obtains professional qualifications or when a successful entrepreneur becomes wealthy. Upward mobility is often associated with improved health status compared with that of the original socioeconomic group, but the relationship is not necessarily causal. See also SOCIAL MOBILITY.

uracil A pyrimidine compound, one of four nucleotide bases in RNA molecules, corresponding to THYMINE in DNA. Some laboratory derivatives of uracil have been designed as experimental antimetabolite drugs for use in cancer chemotherapy.

uranium (U) A heavy metal element that is radioactive, i.e., emits ionized radiation. It has several isotopes, one of which has a half-life of 4.5×10^9 years. Uranium is fissile, and its property of nuclear fission is used in nuclear reactors and nuclear weapons.

urban health The phrase can mean health of people in urban areas or the health of ecosystems in and around urban areas. In the sense of human health in urban areas, the concerns include the social well-being and the health problems of populations that may include high proportions of broken families, families living in poverty, isolated old and infirm people, homeless people, and transient and street people. In environmental and ecosystem health terms, high-density urban areas may be afflicted with SMOG and other environmental problems such as INDUSTRIAL WASTE dumps, BROWNFIELDS, and suspect water supplies. Urban and municipal public health departments in Europe and North and South America work in collaboration with other sectors, agencies, and services to minimize adverse outcomes, both for the population and for the urban environment. The result is often that the health indicators of people in urban areas are better than those of rural residents.

urbanization The process by which a rural region or town evolves into a city. The distinction is often ill-defined and is determined partly by population size, partly by the existence of facilities such as a network of public transport, news media, and a sense of identification with the place as a city rather than a community. It may become sociologically and politically significant if associated with a sense of alienation from the evolving city, and there may be adverse health effects if expanding populations outgrow available health care resources and facilities.

urban renewal Policies and programs intended to replace urban slums, decaying or abandoned industrial sites, etc., with new housing and attractive public spaces, such as parks and playing fields, and thereby restore inner city living space. The results vary. Often population health is enhanced by improved housing conditions, but occasionally GENTRIFICATION occurs and low-income people are forced out by rising prices.

urban sprawl The relentless extension of built-up areas around virtually every city on earth as the combination of rising population and rising prosperity apply increasing economic pressure on agricultural and pastoral land, making it difficult or impossible to preserve it for agricultural use. Many cities both in the rich industrial nations and in low-income countries are surrounded by widening zones of suburban housing or, in low-income countries, SHANTYTOWNS.

urea A nitrogenous end product of protein metabolism excreted in the urine. In some renal and metabolic diseases and circulatory failure, urea accumulates in the blood and can cause UREMIA.

uremia Excessive accumulation of urea and other nitrogenous end products, notably creatinine, in the blood, as a consequence of advanced renal or circulatory failure. The usual natural course is lethargy, convulsions, coma, and death, unless the toxic accumulation of nitrogenous metabolic products is reversed by dialysis or renal transplant.

urethane A toxic volatile organic solvent, foaming agent, and sealant derived from toluene. It is used as polyurethane varnish and has many industrial applications. It is toxic and a respiratory irritant.

urethritis Inflammatory disease of the urethra. In females, with a short urethra within a moist vulva, infection is frequent, can have many causes, and is often difficult to treat successfully. In males, sexually transmitted diseases, notably gonorrhea, are a common cause.

uric acid A white crystalline solid, the end product of purine metabolism that accumulates in GOUT and sometimes forms renal calculi.

urology The medical and surgical specialty dealing with diseases of the genitourinary system.

URTI The usual acronym for a nonspecific UPPER RESPIRATORY TRACT INFECTION, also known as upper respiratory infection, or URI.

urticaria An allergic condition affecting the skin and mucosal membranes, producing swelling, redness, and sometimes a rash. When the swelling occurs in the mucosa of the larynx or trachea in the condition of anaphylactic shock, it can be fatal. It can be occupational in origin.

USAID See AGENCY FOR INTERNATIONAL DEVELOPMENT.

USDA See UNITED STATES DEPARTMENT OF AGRICULTURE.

user fee A charge levied for use of health or social services that, although intended to help cover the cost of the service, usually has a deterrent effect and may deter those most in need of help.

USPHS See UNITED STATES PUBLIC HEALTH SERVICE.

uterine cancer A common female malignancy. Cancer of the cervix is often—perhaps usually, or even always—a sexually transmitted disease and can usually be detected early by PAP SMEAR. Infection with HUMAN PAPILLOMA VIRUS (HPV) is a necessary cause. Cancer of the body of the uterus is weakly associated with HORMONE REPLACEMENT THERAPY (HRT).

utilitarianism The philosophy associated with John Stuart Mill (1806–1873) that can be summed up in the phrase "greatest good for the greatest number." It is the guiding principle for many of the decisions and actions of public health professionals.

utility In economics, a synonym for individual welfare or well-being. Health economists use the term to mean the value of a specified health state, often expressed on a scale from 0 to 1, and use it to determine QUALITY-ADJUSTED LIFE YEARS (QALYs) and HEALTH-ADJUSTED LIFE EXPECTANCY (HALE). Utility is based on preferences that individuals express about alternative outcomes likely to follow their treatment choices.

utilization review In the evaluation of health care, the process of assessing how services are used, by whom, under what circumstances, and with what outcomes.

UV, UVL, UVR Acronyms for ultraviolet light and ULTRAVIOLET RADIATION. Ultraviolet radiation is subdivided according to wavelength into UVA, UVB, and UVC.

V

vaccination The word "vaccination" derives from Latin *vacca*, meaning cow, and originally referred to the process used by the British physician Edward Jenner (1749–1823), who coined the word to describe his method of inoculating cowpox lymph to provide immunity from smallpox, which he based on observations of a local farmer, Benjamin Jesty, who told him that milkmaids who got cow-pox never got smallpox. Jenner's original meaning has broadened to include all forms of IMMUNIZATION against infectious pathogens, including oral, as well as injected, VACCINES.

vaccine The biologically active antigen, usually in liquid solution or colloid suspension that is injected or taken orally to immunize (vaccinate) individuals against communicable diseases. It may be prepared from a culture of live attenuated or killed organisms or from organisms with antigenic properties closely similar to those of the pathogen from which the vaccine is intended to provide protection.

vaccine efficacy and safety The safety and efficacy of vaccines are usually evaluated in PHASE II and PHASE III CLINICAL TRIALS. Efficacy can be measured by the postvaccination antibody titer and by the reduction, preferably to zero, in incidence of cases of the infectious disease against which the vaccine provides protection, and safety is assessed from the occurrence rate of adverse reactions among persons receiving the vaccine.

vaccine-preventable disease A disease that can be prevented or controlled by vaccination. The term is usually applied to the infectious diseases that were formerly commonplace among infants and children, i.e., diphtheria, pertussis, tetanus, polio, measles, mumps, rubella, and, in high-risk groups, hepatitis B, tuberculosis (using BCG vaccine), and *Haemophilus influenza* Type b. Public health authorities aspire to vaccinate all vulnerable infants and children against most of these diseases. Other vaccine-preventable diseases include smallpox, typhoid, yellow fever, typhus, plague, relapsing fever, Japanese B encephalitis, and several others. For current CDC recommendations, see http://www.cdc.gov/nip/diseases/child-vpd.htm.

vaccinia virus The virus that causes cowpox that, when inoculated into the skin of humans, gives rise to development of antibody that confers immunity to SMALLPOX. In antigenic structure and immunological properties, vaccinia virus resembles the smallpox virus.

vacuum packed foods A safe and effective method of food preservation, achieved by enclosing the food in an airtight package and exhausting all the air in the package. The method is most suitable for dried and dehydrated food.

vaginal pouch See FEMALE CONDOM.

vaginal smear A swab taken from vaginal secretions to test for the presence of pathogens, including especially those responsible for SEXUALLY TRANSMITTED DISEASES. Not to be confused with a CERVICAL SMEAR or PAP TEST.

vaginitis Inflammation of the vagina, commonly due to infection, either a sexually transmitted disease or other reproductive tract infection, such as TRICHOMONIASIS, or a fungus infection, such as candida.

valid From the Latin *validus* (meaning strong), this adjective refers to an entity, measurement, or set of findings that means what it purports to mean, measures what it claims to measure, is a true statement of the reality.

validity The extent to which a measurement actually measures what it purports to measure or an entity actually is what it purports to be. There are several kinds of validity. Criterion validity is the extent to which a measured variable or an entity correlates with an external criterion of the phenomenon under study. This has two aspects: concurrent validity means that the measurement and the criterion refer to the same time and place; predictive validity is the ability to predict the criterion. Construct validity is the extent to which measurements conform to theoretical concepts or constructs. Content validity is the extent to which measurements incorporate the domain of the phenomenon under study. Study validity is the degree to which the inferences from a scientific study are warranted, taking into account the strengths and weaknesses of the study design. This has two aspects: internal validity, the degree to which observations may be attributed solely to the hypothesized effect that is being studied, and external validity, which is the extent to which the findings of a study can be generalized.

value neutral The situation in which a participant in a controversial situation is impartial and not influenced by personal beliefs, attitudes, or values, a situation that may often be more theoretical than real. Philosophers of science have long debated the question of whether science can ever be truly value neutral, starting from the premise that the scientific approach to problem solving in itself requires values that accept the importance and relevance of so doing, in addition to the values implied in the search itself, such as the definition of truth. Beyond this, the ethical and moral choices that biological and health scientists must frequently make will always require them to hold certain values.

values 1. In sociology, the beliefs, traditions, and social customs that are held dear and upheld by individuals and society. Values influence the behavior of individuals, families, groups, and entire nations. They include MORAL VALUES that are deeply believed, are often grounded in religious beliefs, and are almost immutable social values, such as attitudes toward the roles and functions of women in society, which are more flexible and sometimes change rather quickly, as values regarding marriage in many Western societies did after about the 1970s. Moral and social values influence public health policies, priorities, and actions, such as the provision of health promotion programs. 2. In statistics and the physical sciences, values are the magnitude of measurements.

vapor pressure The atmospheric pressure exerted by a vapor in the presence of the liquid form of the same substance at specified temperature. It is an indicator of the VOLATILITY of the liquid.

variable Any quantitative measurement of an entity, attribute, or phenomenon that can vary. In epidemiological and other scientific studies, the aim is often to assess how variables relate to one another. For this purpose, a distinction is made between independent and dependent variables. An independent variable is one that is assumed to remain constant or uninfluenced by changing conditions or circumstances during a study. A dependent variable changes in ways that are determined by the influence of attributes or external factors. The aim of a research study is often to identify how these attributes or factors influence the behavior of a dependent variable or variables, preferably to develop a generalizable model or mathematical rule to explain and predict the relationship.

variance The extent or range by which a set of measurements of an entity, attribute, or phenomenon varies. It is defined as the sum of the squares of the deviation from the mean, divided by the number of DEGREES OF FREEDOM in the set of observations, usually the number of observations minus 1.

variant Creutzfeldt-Jakob disease (vCJD) The clinically, epidemiologically, and histologically distinct form of Creutzfeldt-Jakob disease that has been confirmed to be caused by the same PRION that is responsible for BOVINE SPONGIFORM ENCEPHALOPATHY (mad cow disease). The weight of evidence, including DNA typing, suggests that vCJD is a prion disease that has "jumped species" from cattle to humans. By May 2006, 155 confirmed cases had been reported, mainly in the United Kingdom, suggesting that if the cause is transmission of prions via ingested cattle meat, the risk is probably low. No cases of person-to-person transmission have been reported. The course is rapid, progressive, and fatal. See http://www.cdc.gov/ncidod/dvrd/vcjd/ and http://www.cjd.ed.ac.uk/figures.htm.

varicella Syn: chickenpox. Highly contagious virus disease caused by the varicella-zoster virus, human herpes virus 3. It is primarily a disease of children and is usually innocuous but can be serious in persons with compromised immune systems. The varicella-zoster virus apparently may remain dormant when the infection has resolved, but may reactivate in later life after re-exposure to infection, such as contact with a case of chickenpox, when it can cause HERPES ZOSTER.

variola The Latin scientific name for SMALLPOX. Two varieties of smallpox were clinically defined. Variola major was a dangerous disease with very severe symptoms, extensive rash that could be hemorrhagic, and a case fatality ratio of 30% to 40%. Variola minor, alastrim, was less severe clinically, had a less extensive and nonhemorrhagic rash, and had a case fatality rate of 5% or less. The World Health Assembly of 1980 declared smallpox eradicated from the world.

variolation The practice invented in China about 1,000 years ago of inoculating or insufflating into the nose a small quantity of dried secretions from a smallpox vesicle. This provided some immunity to smallpox, although it apparently caused death in as many as 1 in 100 cases. The practice spread across Asia along the silk route, reaching Constantinople by the 17th century. Lady Mary Wortley Montagu (1689–1762), the wife of the British ambassador to Constantinople, observed the practice, was persuaded of its efficacy, and introduced it in England when she returned home. It was the model for Edward Jenner's method of VACCINATION.

vasectomy A surgical procedure in which the vas deferens is ligated and a small segment of it is excised in order to prevent the passage of spermatozoa from the testes to the seminal vesicles, and therefore to the ejaculate in semen. This is a reliable method of male sterilization, but as viable spermatozoa are stored for a considerable time in the seminal vesicles, multiple ejaculations are required before semen is cleared of spermatozoa capable of fertilizing an ovum.

vCJD See VARIANT CREUTZFELDT-JAKOB DISEASE.

vector 1. In infectious disease epidemiology, a living creature, usually an insect, that carries an infectious pathogen to a susceptible human host. In many vector-borne diseases, the pathogen undergoes a developmental stage in the vector; in others the vector acts merely as a passive carrier. 2. In statistics, an ordered set of numerical values. 3. In physics and mathematics, the graphical representation of the magnitude and direction of a force.

vector-borne diseases A large and miscellaneous class of diseases that are transmitted to humans by vectors, predominantly insects. They include mosquito-borne diseases caused by viruses, bacteria, protozoa, and helminths; diseases spread by blackflies and other biting and blood-sucking flies, ticks, lice, fleas, etc.; and diseases in which the intermediate hosts are fish, freshwater snails, and mammals. Those of current concern in North America are described and discussed at http://www.cdc.gov/ncidod/dvbid/.

Vedic healing See AYURVEDIC MEDICINE.

vegan An extreme VEGETARIAN who refrains from ingesting all animal products, including milk, milk products, and eggs. Vegans are at risk of iron deficiency anemia and protein deficiency.

vegetarian A person who does not eat animal meat or meat products. Some vegetarians take avoidance of meat one stage further and avoid eating fish or other seafood, but many include seafood in their diet. Followers of several religions, notably Hindus and some members of Christian sects such as Mormons and Seventh Day Adventists, include a vegetarian diet among their practices, and comparative studies have demonstrated that their health is in no way impaired as a result. In some ways, such as reduced risk of coronary heart disease and some cancers, their health status is superior to that of otherwise comparable populations who eat meat. However, vegetarians are more vulnerable than meat eaters to iron deficiency anemia, for example, caused by postpartum blood loss or heavy menstrual loss. Variations include lactovegetarians, who eat dairy products; lacto-ovo-vegetarians, who eat dairy products and eggs; and fruitarians, or vegans, who eat only fruits and vegetables.

vegetative state The neurophysiological condition in which autonomic physiological functions such as respiration and heart beat are retained but consciousness and voluntary muscle activity are suspended. A persistent vegetative state exists when this condition is prolonged and the prognosis is that consciousness will not return.

vehicle The medium whereby infectious pathogens are conveyed. The vehicle of transmission may be water, milk, food, air, or contaminated blood or blood products. Water-borne diseases are predominantly fecal-oral infections causing diarrhea and/or vomiting. Milk- and food-borne infections include other conditions, such as poisoning by bacterial or chemical toxins. Moisture-laden air that has passed through a contaminated water-cooled air conditioning plant is the vehicle for infection with the legionella that causes LEGIONNAIRES DISEASE. Contaminated blood and blood products are the vehicle for HIV, hepatitis C, and occasionally other infections.

venereal diseases An obsolete name for SEXUALLY TRANSMITTED DISEASES.

Venn diagram A useful diagrammatic way to display the extent to which two or more entities, concepts, or distributions are mutually inclusive or exclusive, invented by the English logician John Venn (1834–1923).

ventilation An important determinant of individual and population health is the extent to which fresh, pollution-free air is available in dwellings, workplaces, and public buildings. The nature and quality of ventilation are therefore important criteria for specialized engineers and architects to ensure when designing and equipping homes, workplaces, and public spaces, and for sanitarians to monitor. In hot and cold climate regions, a balance has to be struck between preserving indoor air quality and maintaining a comfortable temperature. Inadequate ventilation in these circumstances is a cause of the SICK BUILDING SYNDROME.

Venturi effect The Italian physicist Giovanni Venturi (1746–1822) described the phenomenon of increased flow rate and reduced pressure when fluid or air flows through a constriction in a tube. This effect is observed when airways are constricted by disease such as asthma, when large blood vessels have a region of constriction, in mine shafts of varying size, and in many other situations.

verbal autopsy Syn: psychological autopsy, social autopsy. An attempt to ascertain the cause of otherwise unexplained death by asking questions about antecedent conditions and experiences that the deceased person has had. When death is manifestly due to suicide, a verbal autopsy is a method of investigation that can sometimes reveal why a person committed suicide. A similar approach is used at the population level in rural villages in low-income countries lacking adequate medical care to construct a profile of common causes of death in particular villages. This has been applied to the study of infant mortality. This can be done in a standardized manner using predetermined questions that have been validated by observed diagnoses in comparable populations. Deaths are classified in groups according to leading signs such as fever and skin rash, diarrhea, coma, cough, breathlessness.

verruca A wart. The word is often reserved to describe the painful and troublesome variety of plantar wart, verruca vulgaris, caused by the human papilloma virus and acquired by walking barefoot on an infected surface, typically the warm wet surface of a public swimming pool.

vertical transmission Syn: mother-to-fetus transmission, mother-to-child transmission. A term usually applied to diseases transmitted by infected blood or body fluids in which an infected mother infects a fetus, either by transplacental transmission of pathogens or by way of abrasions, etc., sustained during childbirth. This is one of the ways maternal infections, including hepatitis B, HIV, syphilis, and toxoplasmosis. can be transmitted.

vertigo Dizziness or giddiness caused by disturbance of the semicircular canals, sometimes by cerebellar disease. This is a transient phenomenon that most people experience immediately after rotational movements of the body, e.g., on fairground rides. Ménière's disease, named for the French physician Prosper Ménière (1799–1862), is a persistent, sometimes recurrent and disabling form of vertigo caused by inflammation of the semicircular canals, often associated with middle ear disease or arteriosclerosis and hypertension.

very high density lipoprotein (VHDL) A plasma lipoprotein with density of 1.28 kg/liter made up of 57% protein, 21% phospholipid, 17% cholesterol, and 5% triglycerides. It is the most efficient lipid to transport cholesterol from the intestine to the liver; the concentration of VHDL is inversely related to the risk of severe atherosclerosis.

very low birth weight A birth weight less than 1,500 grams. Neonates in this weight category account for about half of all neonatal deaths.

very low density lipoprotein A lipoprotein with a density of 0.950 to 1.006 kg/liter that consists of 6% to 10% protein, 15% to 20% phospholipids, 20% to 30% cholesterol, and 45% to 65% triglycerides. It is implicated in the pathogenesis of atheroma.

Veterans Administration The US federal government agency responsible for administering all aspects of publicly funded services for veterans, including their health care.

veterinary epidemiology The use of epidemiological methods in veterinary practice and research has enhanced understanding and management of many human diseases of public health importance and aided in the discovery of ways to protect and maintain good health of livestock—cattle, sheep, pigs, poultry, and some wild animals, e.g., in parks. Some methods developed in veterinary epidemiology and wildlife biology, e.g., CAPTURE–MARK–RECAPTURE METHOD and the NEAREST NEIGHBOR METHOD, have some useful applications in epidemiological studies of human populations.

veterinary medicine The science and practice of medicine in which animals rather than humans are the patients. Usually this means domestic animals, farm livestock, and pets. It is an important aspect of public health because many diseases can pass from animals to humans and vice versa.

veterinary public health An aspect of public health services, often maintained at a national level in recognition of its importance, the main aims of veterinary public health are to protect humans from ZOONOTIC DISEASES and to protect livestock

herds from epidemic disease by enforcing strict animal quarantine and, where feasible, the use of vaccines. High-intensity livestock management, use of animal feed fortified with animal protein, confinement of herds in feedlots, factory farming, and transport of live animals to distant markets have all increased the risks of epidemics in livestock. Outbreaks of foot-and-mouth disease, BOVINE SPONGIFORM ENCEPHALOPATHY, avian influenza on large poultry farms, and other outbreaks in recent years have all underscored the economic importance of this specialty. The possibility of bioterrorist attacks on animal herds adds a further dimension to its importance.

VI antigen The capsular antigen of salmonella species, especially *S. typhi*, which was formerly thought to be associated with the virulence of the organism. Its main laboratory use is in typing the organism precisely.

vibration syndrome A vascular disorder that is a form of Raynaud's disease, presumed to be a chronic vasospasm triggered by the trauma of repeated coarse vibrations of the hands. It is an occupational disease of people whose work requires prolonged operation of a pneumatic drill.

victim-blaming A rather frequent and deplorable attitude and practice of some health care workers when dealing with certain conditions, especially those that carry a stigma, in which, subconsciously or deliberately, sick people are given substandard or inadequate care because they are regarded as responsible for causing their own diseases. Persons with alcohol or substance abuse problems are frequent targets. An overt manifestation of victim-blaming was the widely publicized refusal of a cardiothoracic surgeon to perform a coronary artery bypass operation on a patient who was overweight and a compulsive cigarette smoker. Many lesser varieties are more subtle and covert but can nonetheless be hurtful to patients who seek help, rather than criticism, from their medical and nursing attendants.

video display terminal (VDT) A computer screen. Operators of computer keyboards are at risk of ERGONOMIC conditions, such as carpal tunnel syndrome, repetitive strain injury, cervical soft-tissue pains, and disturbances of vision. The incidence and prevalence of all these conditions have risen sharply since the advent of computers in office and commercial work.

vinyl chloride The monomer chemical compound that is converted to polyvinylchloride (PVC) by gently heating the liquid to about 70°C. PVC is well known as a plastic compound with many uses. Vinyl chloride fumes have adverse effects on health, including narcosis, acro-osteolysis, hepatitis, and angiosarcoma.

violence The simplest definition of violence is behavior causing harm by the use of force. Two types are unintentional violence, which occurs in the workplace or domestic settings, or may be traffic-related or recreational; and intentional violence, self-harm, and harm caused by others. The latter includes DOMESTIC VIOLENCE and violence at the hands of strangers, assault, robbery with violence, violence as part of civil disturbances such as riots, sports-related hooliganism, etc. An additional large category includes all forms of WAR and violent armed conflicts.

Virchow, Rudolf (1821–1902) This German physician was a towering figure in 19th century pathology, public health, and social reform. He investigated an epidemic of typhus, about which he wrote a critical report that correctly attributed the outbreak to deplorable social conditions; he founded *Archiv für pathologische Anatomie und Physiologie* (Virchow's Archives). In his speeches and writings, he repeatedly drew attention to the importance of social conditions as causal factors of diseases and epidemics. He was a founding figure in German SOCIAL MEDICINE.

virgin population A population that has not previously been exposed to a specific infectious pathogenic microorganism and in which, therefore, there is no herd immunity. Consequently, an epidemic affects virtually everyone, regardless of age, and sometimes has high case fatality rates. Historical examples include the original indigenous populations of the Americas, who suffered devastating epidemics of smallpox, measles, and tuberculosis when first in contact with European colonizers who brought these pathogens with them.

virtue-based ethics Aristotle's *Ethics* (4th century BCE) is a philosophical account of the role of virtues such as truth, integrity, honesty, and altruism in achieving a good life. These and other virtues are the basis for virtue-based ethics and form part of the foundation of public health ethics. Contrast principle-based and rule-based ethics. See also ETHICS.

virulence The potential for degree of pathogenicity or severity of agents that cause disease. It can be measured quite precisely in experimental animals and often can be inferred from available clinical evidence in human infection, but with caution, because the occurrence of subclinical, mild, serious, or overwhelming infection is also influenced by susceptibility or resistance of the individual human host.

virus Small living organism, size 20 to 400 nm, visible only by electron microscopic analysis, consisting mainly of DNA and RNA. Viruses are ubiquitous and infect animals (including humans), plants, and bacteria. They are obligate parasites that invade host cells. In humans they cause some of the most dangerous and deadly human epidemic diseases, including influenza, smallpox, HIV/AIDS, yellow fever, and viral hemorrhagic fevers.

viscose rayon One of the oldest synthetic fibers, widely used in textiles since the 1930s. Viscose rayon manufacture may expose workers to volatile toxic solvents and to carbon disulfide, which can cause polyneuritis and increased cardiovascular disease risk.

visible minority A term for members of specific ethnic, racial, or cultural groups or persons who "look different" from the "majority" in the United States, United Kingdom, and other English-speaking nations, because their skin color, hair, facial features, and mode of dress differ conspicuously in appearance from those of the rest of the population.

visible radiation Electromagnetic radiation in the wavelengths that stimulate the light-sensitive retinal rods and cones, the cells that are end organs of sight. This radiation extends from violet, with a wavelength of 390 to 425 nm, to red, with a wavelength of 620 to 740 nm.

visioning A method of long-range planning that is based on the concept of a realizable "ideal" future and formulation of realistic plans to achieve this. Visioning is a practical method of long-range planning, not an unrealistic or idealistic approach. As applied in long-range planning, the method considers the range of possible futures, selects the most desirable and realistic, and develops a systematic set of plans, methods, and procedures most likely to achieve this future.

vis medicatrix naturae Literally, the curative strength of nature; cure brought about by the force of nature or natural healing. This can effectively deal with minor injuries and many illnesses.

visual aid A collective name for all forms of corrective lenses for refractive errors and for many devices to magnify small objects or small print. The term is also used to describe the audiovisual devices that speakers can use to illustrate a lecture or other oral presentation.

visual impairment Inability to see adequately or difficulty with necessary aspects of vision, such as inability to read the newspaper, recognize the face of a friend across the street, or read traffic signs, that are indicators of refractive errors.

vital capacity The total amount of air that can be exhaled after inspiring the maximum possible. Measuring vital capacity is a basic feature of respiratory function tests.

vital record A record, commonly a certificate recording a vital event, that is, an event relating to "a matter of life and death." This is a birth, marriage, divorce, or death certificate, and in some nations a certificate recording some other event of national importance, such as military service.

vital signs Three basic vital signs are heart beat, usually assessed by feeling the pulse, preferably in the carotid artery; respiration; and reaction of the pupil, i.e., the iris, to light. Other vital signs include body temperature and blood pressure and reaction to speech, heat, cold, pain, etc.

vital statistics The word "statistics" derives from "state," and vital statistics are the data on "vital events," that is, births, deaths, and civil activities that relate to births and deaths, namely marriage and divorce. Vital statistics are compiled by public authorities at the national, regional, and sometimes local level, and in most nations are routinely published in annual reports. There is an overlapping area belonging both to vital statistics and DEMOGRAPHY and another large overlap with epidemiology. Indeed, WILLIAM FARR (1807–1883), a founding father of vital statistics, was also an innovator in the emergence of epidemiology as a rigorous scientific method of studying disease distribution. One of his aphorisms was "Death is a fact. All else is inference." Farr was a master of the art of inference from mortality statistics. Vital statistics provide essential information in public health, by identifying problems and measures of progress or lack of progress in dealing with these problems.

vitamin A Syn: carotene, retinol. A fat-soluble vitamin occurring in high concentration in certain vegetables. It is essential for fetal development, cell differentiation, and chemical changes that facilitate vision in poor illumination. Severe vitamin A deficiency causes XEROPHTHALMIA, formerly a common cause of blindness among children in some low-income countries. Vitamin A intoxication affecting the liver may rarely occur, for instance in Inuit people who eat excessive quantities of polar bear and other carnivore liver. The NIH Clinical Research Center has a useful fact sheet on vitamin A content of common foods, recommended dietary allowances, and other information, at http://ods .od/nih.gov/factsheets/vitamina.asp.

vitamin B group A miscellaneous group of water-soluble chemical compounds that have been demonstrated to be essential for growth, development, or specific metabolic processes in humans and/or animals. They include THIAMIN (vitamin B_1); RIBOFLAVIN (vitamin B_2); PYRIDOXINE (vitamin B_6); FOLIC ACID (sometimes called vitamin B_c); NIACIN or nicotinic acid (vitamin B_5); cobalamine or intrinsic factor (VITAMIN B_{12}) and several others of uncertain importance for human health. Vitamin B intoxication causes arthritis but very rarely occurs.

vitamin B_2 (riboflavin) deficiency Riboflavin (vitamin B_2) is an essential coenzyme for carbohydrate metabolism. Deficiency, commonly due to insufficient dietary intake of animal protein such as milk and milk products, presents clinically with fissures at the corners of the mouth and lips, which become deeply pigmented. More serious deficiency causes vascular changes in the cornea, leading to visual impairment and ultimately blindness.

vitamin B_{12} Syn: cobalamin, because it contains cobalt. With intrinsic factor, a glycoprotein secreted in gastric juices, this is reabsorbed in the ileum. Deficiency causes SPRUE or MALABSORPTION SYNDROME and anemia. Recommendations and cobalamin content of various foods are available at http://ods.od.nih.gov/factsheets/vitaminb12.asp.

vitamin C Syn: ascorbic acid. This occurs in fresh vegetables and fruit, with especially high concentration in citrus fruits, rose-hip syrup, etc. It plays an essential role in tyrosine metabolism, bone and cartilage metabolism, integrity and function of mesothelium, and adrenal gland function. Deficiency causes SCURVY, which was the first vitamin deficiency disease identified (see JAMES LIND). Vitamin C is excreted by the kidneys, and overdosage can cause renal calculus.

vitamin D Fat-soluble sterols, calciferol, and related substances are produced in the skin by the action of solar radiation. These are essential enzymes in calcium metabolism and in the formation and continuing integrity of bone structure. Deficiency causes RICKETS and osteomalacia. For dietary requirements and other information, see http://ods.od.nih.gov/factsheets/vitamind.asp.

vitamin deficiency diseases A miscellaneous group of specific diseases having in common the fact that they are caused by deficiency of a particular vitamin. Some are listed in the text in separate discussion of particular vitamins. Vitamin deficiency diseases occur during periods of famine or severe food shortage or are associated with unusual circumstances leading to deficiency of specific vitamins, for instance, the occurrence of scurvy in children in inland Australia or among isolated old people deprived of fresh vegetables until these dietary deficiencies were recognized as a public health problem and corrected.

vitamin E Syn: α-tocopherol. The essential nature of this vitamin remains debatable, but it probably plays a role in metabolism of sterols and steroids, may boost immune reactions, and may facilitate healing of wounds and ulcers. The NIH Clinical Research Center has a fact sheet giving relevant information, at http://ods.od.nih.gov/factsheets/vitamine.asp.

vitamin K A fat-soluble substance produced in the gut by the action of normal intestinal flora that is absorbed in the small intestine and plays an essential role in the blood clotting mechanism.

vitamins A miscellaneous class of chemical compounds of varying complexity and solubility in water or fats having in common the fact that all are essential to maintenance of some metabolic function required for good health. Vitamins do not occur naturally in the body, and most are not synthesized by body functions but must be ingested and absorbed. Most vitamins are ingredients of normal balanced diets of carbohydrates, fats, and proteins derived from vegetable and animal origins. Vitamin D is manufactured partly by the interaction of solar radiation with cells in the skin, and vitamin K is manufactured by commensal organisms in the gut. Most vitamins can be designated by alphabet letters, as listed above, but they have chemical identifying names, and it is often preferable to use these. It is possible to overdose with some vitamins, notably vitamins A and C, but it is rare and usually innocuous.

vitreous humor A translucent gelatinous material that fills the space in the globe of the eye between the lens and the retina.

vocational guidance A program that is part of routine activity in many school systems, to provide information and advice to school children and school leavers about possible careers and occupations that fit well with their abilities and interests. Vocational guidance is credited with helping to prevent frustration and psychological disturbances due to dissatisfaction with work. It is also often a feature of adult rehabilitation services after serious illness or injury. It is one of the ways in which school teachers can help health professionals by identifying children and youth at risk, for instance, because of emotional, personality, and psychiatric disorders.

vocational rehabilitation Actually a form of OC-CUPATIONAL THERAPY aimed at equipping people who are physically or mentally impaired with skills that enable them to take part in work and achieve gainful employment.

volatile organic compounds (VOCs) A miscellaneous group of organic substances that are either liquid or solid and readily vaporize on contact with air. They include formaldehyde, carbon tetrachloride, chloroform, benzene, tetrachlorethylene, toluene, etc,, many of which are toxic; some are narcotic and some asphyxiant. VOCs are sometimes a component of urban air pollution.

volatility The property of liquids and some solid substances that vaporize readily.

volt The SI unit of potential electromotive force named for the Italian physicist Alessandro Volta (1745–1827).

voluntarism The concept of meeting the medical, social, fiscal, psychological, and spiritual needs of individuals, defined groups, or society as a whole without financial recompense. Many people do this from a spirit of altruism, alone or as members of voluntary organizations.

voluntary agency A community agency that is staffed mainly or entirely by unpaid volunteers. It may or may not be part of a larger voluntary organization and may or may not be supported by charitable contributions.

von Economo's encephalitis Syn: encephalitis lethargica. The eponym honors the German neurologist Constantin von Economo (1876–1931). A presumed virus disease that occurred in worldwide low-grade epidemic form in the 1920s, and was followed in a high proportion of cases by a late sequel of postencephalitis Parkinson's disease.

von Hohenheim, Theophrastus Bombastus See PARACELSUS.

voodoo A form of WITCHCRAFT linked to religious beliefs, indigenous to certain African tribal groups that were taken to the West Indies, principally Haiti, by African slaves in the 16th and 17th centuries. It is associated with the use of charms either to harm others or to heal their illnesses.

voucher system A method used in some countries, including the United States, to augment assistance for persons and families on welfare and in receipt of old age and invalid pensions by providing vouchers that can be exchanged for specific food items, and in some countries for clothing for children. Vouchers are employed rather than cash handouts on the basis of a belief that cash would very likely be spent on nonessentials such as tobacco and alcohol. This implication is often resented by people in poverty, and the voucher system is opposed by advocates for the poor. Vouchers are also used in the United States for educational services provided by schools other than the public system, including many linked to specific religious faiths and denominations.

vulnerable groups This term is applied to any designated group identified by epidemiological or other studies as being at higher risk than the general population either for specific conditions such as coronary heart disease and HIV/AIDS or for a broad class of conditions such as childhood infectious diseases. Vulnerability implies more than merely being at risk because it reflects that the impact of disease may be aggravated by other factors, such as poverty or malnutrition. Terms such as "vulnerable group" and "high-risk group" must be used carefully to avoid stigmatizing members of the designated group.

W

---

waist-to-hip circumference ratio An indicator of obesity when waist circumference exceeds hip circumference, also known as "upper body obesity," this is a useful prognostic indicator of future morbidity and mortality from coronary heart disease, stroke, and non-insulin-dependent diabetes. Recent studies have indicated that it is a better indicator than body mass index.

war A violent conflict between armed forces, usually involving two or more nations or hostile forces within a nation (civil war). It is one of the worst, most intractable public health problems. In the 20th century, two world wars and about 250 local and regional wars had a combined death toll of more than 110 million people, and at least three to four times that number were permanently maimed. Since the end of World War II (1945), more than 150 regional and local wars, civil wars, "low-intensity" wars, proxy wars, and guerilla wars have killed as many people as the two world wars. Wars do not harm only the combatants: 75% or more of all those killed and maimed in wars since 1945 have been noncombatant children, women, and the elderly. Wars draw national wealth away from expenditure on health, education, and other socially desirable causes; lead to much environmental damage; and destroy or disrupt water and food supplies, essential infrastructure, transport and communication networks, schools, clinics, hospitals, and organized political life, all of which have detrimental effects on population health. In the last few decades of the 20th century war was increasingly recognized as a public health and social and cultural concern, and serious scholarly research began on the causes and prevention of violent armed conflict.

warfarin An anticoagulant that inhibits production by the liver of prothrombin and several factors involved in blood clotting mechanisms. It is used to treat and prevent recurrence of coronary and cerebral thrombosis and as a RODENTICIDE. The name derives from the agency that funded original developmental work on it, the Wisconsin Alumni Research Foundation (WARF).

warning labels A standardized system used worldwide to identify hazardous substances by means of recognizable labels on their containers. There are distinctive pictographs (LABELS) for toxic and poisonous substances, biological hazards, live electrical cables, and radioactive compounds. A skull and crossbones symbol indicates poisonous substances, a stylized flash of lightning indicates high-voltage electricity, and three equidistant bars radiating from a circle indicate hazardous radioactivity.

wart Horny or scaly localized small cutaneous tumor or excrescences, slow growing, solitary or occurring in clusters, usually caused by a PAPILLOMA VIRUS. Other causes include fungus infections and premalignant hyperkeratosis induced by solar or other ionizing radiation exposure. Warts vary considerably in response to treatment. Some disappear spontaneously, others require treatment with liquid nitrogen or cautery or sometimes can be "charmed," that is, they disappear under the influence of a "magic spell" or the power of suggestion.

washer Syn: wet scrubber. A dust or emission particle collector or gas purifier that works by spraying airborne particles or water-soluble toxic gases and collecting the suspended particles or dissolved gases in a slurry that runs into gutters for collection, cleaning, or safe disposal.

washout phase The phase of a clinical trial after stopping the test medication when its effects are wearing off. It is comparable to "drying out" after acute or chronic alcohol intoxication, but the washout phase varies in duration, according to the metabolic half-life of the medication.

Wassermann reaction Known in Belgium and France as the Bordet-Wassermann reaction because the Belgian physician Jules Bordet (1870–1961) was codiscoverer with the German microbiologist A. P. von Wassermann (1866–1925), this test has been used since the 1920s to detect antibodies to *Treponema pallidum*, the agent causing syphilis. It relies on a nonspecific reaction that leads to both false-positive and false-negative results and has been superseded by more reliable tests, such as the rapid plasma reagin (RPR) and fluorescent treponemal antibody absorbed (FTA-Abs) tests.

waste Material or substances discarded during or at the completion of industrial, commercial, or domestic processes and activities. Waste is classified as industrial, commercial, domestic, or street waste, organic matter that will decompose and inorganic material that will not. Domestic waste is increasingly often sorted into material that can be recycled or reused, organic matter suitable for composting, and material that must be disposed in waste sites. The distinction between domestic and commercial waste is important for financial reasons because collection and WASTE DISPOSAL by public authorities or private companies are paid from different budgets. Waste accumulates in prodigious quantities in rich industrial nations and has given rise to a large, diversified system of WASTE MANAGEMENT.

waste disposal An increasingly difficult, almost insoluble problem in modern industrial societies, disposal methods are best based on separation of waste into components that can be recycled or reused; composted, compacted, or combusted, leaving only a residue of TOXIC WASTE; industrial waste such as dead automobiles, large machinery, and parts; "white waste" (defunct kitchen appliances); and disused industrial buildings, warehouses, and the like, occurring in BROWN-FIELDS. An important large category is obsolete electronic equipment, notably computers and screens, which contain toxic material and trace amounts of costly compounds that can often be salvaged and recycled.

waste management The method and procedure used to dispose of waste. The administrative and economic basis for methods of waste disposal deals with the logistics, provision of special vehicles for street sweeping, movement of domestic waste, provision for disposing of it in LANDFILL, incineration, dumping at sea, etc., and determining the charges payable by industrial and commercial organizations and by private citizens to municipal authorities for waste disposal services. This is a large, complex, and essential feature of all societies, paid for usually by local taxation, and taken for granted by almost everybody unless or until the system breaks down, for instance, as a result of industrial disputes involving

the usually low-paid workers who do this dirty work.

waste sites Large quantities of waste are dumped in waste sites, which fall into several categories, including garbage dumps, landfill, toxic waste sites, radioactive waste sites, etc. Most troublesome are toxic waste sites containing poisonous chemicals and radioactive waste. These are ultimately the most costly and dangerous because of the extremely long half-life of some radioactive waste. There are an estimated 100,000 toxic waste sites in the United States. Many are poorly documented, unsupervised, and unregulated.

wastewater Liquid domestic, commercial, and industrial waste that includes sewage, storm water, and liquid industrial effluent. In some sewage disposal systems, no distinction is made, but in those in which surplus water or toxic effluent could inactivate the system, these varieties of wastewater must be segregated. Many cities with sewerage systems have separate drains for storm water for this reason, especially if the areas are subject to torrential rainstorms. Wastewater from public and domestic toilets is always polluted and is referred to as "black water." Water from domestic baths, kitchens, laundries, etc., is nonpotable, but usually it may be used for irrigation. This is referred to as "gray water."

wastewater treatment Water that has been used for industrial purposes is often contaminated with toxic chemicals requiring special detoxification to render it harmless. Domestic wastewater (GRAY WATER) containing detergents and soapsuds can damage the biological filtration methods of some sewage disposal systems, so it too may require special treatment.

water H_2O, the oxide of hydrogen, the most plentiful substance on earth, although only about 2% of it is fresh water suitable for drinking and irrigation. Almost half of all humans lack access to adequate supplies of safe drinking water. Water is absolutely essential to life and has always been regarded as part of the GLOBAL COMMONS (along with the air that we breathe). But access to drinking water is increasingly being privatized, notably in some low-income countries. The minimum daily intake is about 1 to 1.5 liters, more in hot weather or sweaty conditions; an additional 0.5 liters is ingested as water content of food. The daily requirement rises in warm and hot environments where fluid loss in sweating is greater.

water-borne diseases A miscellaneous group of communicable diseases transmitted in water that has been contaminated by pathogens of viral, bacterial, protozoan, and helminthic origin. Chemical toxins such as arsenic and heavy metals can also cause water-borne disease. The most important are listed at http://www.cdc.gov/ncidod/diseases/list_waterborne.htm.

water hardness "Hard" water contains a high concentration of dissolved salts, notably calcium or magnesium salts, which inhibit the action of soap and therefore its cleansing quality. The geological composition of the catchment area determines the hardness or softness of the water supply from a particular source. Epidemiological evidence suggests that there may be an association between hardness or softness of drinking water supplies and the prevalence of certain conditions, e.g., cardiovascular disease, but the evidence is inconsistent and disputed.

water pollution Contamination of fresh water by pollutants, i.e., human and/or animal wastes, agricultural pesticides and fertilizers, industrial toxic waste, etc. Each presents particular risks to the environment, ecosystems, and human health. Human waste carries fecal-oral infections, such as gastrointestinal infections, polio, and hepatitis A; animal waste carries Giardia, Cryptosporidium, Escherichia coli O157, etc. Agricultural fertilizers can cause severe disruption of ecosystems, e.g., choking rivers and lakes. Industrial toxic wastes can be any of a wide range of substances, some of which are extremely dangerous to human health. Control of water pollution is an essential public health function, preferably conducted in collaboration with environmental and often agricultural experts because the problem is basically one of ecosystem management.

water quality criteria POTABLE water, water fit for drinking, must be free of pathogens, toxic chemicals, and excessive or harmful concentrations of dissolved salts. Pathogens, especially fecal-oral pathogens, should be detected by routine tests that are best conducted by professionally qualified staff in an authorized laboratory. Public health and environment departments often work in collaboration to monitor and maintain surveillance of drinking water quality. When budget cuts force reductions in rigorous surveillance, outbreaks of water-borne diseases almost invariably occur. Irrigation water may contain some pathogens, and its chemical content should not cause buildup of harmful salts in the soil. Industrial water is often heated and cooled again, so it must be free of dissolved salts that could crystallize out. The criteria applicable in the United States are available at http://www.epa.gov/water science/standards/. Those in other countries are similar.

water, recreational See RECREATIONAL WATER.

watershed The mountains, hills, sloping land that collect snow-melt, rainwater, etc., which runs into rivers, lakes, and the sea. See also CATCHMENT AREA.

water table The soil or subsoil level, or the geological strata, at and below which the ground is saturated with water. The water table level must be taken into account when constructing a pit privy or septic tank close to a shallow well used for drinking water supplies. In many heavily populated parched regions, such as northern China and the southwestern United States, the water table is sinking and shrinking, with serious implications for sustainability in the near future.

water treatment In public health, this means treating water to make it POTABLE, safe to drink. Reservoir water may be treated systematically to eliminate suspended solid particles, using alum to encourage flocculation, followed by filtration through gravel and sand beds, then water weeds and algae to provide a biological filter before further purification by chlorination, and sometimes augmenting fluoride content to correct a deficiency that promotes dental caries. Not all these processes are routinely used everywhere.

watt The SI unit of electric power, determined by the product of voltage and amperage. The name honors the memory of the British scientist James Watt (1736–1819).

weaning An infant in transition from breast (or bottle) feeding to solid food.

weaning diarrhea A common condition among infants shortly after the end of breast feeding, usually caused by poor hygiene in the preparation of infant formula, therefore especially common in slums and poverty-stricken communities, that leads to contamination with pathogenic organisms.

weapons of mass destruction (WMD) A collective name for several classes of lethal weapons having in common the fact that when deployed they can cause death and injury indiscriminately among large numbers of people. Three classes of WMD are biological, chemical, and nuclear weapons. All have been used in conventional war, and two (biological and chemical weapons) have been used in terrorist attacks. WMDs have considerable potential and often actual public health implications, as well as their immediate impact. Nuclear weapons cause death and injury on a massive scale and also are extremely destructive to infrastructure and human habitat. In 1947, the UN Security Council defined WMDs as atomic explosive weapons, radioactive material weapons, lethal chemical and biological weapons, and any weapons developed in the future that have characteristics comparable in destructive effect to those of the atomic bomb or other weapons mentioned.

weather The variations in climate that occur in small defined localities over a short time. It is possible to forecast weather with reasonable reliability for a few days, but beyond a week or so the complex operation of CHAOS THEORY reduces reliability to near zero. Weather has been recognized as a determinant of health since the Greek "father of medicine," Hippocrates (c. 460–377 BCE), described it in *Airs, Waters, Places*.

Web site A set of texts and/or images usually sharing a common theme, accessible via the Internet by keying in the address of the site, known as a uniform (or universal) resource locator (URL), or by using a hyperlink from another site. See WORLD WIDE WEB.

Wechsler scales This term describes several survey instruments to assess intelligence levels in adults and children. The Wechsler-Bellevue scale was developed in the 1950s by the American psychologist David Wechsler (1896–1981) to assess adult intelligence. It is a set of standardized questions on aspects of verbal, numerical, social, and perceptual intelligence. Wechsler and his colleagues developed modified forms to assess the intelligence of children. Details of the scales can be seen at http://www.wilderdom.com/personality/intelligenceWAISWISC.html.

Weekly   Epidemiological   Record/Relevé épidémiologique hebdomadaire The bilingual weekly publication in print and online that is produced by the World Health Organization. It contains statistical summaries of surveillance epidemiology, information about the global health situation, and articles on public health problems of current concern. It can be seen at http://www.who.int/wer/en/.

weighting A method of adjustment to allow for differences between a study population and a "standard" one, between two or more populations that are being compared, or among any set of variables in which confounding factors might otherwise invalidate comparisons. It can be done in several ways, often by taking different predetermined proportions from several parts of the study population or set of variables, to ensure that numbers in each are sufficient to yield stable rates.

Weil-Felix reaction A serological test to identify rickettsial organisms, using agglutinins from nonmotile strains of *Proteus vulgaris*, with which rickettsia share a nonspecific agglutinin reaction.

The test varies in sensitivity and is relatively nonspecific but is sometimes useful for screening purposes. It must be followed up by specific tests to confirm the presence of rickettsial infection, such as scrub typhus. The test was invented by the Austrian physician Edmund Weil (1880–1922) and the Polish microbiologist Artur Felix (1887–1956)

Weil's disease Syn: leptospirosis, sewer-worker's disease. A serious potentially fatal zoonosis affecting the liver and kidneys, caused by a spirochete, *Leptospira ictohemorrhagica*. It is a disease of rats that is spread to humans in infected rat urine or feces. It was identified by the German physician Adolf Weil (1848–1916).

welding The industrial process of joining two metals together by heating the juxtaposed surfaces to above their melting points in order to mix and fuse them. Methods of welding expose welders to several health risks. Oxyacetylene welding uses the hot flame of acetylene gas, which generates toxic fumes. Arc welding uses direct electric current, and the white-hot metals radiate ultraviolet radiation, which can cause retinal burns and blindness.

welfare Provision of publicly funded financial support, usually from tax revenue, for persons and families who are experiencing financial hardship. These persons include long-term unemployed, single-parent, mother-led families in which the mother cannot work because she must care for infant(s) and child(ren) and persons receiving invalid pensions, etc. Welfare support is intended to pay for shelter, clothing, and food, but it is seldom adequate.

welfare state A system of political economy in which taxes are raised to pay for universal coverage of all or substantial parts of health care costs, old age and invalid security pensions, income maintenance (welfare), housing subsidies, and support for universal education. There is much variation among high-income countries in the proportion of national income used for social transfers of this kind, ranging from around 30% in the Scandinavian countries to less than half this in the United States, Japan, and Greece. These figures do not include government spending on education, which tends to be redistributive. The level of government spending on health services is around 7% of gross domestic product (GDP) in all high-income countries. The United States differs from other Organization for Economic Cooperation and Development (OECD) countries in not providing universal entitlement to a publicly funded system of health care services.

well-baby care Primary health care services for infants that aim to protect and preserve their health by providing preventive immunizations, advice on nutrition and feeding schedules, and routine monitoring of growth and development. In low-income countries, distinction between a "well baby" and one with ailments (common or otherwise) is usually not practical, and care of both is often best provided by integrated forms of primary care, such as mother and child clinics.

wellness A word used by behavioral scientists to describe a state of dynamic physical, mental, social, and spiritual well-being that enables a person to achieve full potential and an enjoyable life.

Wernicke's syndrome A neuropsychiatric disorder with peripheral neuropathy, memory loss, and progressive dementia, caused by thiamine deficiency, characteristically seen in advanced stages of chronic alcoholism. It was identified by the Polish-German physician Carl Wernicke (1848–1905).

Western blot An electrophoretic test for protein antibody reaction that is used to test for the presence of HIV infection. The test actually determines the molecular weight of specific proteins, and HIV is thus inferred to be present. The first such test, the SOUTHERN BLOT, was named for its discoverer; similar tests are named for the points of the compass.

western equine encephalitis (WEE) An arbovirus infection first identified in horses but also capable of causing human disease, spread by culicine mosquitoes, e.g., *Culex tarsalis*, indigenous to the western regions of North America. A similar disease, eastern equine encephalitis (EEE), occurs in the northeastern United States and adjacent regions in Canada and is transmitted mainly by *Culex pipiens*. See http://www.cdc.gov/ncidod/dvbid/arbor/weefact.htm.

West Nile virus An arbovirus that is indigenous to North Africa. It is a flavivirus that primarily infects birds, but mosquitoes can transmit it to humans and large mammals, such as horses, as well as to birds. It is not transmissible from person to person. It was introduced to North America either in infected birds or in mosquitoes, or perhaps both, in the 1990s, and has caused small epidemics in several recent years, with a few deaths, but many human cases appear to be mild or subclinical. It has had more damaging effects on birds, reducing some rare species to near extinction. Efforts to control the human disease included overreaction by politicians and public health officials in some jurisdictions, with extensive and inappropriate use of insecticides to control mosquitoes. It is a blood-borne infection, so it is important to safeguard blood supplies by excluding infected persons from blood banks. See http://www.cdc.gov/ncidod/dvbid/westnile/ for details.

wetlands Open water habitat, e.g., in coastal tidal zones or inland marshes and waterlogged country adjacent to lakes and rivers. Wetlands are an essential component of flood control because they are a safety zone for inhabited regions at times of flood and tidal surges, and are ecologically important for several reasons: coastal wetlands play an essential role in food chains that sustain coastal and sometimes also ocean fisheries; and often they provide seasonal habitat for migratory birds. Unfortunately, many wetlands were lost to urban and suburban development and landfill sites before their ecological importance was understood. Development frequently continues to threaten them.

wheat Probably the first grain crop to be cultivated when the concept of agriculture was invented about 10,000 BCE, perhaps by observant women in Mesopotamia, the fertile region in what is now Iraq. The discovery that grains of wheat could be crushed to yield flour and that this could be cooked to produce bread led to the transformation of hunter gatherers into agriculturalists and made human settlements possible, thus leading to the birth of civilization.

wheat germ Embryonic wheat that contains most of the fat, 60% of the vitamin B_1, and 20% to 25% of the vitamin B_2 and vitamin B_6 in mature wheat grains. Milled grain to make white flour removes most of these ingredients, so wheat germ is regarded as a superior, "natural" health food.

whiplash A soft-tissue injury to the ligaments and joints of the spinal column, most commonly caused by rear-end automobile collisions in which the occupants of the car that is hit from behind are suddenly and violently jerked forward and backward. The resulting painful stiff neck can persist for months, requiring physiotherapy or chiropractic treatment to relieve it. SHAKEN BABY SYNDROME is a variation of whiplash, in which violent shaking of an infant by an irritated caregiver can cause severe damage to the neck, as well as intracranial hemorrhage.

whipworm A nematode worm, *Trichuris trichiura*, the most common nematode worm infection in the world, spread from person to person by the fecal-oral route, sometimes by fecal-feeding flies. It is common in communities with poor sanitation and poorly maintained summer camps, and it is almost universal in some low-income nations with poor sanitation.

whistle-blower A person in a government agency or a private sector corporation who reports malfeasance to responsible authorities or the media, thus allowing information that would otherwise have been concealed to enter the public domain. Whistle-blowers perform a valuable public service, but they are often victimized, and in some jurisdictions it has been found useful to enact legislation to protect them.

white coat hypertension Elevation of blood pressure stimulated by anxiety that some people experience when the doctor (who wears a white coat) checks their blood pressure.

white-collar worker A clerical, rather than manual, worker. The term is usually restricted to persons occupying lower echelons of clerical work in organizations such as banks, insurance companies, and government departments.

Whitehall study A long-term COHORT STUDY of British civil servants that was started in 1967. The aim of the first phase was to explore the relationship of cardiovascular disease to stress, social status, individuals' location in the hierarchical administrative structure of the civil service, access to and use of leisure facilities, and numerous other social and behavioral variables. This is summarized at http://www.workhealth.org/projects/pwhitew .html. The second phase focused on stress, perceived status, and self-esteem. The progress of this study of work and health is reported at http:// www.ucl.ac.uk/whitehallII/. These studies and others have demonstrated the importance of social and psychosocial factors as determinants of health.

whole grains Wheat, corn, oats, or rice that retains the outer husk, i.e., is unmilled. It retains the fiber and some mineral and vitamin content that is lost in milling and refining and is therefore considered to be a "healthier" food than milled grain. It is a popular food item in health food stores and the basis for some popular commercially manufactured breakfast cereal products.

whooping cough See PERTUSSIS.

WIC (women infants and children) program A US government funded program to help ensure that pregnant women on welfare and with low incomes receive an adequate diet. The program provides vouchers to enable these women and their infants and children to receive nutritious food supplements and also offers information, suggestions, etc., about sensible diets.

Widal test A serological agglutination reaction to detect serum agglutinins to *Salmonella typhi* and related organisms. It has limited sensitivity and specificity. It is being phased out and replaced as a diagnostic test, but it remains a useful prognostic test for TYPHOID and related salmonelloses, as the titer declines during recovery. The test was developed by the French bacteriologist Georges Widal (1862–1929).

witchcraft Occult practices such as BLACK MAGIC that have existed for millennia in traditional societies and persist today in some strata and subcultures of even sophisticated and well-educated modern industrial societies. Generally witchcraft is harmless, but occasionally its practices can harm health. There is a connection between witchcraft and traditional folk remedies, some of which are efficacious and many of which have not yet been evaluated.

withdrawal symptoms The symptoms associated with absence of the metabolic or psychological effect of a drug or other substance, such as alcohol, to which a person has become physiologically or psychologically habituated or dependent. The symptoms vary with the substance but generally include irritability, sleeplessness, headaches, and malaise. In the case of severe alcohol addiction, withdrawal can precipitate delirium tremens (DTs).

Women's Christian Temperance Union (WCTU) A Protestant Christian social and political movement founded in the 19th century to combat widespread public drunkenness. It helped lead the political pressures for Prohibition, the constitutional amendment banning alcohol in the United States in the 1920s that became a failed social experiment. See TEMPERANCE MOVEMENT. Although it is now a low-key organization, the WCTU remains active. See http://www.wctu.org.

women's health A broad category of illnesses and health conditions associated with being female. The rise of the feminist movement in the second half of the 20th century gave a boost to assertive approaches, increasingly by women physicians and women patients who sought to eliminate the tendency to "medicalize" the normal physiological functions of menstruation, pregnancy, and menopause. By the late 20th century, women's health care was increasingly being provided by women physicians in all the English-speaking nations, where until early in the 20th century medicine was an almost exclusively male profession. The same trends affected the Scandinavian nations and the Netherlands a little earlier, and in some nations, such as India and Pakistan (where the term "lady doctor" is official terminology) and, more recently, orthodox Islamic nations, women's health care was a virtually exclusive preserve of female physicians. A comparable but lower-profile specialty of men's health has evolved, partly from genitourinary surgery, since the 1980s. Much useful information is available at http:// www.4woman.gov/.

women's liberation movement A social and political movement with origins in the writings of early feminists, such as the English woman Mary Wollstonecraft (1759–1797), that gained much momentum in Western democracies in the 1950s, seeking equal social and political rights, equity in job opportunities, freedom from male domination, and freedom of reproductive choice. Now usually called the women's movement, it emphasizes general health concerns, as well as aspects of health that relate directly to reproduction and birth control.

wool-sorter's disease See ANTHRAX.

worker education A social and political movement initiated by the British activists Beatrice (1858–1943) and Sidney (1859–1947) Webb, who believed that educated workers would be more effective, happier, and healthier than ignorant workers. They established the Workers' Education Association (WEA), a network of educational programs, bookshops, and recreational facilities with emphasis on promoting improved health.

workers' compensation Insurance programs financed by contributions from employers, e.g., in a payroll tax, to pay for medical care and rehabilitation of workers who are incapacitated by work-related injury or illness. Compensable work-related illnesses vary from one jurisdiction to another, and eligibility is often contested by employers. Currently, compensable illnesses in most jurisdictions include pneumoconioses and poisoning caused by workplace exposure to lead, other heavy metals, and some toxic chemicals. Work-related injury for which compensation claims are made may be quite straightforward but includes one common category, back injuries, in which the objective evidence may be elusive.

workforce A word that has replaced the sexist term "manpower" to describe the size of the population employed in a specified occupation and to describe the total population of a country who are employed and looking for employment.

workhouse A system of providing shelter for the destitute in return for work that was used in many industrial nations in the 19th century. Workhouses were usually run by private individuals and often exploited the people obliged by necessity to use them. They were replaced in the late 19th or early 20th century by more humane approaches, such as SHELTERED WORKSHOPS, to provide support for those unable to join the workforce available for fit and healthy people.

working class Loosely, those engaged in heavy manual labor. A term popularized by 19th century socialist philosophers such as Karl Marx (1818–1883) and Friedrich Engels (1820–1895). Engels used it in the title of his book *The Condition of the Working Class in England* (1845), which, like Marx's *Das Kapital* (1867), emphasized the inequities as well as inequalities in income, education, and opportunity—and health status—that separated the working class from others. Other 19th century writers, notably Edwin Chadwick (1800–1890), documented the discrepancies and disparities that persisted through the end of the 20th century and got even more pronounced in the late 20th century than they had been in the middle years.

working poor People who are working for low wages, often in precarious working conditions where they do not earn enough even to reach the officially designated poverty level (a "living wage") and require assistance, such as subsidized housing and food aid or VOUCHERS.

workplace inspection A routine or sometimes ad hoc procedure in which industrial safety officials and/or sanitarians (health inspectors) carry out inspections to ensure that working conditions are safe and do not expose workers to needless risk of harm. The nature and frequency of the inspection vary. For instance, inspections of underground mines are usually conducted more frequently and with greater rigor than are inspections of a textile or tailoring factory.

workshop 1. A place where articles are made or repaired. It may be a large factory floor, a modest establishment with one or a handful of artisans, or a basement hobby room. Each of these can be safe or hazardous to workers and perhaps others in many ways. 2. A descriptive term for a gathering of people whose aim is to discuss and perhaps attempt to solve a social, medical, philosophical, or intellectual problem.

worksite health promotion A program of health promotion at the work place, often sponsored and wholly or partly funded by employer/employee partnerships, usually with participation of organizations, such as coalitions of management and labor organizations. Such programs typically provide or sponsor early detection programs, such as Pap tests and mammography, as well as fitness regimens led by trained professionals. In some Scandinavian programs, workers' families are included in the service.

World Bank The popular name for the United Nations agency established in 1945, with the official name of International Bank for Reconstruction and Development. The World Bank mainly provides long-term loan support, whereas the INTERNATIONAL MONETARY FUND provides crisis intervention short-term loan support. In the 1970s, the World Bank began to play an increasingly assertive and prominent role in world health, investing in and assuming a leadership role in research on effective ways to control tropical diseases such as malaria that were impeding the economic development of many tropical low-income nations. However, the STRUCTURAL ADJUSTMENT policy required by wealthy donor nations has had a negative effect on health in some low-income countries. Regionally, the African Development Bank, the Asia Development Bank, Banca Interamericana de Desarolla (Inter-American Development Bank), and others fulfill similar functions. See http://www.worldbank.org/ for information on the range and scope of the World Bank's activities.

World Bank classification of nations See IN-COME LEVELS, WORLD BANK CLASSIFICATION.

World Commission on Environment and Development Chaired by the former Norwegian prime minister Gro Harlem Brundtland (b. 1939), who was director general of the World Health Organization in 1998–2003, the Brundtland Commission produced a report, *Our Common Future* (1987), on the relationship of environment and development that was the basic working document for the World Summit on Environment and Development in Rio de Janeiro in 1992. The public health relevance of the Rio Summit was that it drew attention to the problem of GREENHOUSE GASES and paved the way for the KYOTO PROTOCOL. The Report is available in summary form at http://www.un.org/documents/ga/res/42/ares42-187.htm.

World Federation of Public Health Associations (WFPHA) This is an international, nongovernmental organization of health workers throughout the world, founded in 1967. It aims to achieve professional exchange, collaboration, and action on public health issues. It includes about 70 national and regional public health societies whose members include nurses, sanitarians, administrators, physicians, health educators, pharmacists, anthropologists, researchers, and others interested in public health. WFPHA membership also includes regional associations of schools of public health, formalizing a link with academic public health. See http://www.wfpha.org for details.

World Food Programme Established in 1963 as a branch of the UN FOOD AND AGRICULTURE ORGANIZATION, this United Nations agency provides food aid, and often other humanitarian assistance, to populations who are experiencing FAMINE or severe food shortages as a result of natural or manmade disasters. Often the program facilitates other humanitarian assistance, such as emergency public health services to the same populations at the same time. Since 1996, the World Food Programme has been governed by an executive board of 36 member states, chaired by an executive director appointed by the UN Secretary General and the Director-General of the Food and Agriculture Organization. See http://www.wfp.org/english/ for details.

World Health Organization (WHO) Founded in 1948 as the successor to the Health Office of the League of Nations, the World Health Organization is among the most important of the United Nations agencies. Its wide responsibilities include surveillance and control of health problems affecting the world's people, especially the people in tropical and low-income countries where pervasive and intractable health problems persist. It conducts and sponsors health research and is a standard-setting, information-disseminating, and educational organization. The achievements of WHO include coordination and direction of efforts to eliminate malaria and pervasive bacterial and parasitic disease from much of the tropical and subtropical world, control of many pandemic communicable diseases, and, probably its most spectacular achievement, the worldwide eradication of smallpox, which was proclaimed by the World Health Assembly in 1980. Control of many tropical diseases has been at least partially successful, and malaria has been reduced or even eliminated in a few places, but generally efforts to control malaria have had only limited or no success. WHO headquarters are in Geneva, and regional offices are located in Brazzaville for the African Region, Cairo for the Eastern Mediterranean Region, Copenhagen for the European Region, New Delhi for the South-East Asian Region, Manila for the Western Pacific Region, and Washington, D.C., for the Americas. Details of the work of the WHO are contained in its annual reports and in many serial and occasional publications, and many are retrievable at http://www.who.int.

World Resources Institute A private nonprofit organization based in Washington, D.C., that provides advice and technical assistance to developing countries and to nongovernmental organizations in order to help them manage resources in a sustainable manner. It publishes periodic reports that contain useful statistical summaries of living conditions, potential for sustainable development, and other information from low-income nations. See http://www.wri.org/ for details.

World Summit on Children Convened by UNICEF, this Summit conference was held at UN headquarters in New York in 1990 and attended by 71 heads of state and many national ministers of relevant government departments. The Summit approved a declaration on the survival, protection, and development of children, the "Declaration on the Rights of the Child," which has been ratified by all nations except the failed state of Somalia and the United States. See http://www.unicef.org/wsc/ for details.

World Summit on Sustainable Development Syn: The Johannesburg Summit. A conference of heads of state and delegations of member nations of the United Nations convened in 2002 in Johannesburg, South Africa, to discuss the global environmental, demographic, climatic, and health condition, under the auspices of UN agencies, including WHO, UNEP, and UNDP. The report of the Johannesburg Summit is available at http://www .johannesburgsummit.org/.

World Trade Organization The World Trade Organization (WTO) was founded after the Uruguay Round of the General Agreement in Tariffs and Trade (1986–1994). On the basis of negotiations in 1993, led by the United States and the European Union, WTO gave itself enhanced power to determine the conditions for "free" trade among autonomous nations in goods and services, including many with implications for health, education, and environmental protection. WTO has some power to impose sanction on nations that resist attempts by foreign companies to introduce private health care services that "compete" with tax-supported or government-subsidized services, but member states sign on to specific agreements. The Doha agreement allows low-income countries to make exceptions to drug patent law in the face of public health emergencies, such as the HIV/AIDS epidemics in Sub-Saharan Africa, Latin America, and Asia. For information, see http://www.wto.org.

World Wide Web Syn: the Web. An electronic search and retrieval system originally developed at le Conseil Européen pour la Recherche Nucléaire (CERN), the high-energy particle physics laboratory near Geneva, Switzerland. It was the creation of Tim Berners-Lee (b. 1955), a British scientist who did not patent it, thus leaving it freely available to all. It uses the Internet, search engines, and a system of uniform resource locators (URLs) to identify and retrieve on the recipient's computer terminal any or all of the information that is indexed and electronically accessible in text, graphical form, audio, or moving images. The explosive growth of this information resource since the early 1990s has been the most remarkable advance in information technology since the invention of printing. Entire library indexes and abstract summaries of individual articles, such as those in the US National Library of Medicine, are accessible on the Web. Project Gutenberg aims to store the texts of all works in some of the world's most comprehensive libraries in retrievable electronic form. The World Wide Web is an immensely valuable resource for all forms of scholarly activity. Several SEARCH ENGINES have been developed to facilitate navigating it, but users must beware of experiencing information overload and of accepting misleading information.

worm count As estimate of the burden of intestinal worms, usually based on counts of the number of eggs excreted per cubic milliliter of feces and therefore more precisely called an egg count.

worms A general word that describes many varieties of intestinal and tissue parasites that humans can harbor. About half the human race plays host to one or more kinds of worms: roundworms, pinworms, tapeworms, nematodes, blood flukes, etc. Most are harmful because they, rather than their human host, consume nutriment that the host requires for healthy growth, development, and sustenance. Some do worse, for instance, hookworms, which suck the host's blood and cause serious anemia. Many worms can be killed by suitable orally administered drugs, but some are resistant and persistent, and some, such as pinworms, easily reinfect the host because their eggs survive in bedding and clothing and on the toys of the children who are their usual hosts.

wrongful death A death for which someone, such as an attending physician or an agency of the health care system, can be held legally accountable and therefore can be charged in a court of law or sued for damages by next of kin.

X

X axis The name for the horizontal axis on a two-dimensional graph. The other is the vertical or Y axis. The two are called the CARTESIAN COORDINATES.

X chromosome One of the sex chromosomes. Females have two X chromosomes, males have an X and a Y chromosome. The X chromosome is unusually large and carries many genes for sex-linked (or X-linked) characteristics.

xenobiotic Literally a substance that is foreign to the living body or other living organism. A chemical that does not normally occur in but interacts with one or more metabolic pathways of an organism, often in a way that has adverse effects on health.

xenodiagnosis The procedure of feeding laboratory-reared insects on the blood of patients who are suspected of infection with pathogens, typically CHAGAS DISEASE, and examining the insects or, in the case of Chagas disease, their feces, for evidence of the intermediate stage of the pathogen.

Xenopsylla cheopis The rat flea, which, when it feeds on a rat infected with the PLAGUE bacillus, *Yersinia pestis*, transmits the pathogen to new mammalian hosts: other rats or humans.

xerophthalmia A condition caused by vitamin A deficiency in which the sclera and cornea become thickened, dry, and ulcerated. This leads to irreversible blindness. It is one of the main causes of blindness in some low-income countries where vitamin A deficiency is common.

X-linked disease An inheritable disease caused by a gene on the X chromosome. Most X-linked characteristics are recessive. A male with a recessive gene on his X chromosome passes his X chromosomes to his daughter, where the chromosomes will be masked if the daughter does not have the same gene or be expressed if his female partner carries the same gene.

x-rays Ionizing electromagnetic radiation produced by bombarding atoms of a heavy metal such as tungsten with a beam of high-energy electrons produced by a high-voltage electric charge. The phenomenon was discovered by the Dutch-German physicist Wilhelm Röntgen (1845–1923) in 1895. The radiation penetrates soft tissues and produces an image on a photographic plate. This phenomenon has been an immensely useful diagnostic testing method for the last 100 years, during which the hazards and harms due to needless exposure to x-rays have been effectively minimized.

XXX syndrome The most common chromosomal abnormality of females, associated with visible stigmata, including tallness and enlarged epicanthic folds similar to those of Down syndrome. Girls with XXX syndrome usually have normal intelligence but may be emotionally unstable and have learning difficulties. They are fertile, but their offspring have a higher than average incidence of congenital abnormalities. Several rare variations of female chromosome anomalies have been identified, including XXXX syndrome ("superwoman"), which causes mild mental retardation, and XXY, or Klinefelter's, syndrome

xylene A colorless, flammable, sweet-smelling liquid distilled from petroleum or coal tar, used as a chemical solvent, e.g., in medical laboratories. It is toxic, irritating to skin and mucosal surfaces, and a renal, hepatic, and neurological toxin. Most of its toxic effects are reversible.

Y

yaws A tropical infectious disease now confined mainly to central Africa and the West Indies, with scattered foci in India, Southeast Asia, and some Pacific islands, caused by a spirochete, *Treponema pallidum* subspecies *pertenue*, an organism closely related to the spirochete of syphilis. It causes skin lesions that ulcerate and is transmitted by contact with the seropurulent discharge. It is a chronic disease but, unlike syphilis, it does not attack the central nervous system. The word comes from a Carib Indian dialect word, *yaya*, meaning a sore.

Y axis The vertical axis of a graph, one of the two Cartesian coordinates, the other being the horizontal or X axis.

Y chromosome The small sex chromosome associated with male sex; females have two X chromosomes, males have one X and one Y chromosome.

years of potential life lost (YPLL) See POTENTIAL YEARS OF LIFE LOST (PYLL).

yeast Unicellular fungus organisms that are widely distributed in nature. Most are harmless; a few are commercially very important, generating carbon dioxide by their metabolism, responsible for aerating bread and other grain-based carbohydrates when cooked and for fermentation of sugar solutions in beer and wine making. Some varieties of yeast, notably *Candida albicans*, are pathogenic, causing several kinds of yeast infection, in particular vulvovaginitis.

yeast infection Infection with yeast organisms can affect the oropharynx, vagina, penis, rectum, and sometimes, especially in immunocompromised persons, the respiratory and gastrointestinal tract. Yeast infections may complicate advanced stages of HIV/AIDS. See also CANDIDIASIS.

yellow fever An acute, severe viral disease transmitted by culicine mosquitoes such as *Aedes aegypti*. The name is given because, in severe infection, liver and renal failure cause jaundice. It is a zoonosis that occurs in several varieties of jungle monkeys in West Africa and infects humans who come into contact with mosquitoes, typically when clearing jungle forests. Mosquitoes can spread from human to human in urban epidemics because the virus does not require a developmental stage in mosquitoes. The disease originated in tropical Africa, where it is still endemic, with an ever-present threat of major urban epidemics. It was imported to the Americas by African slaves, causing epidemics primarily by person-to-mosquito-to-person spread, but also became established in monkeys in Central and South America and some Caribbean islands. Currently, there are a few hundred cases annually in affected regions. Indigenous yellow fever has never been reported from Asia, Europe, or Oceania. It can be prevented by mosquito control and vaccination. Information is available at http://www.who.int/csr/disease/yellowfev/en/ and http://www.cdc.gov/ncidod/dvbid/yellowfever/.

yellow fever vaccine A safe, effective attenuated live virus vaccine that is required for travel to countries where yellow fever is endemic. It confers long-term, possibly lifelong, protection, but booster doses are recommended. See http://www.who.int/vaccines/en/yellowfever.shtml and http://www.cdc.gov/ncidod/dvbid/yellowfever/ for further information.

Yersinia enterocolitica A fecal-oral Gram-negative pathogen that causes enterocolitis and mesenteric adenitis with symptoms often indistinguishable from those of acute appendicitis.

yersiniosis An obsolete term for PLAGUE. The word is now rather confusedly used to describe diseases caused by *Yersinia.*

yoga A spiritual development and health maintenance system derived from Ayurvedic medicine in which the aim of exercises and meditation is to condition the mind and body, including the autonomic system, to minimize or even eliminate the effects of external stresses and, if possible, to reverse or retard the effect of chronic and progres-sive diseases such as hypertension and cancer. Clinical trials have provided weak supporting evidence of efficacy in controlling severe hypertension, although the effect of confounding variables is hard to eliminate.

yogurt A fermented milk product produced by culturing *Lactobacillus acidophilus* and other bacteria in milk, causing it to thicken to a jelly-like consistency. It is widely regarded as a health-promoting food and does have some therapeutic value, e.g., in restoring intestinal flora to normal after disruption and reducing the incidence and severity of some vaginal yeast infections.

young offender A person below the legal age of consent who has committed an indictable offense that comes to trial and, because of the defendant's age, is tried before a juvenile court. This has the advantage that in many jurisdictions there are more effective rehabilitation measures available than in the adult criminal justice system. The age range for young offenders varies according to the jurisdiction and sometimes is adjusted according to the severity of the offense.

youth A young person or a collective noun for young people. The age definition varies from one jurisdiction to another and according to the circumstances in which the designation "youth" is applied. It differs for voting, military service, purchasing alcohol and tobacco, driving a car, and, especially for females, obtaining contraceptive advice and access to supplies, receiving medical and public health interventions, and marrying without parental consent. Public health officials must be familiar with the legal definitions and limitations on autonomy of youth in the jurisdictions where they work.

yuppie disease See CHRONIC FATIGUE SYNDROME, for which it is an alternative name when it affects "yuppies," i.e., young urban professional people.

Yusho disease The name for an epidemic of CHLO-RACNE that affected people exposed to PCBs in Yusho, Japan, in 1968.

Z

zen macrobiotic diet See MACROBIOTICS.

zero-based budget A method of preparing annual budgets that begins each fiscal period without regard for the previous year's experience and available facts about assets, liabilities, income, and expenses in previous years. Instead, the treasurer and other financial officers are required to estimate anew their expectations for each line item in their proposed budget. Conservative elected officials often favor this approach because they believe it leads to reduced expenditure.

zero population growth A situation in which a population has ceased to increase by producing through births to its members larger numbers of new members than the number dying from natural causes; i.e., births and deaths are evenly balanced. This usually occurs with a TOTAL FERTILITY RATE of approximately 2.1.

zero report A term used in surveillance systems to designate an unequivocal report that no cases of a designated disease of interest occurred during the reporting period. When correctly implemented, zero reporting is important and valuable because it eliminates the possibility that the report was simply not completed or sent.

zero-sum game A situation in which gains to one group or individual can occur only at the expense of losses to another group or individual.

zero tolerance An expression for official policies that allow no scope of equivocation, e.g., about allegations of HATE CRIMES or other manifestations of bigotry.

zidovudine Syn: AZT. The first effective antiviral agent that slows the rate of progression from HIV infection to AIDS, and the progress of AIDS itself. It is a reverse transcriptase inhibitor that acts by stopping HIV from infecting uninfected body cells. It can retard the progress of HIV disease but cannot cure it. Long-term use may lead to bone marrow depression, mucosal ulcers, debility, muscle weakness, nausea, and vomiting. It is usually taken as part of a complex regimen that includes other drugs to minimize the adverse effects.

Ziehl-Neelsen stain A staining technique for the presence of *Mycobacterium tuberculosis* in sputum or other body fluid, based on alcohol solubility of the unstained tissues, that reveals the presence of tubercle bacilli. It was developed by the bacteriologist Franz Ziehl (1859–1926) and the pathologist Friedrich Neelsen (1854–1894), both German.

zinc A metallic element that is an essential dietary ingredient in trace amounts for many human enzyme systems. Zinc deficiency causes immune disruption, skin disease, and stunted growth in children.

zoning Allocation of designated sectors or portions in a city, municipality, or sometimes larger regions for residential, commercial, industrial use, public space, etc. Zoning should be coordinated with arrangements for provision of suitable infrastructure according to the designated uses of the zone.

zoology The branch of biological sciences that deals with the scientific study of species in the animal kingdom, often specialized, such as the study of specific species or animal behavior. Its relevance to human health, including public health, has been re-emphasized since the late 1990s by the emergence of SEVERE ACUTE RESPIRATORY SYNDROME (SARS) and AVIAN INFLUENZA, demonstrating the importance to human health of the behavior, as well as health, of wild and feral species and domestic livestock.

zoonosis A disease that is transmissible from animals to humans; usually a disease that causes disease also in animals, although the degree of severity may vary between the species. The animal hosts include rats, bats, dogs, foxes, bears, cats, pigs, goats, sheep, cattle, primates, birds, and many other species; the pathogens include viruses, bacteria, protozoa, and worms. Some infectious pathogens probably evolved from zoonotic infections to become human diseases, for example influenza, plague, typhus, measles, and possibly AIDS, and others may be in the process of doing so, for example Marburg and Ebola virus diseases and SEVERE ACUTE RESPIRATORY SYNDROME (SARS).

zooplankton Microscopic, single-cell, and other very small aquatic organisms at the base of the animal kingdom, corresponding to phytoplankton at the base of the plant kingdom. Zooplankton include, among other species, those responsible for proliferations that cause RED TIDE and the related episodes of shellfish poisoning, etc.

zoster See HERPES ZOSTER.

zygote A fertilized ovum.

Zyklon B A gaseous compound of cyanide and tear gas that was developed and used by the Nazi regime in its extermination camps to kill large numbers of concentration camp inmates, mainly members of the European Jewish community.

BIBLIOGRAPHY AND REFERENCES

Abercrombie N, Hill S, Turner BS: The Penguin dictionary of sociology. London: Penguin, 1984

Allaby M: Oxford dictionary of ecology. Oxford: Oxford University Press, 1998

American Public Health Association: Healthy communities 2000—Model standards, 3rd ed. Washington, DC: American Public Health Association, 1991

Atmospheric Air Quality Glossary, http://www.shsu.edu/~chemistry/Glossary/glos.html

Barker RL: The social work dictionary, 5th ed. Washington, DC: NASW Press, 2003

Bender AE, Bender DA: Dictionary of food and nutrition. Oxford: Oxford University Press, 1995

Bentzen N (Ed): WONCA dictionary of general/family practice. Copenhagen: Laegeforingens Forlag, 2003

Black J (Ed): Oxford dictionary of economics, 2nd ed. Oxford: Oxford University Press, 2002

Breslow L, Goldstein BD, Green LW, Keck CW, Last JM, McGinnis M (Eds): Encyclopedia of public health. New York: Macmillan Reference, 2002

Campbell RJ: Psychiatric dictionary, 8th ed. New York, Oxford, Toronto: Oxford University Press, 2004

Davidson A: The Oxford companion to food. Oxford, New York, Toronto: Oxford University Press, 1999

Detels R, McEwen J, Beaglehole R, Tanaka H (Eds): Oxford textbook of public health, 4th ed. Oxford, New York, Toronto: Oxford University Press, 2002

Gosling PJ: Dictionary of biomedical sciences. London, New York: Taylor and Francis, 2002

Grad FP: The public health law manual, 3rd ed. Washington, DC: American Public Health Association, 2004

Green LW: Community health. St. Louis: Mosby, 1990

Gunton T: Dictionary of information technology. London: Penguin Books, 1993

Heymann D (Ed): Control of Communicable Diseases Manual, 18th ed. Washington, DC: American Public Health Association, 2004.

Hogarth J: Glossary of health care terminology. Copenhagen: World Health Organization, Regional Office for Europe, 1978

Honderich T (Ed): Oxford companion to philosophy. Oxford: Oxford University Press, 1995

Institute of Medicine: The future of public health. Washington, DC: National Academy Press, 1988

International Programme on Chemical Safety: Glossary of terms on chemical safety for use in IPCS publications. Geneva: UNEP, ILO, and WHO, 1989

Isaacs A, Daintith J, Martin E (Eds): Oxford dictionary of science. Oxford: Oxford University Press, 2003

Jewell EJ, Abate F (Eds): The new Oxford American dictionary. New York: Oxford University Press, 2001

Kennedy H: Dictionary of GIS terminology. Redlands, Calif.: ESRI Press, 2003

Kerr C, Taylor R, Heard G (Eds): Handbook of public health methods. Sydney, New York, San Francisco, London: McGraw-Hill, 1998

Khoury MJ, Burke W, Thomson EJ: Genetics and public health in the 21st century. New York: Oxford University Press, 2000

King RC, Stansfield WD: A dictionary of genetics, 5th ed. New York: Oxford University Press, 1997

Kishore J: A dictionary of public health. Delhi Century Publications, 2002

Last JM (Ed): A dictionary of epidemiology, 4th ed. New York: Oxford University Press, 2000

Last JM, Wallace RB (Eds): Maxcy-Rosenau-Last public health and preventive medicine, 13th ed. Stamford, Conn.: Appleton & Lange, 1992

Levy BS, Wagner GR, Rest KM, Weeks JL: Preventing occupational disease & injury, 2nd ed. Washington, DC: American Public Health Association, 2004

Lippmann M, Cohen BS, Schlesinger RB: Environmental health science. New York: Oxford University Press, 2003

Lock SP, Last JM, Dunea G (Eds): Oxford illustrated companion to medicine. Oxford, New York, Toronto: Oxford University Press, 2001

Marshall G (Ed): Oxford dictionary of sociology. Oxford, New York: Oxford University Press, 1998

Martin E, Hine RS (Eds): Oxford dictionary of biology, 4th ed. Oxford: Oxford University Press, 2000

Mayhew S: Oxford dictionary of geography. Oxford: Oxford University Press, 1997

McLean I, McMillan A: Oxford concise dictionary of politics, 2nd ed. Oxford: Oxford University Press, 2003

Medawar PB, Medawar JS: Aristotle to zoos: A philosophical dictionary of biology. Cambridge, Mass.: Harvard University Press, 1983

Meinert CJ: Clinical trials dictionary. Baltimore: Johns Hopkins Center for Clinical Trials, 1996

Millar DIJ, Millar MT: The Cambridge dictionary of scientists. Cambridge: Cambridge University Press, 1996

Modeste NN: Dictionary of public health promotion and education. Thousand Oaks, Calif.: Sage Publications, 1996

Oxford English Dictionary, 2nd ed. on CD-ROM. Oxford: Oxford University Press, 2000

Oxford Reference Online, http://www.oxfordreference.com/pub/views/home.html

Pearce DW (Ed): The MIT dictionary of modern economics. Cambridge MA: MIT Press, 1999

Pencheon D, Guest C, Melzer D, Gray JAM (Eds): Oxford handbook of public health practice. Oxford, New York, Toronto: Oxford University Press, 2001

Raffle PAB, Lee WR, McCallum RI, Murray R (Eds): Hunter's diseases of occupations. Boston: Little, Brown & Co, 1987

Rom WN (Ed): Environmental and occupational medicine. Boston: Little, Brown & Co., 1983

Schottenfeld D, Fraumeni DS (Eds): Cancer epidemiology and prevention, 2nd ed. New York: Oxford University Press, 1996

Schwandt TA: Dictionary of qualitative inquiry. Thousand Oaks, Calif.: Sage Publications, 2001

Scutchfield FD, Keck CW (Eds): Principles of public health practice, 2nd ed. Albany, N.Y.: Delmar, Thomson, 2003

Segen JC: Dictionary of alternative medicine. Stamford, Conn.: Appleton & Lange, 1998

Segen JC: Dictionary of modern medicine. Park Ridge. N.J.: Parthenon, 1992

Slee V, Slee D, Schmidt H: Health care terms, 4th ed. St. Paul, Minn.: Tringa Press, 2001

Society for Risk Analysis: Glossary of risk analysis terms. http://www.sra.org/glossary .htmhttp://www.sra.org/resources_glossary .php

Stedman's medical dictionary, 27th ed. Philadelphia: Lippincott Williams & Wilkins, 2000

Stedman's medical eponyms. Baltimore: Williams & Wilkins, 1998

Wallace RB (Ed): Maxcy-Rosenau-Last public health and preventive medicine, 14th ed. New York: McGraw-Hill, 1998

Warren KS, Mahmoud AAF (Eds): Tropical and geographical medicine. New York: McGraw-Hill, 1984

Weeks JL, Levy BS, Wagner GR: Preventing occupational disease and injury. Washington, DC: American Public Health Association, 1991

Westheimer R: Dr. Ruth's encyclopedia of sex. New York: Continuum, 1994

Wigle DT: Child health and the environment. New York: Oxford University Press, 2003

Wikipedia, the online encyclopedia, http://en .wikipedia.org

Winger G, Woods JH, Hofmann FG: A handbook on drug and alcohol abuse, the biomedical aspects, 4th ed. Oxford, New York, Toronto: Oxford University Press, 2004

World Health Organization: Glossary of terms used in the 'Health for All' series. Geneva: WHO, 1984

World Health Organization, Regional Office for Europe: Glossary on air pollution. Copenhagen, 1980

World Health Organization, Regional Office for Europe: Glossary on solid waste. Copenhagen, 1980

Worthington D: Dictionary of environmental health. London, New York: Taylor & Francis, 2003

Yassi A, Kjellstrom T, de Kok T, Guidotti TL: Basic environmental health. Oxford, New York, Toronto: Oxford University Press, 2001

Zenz C (Ed): Occupational medicine: principles and practical applications. Chicago: Year Book Publications, 1988

Serial publications, journals of public health, epidemiology, environmental health, etc., included, but were not limited to, the following:

American Journal of Epidemiology
American Journal of Preventive Medicine

American Journal of Public Health
Annals of Epidemiology
British Medical Journal
Bulletin of the World Health Organization
Canadian Journal of Public Health
Environmental Health Perspectives
Epidemiology
European Journal of Public Health
International Journal of Epidemiology
Journal of Epidemiology and Community
  Health
Journal of the American Medical Association
Journal of Occupational Medicine
Lancet
Morbidity and Mortality Weekly Reports
New England Journal of Medicine

Public Health (UK)
Weekly Epidemiological Record
Electronic references
UK Public Health Electronic Library
  http://www.phel.gov.uk/glossary/glossary.asp
Agency for Toxic Substances and Disease
  Registry, glossary of terms and common
  important toxic substances
  http://www.atsdr.cdc.gov/glossary.html
Medline Plus Encyclopedia
  http://www.nlm.nih.gov/medlineplus/encyclo
  pedia.html
National Center for Health Statistics Fast Facts
  (statistical tables and glossary of definitions)
  see http://www.cdc.gov/nchs/fastats/Default
  .htm